W9-BZB-870

Psychosocial Interventions
for Cancer

Psychosocial Interventions for Cancer

Edited by
**Andrew Baum and
Barbara L. Andersen**

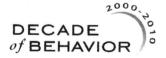

DECADE
of BEHAVIOR

American Psychological Association
Washington, DC

Published by
American Psychological Association
750 First Street, NE
Washington, DC 20002

Copies may be ordered from
APA Order Department
P.O. Box 92984
Washington, DC 20090-2984

In the U.K., Europe, Africa, and the Middle East, copies may be ordered from
American Psychological Association
3 Henrietta Street
Covent Garden, London
WC2E 8LU England

Typeset in Berkeley Book by Automated Graphic Systems, Inc., White Plains, MD

Printer: Sheridan Books, Ann Arbor, MI
Cover Designer: Naylor Design, Washington, DC
Technical/Production Editor: Jennifer L. Macomber

The opinions and statements published are the responsibility of the authors, and such opinions and statements do not necessarily represent the policies of the APA.

Library of Congress Cataloging-in-Publication Data
Psychosocial interventions for cancer / edited by Andrew Baum and Barbara L. Andersen.
    p. cm.
  Includes bibliographical references and index.
  ISBN 1-55798-734-3 (alk. paper)
    1. Cancer—Psychological aspects. 2. Cancer—Social aspects. 3. Stress management.
  4. Adjustment (Psychology). I. Baum, Andrew. II. Andersen, Barbara L.
RC262.P7837   2001
616.99′4′0019—dc21   00-048516

British Library Cataloguing-in-Publication Data
A CIP record is available from the British Library.

Printed in the United States of America
First Edition

To my father, whom I always aspired to be (AB)

To my parents, Edgar and Gladys Andersen (BA)

and to those who triumph in the face of this disease

APA Science Volumes

Attribution and Social Interaction: The Legacy of Edward E. Jones

Best Methods for the Analysis of Change: Recent Advances, Unanswered Questions, Future Directions

Cardiovascular Reactivity to Psychological Stress and Disease

The Challenge in Mathematics and Science Education: Psychology's Response

Changing Employment Relations: Behavioral and Social Perspectives

Children Exposed to Marital Violence: Theory, Research, and Applied Issues

Cognition: Conceptual and Methodological Issues

Cognitive Bases of Musical Communication

Cognitive Dissonance: Progress on a Pivotal Theory in Social Psychology

Conceptualization and Measurement of Organism–Environment Interaction

Converging Operations in the Study of Visual Selective Attention

Creative Thought: An Investigation of Conceptual Structures and Processes

Developmental Psychoacoustics

Diversity in Work Teams: Research Paradigms for a Changing Workplace

Emotion and Culture: Empirical Studies of Mutual Influence

Emotion, Disclosure, and Health

Evolving Explanations of Development: Ecological Approaches to Organism–Environment Systems

Examining Lives in Context: Perspectives on the Ecology of Human Development

Global Prospects for Education: Development, Culture, and Schooling

Hostility, Coping, and Health

Measuring Patient Changes in Mood, Anxiety, and Personality Disorders: Toward a Core Battery

Occasion Setting: Associative Learning and Cognition in Animals

Organ Donation and Transplantation: Psychological and Behavioral Factors

Origins and Development of Schizophrenia: Advances in Experimental Psychopathology

The Perception of Structure

Perspectives on Socially Shared Cognition

Psychological Testing of Hispanics

Psychology of Women's Health: Progress and Challenges in Research and Application

Researching Community Psychology: Issues of Theory and Methods

The Rising Curve: Long-Term Gains in IQ and Related Measures

Sexism and Stereotypes in Modern Society: The Gender Science of Janet Taylor Spence

Sleep and Cognition

Sleep Onset: Normal and Abnormal Processes

Stereotype Accuracy: Toward Appreciating Group Differences

Stereotyped Movements: Brain and Behavior Relationships

Studying Lives Through Time: Personality and Development

The Suggestibility of Children's Recollections: Implications for Eyewitness Testimony

Taste, Experience, and Feeding: Development and Learning

Temperament: Individual Differences at the Interface of Biology and Behavior

Through the Looking Glass: Issues of Psychological Well-Being in Captive Nonhuman Primates

Uniting Psychology and Biology: Integrative Perspectives on Human Development

Viewing Psychology as a Whole: The Integrative Science of William N. Dember

APA Decade of Behavior Volumes

Computational Modeling of Behavior in Organizations: The Third Scientific Discipline

The Nature of Remembering: Essays in Honor of Robert G. Crowder

New Methods for the Analysis of Change

Personality Psychology in the Workplace

Psychosocial Interventions for Cancer

Unraveling the Complexities of Social Life: A Festschrift in Honor of Robert B. Zajonc

Contents

Contributors   xiii

Foreword   xvii

Acknowledgments   xix

CHAPTER 1   Psychosocial Intervention and Cancer: An Introduction
              Andrew Baum and Barbara L. Andersen   3

PART 1: Bases of Adjustment to Living With Cancer

CHAPTER 2   Adapting to Cancer: The Importance of Hope and Purpose
              Michael F. Scheier and Charles S. Carver   15

CHAPTER 3   General and Specific Measures of Quality of Life in Younger
                  Women With Breast Cancer
              Joan R. Bloom, Susan L. Stewart, Monica Johnston, and
                  Priscilla Banks   37

CHAPTER 4   Quality-of-Life Measurement in Oncology
              David Cella   57

CHAPTER 5   Long-Term Adjustment in Cancer Survivors: Integration of
                  Classical-Conditioning and Cognitive-Processing Models
              William H. Redd, Katherine N. DuHamel, Suzanne M. Johnson
                  Vickberg, Jamie L. Ostroff, Meredith Y. Smith, Paul B.
                  Jacobsen, and Sharon L. Manne   77

CHAPTER 6   A Social–Cognitive Processing Model of Emotional Adjustment
                  to Cancer
              Stephen J. Lepore   99

PART 2: Bases of Intervention: Targets and Processes

CHAPTER 7   A Biobehavioral Model for Psychological Interventions
              Barbara L. Andersen   119

CHAPTER 8   Group Processes in Therapeutic Support Groups
              Paul B. Paulus   131

CHAPTER 9   Traumatic Stress as a Target for Intervention With Cancer Patients
             Andrew Baum and Donna M. Posluszny   143

CHAPTER 10   Assessing the Important Effector Mechanisms in the Immune
             Response Against Cancer
             Olivera J. Finn   175

CHAPTER 11   Immune System Versus Tumor
             Pierre L. Triozzi   193

PART 3: Prevention and Intervention

CHAPTER 12   Psychosocial Interventions in Cancer: Group Therapy Techniques
             David Spiegel and Susan Diamond   215

CHAPTER 13   Psychoeducational Intervention Programs for Patients
             With Cancer
             Fawzy I. Fawzy, Nancy W. Fawzy, and Andrea L. Canada   235

CHAPTER 14   Group Support Interventions for People With Cancer:
             Benefits and Hazards
             Vicki S. Helgeson, Sheldon Cohen, Richard Schulz, and
             Joyce Yasko   269

CHAPTER 15   Psychosocial Interventions for Women at Increased Risk for
             Breast Cancer
             Marc D. Schwartz, Caryn Lerman, and Barbara Rimer   287

CHAPTER 16   Interventions for Healthy Individuals at Familial Risk for Cancer:
             Biobehavioral Mechanisms for Health Benefits
             Dana H. Bovbjerg and Heiddis B. Valdimarsdottir   305

CHAPTER 17   Targets for Interventions to Reduce Cancer Morbidity
             Lorenzo Cohen and Andrew Baum   321

PART 4: Conclusions

CHAPTER 18   Tailoring Psychosocial Interventions to the Individual's Health
             Information-Processing Style: The Influence of Monitoring
             Versus Blunting in Cancer Risk and Disease
             Suzanne M. Miller, Carolyn Y. Fang, Michael A. Diefenbach, and
             Christina B. Bales   343

CHAPTER 19   Preventive Psychosocial Intervention in Cancer Treatment:
             Implications for Managed Care
             Gerald P. Koocher and Irene S. Pollin   363

CHAPTER 20   Speculations on the Relationship of Behavioral Theory to
             Psychosocial Research on Cancer
             Howard Leventhal and Sasha Carr   375

Author Index   401
Subject Index   431
About the Editors   445

Contributors

Barbara L. Andersen, PhD, Department of Psychology, The Ohio State University, Columbus

Christina B. Bales, BA, Fox Chase Cancer Center, Cheltenham, PA

Priscilla Banks, MA, Northern California Cancer Center, Union City

Andrew Baum, PhD, Department of Psychiatry and Psychology, University of Pittsburgh, and Behavioral Medicine and Oncology, University of Pittsburgh Cancer Institute

Joan R. Bloom, PhD, School of Public Health, University of California, Berkeley

Dana H. Bovbjerg, PhD, Ruttenberg Cancer Center, Mount Sinai School of Medicine, New York

Andrea L. Canada, PhD, Department of Psychiatry and Behavioral Sciences, UCLA School of Medicine

Sasha Carr, MS, Health Behavior Program, Institute on Health Policy and Aging, Rutgers University, New Brunswick, NJ

Charles S. Carver, PhD, Department of Psychology, University of Miami

David Cella, PhD, Institute for Health Services Research and Policy Studies, Northwestern University and Center on Outcomes Research and Education, Evanston, IL

Lorenzo Cohen, PhD, Department of Behavioral Sciences, University of Texas, M. D. Anderson Cancer Center, Houston

Sheldon Cohen, PhD, Psychology Department, Carnegie Mellon University, Pittsburgh

Susan Diamond, MSW, Department of Psychiatry and Behavioral Sciences, Stanford University School of Medicine, Stanford, CA

Michael A. Diefenbach, PhD, Psychosocial and Behavioral Medicine Program, Fox Chase Cancer Center, Cheltenham, PA

Katherine N. DuHamel, PhD, Ruttenberg Cancer Center, Mount Sinai School of Medicine, New York

Carolyn Y. Fang, PhD, Division of Population Science, Fox Chase Cancer Center, Cheltenham, PA

Fawzy I. Fawzy, MD, Department of Psychiatry and Behavioral Sciences, UCLA School of Medicine

Nancy W. Fawzy, RN, DNSc, John Wayne Cancer Institute, Saint John's Health Center, Santa Monica, CA

Olivera J. Finn, PhD, Department of Molecular Genetics and Biochemistry, University of Pittsburgh School of Medicine and University of Pittsburgh Cancer Institute

Vicki S. Helgeson, PhD, Psychology Department, Carnegie Mellon University, Pittsburgh

Paul B. Jacobsen, PhD, Moffit Cancer Center, South Florida University, Tampa

Monica Johnston, BA, Department of Statistics, Stanford University, Stanford, CA

Gerald P. Koocher, PhD, Department of Psychology, Harvard Medical School, Boston, MA

Stephen J. Lepore, PhD, Department of Psychology, Brooklyn College and the Graduate Center of City University of New York

Caryn Lerman, PhD, Lombardi Cancer Center, Georgetown University School of Medicine, Washington, DC

Howard Leventhal, PhD, Institute for Health, Rutgers University, New Brunswick, NJ

Sharon L. Manne, PhD, Fox Chase Cancer Center, Cheltenham, PA

Suzanne M. Miller, PhD, Fox Chase Cancer Center, Cheltenham, PA

Jamie L. Ostroff, PhD, Memorial Sloan-Kettering Cancer Center, New York

Paul B. Paulus, PhD, Psychology Department, University of Texas at Arlington

Irene S. Pollin, MSW, Harvard Medical School, Boston, MA

Donna M. Posluszny, PhD, Behavioral Medicine and Oncology, University of Pittsburgh Cancer Institute

William H. Redd, PhD, Ruttenberg Cancer Center, Mount Sinai School of Medicine, New York

Barbara Rimer, Dr PH, Division of Cancer Control and Populations Sciences, National Cancer Institute, Rockville, MD

Michael F. Scheier, PhD, Department of Psychology, Carnegie Mellon University, Pittsburgh

Richard Schulz, PhD, Department of Psychiatry, University of Pittsburgh

Marc D. Schwartz, PhD, Lombardi Cancer Center, Georgetown University School of Medicine, Washington, DC

Meredith Y. Smith, PhD, Ruttenberg Cancer Center, Mount Sinai School of Medicine, New York

David Spiegel, MD, Department of Psychiatry and Behavioral Sciences, Stanford University School of Medicine, Stanford, CA

Susan L. Stewart, PhD, Northern California Cancer Center, Union City

Pierre L. Triozzi, MD, Division of Hematology and Oncology, The Ohio State University Medical Center, Columbus

Heiddis B. Valdimarsdottir, PhD, Ruttenberg Cancer Center, Mount Sinai School of Medicine, New York

Suzanne M. Johnson Vickberg, PhD, Ruttenberg Cancer Center, Mount Sinai School of Medicine, New York

Joyce Yasko, PhD, University of Pittsburgh School of Nursing and University of Pittsburgh Cancer Institute

Foreword

In early 1988, the American Psychological Association (APA) Science Directorate began its sponsorship of what has become an exceptionally successful activity in support of psychological science—the APA Scientific Conferences program. This program has showcased some of the most important topics in psychological science, and the conference participants have included many leading figures in the field.

As we enter a new century, it seems fitting that we begin with a new face on this book series—that of the Decade of Behavior (DoB). The DoB is a major interdisciplinary initiative designed to promote the contributions of the behavioral and social sciences to address some of our most important societal challenges and will occur from 2000 to 2010. Although a major effort of the initiative will be related to informing the public about the contributions of these fields, other activities will be put into place to reach fellow scientists. Hence, the series that was the "APA Science Series" will be continued as the "Decade of Behavior Series." This represents one element in APA's efforts to promote the DoB initiative as one of its partner organizations.

Please note the DoB logo on the inside jacket flap and the full title page. We expect this logo will become a familiar sight over the next few years. For additional information about DoB, please visit http://www.decadeofbehavior.org.

As part of the sponsorship agreement with APA, conference organizers commit themselves not only to the conference itself but also to editing a scholarly volume that results from the meeting. This book is such a volume. Over the course of the past 12 years, we have partnered with 44 universities to sponsor 60 conferences on a variety of topics of interest to psychological scientists. The APA Science Directorate looks forward to continuing this program and to sponsoring other conferences in the years ahead.

We are pleased that this important contribution to the literature was supported in part by the Scientific Conferences program. Congratulations to the editors and contributors on their sterling effort.

Richard McCarty, PhD
Executive Director for Science

Virginia E. Holt
Assistant Executive Director for Science

Acknowledgments

As with any project of this size, we are indebted to many others who played key roles in pulling this volume together. The American Psychological Association (APA) Science Directorate, most notably Virginia Holt, provided support, encouragement, advice, and important guidance throughout, as did their colleagues at APA Books, including Susan Reynolds and Ed Meidenbauer. The University of Pittsburgh Cancer Institute also provided support for the meeting on which this book is based. Several colleagues provided valuable input on the plans for the conference and for this book, and Michele Hayward, Lori McBurney, and Beth Visnich provided outstanding and critical expertise and assistance in these endeavors. We are very grateful for all of this assistance and hope that it has helped produce an important volume on the decades-long war on cancer.

Psychosocial Interventions
for Cancer

CHAPTER 1

Psychosocial Intervention and Cancer

An Introduction

Andrew Baum

Barbara L. Andersen

This book is about cancer and about the research in psychosocial and biobehavioral oncology that is underway to help control it. It is about the advent, implementation, and evaluation of interventions to modify behaviors, beliefs, and risk factors associated with the onset, progression, and recurrence of cancer. It is also about the underlying excitement of discovery and purpose, about working side by side with men and women from strangely different disciplines who speak in unfamiliar scientific and clinical languages. Ultimately, it is a shot across the bow of this monster disease, a confident prediction that the broad influences of psychosocial and biobehavioral variables can and will be harnessed to modify and enhance treatment and quality-of-life outcomes. As this new field grows and our knowledge of cancer and its causes develops, psychosocial interventions will become more targeted and more successful. The rapidly growing literature on psychosocial interventions and cancer strongly indicates that behavioral phenomena and modification of them can affect whether people develop cancer, how they respond to treatment, and (in some cases) how long they live.

Cancer as a Major Health Problem

A good deal of the work in psychosocial intervention is focused on cancer, for several reasons. Cancer is an important medical and public health problem. Each year, more than 1.2 million individuals in the United States are diagnosed with the disease and more than 500,000 die from it (Garfinkel, 1995). Cancer is the second leading cause of death in the United States (after heart disease) and a major source of premature mortality among both men and women (Garfinkel, 1995). Although it is associated with age and appears to be associated with lower socioeconomic status, it strikes all ages and all social, ethnic, religious, and cultural strata. At the turn of the 20th century, cancer was the eighth leading cause of death, far behind infectious illness (e.g., pneumonia, tuberculosis, diarrhea–enteritis), heart disease, and stroke, accounting for about 3% of deaths in the United States (Institute for the Future, 2000). Now cancer accounts for approximately 23% of deaths in the United States, more than the toll of chronic lung diseases, injuries, infectious diseases (pneumonia and influenza), HIV infection, diabetes, suicide, and liver disease combined (Hoyert, Kochanek, & Murphy, 1999).

Cancer is also a complicated disease, representing a collection of more than 100 local syndromes that are characterized by progressive weakening of cellular restraints on proliferation, by inactivation of apoptotic mechanisms (processes that lead defective cells to "commit suicide" by destroying themselves), and by the developing capacity to be malignant (i.e., to spread to other locations and tissues). Some cancers (e.g., pancreas, liver, and stomach) are relatively rare, each accounting for fewer than 10 deaths per 100,000 population in 1990; others (e.g., prostate) are more common, accounting for 128.9 per 100,000 population in 1990 (Garfinkel, 1995). Causes or promoters of disease, survival rates, treatment costs, treatments, disability, and availability of early detection and prevention options vary with disease site and by type of cancer. Research on these aspects of cancer is hampered by its very long development and the lack of good biomarkers or intermediate outcomes that allow us to trace early stages of disease in humans.

Cancer also affects and is affected by a variety of social, cultural, and psychological factors. For several reasons cancer is greatly feared and arouses distress among many who are at risk or are just worried about getting it. Research has suggested that risk status is associated with stable distress that features expression of anxiety and worry and that may interfere with surveillance and early detection of disease. Other studies have identified fear and worry about cancer in the general population and have documented stressful aspects of cancer diagnoses, treatments, and survival. The success of psychotherapeutic interventions for cancer and the apparent fact that reductions in distress are associated with better disease or treatment outcomes (topics that are covered in some detail in this volume) underscores the psychological significance of cancer and the potentially modifiable variance associated with stress and emotions. Social stigma has also been attached to the disease, and many of the side effects or direct products of treatment (e.g., disfiguring surgery, hair loss from adjuvant therapy) produce social strains and may require alteration of family, neighborhood, and community roles. Shared beliefs about cancer; about cancer care; and about body image, death, or survival also play important roles in cancer treatment and survival.

These psychosocial aspects of cancer and cancer control are the focus of this volume and reflect growing interest in biobehavioral mediation of disease processes and the centrality of lifestyle factors in pathophysiology. Some aspects of this perspective have received relatively little research attention, but others have generated substantial effort and several important findings. Stress has been a primary focus, in part because of interest in it as a broadly generalized response modifier across several systems and diseases. Stress may play a role in the development of malignancies or in the nature and speed of disease recurrence after treatment for initial manifestations of disease. Some evidence of this has been reported, but the long periods of slow growth and currently undetectable cellular changes that are characteristic of most tumors introduce issues of timing and measurement that limit conclusions that can be drawn from this literature. However, some circumstantial evidence supports the notion that stress contributes to cancer pathobiology, and some mechanisms by which stress could affect early disease-related events have been studied (e.g., Forlenza, Latimer, & Baum, 2000; Kiecolt-Glaser, Stephens, Lipetz, Speicher, & Glaser, 1985). Discovery of new biomarkers and development of new technologies will permit better measurement of cancer pathogenesis and foster new and more successful studies of biobehavioral modulation of cancer etiology and progression.

Research on Psychosocial Issues Related to Cancer and Cancer Treatment

Substantial and credible evidence exists for the idea that behavior, emotion, and stress affect the progression and course of cancer once it has been established. This appears to be particularly the case after diagnosis of cancer is made and may reflect the sharp upturn in stress and mental health problems that occurs when the disease is identified and treatments are initiated. Again, limitations on the design and conduct of much of this work reduces the strength of the conclusions that can be drawn, but evidence clearly favors the hypothesis that stress broadly affects biological and behavioral systems that govern or contribute to disease course (Baum, in press). Research targeting these biobehavioral systems and working on broad influences like stress or more sharply focused influences such as diet, exercise, tobacco use, and sun-protective behaviors will yield effective nonmedical means of reducing cancer morbidity and mortality.

The rapid growth of this research and clinical activity and the importance of answering relevant questions make the systematic review and integration of research in this area important and timely. The scientific underpinnings of this research and application of its findings have become clearer as research on mechanisms and moderators of biological systems and on targeting and implementation of interventions has increased. The clinical significance of these programs is also much clearer, and policy and practice issues have joined efficacy and mechanism studies as active research areas. There is still a great deal that we do not yet know and that probably is more complicated than we currently expect. Periodic pauses for reevaluation and integration, particularly after a major initial burst of scientific activity, can only advance further our understanding of how psychotherapeutic interventions work, what they can accomplish, and how they can be improved.

The following principles guided us in selecting the topics to be covered in this volume. First, it seemed important not to limit the scope of the volume to one or another "stage" of cancer care. Psychosocial influences are readily apparent in prevention and in early detection of cancer. Motivation and cost–benefit analyses that broadly consider emotional as well as physical health outcomes appear to be strong determinants of behavior oriented toward preventing or monitoring signs of cancer. As we noted earlier, people who view themselves as likely to get cancer or are at high risk because of familial or other factors experience stress and worry as a result. Several studies suggest that people who believe they are at risk for cancer overestimate that risk and are upset by several aspects of screening or surveillance (Black, Nease, & Tosteson, 1995; Dolan, Lee, & McDermott, 1997; Smith et al., 1996). Being at risk for cancer appears to engender a stable, chronic stress burden that may affect prevention or early detection efforts. For example, women who are at elevated risk for breast cancer appear to experience more chronic stress than do women at average risk (e.g., Kash, Holland, Halper, & Miller, 1992) and to exhibit lower levels of natural killer cell activity (see chapter 16). Stress may also interfere with practice of early detection activities in this population. At the same time, women at the highest levels of risk sometimes adhere less to recommendations for mammography or self-examination than women with fewer risk factors, and women who do not have mammography appear to be overrepresented among women with advanced breast cancer (e.g., Posluszny, McFeeley, Hall, & Baum, 2000; Wu, Weissfeld, Weinberg, & Kuller, 1999). Fear, stress, and coping are likely culprits in this breakdown of seemingly rational screening activities, and because they are modifiable they offer appealing targets for intervention. Clearly, management of distress alone does not necessarily produce meaningful changes in prevention activities and lifestyle, and issues related to education, persuasion, message framing, and other issues not covered centrally in this volume also are important. In particular, prevention and early detection activities can be enhanced by better understanding the psychological aspects of disease risk.

At the same time, health psychologists and behavioral scientists have targeted the stressful postdiagnosis phase of cancer, supplementing this traditional behavioral emphasis on prevention and surveillance and extending it to those battling the disease as well as to those surviving it. This effort quickly has gained momentum, focusing primarily on group interventions, skills, acquisition, stress management, and support. Quality of life can be enhanced and distress reliably reduced, and some data point to gains in treatment outcomes or survival as well. These interventions are a prominent focus of this volume and offer a remarkable opportunity to meaningfully deflect distress and slow progression of the disease as well as better understand the contributions of psychosocial or behavioral variables and disease course.

These considerations suggest that effective interventions must necessarily span several stages of cancer care and of disease. Some interventions or components of interventions are designed for people soon after diagnosis and others for patients approaching the completion of treatment, typically for primary-stage disease. Several interventions have been designed for people with advanced-stage disease or who have exhausted conventional treatments and are facing the possibility of death. Some are palliative in nature and seek primarily to reduce pain and suffering or to ease the burden on caregivers as they lose their ability to ameliorate patients' symptoms or distress. Across all of these phases of treatment and for patients of varying disease status, postdiagnosis interventions have underscored the importance of attending to the patient's psychological status in coping with and surviving cancer.

The variety of issues and challenges facing current or former cancer patients offer a daunting set of threats and behaviors to overcome or modify. The possibility that one may get cancer is stressful, and the problems associated with this distress include avoidance of screening and poor health behaviors. When individuals have been or are about to be diagnosed with cancer, the intensity and focus of these threats change and can become more emotionally disruptive. The primary issues of concern to this group of patients are clearly different from those characterizing "at-risk" populations or those who have had time to adjust to the diagnosis but have not experienced the demands and disruption associated with cancer treatments. During treatment existential concerns about life and death or about the randomness of the world may be replaced with specific fears about surgery or adjuvant therapy and the side effects and consequences of these therapies. Prognosis and severity of treatments are important determinants of response among all those patient groups, and the specific stressors and concerns among primary stage patients with relatively good prognoses should be different from those that are prominent among patients with advanced or metastatic cancer, whose prognosis is poorer. The effects of these variables mingle with psychosocial variables such as coping or with personality or styles such as optimism, producing variable but predictable reactions to cancer and cancer treatment.

The likelihood that different phases of treatment and stages of disease dictate different concerns and make different threats salient argues strongly for a perspective that considers these and other variables in the design and implementation of interventions. Some interventions may be directed acutely at specific aspects of treatment such as surgery or chemotherapy, others at larger channels of the cancer experience, and still others at prevention or palliation. At the same time, some interventions address concerns of primary cancer patients, others of advanced patients, and still others of family members or caregivers. By appropriately targeting groups along continua of stage of disease and phase of care, the likelihood of achieving meaningful changes in disease course and life quality should be enhanced (see Figure 1.1).

Addressing psychological variables as part of medical treatment is not a new idea, and behavioral scientists have been studying cancer and cancer-related issues for several decades. This enterprise did not spring full-blown into the cancer research arena, however, and the extent to which previous research in mental health and consultation–liaison settings, in cancer populations, or in other medical populations has laid the bases for current research is undeniable but often unappreciated. Present-day interventions aimed at minimizing stress and complications from prostate surgery

FIGURE 1.1

By considering interactions of stage of disease and stage of treatment, variable demands and difficulties may be identified as prominent and pressing.

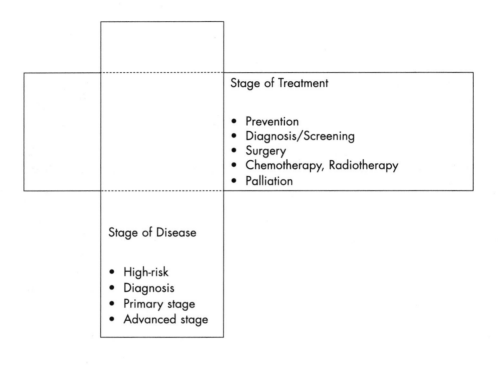

Stage of Treatment

- Prevention
- Diagnosis/Screening
- Surgery
- Chemotherapy, Radiotherapy
- Palliation

Stage of Disease

- High-risk
- Diagnosis
- Primary stage
- Advanced stage

or during aversive medical examinations are clearly based in a literature growing out of research by Janis (1958) on the "work of worrying" and Leventhal (e.g., Johnson & Leventhal, 1974; Leventhal, 1980; see this volume, chapter 20) on fear-arousing persuasion, cognitive control, and processing of emotions. Social support, cognitive–behavioral stress management, and other key components of many cancer patient interventions have been studied in the context of stress inoculation therapy, disasters, traumatic events, and exposure therapies and have been shown to be effective in HIV-positive populations as well (e.g., Schneiderman, 1999; Turk, Meichenbaum, & Genest, 1983). At the same time, there are extensive histories and scientific literatures on group therapy and group dynamics. To a large extent these theoretical undercurrents and contexts for contemporary care are underappreciated and are not well exploited. Systematic consideration and integration of these theories and literatures should enhance the value of intervention.

Plan for This Volume

The chapters in this volume are arranged in four general parts roughly paralleling the organization of these introductory remarks. Part I deals with the bases of adjustment to living with cancer, the reasons why one might predict that interventions would be useful, and the channels through which they may operate. Scheier and Carver (chapter 2) consider the role of hope and purpose in adjusting to cancer and its treatment, providing some psychosocial bases for intervention programs and how the threats and harm associated with cancer translate into psychoactive stressors. Bloom, Stewart, Johnston, and Banks (chapter 3) and Cella (chapter 4) address some primary outcomes of intervention and provide detailed and systematic analyses of quality of life in cancer. Redd, DuHamel, Vickberg, Ostroff, Smith, Jacobsen, and Manne (chapter 5) describe an important integration of approaches to behavior change and to enhancing long-term adjustment among cancer survivors. Lepore (chapter 6) offers a new model of adjustment in which social constraints and cognitive processing affect emotional adjustment to cancer.

Part II includes chapters dealing with processes and targets for intervention and prevention. Andersen (chapter 7) offers a broad conceptualization of the bases of interventions and some of the pathways by which they work. She considers the initial results of a major intervention trial as evidence of a biobehavioral model of cancer. Emphasis on this single major study provides some new insight into the operation of systems that seem to be critical for successful intervention. Baum and Posluszny (chapter 9) similarly consider aspects of stress that offer important targets for intervention, including psychological trauma associated with cancer. Paulus (chapter 8) discusses key aspects of group dynamics that provide unique information for those seeking to intervene. Finn (chapter 10) and Triozzi (chapter 11) address the immunologic and tumor-related aspects of such an approach in their chapters, describing biological pathways through which these interventions may operate.

Part III details several intervention programs and reviews data from studies of preventive and treatment-oriented interventions. One emphasis is on intervention programs for cancer patients at various stages of the disease. Pioneering efforts in these areas are the focus of chapters by Spiegel and Diamond (chapter 12) and by Fawzy, Fawzy, and Canada (chapter 13). These chapters describe the rationale for psychosocial patient intervention as well as theories and approaches that underlie these efforts. Treatment techniques and evidence for these techniques are also considered. Helgeson, Cohen, Schulz, and Yasko (chapter 14) consider important issues related to stage and variation in concerns across disease sites and stages, arguing that some intervention approaches may not always produce clear benefits. This section includes two chapters (chapter 15 by Schwartz, Lerman, & Rimer; and chapter 16 by Bovbjerg & Valdimarsdottir) that discuss risk management and distress in high-risk breast cancer populations. Chapter 17 (by Cohen & Baum) more generally targets prevention interventions and suggests that the overall payoff in reduced morbidity and mortality should more than justify intensive efforts in this area of cancer education and control. These chapters provide a broad impression of this large and well-established area of scientific activity and suggest new ways to increase early detection and prevention activities.

Part IV includes chapters that integrate and critically evaluate some implications of various approaches to intervention populations. These chapters address questions relating to how clinicians and researchers target various groups or subgroups or stages of disease or treatment and how we design interventions. Miller, Fang, Diefenbach, and Bales (chapter 18) describe a complex model of relationships among cognitive variables that underlies tailoring of interventions to fit personality or information-processing styles. Broader issues are also important, including the manner in which patient-centered research and care fit in evolving social and health care environments. Koocher and Pollin (chapter 19) evaluate implications of psychological interventions in managed care. Leventhal and Carr (chapter 20) speculate on the importance and nature of the relationships of behavioral and psychosocial variables and cancer. All of these chapters address the importance of behavioral and psychosocial issues in the quality and effectiveness of intervention at a number of points in the disease process.

Although the evidence is not always available in the strongest possible form, the data are clear and suggest that behavioral or psychosocial factors affect cancer in many important ways. There are indisputable causes of cancer that have major behavioral components, such as tobacco use and diet or obesity; stress, emotional expression, and psychophysiological arousal affect everything from endocrine profiles to decision making, from immune system surveillance for nascent tumor cells to adherence to treatment or chemoprevention regimens. Implementing interventions to modify behaviors that constitute risks or that minimize or help to manage distress also seems to have far-reaching effects, many of which are still under study and are the focus of chapters included in this volume. Although not all of this exciting and innovative work is covered in this book, we have provided a comprehensive view and have touched on the major theoretical and applied developments in this emergent field. This work is becoming more complex and more ambitious all the time, and the glimpse that is offered in this book is a benchmark of work at the close of the 20th century, allowing us to "take stock" of what we know and need to learn.

There is some overlap among the chapters in these parts, reflecting the interlocking constructs and shared theories that characterize intervention and prevention efforts. Present research and theory in this area overlap as well, as partial replications and extensions, integration of seemingly disparate findings, and examination of mechanistic and holistic aspects of interventions continue to move our knowledge ahead. Although the overall approaches and interests may vary, most of these efforts depend on similar literatures and theories, each viewed from a different perspective. Consequently, we have not asked that this overlap be removed or reduced, in part to preserve the differences in perspective that can be seen in these chapters and in part to maintain the contexts in which they were written. We hope that this editorial division does not affect how the chapters read; cross-referencing and referral among them should minimize redundancy without disrupting the general bases for work that is described.

Given the coming changes in health care (such as the continued dominance of HMOs, growth of minority and elderly populations, and growth of long-term home care) and the likely continuation of a shift toward research on chronic, disabling diseases that are complex and costly to manage and treat, the advent and expansion of behavior change and psychotherapeutic interventions is a major public health development. The U.S. population is changing, and insurance or medical coverage is changing as well. Our population has shown steady increases in education over the past 50 years, and as the baby boomers age there will be a dramatic increase in the number of older Americans as a group and as a proportion of the population. Similarly, family incomes have increased, and Americans have shown dramatic increases in HMO membership over the past 5 years (Institute for the Future, 2000). The "shifting burden of disease," reflecting the growing importance of chronic diseases, mental health, and lifestyle behaviors, is due in part to better life expectancies and control of infectious diseases and in part to advances in the care and management of these chronic diseases. This shift denotes a change in the causes of premature disability and mortality, and these changes will continue to strain health care systems (Institute for the Future, 2000). Some of the best strategies for managing these changes, for meeting increasing demand for care, and for dealing with escalating costs in the face of decreasing numbers of inpatient beds and falling hospital occupancy lie in the development and implementation of behavioral or psychosocial interventions that help manage disease risk, decrease stress and negative emotions in the face of cancer diagnosis and treatment, and enhance quality of life and decision making.

References

Baum, A. (in press). Behavioral and psychosocial interventions to modify pathophysiology and disease course. In B. D. Smedley & S. L. Syme (Eds.), *Promoting health: Intervention strategies from social and behavioral research.* Washington, DC: National Academy Press.

Black, W. C., Nease, R. F., Jr., & Tosteson, A. N. (1995). Perceptions of breast cancer risk and screening effectiveness in women younger than 50 years of age. *Journal of the National Cancer Institute, 87*(10), 720–731.

Dolan, N. C., Lee, A. M., & McDermott, M. M. (1997). Age-related differences in breast carcinoma knowledge, beliefs, and perceived risk among women visiting an academic general medicine practice. *Cancer, 80*(3), 413–420.

Forlenza, M. J., Latimer, J. J., & Baum, A. (2000). Stress and DNA repair [Abstract]. *Psychosomatic Medicine, 62*(1), 117.

Garfinkel, L. (1995). Cancer statistics and trends. In G. P. Murphy, J. W. Lawrence, & R. E. Lenhard (Eds.), *American Cancer Society textbook of clinical oncology* (pp. 1–11). Washington, DC: American Cancer Society.

Hoyert, D. L., Kochanek, K. D., & Murphy, S. L. (1999). Deaths: Final data for 1997. *National Vital Statistics Reports, 47*(19), 1–113.

Institute for the Future. (2000). *Health and healthcare 2010: The forecast, the challenge.* San Francisco: Jossey-Bass.

Janis, I. L. (1958). *Psychological stress.* New York: Wiley.

Johnson, J. E., & Leventhal, H. (1974). Effects of accurate expectations and behavioral instructions on reactions during a noxious medical examination. *Journal of Personality and Social Psychology, 29*, 710–718.

Kash, K. M., Holland, J. C., Halper, M. S., & Miller, D. G. (1992). Psychological distress and surveillance behaviors of women with a family history of breast cancer. *Journal of the National Cancer Institute, 84*, 24–30.

Kiecolt-Glaser, J. K., Stephens, R. E., Lipetz, P. D., Speicher, C. E., & Glaser, R. (1985). Distress and DNA repair in human lymphocytes. *Journal of Behavioral Medicine, 8*, 311–320.

Leventhal, H. (1980). Emotions: A basic problem for social psychology. In C. Nemeth (Ed.), *Social psychology: Classic and contemporary integrations* (pp. 1–51). Chicago: Rand McNally.

Posluszny, D. M., McFeeley, S., Hall, L., & Baum, A. (2000). *Stress, breast cancer risk, and surveillance: Chronic effects of risk and worry.* Manuscript submitted for publication.

Schneiderman, N. (1999). Behavioral medicine and the management of HIV/AIDS. *International Journal of Behavioral Medicine, 6*(1), 3–12.

Smith, B. L., Gadd, M. A., Lawler, C., MacDonald, D. J., Grudberg, S. C., Chi, F. S., Carlson, K., Comegno, A., & Souba, W. W. (1996). Perceptions of breast cancer risk among women in breast center and primary care settings: Correlation with age and family history of breast cancer. *Surgery, 120*(2), 297–303.

Turk, D. C., Meichenbaum, D., & Genest, M. (Eds.). (1983). *Pain and behavioral medicine: A cognitive–behavioral perspective.* New York: Guilford Press.

Wu, Y., Weissfeld, J. L., Weinberg, G. B., & Kuller, L. H. (1999). Screening mammography and late-stage breast cancer: A population-based study. *Preventive Medicine, 28*, 572–578.

PART 1

Bases of Adjustment to Living With Cancer

CHAPTER 2

Adapting to Cancer

The Importance of Hope and Purpose

Michael F. Scheier
Charles S. Carver

Hope makes us live. (Haitian proverb)

* * *

Formula of my happiness: A yes, a no, a straight line, a *goal*. (Friedrich Nietzsche, *Twilight of the Idols/The Anti-Christ,* p. 37, italics in original)

* * *

Without a mountain to climb, a stream to cross, a goal to reach, there is no reason to live. (Richard M. Nixon)

A cancer diagnosis is life-disrupting on many levels, and people react to the diagnosis and treatment of cancer differently. Some people adapt relatively well to the adversity, whereas others adjust with more difficulty. Although everyone is buffeted by the physical and psychological threats that permeate the experience of the cancer patient, some people negotiate the rapids in fine order, emerging from the ordeal reasonably intact—indeed, sometimes they are psychologically better off than they were before their diagnosis (cf. Collins, Taylor, & Skokan, 1990; Dow, Ferrell, Leigh, Ly, & Gulasekaram, 1996; Fromm, Andrykowski, & Hunt, 1996; Kahn & Steeves, 1993; Kurtz, Wyatt, & Kurtz, 1995; Wyatt, Kurtz, Friedman, Given, & Given, 1996). For others, however, the toll is more severe. Their lives never return to a semblance of order, and their emotional scars last throughout their lives.

What accounts for these differences in reactions? In this chapter we argue that people who respond well to cancer diagnosis and treatment are those who maintain hopefulness and continue to find purpose in living during and after their encounter

Preparation of this chapter was facilitated by National Cancer Institute Grants CA64710, CA62711, and CA84944 as well as Grants HL65111 and HL65112 from the National Heart, Lung, and Blood Institute.

with the disease. In the same vein, we believe that intervention efforts that successfully help people adjust to their cancer are successful partly because they foster hopefulness and help patients remain engaged with life.

Our beliefs concerning the importance of hope and purpose derive from a larger view of what it means to be alive and to be immersed in the process of living. Consequently, we begin our story with a brief discussion of this larger theoretical framework. Following this discussion, we review some evidence linking hope and purpose to psychological and physical well-being. We then turn our attention to a consideration of the nature of successful cancer interventions and discuss why we think these work by influencing purpose and hope. We close the chapter with a discussion of several issues related to the process of goal engagement and disengagement.

Conceptual Framework

For the past two and a half decades, we have worked with a particular model of behavioral self-regulation (Carver & Scheier, 1981, 1990, 1998). Central to our view is the notion that people live by identifying goals for themselves and working and behaving in ways to attain these goals (Figure 2.1, Loop 1). The goals themselves can take a variety of forms. Some of the goals that people pursue reflect biological programming (e.g., finding and drinking water when thirsty); others stem from dreams and fantasies of what might be (e.g., catching the biggest steelhead in Pennsylvania). Some goals are very concrete (e.g., taking out the garbage); others are more abstract and ephemeral (e.g., being a successful psychologist). Some goals arise recurrently (e.g., desiring sleep); others remain constant fixtures in the person's life (e.g., being a good parent). Regardless of their origin and nature, goals are seen in this view as providing the structure that define people's lives, imbuing lives with meaning, both in the short run and in the long run (see also Leventhal & Carr, this volume, chapter 20). Indeed, we have even suggested that goal-engagement is a *necessity* of life (Carver & Scheier, 1998).

In our view, two factors are important in goal engagement. First, a person must be able to identify goals that are valued. People do not take up goals that do not matter to them, and if they did, they would not persist at them very long when things got difficult. Valued goals provide the purpose for living. The second important factor is the sensed attainability of the goal. If a goal seems unattainable at the outset, effortful behavior never even begins. If people continually fail to make progress toward goals they have committed themselves to, they will begin to withdraw effort and start to perceive those goals as out of reach. In contrast, hope enables one to hold onto valued goals, remain engaged in the process of goal striving, and stay committed to the attempt to move forward (Figure 2.1, Loop 2).

These general themes are those of generations of expectancy-value models of motivation (Atkinson, 1964; Feather, 1982; Shah & Higgins, 1997; Vroom, 1964).

FIGURE 2.1

A model for self-regulation. Successful self-regulation is a continuing process of identifying goals, pursuing them, attaining them, and identifying further ones (Loop 1). Given adversity, a step of evaluating chances of success may be added (Loop 2), but sufficient confidence places the person back into the first loop. If confidence is low, the person may seek an alternative goal (Loop 3); if available, this alternative goal returns the person to goal pursuit and attainment. If, however, the original goal is seen as unattainable and no alternative is available, the person may disengage completely. From On the Self-Regulation of Behavior *(p. 349), by C. S. Carver and M. F. Scheier, 1998, New York: Cambridge University Press. Copyright 1998 by Cambridge University Press. Reprinted with permission.*

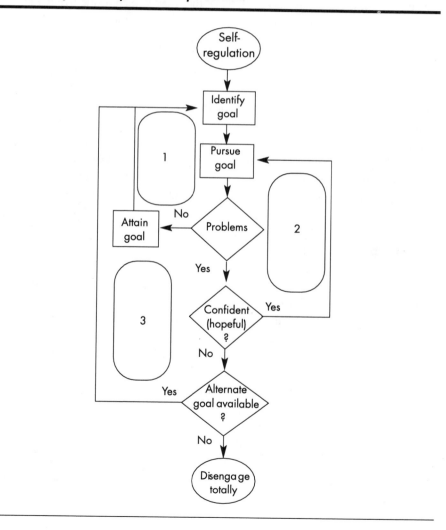

In such models, engagement of effort occurs when a goal matters enough to try to reach it (value) and the person has sufficient confidence about its eventual attainment (expectancy). Our view on behavior is one such model.

How do these principles apply to illness episodes? In some respects illness is no different from any other obstacle to goal attainment (what is labeled in Figure 2.1 as *Problems*). Illness is one of a host of adversities that a person might encounter on the way to goal attainment. On the other hand, episodes of serious illness have a particularly pernicious role. Major illnesses explicitly and directly threaten the desire to stay alive and be healthy (valued goals in their own right). They also indirectly undermine other ongoing goal pursuits. Thus, people diagnosed with a disease such as cancer suffer two sorts of disruption, potentially undermining two classes of hopes: They may lose confidence that they will continue living, and they may also confront the loss of hope of achieving major life ambitions.

One final part of the overall picture is that the loss of engagement in a goal does not necessarily lead to a vacuum of goal-lessness. Elsewhere, we have discussed the ebb and flow of engagement and disengagement in terms of competition among goals (Carver & Scheier, 1998). We suggested that disengagement from one goal may reflect a weakening of commitment to it. Because people usually have many goals at once, however, this weakening of commitment permits another goal to become prepotent and thus permits behavior to shift toward its pursuit. Thus, the loss of one goal is often followed directly by pursuit of another one.

Sometimes this means scaling back to a less ambitious goal in the same domain as the abandoned goal. By taking up an attainable alternative, the person remains engaged in goal pursuit and forward movement (Figure 2.1, Loop 3). This is particularly important when the blocked path concerns a value central to the self. People need multiple paths to these core values (cf. Linville, 1985, 1987; Showers & Ryff, 1996; Wicklund & Gollwitzer, 1982). If one path is barricaded, people need to be able to jump to another one. Consider a cancer patient who has great personal investment in family ties. If chemotherapy destroys the ability to have children, positive family experiences can be obtained in other ways (cf. Clark, Henry, & Taylor, 1991). If long-term career ambitions are threatened by a potentially fatal illness, those ambitions might be realized in smaller ways in the time that remains. Alternatively, the person might reprioritize various aspects of life and spend less time working and more time in close relationships.

It seems likely that substituting a new path for an obstructed one is made easier by having clearly specified goals at a more abstract level. Someone who understands that his or her core desire is to experience closeness can more readily recognize that there are many ways to do this than can someone who is less clear about the nature of the higher level goal. Similarly, it seems likely that a person who already recognizes the multiple paths that exist to a given goal will be better prepared to make such shifts as necessary.

In any case, it seems apparent that the ability to shift to a new goal or to a new path to a continuing goal is a very important part of remaining goal-engaged. What happens if there's no alternative to take up? In such a case disengagement from an unattainable goal is not accompanied by a shift, because there's nothing to shift to. This is the worst situation; there is nothing to pursue, nothing to take the place of what is seen as unattainable (cf. Moskowitz, Folkman, Collette, & Vittinghoff, 1996). If commitment to the unattainable goal remains, the result is considerable distress. If the commitment wanes, the result is emptiness. There is reason to suspect that such a state might also be implicated in premature death (i.e., not surviving as long as the physical condition would suggest) (Carver & Scheier, 1998).

Purpose, Hopefulness, and Well-Being

In this section we review some of the research that ties purpose and hope to health and well-being. Most of the research in this domain has focused on the beneficial effects of hope and positive expectancies rather than on the beneficial effects of purpose. To some degree, the neglect of purpose is due to the tendency of researchers (ourselves included) to use such qualities as hope, confidence, and optimism as proxies for purpose, and indeed as proxies for goal engagement more generally (in that these qualities seem to imply the existence of valued goals toward which one continues to strive).

The relative absence of data is also due to investigators' tendency to embed the study of purpose within larger theoretical frameworks. Antonovsky (1987), for example, has explicitly discussed the critical role played by purpose (or what he calls *meaningfulness*) in the development of a sense of coherence.[1] Similarly, Kobasa (1979; Kobasa & Maddi, 1981) has described how a sense of commitment to goals and activities combines with feelings of control and challenge to create the "hardy" personality. Studies from these and other research traditions have tended to focus on the composite variable rather than on the individual components from which the composite is derived. As a result, the unique effects of purpose have remained obscured.

---

[1] Theorists vary in what they mean by *finding meaning* in a negative event. Included in most definitions is one or more of the following: the capacity to understand the origin or etiology of the event, the ability to find something beneficial to take from the event, and the attempt to make sense of the event by placing it into a larger existential context (e.g., Bulman & Wortman, 1977; Ersek & Ferrell, 1994; McIntosh, Silver, & Wortman, 1993; Silver, Boon, & Stones, 1983; Thompson, 1985; Thompson & Pitts, 1993). Sometimes they also include a sense of finding meaning through the pursuit of valued goals (Dunn, 1994; Thompson & Janigian, 1988). This latter corresponds most closely to what we have in mind when we talk about finding and maintaining purpose. To avoid confusion, we have tried throughout the present chapter to rely exclusively on the term *purpose*, or some variant of it, to refer to the processes that are of interest to us.

Purpose

Few researchers have directly linked purpose to health and well-being, and even fewer have examined the impact of purpose among people confronting cancer. Nonetheless, the findings that do exist are remarkably consistent in the picture they paint. For example, across three separate studies Ryff and her colleagues (Ryff, 1989; Ryff & Keyes, 1995; Ryff, Lee, Essex, & Schmutte, 1994) found positive associations between a sense of purpose in life and measures of life satisfaction, positive mood states, and happiness. These same studies also uniformly showed purpose in life to be negatively associated with depression. Others have shown that people with a sense of purpose report better self-rated health and less emotional distress across the course of the life span (Holahan, 1988; Reker, Peacock, & Wong, 1987). Finally, Lewis (1982) found that purpose in life among a group of late stage cancer patients was strongly associated with lower self-reported anxiety. Taken together, these various studies begin to make the case that people with a strongly felt purpose in life experience more positive states of psychological well-being.

Conceptually similar findings emerge if one moves beyond purpose per se and examines studies investigating goal engagement more generally. For example, studies show positive relationships between pursuit of goals and life satisfaction (Brand-stadter & Renner, 1990; Harlow & Cantor, 1996; Palys & Little, 1983; Ruehlman & Wolchik, 1988) and happiness (Smith, Haynes, Lazarus, & Pope, 1993), and negative relationships between pursuit of goals and negative affect, depression, and neuroticism (Brandstadter & Renner, 1990; Emmons & King, 1988; Ruehlman & Wolchik, 1988). Indeed, evidence suggests that even people in prisons stay more "sane" and less prone to violence if they are able to pursue long-term educational goals (Worth, 1995).

Hope

Variables such as optimism (Scheier & Carver, 1985), hope (Snyder, 1994), self-efficacy (Bandura, 1986), and optimistic attributional style (Peterson & Seligman, 1984) are central to contemporary theories of self-regulation. In addition, several people have commented on the nature and importance of hope in dealing with cancer in particular (e.g., Bunston, Mings, Mackie, & Jones, 1995; Hickey, 1986; O'Connor, Wicker, & Germino, 1990; Weisman & Worden, 1976–1977). Not surprisingly, more is known about the effects of optimism and hope on health and well-being than is known about the effects of purpose on these outcomes.

The typical study focuses on how positive expectations influence adjustment as people face difficulties in their lives. The range of stressors involved in the research is very broad. Studies have examined the experiences of students entering college (Aspinwall & Taylor, 1992), employees of businesses (Long, 1993), and survivors of missile attacks (Zeidner & Hammer, 1992). Studies have measured the responses of people caring for medical patients of one type or another (Given et al., 1993;

Hooker, Monahan, Shifren, & Hutchinson, 1992; Shifren & Hooker, 1995). Researchers have examined experiences of people dealing with medical procedures such as childbirth (Carver & Gaines, 1987; Park, Moore, Turner, & Adler, 1997), abortion (Cozzarelli, 1993), coronary artery bypass surgery (Fitzgerald, Tennen, Affleck, & Pransky, 1993; Scheier et al., 1989), attempts at in vitro fertilization (Litt, Tennen, Affleck, & Klock, 1992), bone marrow transplantation (Curbow, Somerfield, Baker, Wingard, & Legro, 1993), and the progression of AIDS (Taylor et al., 1992).

It is not our intent to review here all the research documenting the beneficial effects of positive expectations on adjustment (for more comprehensive reviews, see Carver & Scheier, 1999; Peterson & Bossio, 1991; Scheier, Carver, & Bridges, 2001; Seligman, 1991). Rather, we focus on a few illustrative studies that have examined the effects of optimism and hope on reactions to cancer diagnosis and treatment. Two projects have targeted women with breast cancer. In one study (Stanton & Snider, 1993), optimism and mood were assessed on the day prior to biopsy. The mood of women who received a positive cancer diagnosis was then reassessed 24 hours before surgery and again 3 weeks after surgery (subsets of women who received a negative diagnosis were assessed at approximately similar points in time). Optimism was a strong predictor of prebiopsy distress, although it was not predictive of distress at either follow-up point.

The second study (Carver et al., 1993) focused exclusively on women whose biopsy was positive. Patients in this study were interviewed at six times: at the time of their diagnosis, the day before surgery, 7 to 10 days after surgery, and 3, 6, and 12 months later. Optimism was assessed at the time of diagnosis and was used to predict distress levels at the same point in time (i.e., at diagnosis) as well as at each subsequent point in time. Optimism proved to be inversely related to distress levels at all assessment points, controlling for relevant medical and demographic factors. More important, optimism also predicted changes in distress over time. That is, associations between optimism and distress remained significant even when the prior level of distress was controlled (in addition to relevant medical factors). Thus, optimism predicted not just lower distress but also resilience to distress during the year following surgery.

Also relevant here is a study by Christman (1990), which examined adjustment among a group of patients undergoing radiotherapy for a variety of different kinds of cancers. Patients were enrolled in the project at one of three points in time: on the first day of treatment, on the 15th day of treatment, and on the last day of treatment. Multiple assessments were made on those patients who were enrolled prior to their last day of treatment. Hope was negatively related to adjustment problems at all three assessment points, as well as to illness uncertainty at the first and second assessment points. Interestingly, hope was unrelated to preferences for health-related locus of control in this study.

Also noteworthy are findings suggesting that optimism can influence the psycho-logical well-being of patient caregivers, as well as the patients themselves. Given et al. (1993) studied a group of cancer patients and their caregivers and found that caregivers' optimism related to a number of caregiver well-being variables. Higher optimism was associated with lower symptoms of depression, less impact of care-giving on physical health, and less impact on caregivers' daily schedules. Optimists also reported less change in impact on their schedules and less change in health between two time points. Caregiver optimism proved to be independent of patient variables in predicting caregiver reactions to the burdens of caring for a family member with cancer.

The foregoing studies dealt with psychological well-being. There is also evidence that optimism and hope can influence physical well-being. Scheier et al. (1989) examined reactions to and recovery from coronary artery bypass graft surgery. They found that optimism levels assessed prior to surgery inversely predicted clinical signs of myocardial infarction during the course of the surgery. Thus, optimism seemed to buffer patients from the deleterious effects of the operation (see also Leedham, Meyerowitz, Muirhead, & Frist, 1995). More recently, Everson et al. (1996) found that hopelessness was a significant predictor of disease-specific mortal-ity (including cancer mortality) as well as all-cause mortality in a large sample of Finnish men who had been treated for cancer or heart attacks.

There are even data linking pessimism to cancer survival (Schulz, Bookwala, Knapp, Scheier, & Williamson, 1996). Patients in this project, all diagnosed with recurrent cancer, were followed for a period of 8 months, by which time approxi-mately one third had died. Earlier in the study all of the patients had completed a measure of pessimism. Controlling for site of cancer and levels of symptoms at baseline, people with a pessimistic orientation were less likely to be alive at the 8-month follow-up. Furthermore, the findings were specific to pessimism. Depres-sion did not predict mortality in this study. Interestingly, the pessimism finding held only among relatively younger patients in the study (those below 60), a finding that is not without precedent in the research literature more generally (Scheier & Bridges, 1995).

These various observational studies make a persuasive case that goal engagement, in general, and purpose and hope, in particular, confer important psychological and physical benefits to people facing difficult circumstances, including diagnosis and treatment for cancer. In the next section, we consider the beneficial effects of psychosocial interventions and explore the possibility that purpose and hope might mediate those beneficial effects.

Mapping Variables Onto Interventions

Psychosocial interventions for cancer tend to be multifaceted (Andersen, 1992; Fawzy, Fawzy, Arndt, & Pasnau, 1995; Spencer, Carver, & Price, 1998; Trijsburg, van Knippenberg, & Rijpma, 1992). Interventions often include some type of educational component—information about the cancer, its treatment, and the chance of reoccurrence, or information about nutritional considerations or cancer genetics. Most interventions, particularly group interventions, also provide elements of social and emotional support—the opportunity to bond with other similar group members, the context for expressing and clarifying emotions. Interventions also frequently incorporate training in effective coping strategies and problem-solving techniques, thereby providing opportunities for cognitive restructuring and appraisal. Any number of these elements seems capable of augmenting hope and purpose; we first consider their impact on the enhancement of confidence.

Augmenting Hope and Optimism

Hopefulness is maintained when a person believes that desired outcomes will occur, that valued goals will be reached, and that some degree of progress is being made in closing in on goals that matter. In the context of confronting cancer diagnosis and treatment, threatened goals include the person's sense of physical well-being, the ability to keep the consequences of the disease manageable, and the desire not to let the illness interfere with other significant life tasks. Anything that increases the person's confidence in these domains should serve to enhance the person's overall level of hopefulness and optimism.

As noted, explicit training in coping skills and problem-solving techniques is often an important component of interventions. Indeed, training in active-behavioral coping provides the backbone for one of the better known interventions in use with cancer patients today (Fawzy et al., 1990, 1993; see also Fawzy, Fawzy, & Canada, this volume, chapter 13). Moreover, instruction in active coping is frequently combined with relaxation training and training in stress management and pain management techniques, enhancing further the coping arsenal. One effect of all these training experiences should be an increase in the person's confidence in being able to deal effectively with the consequences of the illness. That is, providing coping skills gives the patient something specific to *do* to combat the illness. In the same vein, providing counseling on how to deal effectively with the pain and stress caused by the illness and treatment should make the disease seem more manageable and less likely to interfere with other ongoing life concerns.

What about the provision of information, education, and social support? A reasonable case can be made that these resources might also enhance feelings of confidence and hope. For example, providing patients with information about the genetics of cancer might help to allay any fear arising from erroneous perceptions about the likelihood of passing the disease on to children. Information about the importance of diet, coupled with instruction on how to shop for healthier foods, might create a feeling of empowerment. Counselors and fellow group members can also serve as sources of encouragement and support, bolstering the person's confidence in dealing effectively with the illness in times of uncertainty. Other group members can also serve as positive role models. To see other patients dealing in a functional manner with their illness can increase people's confidence that their own illness can also be managed successfully. Indeed, it is hard to imagine any aspect of psychosocial interventions that could not plausibly be construed as inducing an enhanced sense of hopefulness and optimism.

Augmenting Purpose

Psychosocial interventions can also serve an important function with respect to finding and maintaining a sense of purpose in life. There are at least a couple of ways in which interventions might have such an effect. One route is indirect, operating through enhanced confidence of goal attainment. As we maintained earlier in the chapter, hope and purpose go hand in hand. That is, to the extent that valued goals seem obtainable, they continue to serve as guiding points for action (Figure 2.1, Loop 2). To the extent that interventions produce a sense of hope and optimism about recovering from the cancer, the patient should be less likely to abandon current life goals because of the threat the disease poses for those goals. In this fashion, the interventions might help to keep patients more goal-engaged, especially those with a relatively good prognosis.

On the other hand, cancer or its treatment sometimes cause certain goals to be lost forever. For example, if chemotherapy induces premature menopause, having one's own child becomes impossible. If terminal lung cancer gives the person only a short time to live, that person may not be able to see his or her children complete college. In such circumstances, greater benefit may accrue from abandoning hope for this unattainable goal, giving it up, and trying to identify an alternative goal to take its place (Figure 2.1, Loop 3).

An important factor in moving forward in the search for new goals is the ability to recognize that the previous goal is in fact unattainable. Only by accepting this fact can the person move forward and identify new goals to take the place of the unattainable one. Psychosocial interventions may help to foster this acceptance and guide the person toward alternative goals, perhaps by providing opportunities to see how others have reacted to their experience and moved forward with their lives. Given such experiences, interventions may help the patient to better accept the reality of his or her situation and begin to integrate that reality into a new worldview, from which an alternative sense of purpose might arise (see also Lepore, this volume, chapter 6).

Psychosocial interventions might promote a sense of purpose in another, more direct way. Put simply, the intervention itself may become a purpose for living, an activity that helps give life meaning. This may be particularly likely in group interventions. The point is perhaps best illustrated by Spiegel, Bloom, and Yalom (1981), who documented the beneficial effect of a social support group intervention among women with metastatic breast cancer (see also Spiegel & Diamond, this volume, chapter 12). In discussing mechanisms underlying their findings, the authors were struck by how important the group members had become for each other, and how the act of caring for each other had provided group members with an important reason for living: "being of help to others, even at the very end of life, helped to imbue members with a vital sense of meaningfulness" (Spiegel et al., 1981, p. 532). Thus, for the individual members the group had become an important purpose for life.

Further Considerations

We have made several claims about the importance of hope and purpose in successfully confronting adversity in life, including cancer diagnosis and treatment. Along the way, we passed over a number of complex and possibly controversial issues. Before concluding the chapter, we address some of these issues.

A Cautionary Note: The Potential for Adverse Responses

Many experiences that have the potential for benefit also have the potential for harm. For example, earlier we mentioned that upward social comparison can inspire people, give them goals to strive for, and give them the sense that a better state of affairs is attainable in their own lives. However, the very same sort of upward comparison also has the potential to deflate or discourage people, to lead them to the perception that they are worse off than they really are. Similarly, downward comparisons with worse-off others can produce either positive or negative effects. If people leave the comparison feeling a sense of relief or gratitude that things are not worse for them than they presently are, benefits accrue. If people leave the same comparison feeling a sense of worry or dread that their condition will soon deteriorate, the effect is negative.

Thus, even as simple an act as a mental comparison with someone who is better or worse off than oneself is a double-edged sword. It can motivate, or it can interfere with motivation (Buunk, 1995; Buunk, Collins, Taylor, Van Yperen, & Dakof, 1990; Taylor, Buunk, & Aspinwall, 1990). The key determinant of which happens may be the person's confidence about being able to move toward the upward comparison point or away from the downward comparison point (Bridges, 1998; Carver & Scheier, 1998). Consistent with this position, Bridges (1998) has shown that optimists and pessimists do not differ in the number of upward and downward comparisons they make, but they do differ in how they respond to those comparisons. Optimists are less likely than pessimists to report being frustrated or upset by upward social comparisons. They are also less likely than pessimists to report being worried, fearful, or anxious by downward comparisons.

It is also possible for psychosocial interventions—in the very attempt to provide patients opportunities to enhance their lives—to inadvertently create opportunities for adverse effects. As an illustration, consider a project by Helgeson, Cohen, Schulz, and Yasko (1999; see also Helgeson, Cohen, Schulz, & Yasko, this volume, chapter 14). This project evaluated the relative effectiveness of an educational group intervention versus a support group intervention for women with early stage breast cancer. The education groups produced consistent positive effects on quality of life, both immediately after the intervention and 6 months later. In contrast, participation in the peer support groups had no beneficial effect. In fact, there was even some indication that the support groups increased negative affect. Subsidiary analyses suggested that this negative affect stemmed partly from the tendency of the support group members to engage in more frequent downward social comparisons (compared with participants in the education and control groups) and to come away from those comparisons feeling more distressed.

Thus, whether the patient is making a self-guided attempt to cope or is involved in a systematic intervention, care must be taken to prevent the development of a negative slant on the experience. This can be difficult enough when things are going reasonably well; it is particularly difficult when the patient's condition is worsening.

On the Nature of Acceptance

Another point to consider more fully concerns the role of acceptance in the coping process. We have argued that acceptance is a desirable response, a necessary step in the search for alternative goals and meaning, an indispensable link in the process of reprioritizing life tasks when old goals need to be abandoned. We raise two further issues regarding acceptance.

The first issue concerns our position on denial. That is, saying that acceptance is good seems to imply that denial is bad. As a point of fact, the research literature on the usefulness of denial as a coping strategy is mixed. Some people find that denial is associated with greater distress when confronting stressful circumstances such as cancer (Carver et al., 1993), whereas others have found the effects of denial to be beneficial (Meyerowitz, 1983; Watson, Greer, Blake, & Shrapnell, 1984).

The cause for the inconsistency regarding denial remains unclear. The answer may reside partly in how denial is defined and measured (Spencer et al., 1998). Denial is a difficult construct to measure, and the studies yielding conflicting results operationalized it differently. The duration of denial may also be important. Short-term positive effects are often attributed to denial as providing a psychological breather from the task of coping (Miller, 1990; Repetti, 1992), or as allowing the person to deal with the problem a little bit at a time (Levine et al., 1987; Mullen & Suls, 1982; Suls & Fletcher, 1985). Perhaps denial in the short run can be beneficial, whereas its prolonged use is more uniformly detrimental (Mullen & Suls, 1982).

Why should the prolonged use of denial be maladaptive? Denial (the refusal to accept the reality of the situation) means attempting to adhere to a worldview that is no longer valid. In contrast, acceptance implies a restructuring of one's experience so as to come to grips with the reality of the situation that one confronts. Acceptance thus may involve a deeper set of processes in which the person actively works through the experience, attempting to integrate it into an evolving worldview (see also Tedeschi & Calhoun, 1995).

The active attempt to come to terms with the existence of problems may confer special benefit to acceptance as a coping response. We wish to be very clear, however, about the nature of the acceptance we are talking about (the second issue regarding acceptance). The kind of acceptance we have in mind is a willingness to admit that a problem exists or that an event has happened—even an event that may irrevocably alter the fabric of the person's life. We are *not* talking about a stoic resignation, a fatalistic acceptance of the negative consequences to which the problem or event might lead, no matter how likely those consequences might be. The latter kind of acceptance does not confer a benefit.

Consider, for example, someone dealing with the terminal stages of cancer. The ultimate outcome is death. Yet the person can accept the fact that he or she is terminally ill without simultaneously succumbing to the feeling that he or she is "as good as dead." The latter sort of acceptance, or resignation, may well promote a kind of functional death in which the person prematurely disengages from the opportunities of life. Consistent with this idea, there are findings suggesting that people who react to illness diagnoses with stoic resignation or passive acceptance of their own impending death actually die sooner than those who exhibit less of these qualities (Greer, Morris, & Pettingale, 1979; Pettingale, Morris, & Greer, 1985; Reed, Kemeny, Taylor, Wang, & Visscher, 1994).

In contrast to resignation to the ultimate consequence of the diagnosis, an acceptance of the diagnosis per se has very different consequences. It may cause people to reprioritize their lives, to realistically revise long-term goals, and to use what time they have left in constructive and optimal ways. Stated somewhat differently, by accepting that life may be compromised (but not over), people may be impelled to develop a more adaptive set of parameters within which to live the life they have left (Moskowitz et al., 1996). It is in this spirit that we have suggested that acceptance serves the purpose of keeping the person goal engaged, and indeed "life engaged" (Carver & Scheier, 1998).

The Relative Importance of Purpose and Hope

Our next point concerns the relative importance of purpose and hope. So far, we have treated these two variables as though they were roughly equivalent in importance. While this might be true some of the time, or even most of the time, one can imagine situations in which one might be harder to maintain or more important to maintain than the other. Similarly, there might be certain kinds of people who are more vulnerable to the erosion of hope and others who are more vulnerable to the erosion of purpose. If so, it might be important to direct intervention efforts toward the component that is most at risk.

Consider, for example, two patients in different stages of disease, one early and one late. Realistically, the early stage cancer patient has a better prognosis. Because the disease was caught quickly, medical treatment should be more effective and the odds of cancer-free survival should be higher. Given the enhanced odds of dealing effectively with the disease, the cancer should pose less of a threat to ongoing life tasks, and consequently be less likely to permanently disrupt long-term life projects. For this type of person, maintaining hope may be paramount. What is important is to keep the person optimistic with respect to managing and overcoming the consequences of the disease, and getting on with life. Given the patient's life situation, there may be little objective need to abandon or re-evaluate ongoing life goals.

The situation for someone with advanced disease may be quite different. For this person, ongoing life goals may in fact be objectively threatened. While we think it is important for even this type of person to begin the treatment process with a positive orientation and to maintain that orientation as long as possible, should the treatment begin to falter and the prognosis become less favorable, maintaining a sense of purpose may become the more critical factor. Someone in this situation may begin to sense that lifelong ambitions may go unrealized. As the hope of attaining these long-term goals begins to wane, it is important that the patient find purpose in life elsewhere, either in scaled-back versions of the threatened longer term goals or in alternative, shorter term substitute goals. Thus, as the ability to maintain hope fades, it becomes more important to find renewed purpose (about which it is more realistic to have hope).

Our discussion of the relative importance of hope and purpose provides an interesting perspective on the contradictory findings reported by Helgeson et al. (1999) and Spiegel et al. (1981), regarding the utility of social support interventions (see also each group's contribution to this volume). Helgeson et al. studied early stage breast cancer patients and found that their social support intervention had no positive effect on subsequent adjustment. In contrast, Spiegel et al. (1981; Spiegel et al., 1989) studied later stage metastatic patients and found that their social support intervention enhanced adjustment and increased survival time.

As we just argued, maintaining hope may be most important to early stage patients, whereas maintaining purpose may be more important to later stage patients. Perhaps social support groups have their primary effect on the patient's sense of purpose. If so, the contradictory findings reported by Helgeson et al. (1999) and Spiegel et al. (1981) become more understandable. That is, the later stage patients studied by Spiegel et al. were most vulnerable with respect to the erosion of purpose, and the social support groups helped them to maintain their sense of purpose, perhaps by helping the patients to identify alternative valued goals for living. The early stage patients in the Helgeson et al. study were less in need of finding purpose and more in need of maintaining hope. As a result, the social support groups in that study were less effective in promoting better adjustment, because the group sessions were not giving the patients what they needed most.

It is interesting to note in this regard that the educational groups in the Helgeson et al. (1999) study were effective in enhancing adjustment. Perhaps educational interventions, by providing certain kinds of illness information, function more to enable the patient to maintain hope of overcoming the illness. If so, the pattern of findings reported by Helgeson et al. would underscore even further the importance of matching the "active ingredient" of the intervention to the differential needs of the patients involved.

When to Hold on, When to Move on?

Our final point here concerns the breakpoint between engagement and disengagement. Throughout this discussion there has been a certain tension between opposing forces in the model we presented. On the one hand, we talked about the preservation of hope, the holding on to desired values and goals in the face of adversity. On the other hand, we talked about the importance of accepting that valued goals must at times be abandoned, and the search begun for other, more attainable goals to take their place. Effective self-regulation must embody both sets of processes, holding on and letting go.

The trick to successful living is to know when to do what—when it is right to keep "hanging on" and when it is best to start "letting go" (Pyszczynski & Greenberg, 1992). In the abstract, the choice seems clear. When a goal is truly unattainable, it should be let go. If a cancer patient objectively has only a few weeks or months to live, longer term ambitions should be relinquished and the person should begin disengaging from those goals, spending the time doing things that can be done in the time that remains. When a goal is potentially realizable, on the other hand, even limited giving up can be a mistake. It can keep the person from reaching a goal that might otherwise be attainable and can erode the person's confidence about obtaining similar goals in the future. Thus, hope should be embraced for as long as possible.

How long is "as long as possible"? Unfortunately, there is no definitive answer to this question. With respect to the issues we are raising, our own insight is no better than anyone else's. Our only insight is that questions involving holding on and letting go are critical to the process of successful living. We sense that they are also a critical determinant of the extent to which the therapist is successful in helping cancer patients adjust to their disease.

Conclusion

Designing psychosocial interventions for cancer patients involves many considerations. Theoretical principles are taken into account, and so are intuitions. In addition, interventionists often base procedures on an understanding of the natural course of adjustment to the disease (Spencer et al., 1998). Thus, observational studies can provide springboards for interventions. By noting which cancer patients do better when left to their own devices, interventionists can identify variables to target for their later manipulations. The working assumption is that the coping responses, mind-sets, cognitive tactics, and other personal resources that are useful in the natural adaptation of patients to their disease can be instilled in others for whom the responses do not come as readily. The hope is that the newly acquired responses are as helpful for the patients who have acquired them as the responses are for the patients who use them in the natural course of events.

In this chapter, we have reviewed a number of observational studies showing that people who have hope and purpose in their lives tend to do better when confronting different kinds of adversity. We have also tried to make a plausible case that many of the things that interventionists try to do to help people adjust to cancer diagnosis and treatment have their effects through their impact on hope and purpose. This latter possibility, however, remains somewhat speculative. We think that hope and purpose are central mediators of positive intervention effects, but to date little work has been done to verify that this is so. Rigorous tests of these variables are obviously necessary.

In our view, evaluating the role of hope and purpose in the process of adjusting to cancer is an important and worthy goal. We are very optimistic that these variables are crucial, confident enough to be strongly committed to testing them further. We extend an invitation to others to include measures of these variables in their studies and to join us in the enterprise.

References

Andersen, B. L. (1992). Psychological interventions for cancer patients to enhance the quality of life. *Journal of Consulting and Clinical Psychology, 60,* 552–568.

Antonovsky, A. (1987). *Unraveling the mystery of health: How people manage stress and stay well.* San Francisco: Jossey-Bass.

Aspinwall, L. G., & Taylor, S. E. (1992). Modeling cognitive adaptation: A longitudinal investigation of the impact of individual differences and coping on college adjustment and performance. *Journal of Personality and Social Psychology, 61,* 755–765.

Atkinson, J. W. (1964). *An introduction to motivation.* Princeton, NJ: Van Nostrand.

Bandura, A. (1986). *Social foundations of thought and action: A social cognitive theory.* Englewood Cliffs, NJ: Prentice Hall.

Brandstadter, J., & Renner, G. (1990). Tenacious goal pursuit and flexible goal adjustments: Explication and age-related analysis of assimilative and accommodative strategies of coping. *Psychology and Aging, 5,* 58–67.

Bridges, M. W. (1998). *Social comparison process among amputees: Distinctions between optimists and pessimists.* Unpublished doctoral dissertation, Carnegie Mellon University.

Bulman, R. J., & Wortman, C. B. (1977). Attributions of blame and coping in the "real world": Severe accident victims react to their lot. *Journal of Personality and Social Psychology, 35,* 351–363.

Bunston, T., Mings, D., Mackie, A., & Jones, D. (1995). Facilitating hopefulness: The determinants of hope. *Journal of Psychosocial Oncology, 13,* 79–103.

Buunk, B. P. (1995). Comparison direction and comparison dimension among disabled individuals: Toward a refined conceptualization of social comparison under stress. *Personality and Social Psychology Bulletin, 21,* 316–330.

Buunk, B. P., Collins, R. L., Taylor, S. E., Van Yperen, N. W., & Dakof, G. A. (1990). The affective consequences of social comparison: Either direction has its ups and downs. *Journal of Personality and Social Psychology, 59,* 1238–1249.

Carver, C. S., & Gaines, J. G. (1987). Optimism, pessimism, and postpartum depression. *Cognitive Therapy and Research, 11,* 449–462.

Carver, C. S., Pozo, C., Harris, S. D., Noriega, V., Scheier, M. F., Robinson, D. S., Ketcham, A. S., Moffat, F. L., & Clark, K. C. (1993). How coping mediates the effect of optimism on distress: A study of women with early stage breast cancer. *Journal of Personality and Social Psychology, 65,* 375–390.

Carver, C. S., & Scheier, M. F. (1981). *Attention and self-regulation: A control-theory approach to human behavior.* New York: Springer-Verlag.

Carver, C. S., & Scheier, M. F. (1990). Origins and functions of positive and negative affect: A control-process view. *Psychological Review, 97,* 19–35.

Carver, C. S., & Scheier, M. F. (1998). *On the self-regulation of behavior.* New York: Cambridge University Press.

Carver, C. S., & Scheier, M. F. (1999). Optimism. In C. R. Snyder (Ed.), *Coping: The psychology of what works* (pp. 182–204). New York: Oxford University Press.

Christman, N. J. (1990). Uncertainty and adjustment during radiotherapy. *Nursing Research, 39,* 17–20, 47.

Clark, L. F., Henry, S. M., & Taylor, D. M. (1991). Cognitive examination of motivation for childbearing as a factor in adjustment to infertility. In A. L. Stanton & C. Dunkel-Schetter (Eds.), *Infertility: Perspectives from stress and coping research* (pp. 157–180). New York: Plenum.

Collins, R. L., Taylor, S. E., & Skokan, L. A. (1990). A better world or a shattered vision? Changes in life perspective following victimization. *Social Cognition, 8,* 263–285.

Cozzarelli, C. (1993). Personality and self-efficacy as predictors of coping with abortion. *Journal of Personality and Social Psychology, 65,* 1224–1236.

Curbow, B., Somerfield, M. R., Baker, F., Wingard, J. R., & Legro, M. W. (1993). Personal changes, dispositional optimism, and psychological adjustment to bone marrow transplantation. *Journal of Behavioral Medicine, 16,* 423–443.

Dow, K. H., Ferrell, B. R., Leigh, S., Ly, J., & Gulasekaram, P. (1996). An evaluation of the quality of life among long-term survivors of breast cancer. *Breast Cancer Research and Treatment, 39,* 261–273.

Dunn, D. (1994). Positive meaning and illusions following disability: Reality negotiation, normative interpretation, and value change. *Journal of Social Behavior and Personality, 9,* 123–138.

Emmons, R. A., & King, L. A. (1988). Conflict among personal strivings: Immediate and long-term implications for psychological and physical well-being. *Journal of Personality and Social Psychology, 54,* 1040–1048.

Ersek, M., & Ferrell, B. R. (1994). Providing relief from cancer pain by assisting in the search for meaning. *Journal of Palliative Care, 10,* 15–22.

Everson, S. A., Goldberg, D. E., Kaplan, G. A., Cohen, R. D., Pukkala, E., Tuomilehto, J., & Salonen, J. T. (1996). Hopelessness and risk of mortality and incidence of myocardial infarction and cancer. *Psychosomatic Medicine, 58,* 113–121.

Fawzy, F. I., Cousins, N., Fawzy, N. W., Kemeny, M. E., Elashoff, R., & Morton, D. (1990). A structured psychiatric intervention for cancer patients: I. Changes over time in methods of coping and affective disturbance. *Archives of General Psychiatry, 47,* 720–725.

Fawzy, F. I., Fawzy, N. W., Arndt, L. A., & Pasnau, R. O. (1995). Critical review of psychosocial interventions in cancer care. *Archives of General Psychiatry, 53,* 100–113.

Fawzy, F. I., Fawzy, N. W., Hyun, C. S., Elashoff, R., Guthrie, D., Fahey, J. L., & Morton, D. L. (1993). Malignant melanoma: Effects of an early structured psychiatric intervention, coping, and affective state on recurrence and survival 6 years later. *Archives of General Psychiatry, 50,* 681–689.

Feather, N. T. (Ed.). (1982). *Expectations and actions: Expectancy-value models in psychology.* Hillsdale, NJ: Erlbaum.

Fitzgerald, T. E., Tennen, H., Affleck, G., & Pransky, G. S. (1993). The relative importance of dispositional optimism and control appraisals in quality of life after coronary artery bypass surgery. *Journal of Behavioral Medicine, 16,* 25–43.

Fromm, K., Andrykowski, M. A., & Hunt, J. (1996). Positive and negative psychosocial sequelae of bone marrow transplantation: Implications for quality of life assessment. *Journal of Behavioral Medicine, 19,* 221–240.

Given, C. W., Stommel, M., Given, B., Osuch, J., Kurtz, M. E., & Kurtz, J. C. (1993). The influence of cancer patients' symptoms and functional states on patients' depression and family caregivers' reaction and depression. *Health Psychology, 12,* 277–285.

Greer, S., Morris, T., & Pettingale, K. W. (1979). Psychological response to breast cancer: Effect on outcome. *Lancet, 2,* 785–787.

Harlow, R. E., & Cantor, N. (1996). Still participating after all these years: A study of life task participation in later life. *Journal of Personality and Social Psychology, 71,* 1235–1249.

Helgeson, V. S., Cohen, S., Schulz, R., & Yasko, J. (1999). Education and peer discussion group interventions and adjustment to breast cancer. *Archives of General Psychiatry, 56*(4), 340–347.

Hickey, S. S. (1986). Enabling hope. *Cancer Nursing, 9,* 133–137.

Holahan, C. K. (1988). Relation of life goals at age 70 to activity participation and health and psychological well-being among Terman's gifted men and women. *Psychology and Aging, 3,* 286–291.

Hooker, K., Monahan, D., Shifren, K., & Hutchinson, C. (1992). Mental and physical health of spouse caregivers: The role of personality. *Psychology and Aging, 7,* 367–375.

Kahn, D., & Steeves, R. (1993). Spiritual well-being: A review of the research literature. *Quality of Life: A Nursing Challenge, 2,* 60–64.

Kobasa, S. C. (1979). Stressful life events, personality, and health. *Journal of Personality and Social Psychology, 37,* 1–11.

Kobasa, S. C., & Maddi, S. R. (1981). Personality and constitution as mediators in the stress-illness relationship. *Journal of Health and Social Behavior, 22,* 368–378.

Kurtz, M. E., Wyatt, G., & Kurtz, J. C. (1995). Psychological and sexual well-being, philosophical/spiritual views, and health habits of long-term cancer survivors. *Health Care for Women International, 16,* 253–262.

Leedham, B., Meyerowitz, B. E., Muirhead, J., & Frist, W. H. (1995). Positive expectations predict health after heart transplantation. *Health Psychology, 14,* 74–79.

Levine, J., Warrenburg, S., Kerns, R., Schwartz, G., Delaney, R., Fonatan, A., Gradman, A., Smith, S., Allen, S., & Cascione, R. (1987). The role of denial in recovery from coronary heart disease. *Psychosomatic Medicine, 49,* 109–117.

Lewis, F. M. (1982). Experienced personal control and quality of life in late-stage cancer patients. *Nursing Research, 31,* 113–119.

Linville, P. (1985). Self-complexity and affective extremity: Don't put all of your eggs in one cognitive basket. *Social Cognition, 3,* 94–120.

Linville, P. (1987). Self-complexity as a cognitive buffer against stress-related illness and depression. *Journal of Personality and Social Psychology, 52,* 663–676.

Litt, M. D., Tennen, H., Affleck, G., & Klock, S. (1992). Coping and cognitive factors in adaptation to *in vitro* fertilization failure. *Journal of Behavioral Medicine, 15,* 171–187.

Long, B. C. (1993). Coping strategies of male managers: A prospective analysis of predictors of psychosomatic symptoms and job satisfaction. *Journal of Vocational Behavior, 42,* 184–199.

McIntosh, D. N., Silver, R. C., & Wortman, C. B. (1993). Religion's role in adjustment to a negative life event: Coping with the loss of a child. *Journal of Personality and Social Psychology, 65,* 812–821.

Meyerowitz, B. E. (1983). Postmastectomy coping strategies and quality of life. *Health Psychology, 2,* 117–132.

Miller, S. M. (1990). To see or not to see: Cognitive informational styles in the coping process. In M. Rosenbaum (Ed.), *Learned resourcefulness: On coping skills, self-control, and adaptive behavior* (pp. 95–126). New York: Springer.

Moskowitz, J. T., Folkman, S., Collette, L., & Vittinghoff, E. (1996). Coping and mood during AIDS-related caregiving and bereavement. *Annals of Behavioral Medicine, 18,* 49–57.

Mullen, B., & Suls, J. (1982). The effectiveness of attention and rejection as coping styles: A meta-analysis of temporal differences. *Journal of Psychosomatic Research, 26*, 43–49.

Nietzsche, F. (1990). *Twilight of the idols/The anit-Christ* (R. J. Hollingdale, Trans.). London: Penguin Books. (Original work published 1889)

O'Connor, A. P., Wicker, C. A., & Germino, B. B. (1990). Understanding the cancer patient's search for meaning. *Cancer Nursing, 13*, 167–175.

Palys, T. S., & Little, B. R. (1983). Perceived life satisfaction and the organization of personal project systems. *Journal of Personality and Social Psychology, 44*, 1221–1230.

Park, C. L., Moore, P. J., Turner, R. A., & Adler, N. E. (1997). The roles of constructive thinking and optimism in psychological and behavioral adjustment during pregnancy. *Journal of Personality and Social Psychology, 73*, 584–592.

Peterson, C., & Bossio, L. M. (1991). *Health and optimism.* New York: Free Press.

Peterson, C., & Seligman, M. E. P. (1984). Causal explanations as a risk factor for depression: Theory and evidence. *Psychological Review, 91*, 347–374.

Pettingale, K. W., Morris, T., & Greer, S. (1985). Mental attitudes to cancer: An additional prognostic factor. *Lancet, 1*, 750.

Pyszczynski, T., & Greenberg, J. (1992). *Hanging on and letting go: Understanding the onset, progression, and remission of depression.* New York: Springer-Verlag.

Reed, G. M., Kemeny, M. E., Taylor, S. E., Wang, H. J., & Visscher, B. R. (1994). "Realistic acceptance" as a predictor of decreased survival time in gay men with AIDS. *Health Psychology, 13*, 299–307.

Reker, G. T., Peacock, E. J., & Wong, P. T. P. (1987). Meaning and purpose in life and well-being: A life-span perspective. *Journal of Gerontology, 42*, 44–49.

Repetti, R. L. (1992). Social withdrawal as a short-term coping response to daily stressors. In H. S. Friedman (Ed.), *Hostility, coping, and health* (pp. 151-165). Washington, DC: American Psychological Association.

Ruehlman, L. S., & Wolchik, S. A. (1988). Personal goals and interpersonal support and hindrance as factors in psychological distress and well-being. *Journal of Personality and Social Psychology, 55*, 293–301.

Ryff, C. D. (1989). Happiness is everything, or is it? Explorations on the meaning of psychological well-being. *Journal of Personality and Social Psychology, 57*, 1069–1081.

Ryff, C. D., & Keyes, C. L. M. (1995). The structure of psychological well-being revisited. *Journal of Personality and Social Psychology, 69*, 719–727.

Ryff, C. D., Lee, Y. H., Essex, M. J., & Schmutte, P. S. (1994). My children and me: Midlife evaluations of grown children and self. *Psychology and Aging, 9*, 195–205.

Scheier, M. F., & Bridges, M. W. (1995). Person variables and health: Personality predispositions and acute psychological states as shared determinants for disease. *Psychosomatic Medicine, 57*, 255–268.

Scheier, M. F., & Carver, C. S. (1985). Optimism, coping and health: Assessment and implications of generalized outcome expectancies. *Health Psychology, 4*, 219–247.

Scheier, M. F., Carver, C. S., & Bridges, M. W. (2001). Optimism, pessimism, and psychological well-being. In E. C. Chang (Ed.), *Optimism and pessimism*. Washington, DC: American Psychological Association.

Scheier, M. F., Matthews, K. A., Owens, J. F., Magovern, G. J., Lefebvre, R. C., Abbott, R. A., & Carver, C. S. (1989). Dispositional optimism and recovery from coronary artery bypass surgery: The beneficial effects on physical and psychological well-being. *Journal of Personality and Social Psychology, 57,* 1024–1040.

Schulz, R., Bookwala, J., Knapp, J. E., Scheier, M. F., & Williamson, G. M. (1996). Pessimism, age, and cancer mortality. *Psychology and Aging, 11,* 304–309.

Seligman, M. E. P. (1991). *Learned optimism.* New York: Knopf.

Shah, J., & Higgins, E. T. (1997). Expectancy X value effects: Regulatory focus as determinant of magnitude *and* direction. *Journal of Personality and Social Psychology, 73,* 447–458.

Shifren, K., & Hooker, K. (1995). Stability and change in optimism: A study among spouse caregivers. *Experimental Aging Research, 21,* 59–76.

Showers, C. J., & Ryff, C. D. (1996). Self-differentiation and well being in a life transition. *Personality and Social Psychology Bulletin, 22,* 448–460.

Silver, R. C., Boon, C., & Stones, M. H. (1983). Searching for meaning in misfortune: Making sense of incest. *Journal of Social Issues, 39,* 81–102.

Smith, C. A., Haynes, K. N., Lazarus, R. S., & Pope, L. K. (1993). In search of the "hot" cognitions: Attributions, appraisals, and their relation to emotion. *Journal of Personality and Social Psychology, 65,* 916–929.

Snyder, C. R. (1994). *The psychology of hope: You can get there from here.* New York: Free Press.

Spencer, S. M., Carver, C. S., & Price, A. A. (1998). Psychological and social factors in adaptation to cancer. In J. Holland, W. Breitbart, P. K. Jacobsen, M. Lederberg, M. Loscalzo, M. J. Massie, & R. McCorkle (Eds.), *Psycho-oncology* (pp. 211–222). New York: Oxford University Press.

Spiegel, D., Bloom, J. R., Kraemer, H. C., & Gottheil, E. (1989). Effect of psychosocial treatment on survival of patients with metastatic breast cancer. *Lancet, 2,* 888–891.

Spiegel, D., Bloom, J. R., & Yalom, I. (1981). Group support for patients with metastatic cancer. *Archives of General Psychiatry, 38,* 527–533.

Stanton, A. L., & Snider, P. R. (1993). Coping with breast cancer diagnosis: A prospective study. *Health Psychology, 12,* 16–23.

Suls, J., & Fletcher, B. (1985). The relative efficacy of avoidant and non-avoidant coping strategies: A meta-analysis. *Health Psychology, 4,* 249–288.

Taylor, S. E., Buunk, B. P., & Aspinwall, L. G. (1990). Social comparison, stress, and coping. *Personality and Social Psychology Bulletin, 96,* 569–575.

Taylor, S. E., Kemeny, M. E., Aspinwall, L. G., Schneider, S. G., Rodriguez, R., & Herbert, M. (1992). Optimism, coping, psychological distress, and high-risk sexual behavior among men at risk for acquired immunodeficiency syndrome (AIDS). *Journal of Personality and Social Psychology, 63,* 460–473.

Tedeschi, R. G., & Calhoun, L. G. (1995). *Trauma and transformation: Growing in the aftermath of suffering*. Thousand Oaks, CA: Sage.

Thompson, S. C. (1985). Finding positive meaning in a stressful event and coping. *Basic and Applied Social Psychology, 6,* 279–295.

Thompson, S. C., & Janigian, A. S. (1988). A framework for understanding the search for meaning. *Journal of Social and Clinical Psychology, 7,* 260–280.

Thompson, S. C., & Pitts, J. (1993). Factors relating to a person's ability to find meaning after diagnosis of cancer. *Journal of Psychosocial Oncology, 11,* 1–21.

Trijsburg, R. W., van Knippenberg, F. C. E., & Rijpma, S. E. (1992). Effects of psychological treatment on cancer patients: A critical review. *Psychosomatic Medicine, 54,* 489–517.

Vroom, V. H. (1964). *Work and motivation*. New York: Wiley.

Watson, M., Greer, S., Blake, S., & Shrapnell, K. (1984). Reaction to a diagnosis of breast cancer: Relationship between denial, delay and rates of psychological morbidity. *Cancer, 53,* 2008–2012.

Weisman, A. D., & Worden, J. W. (1976–1977). The existential plight in cancer: Significance of the first 100 days. *International Journal of Psychiatry in Medicine, 7,* 1–15.

Wicklund, R. A., & Gollwitzer, P. M. (1982). *Symbolic self-completion*. Hillsdale, NJ: Erlbaum.

Worth, R. (1995, November). A model prison. *Atlantic Monthly, 276,* 38–44.

Wyatt, G., Kurtz, M. E., Friedman, L. L., Given, B., & Given, C. W. (1996). Preliminary testing of the Long-Term Quality of Life (LTQL) instrument for female cancer survivors. *Journal of Nursing Measurement, 4,* 153–170.

Zeidner, M., & Hammer, A. L. (1992). Coping with missile attack: Resources, strategies, and outcomes. *Journal of Personality, 60,* 709–746.

CHAPTER 3

General and Specific Measures of Quality of Life in Younger Women With Breast Cancer

Joan R. Bloom

Susan L. Stewart

Monica Johnston

Priscilla Banks

Early diagnosis and better treatment methods have resulted in higher rates of cure and long-term overall survival for women diagnosed with breast cancer. In fact, survivors of breast cancer have become the largest identifiable group of cancer survivors. About one-third of all breast cancers are diagnosed in women younger than age 50. This group is of particular concern because (a) breast cancer can be more difficult to detect at earlier stages, when the treatment options are greater; (b) the tumors tend to be more aggressive, which affects the type of treatment offered; and (c) research has indicated that this group is at greater risk for psychological distress than women over 50 (Bloom & Kessler, 1994). This group of women is more likely to have other sources of life stress, including being married, having dependent children, and being employed (Bloom, Stewart, Johnston, & Banks, 1998). To date, few systematic studies of the initial impact of a breast cancer diagnosis have been completed.

This chapter has two objectives. First, we compare quality of life of younger women (50 or younger at diagnosis) with breast cancer with published norms for other groups. Second, we examine general and specific measures of quality of life for this group during the early months following diagnosis. Overall, the findings examine general and specific measures of quality of life as outcomes for assessing

A version of this chapter was presented at the Second International Congress of Psycho-Oncology, held in Kobe, Japan, on October 21, 1995. The efforts of Merilee Morrow and Janine Evans and the financial support of the National Cancer Institute are gratefully acknowledged.

the impact of cancer treatments. Such outcomes are also potentially useful for evaluating psychosocial and educational interventions.

Psychosocial and Functional Outcomes

Longitudinal data suggest that women who have been diagnosed with and treated for breast cancer are psychologically distressed. Over time, the severe distress of the diagnosis dissipates in early stage breast cancer (Stage I and Stage II), and emotions stabilize. By the end of 1 year, their psychological profile is not significantly different from that of women who have received surgical treatment for nonmalignant conditions or for benign breast disease (Bloom et al., 1987; Bloom, Kessler, & Pee, 1992). The results of a study by Ganz and her colleagues (1996) of women of all ages newly diagnosed with breast cancer support these findings. They reported that the total Mood Distress scale of the Profile of Mood States (POMS; McNair, Lorr, & Droppleman, 1971) improved between 1 month and 1 year but that no significant differences were found among the 1-, 2-, and 3-year follow-ups. They also reported improvements in quality of life as measured by the CAncer Rehabilitation Evaluation System (CARES; Schag & Heinrich, 1989), including the global measure as well as interaction with medical providers and psychosocial outcomes during the first year following surgery. Consistent with the findings on the POMS, most of the improvement occurred during the first year following diagnosis and treatment. Both studies excluded women who had preexisting emotional difficulties. However, others have discovered that the presence of previous physical or mental health conditions may exacerbate adjustment difficulties following a breast cancer diagnosis (Maunsell, Brisson, & Deschenes, 1992; Morris, Greer, & White, 1977). In both studies a preexisting history of depression was related to subsequent distress. Following treatment for breast cancer, an estimated 25% of women have significant anxiety or depressed mood (Maguire, 1988) or sexual problems (Shover, 1991).

Sociodemographic factors also contribute to a woman's response to the cancer diagnosis. Younger women (age 50 or under) are more at risk for mood distress than are older women (over age 50) (Penman et al., 1986–1987). Having younger children at home and being divorced are also important predictors of psychosocial risk (Penman et al., 1986–1987). Single women also report problems in dating relationships and sexual relationships and greater preoccupation with worries about recurrence of their cancer, presumably because of their greater isolation and lack of a confidant (Stewart, Fobair, D'Onofrio, & Bloom, 2000; Ganz et al., 1996). Studies comparing breast cancer patients with healthy women do not find that sexual disruption is necessarily related to disturbance in other areas, such as marital relationships (Andersen & Jochimsen, 1985).

Culture and ethnicity affect the ways and the extent to which women express their physical and emotional distress (Aaronson, Cull, Kaasa, & Spangers, 1994).

For example, epidemiological studies comparing African Americans and Whites generally find that after adjustments are made for sociodemographic differences, African Americans report equal or even lower levels of symptoms (Jones-Webb & Snowden, 1993). To date, most studies of psychosocial outcomes of breast cancer have focused on majority populations.

There is relatively little research on physical difficulties accompanying breast cancer. There is evidence, however, that tasks involving upper-body strength are especially problematic 3 months after diagnosis for women older than 55 as compared with women without breast cancer of the same age (Satariano, Rageb, Branch, & Swanson, 1990). Women with breast cancer are twice as likely to report more areas of disability in upper-body strength. Three months after diagnosis, African American women were nearly three times more likely than White women to report great difficulty in lifting items weighing less than 10 pounds. Nine months later, women between ages 55 and 64 had recuperated in all areas except those involving the most strenuous tasks, such as pushing heavy furniture. One year after diagnosis, the odds of severe difficulty were still greater for African American women (odds ratio = 2.4, 95% confidence interval = 1.3, 3.9). Differences in level of upper-body disability seem to be due in large part to racial differences in education, financial resources, stage of disease, and the number of concurrent health conditions (such as diabetes). Deficits in physical functioning have not been studied in women younger than 50. Reductions in physical changes and disruption of daily activity caused by the disease were also found during the first year following breast cancer treatment in the Ganz et al. (1996) study.

The type of treatment that women receive can also affect their levels of distress. Findings with regard to mastectomy versus breast-conserving treatment are fairly consistent: Women who have breast-conserving treatment have better body image (Moyer, 1997). According to Moyer's recent meta-analysis of 40 investigations, modest advantages for breast-conserving surgery also were identified for psychological, marital–sexual, and social adjustment as well as cancer-related fears and concerns. However, women who received chemotherapy had higher levels of psychological distress than women who received radiotherapy (Houghson, Cooper, McArdle, & Smith, 1986; Meyerowitz, Watkins, & Sparks, 1983). Because there is a high correlation between type of surgical treatment and the type of adjuvant therapy the women receives, mastectomy is more often associated with greater body image problems and mood distress. The stage of disease at diagnosis has also been found to affect the women's psychological functioning. Women diagnosed with later stage disease report the greatest distress (Lewis, 1989; Schag et al., 1993).

Quality of Life

The Concept

The notion of quality of life directs attention to the "complete social and psychological being: the individual's performance of social roles, her mental acuity, her emotional state, her sense of well-being and her relationships with others" (Levine, 1987, p. 4). *Quality of life* has been defined as the difference, or the gap, at a particular period of time between the hopes and expectations of the individual and that individual's present life experiences (Calman, 1984, 1987). In other words, the concept encompasses not only the person's objective state, but also the extent to which that objective state and the individual's expectations and hopes are congruent. For example, the objective state may be based on another person's assessment or on an objective measure such as the number of days in the past year a person has stayed in bed. Without the individual's assessment of the meaning of her situation, there is no way of calibrating the experience. Thus, two individuals may have exactly the same objective state of health, but their quality of life might be perceived as being quite different. Recent work by Wan, Counte, and Cella (1997) provides empirical support for the influence of personal expectations on cancer patient's reports of health-related quality of life.

Quality of life changes over time and is modified by age and experience. Older people adjust their perceptions about their health, whereas younger people may hold higher expectations concerning their physical and functional status. This observation was supported by Ganz et al. (1993) and Sarna (1993), who found that quality-of-life scores tend to be better in older compared with younger people.

Quality of life is not unidimensional; it covers a number of life domains. This includes but is not limited to the individual's community, education, family life, friendships, health, housing, work, and marriage or family relationships (Campbell, 1976; Devins et al., 1983). For each domain, quality of life may be perceived differently and may be differentially weighted by the individual.

Measuring Quality of Life

Measuring quality of life is a topic of great importance to research methods in psychosocial oncology and has been a focus of two meetings (April 1983 and December 1989) on research methods sponsored by the American Cancer Society. Whether quality of life should be measured using cross-cultural general measures such as that being developed by the World Health Organization, in terms of health-related quality of life such as Stewart and Ware's (1992) general measure of health status from the Medical Outcome Study (MOS), or by disease-specific measures has been the focus of a long-standing debate (cf. Bloom, 1984; Ware, 1984, 1991). Disease-specific measures might include adjustment to illness and its impact on the patient's life as well as measures that are specific to the type of cancer, age of onset, and its treatment. In contrast, Ware (1991) defined *generic measures* as ones that are non-age and non-disease specific: "Generic measures focus on such basic human values as emotional well-being and the ability to function in everyday life" (p. 774). Moreover, these generic measures are defined as being measures of health-related quality of life, but they have been shown to be highly correlated with overall quality-of-life measures. For example, correlations between MOS Short Form–36 (MOS SF–36) scales and quality of life beyond health, including living arrangements, neighborhood, standard of living, financial situation, family life, and friendships, were positively and significantly correlated in a general population sample (Ware, 1993). Stewart and Ware also have argued that a general measure (and specifically the MOS SF–36) differentiates populations with different disease conditions and may be sufficiently sensitive to differentiate populations that exhibit additional comorbidity (Ware, 1993). More recently, Cella, who developed the Function Assessment of Cancer Therapy (FACT) scale (Cella & Tulsky, 1990), and Aaronson et al. (1994), who developed the European Organization for Research and Treatment of Cancer (EORTC; originally for cancer clinical trials in the European Community), designed their measures so that they could be tailored to certain cancer populations by using a general set of indicators plus a set that was organ specific. Thus, to study the quality of life of younger women with breast cancer, one would use both the set designed for all cancer patients and some items designed for breast cancer.

Additional effort has focused on advocating the importance of quality of life as an endpoint in cancer treatment decisions (Litwin, Hays, Fink, & Ganz, 1995). For example, when treatments appear to be equally efficacious (e.g., limb-sparing treatments for sarcoma or radiation therapy vs. radical prostatectomy for prostate cancer; Litwin et al, 1995; Sugarbaker, Barofsky, Rosenberg, & Gianola, 1982), they can be evaluated in terms of their impact on the individual's functioning and well-being. Such measures are also useful for evaluating intervention outcomes (Barofsky & Cohen, 1984).

It has not yet been determined whether a general measure such as the MOS SF–36 can make within-population discriminations (Bloom, 1984). The impact of alternative treatments on patient functioning and well-being is being evaluated. One clinical application is to better understand the trade-off in functioning and well-being that people are willing to make when treatments appear to be equally efficacious (e.g., in terms of blood pressure control or length of life; Litwin et al., 1995). In a study of osteoarthritis patients following knee replacement, for example, Kantz and his colleagues (Kantz, Harris, Levitsky, Ware, & Davies, 1992) found that knee-specific role function and pain measures were more specific than generic measures among patients with other comorbid conditions, and less so among patients with only knee problems. Recently, Litwin and his colleagues (1995) did not find differences in quality of life between men with localized prostate cancer treated by radiation versus radical prostatectomy on general measures. However, significant differences were found in the CARES Physical Functioning scale and the Sexual scale on cancer-specific quality-of-life measures. However, they found consistent differences in prostate-targeted quality of life, such as sexuality and urinary and bowel problems, on both the "functioning" and "bother" scales of the CARES. In summary, there is some evidence that organ-targeted quality-of-life measures may be superior to more generic measures in predicting quality-of-life outcomes.

To further investigate this issue, we assessed the sensitivity of general as compared with specific measures of health-related quality of life for women age 50 or younger who were treated for breast cancer. First, we compared ratings on the MOS SF–36 with norms for healthy women as well as individuals treated for a nonmalignant medical conditions (clinical depression). Second, we developed regression models to determine whether specific measures of quality of life marginally improve the variance explained by general measures.

Background

The study discussed here is part of a larger project, Breast Cancer in Young Women: A Population-Based Approach, whose purpose was to develop and evaluate psychoeducational support groups targeted to underserved women. In the first phase of the project, we held focus groups and surveyed young women with breast cancer to help specify the approach and topics to be included in the intervention design. To determine the best time for intervention, we included in our sample women who were either within 2 months of diagnosis or 6 to 7 months postdiagnosis. In the second phase, women were randomly assigned to the 10-week psychoeducational support group intervention. The evaluation included assessment at three points: before the groups began, at the end of the intervention, and 3 months following the intervention. Data presented here are from the Phase 1 survey.

Sample

The women interviewed for this study were identified through the Rapid Case Ascertainment (RCA) Procedure of the Greater Bay Area (SEER) Cancer Registry. All of the women identified during a 7-month period (October 1994–April 1995) by the RCA were invited to participate following the usual procedures: (a) The woman's physician was approached; (b) following physician assent, a letter was sent to the woman; and (c) the interviewer contacted the woman by telephone and, if she agreed, an appointment was made for the face-to-face interview. The final sample included 336 women (80% response); half of these women were interviewed within 2 months of treatment, and the other half were interviewed 6–7 months following diagnosis.

Sociodemographic characteristics of the sample indicate that the respondents were young and well educated (41% were younger than age 45, 50% were college graduates, and only 3% had less than a high school education). Most worked (59% full-time and 18% part-time), were married (65%) and had children (63%), and were White (70%). We had expected a majority to have had breast-conserving treatment and were surprised to find that 46% had had a lumpectomy, 47% had had a mastectomy, 3% had had a double mastectomy, and 4% had not had surgical treatment by the time of the interview (Table 3.1).

TABLE 3.1

Sociodemographic and treatment characteristics of sample of women (N = 336)

MEASURE	N	%
Age (years)		
22–44	138	41
45–51	198	59
Marital status		
Married	219	65
Unmarried	117	35
Education		
High school or less	67	20
Some college	102	30
College graduate	166	50
Number of children		
None	126	38
1	95	28
2 or more	115	34
Employment status		
Full-time	199	59
Part-time	61	18
Not working	76	23
Ethnicity		
White	234	70
Non-White (Asian, African American, Latina)	102	30
Type of treatment		
Mastectomy	159	47
Breast-conserving surgery	155	46
Double mastectomy	10	3
No surgical treatment (at interview)	12	4
Time since diagnosis (months)		
1–2	167	50
6–7	169	50
Currently under treatment		
Yes	189	56
No	147	44

Note. From "Intrusiveness of Illness and Quality of Life of Young Women With Breast Cancer," by J. R. Bloom, S. L. Stewart, M. Johnston, and P. J. Banks, 1998, *Psycho-Oncology, 7*, p. 98. Copyright 1998 by John Wiley & Sons Limited. Reprinted with permission.

Measurement

The interview instrument contained general measures of health status, measures of adjustment to illness, and how the cancer was detected; the respondent's knowledge of the treatment and preferences for making treatment decisions; and sociodemographic characteristics, including measures of work history, health insurance, and family composition and relationships. For the current study, the following general and specific measures were collected.

General health-related quality of life was measured using subscales of the MOS SF–36 (Ware, 1993). These scales measure eight health concepts: Physical Functioning (PF), Role Limitations Caused by Physical Problems (RP), Bodily Pain (BP), General Health (GH), Vitality (energy/fatigue; VT), Social Functioning (SF), Role Limitations Caused by Emotional Problems (RE), and Mental Health (MH). PF is a measure of 10 items ranging from limitations in ability to engage in vigorous activities to limitations in activities of daily living. The RP scale is composed of four items measuring whether one's work or other daily activities are affected by one's physical condition. BP is measured by two items that focus on the amount of pain experienced and the extent to which it interfered with normal activity such as work. The GH measure combines the responses to five questions, including a scale rating health from *excellent* to *poor* on a 5-point scale and four single items rating aspects of health. VT is composed of four Likert-scaled items that focus on one's level of energy. RE is measured by three items that ask whether work or other daily activities were affected by one's emotions. SF was measured by two items that focus on the intensity and amount of time that one's physical health and emotions interfered with social activities with family and friends. MH consists of five items assessing how one felt (blue, calm, etc.) in the past 4 weeks. Five scales (PF, RP, BP, SF, and RE) defined health status as the absence of limitation or disability. The data were scored using the RAND method. The highest possible score is 100 when no limitations or disabilities are observed. For the other three scales (GH, VT, and MH), which are "bipolar" and measure a much wider range of positive and negative health states, a score in the midrange is based on a respondent's report of no limitations or disability. Higher scores (closer to 100) mean that a respondent has reported positive states and evaluated her health favorably.

Three of the scales—RP, RE, and SF—reflect a general measure of quality of life in that together they ask respondents how much their physical health and their emotional health affect their work, social, or other daily activities. In fact, these three questions taken together are almost a general equivalent to the dependent measure used for this study, intrusiveness of illness. Therefore, these scales are not included in the initial models for conceptual reasons.

Rosenberg's (1965) scale of self-esteem was also used; it contains 10 Likert-formatted items, which were added together following the procedure suggested by Lewis (1989). Individuals rate themselves as to whether they have good qualities, have a positive attitude, feel useless, and so on. This measure of self-concept is not specific to one's health. It is included in the models as a general measure.

These generic measures were supplemented with several cancer-specific measures. The women's cancer-related concerns were measured by a scale developed by Schain (1979). This scale (Cronbach's α = .85) contains 23 Likert-scaled items. Three factor-derived subscales were developed: Patient–Physician Communication, Self-Image, and Future Concerns (Worry About the Future). Symptom distress caused by sequelae of breast cancer treatment was measured by three measures. Surgical treatment sequelae (Treatment-Related Symptoms) is based on seven items that the women may have experienced in the past 4 weeks, including swelling of the arm, stiffness, problems in healing of the surgical wound, loss of balance, and phantom sensations in the breast area. Women were also asked about five menopausal symptoms they might have experienced since starting treatment, including hot flashes, cessation of menses, and decreased vaginal lubrication. Finally, the women were asked the extent to which they experienced chemotherapy-related side effects, such as nausea and vomiting. We chose to keep these scales conceptually specific even though they were sufficiently intercorrelated to be combined. A specific measure of cancer-related fatigue was also measured, which is highly correlated with VT (r = −.61). Women were asked to rate how fatigued they had felt in the past 4 weeks (0 = *not fatigued at all*; 1 = *activity reduced 25%*; 2 = *activity reduced by 25%–50%*; 3 = *activity reduced more than 50%, cannot work*; and 4 = *unable to care for self*). Intercorrelations of the general and specific measures of quality of life indicate that, as expected, there was substantial correlation between some variable pairs. The correlations were not high enough to be redundant (Table 3.2).

The intrusiveness of breast cancer and its treatment into other life domains was measured using the Intrusiveness of Illness Scale (Devins, 1994). Women were asked to rate on a 4-point scale how breast cancer and its treatment has affected 13 domains of life: health, diet, work, active recreation (sports), passive recreation (reading, listening to music), financial situation, relationship with spouse, sex life, family relations, other social relations, self-expression, religious expression, and community and civic involvement. Because 19% of the women did not have a partner, the sex and spouse items were omitted. The intercorrelations between the three global scales of the MOS SF–36 and intrusiveness of illness were highly correlated, providing empirical evidence that our conceptual concerns were true (Table 3.3).

As described above, we collected information about sociodemographic characteristics, including age, education, ethnicity, marital status, whether the woman had one or two or more dependent children, and whether she worked full- or part-time (see Table 3.1). In addition, information regarding medical treatment was collected. For this study, we were interested in (a) the time postdiagnosis (either less than 2 months or 6–7 months), (b) the type of surgical treatment she received (breast-conserving treatment or mastectomy), and (c) whether she was currently receiving adjuvant treatment or not (either completed treatment or had not started it). We also asked about type of treatment (radiation therapy, chemotherapy, or tamoxifen). In addition, we asked the women how many positive lymph nodes they had, and we used the response as the measure of disease extensiveness for the regression models.

TABLE 3.2

Correlation matrix of variables (N = 314)

VARIABLE	1	2	3	4	5	6	7	8	9	10	11	12	13
1. Physical functioning	—												
2. Lack of bodily pain	.47	—											
3. General health	.38	.26	—										
4. Vitality	.53	.50	.46	—									
5. Mental health	.27	.33	.47	.53	—								
6. Self-esteem	.13	.19	.44	.29	.43	—							
7. Patient–physician communication problems	−.07	−.18	−.28	−.12	−.30	−.23	—						
8. Self-image problems	−.17	−.16	−.36	−.28	−.38	−.33	.26	—					
9. Worry about future	−.11	−.10	−.35	−.22	−.44	−.34	.26	.37	—				
10. Treatment-related symptoms	−.34	−.41	−.19	−.29	−.23	−.22	.18	.22	.12	—			
11. Treatment-related fatigue	−.51	−.43	−.35	−.61	−.42	−.19	.07	.23	.13	.26	—		
12. Chemotherapy side effects	−.18	−.05	−.16	−.28	−.12	−.02	−.04	.18	.07	.00	.43	—	
13. Hormonal side effects	−.16	−.02	−.05	−.22	−.04	.00	−.07	.17	.01	.05	.27	.63	—

TABLE 3.3

Correlation matrix of outcomes (N = 312)

VARIABLE	1	2	3	4
1. Intrusiveness of Illness Scale	—			
2. Social Functioning	− .67	—		
3. Emotional Role	− .46	.46	—	
4. Physical Role	− .45	.48	.34	—

Analytic Strategy

The data analysis consisted of two parts. In the first part, population norms developed by Ware and his colleagues (1993) were compared with those of the sample of young women with breast cancer. In the second part, ordinary least squares (OLS) regression models were designed in which the variables were added in blocks to determine the effect of each. In the first model, the control variables were included. In the second model, five general measures of health-related quality of life were added to the control variables. In Model 3, the breast-cancer-specific measures were added to the control variables. In this way, the amount of variance explained by both the general and the specific measures can be assessed. Finally, in Model 4, all three sets of variables were added to the model. In this model, the marginal effect of the breast-cancer-specific measures can be examined.

Comparisons With Other Populations

We compared our sample of young women with breast cancer with a sample of healthy women of the same age. In the first comparison, a normative sample of women ages 35–44 was compared with a similar-age sample of young women with breast cancer. The sample with breast cancer expressed more limitations than the normative sample on all eight scales. The greatest difference was for RP, whereas little difference was found for PF, GH, and MH (Figure 3.1). With one exception, a similar pattern was noted for women ages 45–54; the sample with breast cancer perceived themselves to be healthier than the general population (GH) (Figure 3.2). The final comparison was with the national norms for clinical depression (Figure 3.3). This comparison was chosen as the sample of women was closer in age (the normative sample had a mean age of 41.6 years, and 75% were female). Women with breast cancer reported fewer limitations than the clinically depressed sample. The one exception was in RP, for which the clinically depressed sample reported fewer limitations.

Generic and Specific Measures of Quality of Life

To test our predictions about the effects of general and specific measures of quality of life, we developed an OLS regression model in which variables were grouped

Health-related quality of life (as measured by the Medical Outcome Study, Short Form 36): National (Natl) norms for women ages 35–44 years (N = 264) compared with women with breast cancer (BC; N = 120). PF = physical functioning, RP = role limitations caused by physical problems, BP = bodily pain, GH = general health, VT = vitality, SF = social functioning, RE = role limitations caused by emotional problems, and MH = mental health. National norms data are from Ware (1993).

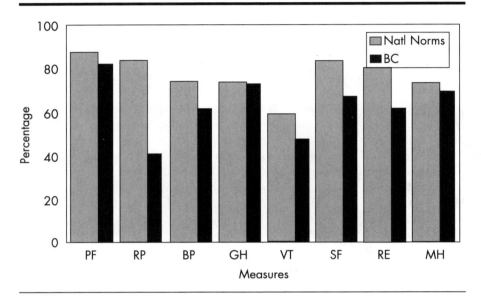

and entered in blocks (Table 3.4). In the first block (Model 1), the control variables were entered (specifically, sociodemographic and treatment-related variables). Four of the control variables were statistically significant ($p < .05$): Having two or more children, being on chemotherapy, and having one or more lymph nodes positive for breast cancer increased the intrusiveness of the illness, whereas being non-White reduced illness intrusiveness. The model was statistically significant and explained 13% of the adjusted variance.

In the second block (Model 2), the five generic measures taken from the MOS SF–36 Scale and Rosenberg's (1965) measure of self-esteem were added to the equation. Scores on PF, GH, and VT were statistically significant; fewer limitations in PF and higher perceived GH and VT were related to less intrusiveness of illness. One of the sociodemographic variables—having two or more children—had marginal significance ($p = .057$). The adjusted variance explained increased to 48%, and the equation was statistically significant.

In the third block (Model 3), the specific measures of quality of life were added to Model 1. Of the seven specific measures, four were statistically significant.

FIGURE 3.2

Health-related quality of life (as measured by the Medical Outcome Study, Short Form 36): National (Natl) norms for women ages 45–54 years (N = 193) compared with women with breast cancer (BC; N = 198). PF = physical functioning, RP = role limitations caused by physical problems, BP = bodily pain, GH = general health, VT = vitality, SF = social functioning, RE = role limitations caused by emotional problems, and MH = mental health. National norms data are from Ware (1993).

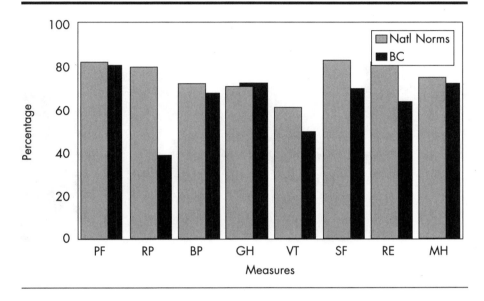

Treatment-related fatigue, treatment-related symptoms, self-image problems, and worry about the future increased intrusiveness of illness. One of the control variables, being on chemotherapy, is no longer statistically significant. The model is statistically significant and explains 48% of the adjusted variance.

In Model 4, all three blocks of variables were combined. Two of the control variables remained significant: the ethnicity of the women and the presence of positive lymph nodes. Having two or more children was marginally significant ($p = .052$). VT and PF were the only generic measures that were statistically significant. The women's perception of their general health was marginally significant ($p = .052$). The higher the ratings on all three, the less intrusive the breast cancer diagnosis and treatment were rated. Of the specific measures, symptom-related concerns, treatment-related fatigue, and Worry About the Future increased the intrusiveness of breast cancer on more domains of one's life. The Self-Image Problems scale is marginally significant ($p = .074$). The model is significant and explains 53% of the adjusted variance.

FIGURE 3.3

Health-related quality of life (as measured by the Medical Outcome Study, Short Form 36): National (Natl) for clinical depression compared with women with breast cancer (BC; N = 336). PF = physical functioning, RP = role limitations caused by physical problems, BP = bodily pain, GH = general health, VT = vitality, SF = social functioning, RE = role limitations caused by emotional problems, and MH = mental health. National norms data are from Ware (1993).

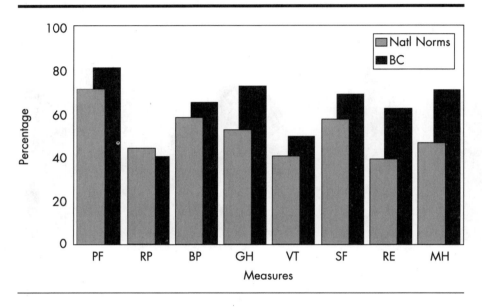

Discussion

Young women with breast cancer reported more limitations than did a national normative sample stratified by age, but they reported fewer limitations than did a group composed mostly of women of comparable age with clinical depression. Most dramatic are the physically based role limitations (RP) reported by the sample of women with breast cancer. On this measure the women with breast cancer reported twice as many limitations than did the healthy group and reported more limitations than did the clinically depressed sample. These data suggest that health-related quality of life as measured by the MOS SF–36 is sufficiently sensitive to differentiate among breast cancer, a clinically depressed population, and two age groups of healthy women. These findings contrast with those reported by Ganz and her colleagues (1996), who compared breast cancer survivors 2 and 3 years from treatment and found that the women had higher scores on all eight scales from the MOS SF–36.

The regression models indicate that general (Model 2) and specific measures of quality of life (Model 3) both explain the same amount of variance. When both

TABLE 3.4

The effects of general and specific measures of quality of life on intrusiveness of illness in women 50 years of age and younger with breast cancer

QUALITY-OF-LIFE MEASURE	MODEL 1 (N = 322)	MODEL 2 (N = 322)	MODEL 3 (N = 314)	MODEL 4 (N = 314)
Demographic–treatment factors				
Non-White ethnicity	−.15	−.17	−.15	−.16
Having 2+ children	.16	NS	.10	NS
On chemotherapy	.17	.09	NS	NS
Positive lymph nodes	.22	.17	.13	.14
General measures				
Physical functioning		−.18		−.11
General health		−.15		NS
Vitality		−.30		−.22
Specific measures				
Treatment-related symptoms			.20	.15
Treatment-related fatigue			.42	.22
Self-image problems			.11	NS
Worry about future			.14	.09
Adjusted R²	.13	.48	.48	.53

Note. Standardized estimates of parameters are significant at the .05 level. NS = not significant.

models are combined, the explained variance increases slightly. The relationships demonstrated in Model 4 also suggest that both generic and specific measures have independent effects on how much breast cancer compromises quality of life. These findings are consistent with other studies using both general and specific measures of quality of life (Litwin et al., 1995), albeit the general measures were as strong as the specific measures. The findings are also consistent with the measurement strategy used by Cella and Tulsky (1990) and Aaronson et al. (1994), who have more recently developed cancer-specific measures of quality of life that contain general and organ-specific measures.

We also considered a more extended version of Model 2 in which the three more general measures of the MOS SF–36 (RP, RE, and SF) were added to Model 2 and Model 4. Including these three general measures of quality of life in the models increases the strength of the model whether or not the specific measures are included. Furthermore, the independent effect of the specific measures remain. However, their inclusion is potentially problematic from a conceptual viewpoint. Are these three measures predictors of intrusiveness of illness, or are they more general measures of the same concept? Because we believed that they captured the same elements of compromised functioning in different arenas of life, we initially excluded them from our models. However, the answer to this question brings us full circle: How should we define *quality of life*? Should it be defined in terms of compromised functioning, as we have defined the outcome for this study, or should it be defined purely from the participant's viewpoint by asking the participant to rate her quality of life—in other words, asking her to calibrate each of the life domains to provide one overall measure? In this study, we did this for her and assumed that each domain of life was of equal weight.

Some of the variables had consistent effects in each of the models—the individual's ethnicity, the severity of her illness (number of positive lymph nodes), Vitality, Symptom Concerns, and Worry About the Future. Others, such as having two or more children, PF, and Self-Image, were important in some of the models, but they were not important in Model 4.

It is puzzling why the women of color were less likely to report that the cancer experience was intrusive than were the White women. One explanation is that the illness in women of color has a different priority in their lives than it does for White women. If the women of color are poorer and less educated than are the White women, this might be a plausible explanation; however, we adjusted the responses for sociodemographic differences. An alternative explanation is that women from other cultures are less likely to report that the breast cancer diagnosis and treatment are intrusive. Because the measure combined Chinese, Japanese, Filipino, and other Asian women with Hispanic and African American women, differences in cultural responses are a more plausible explanation. Further analyses of the dependent variable reveal that all of the ethnic groups reported lower intrusiveness scores; this finding is consistent with the study by Jones-Webb and Snowden (1993). White women were more likely to report intrusiveness in all life domains sampled, but they were significantly more likely to report that family relations, other social relations, community involvement, and diet were affected by the breast cancer diagnosis and treatment than were women of color. Further analyses might help us determine whether this finding reflects a measurement issue or a difference in the women's support system.

The consistency in the findings for severity of illness, concerns for the future, vitality, and treatment-related symptoms suggests that there are two issues of great concern to women newly diagnosed with breast cancer: (a) the women's experience with adjuvant chemotherapy, which included symptom concerns, fatigue, and lack of vitality, and (b) the women's response to the severity of their illness and its effect on the uncertainty about the future. These findings are consistent with earlier studies that also indicated that women's initial response was to confront their own mortality and meet the challenges of their treatment regimen (Bloom, Ross, & Burnell, 1978; Penman et al., 1986–1987).

Health-related quality of life also differentiates between subgroups within our sample of women recently diagnosed with breast cancer. PF has independent effects in both Models 2 and 4. When RP is added to the model, the effect of PF is reduced significantly, probably as a result of the intercorrelation between the two measures.

This finding persists irrespective of the type of surgical treatment received and the presence or absence of adjuvant chemotherapy. In our analysis of the PF measure, we found that the most predictive items in the scale were ones relating to the women's ability to bend, kneel, or stoop. Women who had received grafts because of breast reconstruction were most likely to report these limitations. In fact, the PF measure does not focus on upper-body strength. However, interviewer-rated mobility of the arms indicated that this sample of young women had excellent range of motion. This finding is contrary to the finding of Satariano and his colleagues (1990) of decrements in range of motion in older women.

Of the specific measures, the Self-Image scale from the Problems Checklist was only important in Model 3 (control and specific variables are included). Including the general measures reduced the effect of the Self-Image scale. Higher self-image has been a consistent effect in studies differentiating women who received breast-conserving surgery from women who had a mastectomy. These studies have also found that women who had reconstruction reported intermediate scores. A large proportion of the women receiving a mastectomy in this study also had reconstruction, which may have reduced the differences others have found between groups having either of the two procedures (Moyer, 1997).

Conclusion

In conclusion, general quality-of-life measures are sufficiently sensitive to differentiate between women with cancer and depressed or healthy women. With regard to the differential sensitivity of general and specific measures of quality of life, we found that generic health-related quality-of-life measures were equally sensitive to specific measures in predicting intrusiveness of breast cancer on quality of life. In the final model, where both the general and specific measures were included, we found both to make independent contributions.

References

Aaronson, N. K., Cull, A., Kaasa, S., & Spangers, M. A. G. (1994). The European Organization for Research and Treatment of Cancer (EORTC) modular approach to quality of life assessment in oncology. *International Journal of Mental Health, 23*(2), 75–96.

Andersen, B. L., & Jochimsen, P. R. (1985). Sexual functioning among breast cancer, gynecological cancer, and healthy women. *Journal of Consulting and Clinical Psychology, 53*, 25–32.

Barofsky, I., & Cohen, S. (1984). *Quality of life assessment and the practice of medicine.* Unpublished manuscript.

Bloom, J. R. (1984). Bring the patient back in: Response to Ware's "Conceptualizing disease impact and treatment outcomes." *Cancer, 53*, 2323–2326

Bloom, J. R., Cook, M., Flamer, D. P., Fotopolis, S., Holland, J. C., Gates, C., Muenz, L., Murowski, B., Penman, D., & Ross, R. D. (1987). Psychological response to mastectomy. *Cancer, 59,* 189–196.

Bloom, J. R., & Kessler, L. (1994). The risk and timing of counseling and support interventions for younger women with breast cancer. *Journal of the National Cancer Institute,* Monograph No. 16, 99–106.

Bloom, J. R., Kessler, L., & Pee, D. (1992). Psychosocial assessment of the recovery from mastectomy: A comparison of static and dynamic modeling. *Psychology and Health: An International Journal, 10,* 1–16.

Bloom, J. R., Ross, R. D., & Burnell, G. M. (1978). The effect of social support on patient adjustment following breast surgery. *Patient Counselling and Health Education, 1*(2), 50–59.

Bloom, J. R., Stewart, S. L., Johnston, M., & Banks, P. J. (1998). Intrusiveness of illness and quality of life of young women with breast cancer. *Psycho-Oncology, 7*(2), 89–100.

Calman, K. C. (1984). Quality of life of cancer patients—An hypothesis. *Journal of Medical Ethics, 10,* 124–127.

Calman, K. C. (1987). Definitions and dimensions of quality of life. In N. K. Aaronson & J. Beckmann (Eds.), *Quality of life of cancer patients* (pp. 1–10). New York: Raven Press.

Campbell, A. (1976). Subjective measures of well-being. *American Psychologist, 31,* 117–124.

Cella, D. F., & Tulsky, D. S. (1990). Measuring quality of life today: Methodological aspects. *Oncology, 4*(5), 29–38.

Devins, G. M. (1994). Illness intrusiveness and the psychosocial impact of lifestyle disruption in chronic life-threatening disease. *Advances in Renal Replacement Therapy, 1*(3), 251–264.

Devins, G. M., Binik, Y. M., Hutchinson, T. A., Holomby, D. J., Barre, P. E., & Guttman, R. D. (1983). The emotional impact of end-stage renal disease: Importance of patients' perceptions of intrusiveness and control. *International Journal of Psychiatry in Medicine, 13,* 327–343.

Ganz, P. A., Coscarelli, A., Fred, C., Kahn, B., Polinsky, M. L., & Petersen, L. (1996). Breast cancer survivors: Psychosocial concerns and quality of life. *Breast Cancer Research and Treatment, 38,* 183–199.

Ganz, P. A., Hirji, K., Sim, M. S., Schag, C. A. C., Fred, C., & Polinsky, M. L. (1993). Predicting psychosocial risk in patients with breast cancer. *Medical Care, 31,* 419–431.

Houghson, A. V., Cooper, A. F., McArdle, C. S., & Smith, D. C. (1986). Psychological impact of adjuvant chemotherapy in the first two years after mastectomy. *British Journal of Clinical Research, 293,* 1268–1271.

Jones-Webb, R. J., & Snowden, L. R. (1993). Symptoms of depression among Blacks and Whites. *American Journal of Public Health, 83*(2), 240–244.

Kantz, M. E., Harris, W. J., Levitsky, K., Ware, J. E., & Davies, A. R. (1992). Methods for assessing condition specific and generic functional status outcomes after total knee replacement. *Medical Care, 30*(Suppl.), 240–252.

Levine, S. (1987). The changing terrain of medical sociology: Emergent concern with quality of life. *Journal of Health and Social Behavior, 28*(1), 1–7.

Lewis, F. M. (1989). Attributions of control, experienced learning and psychosocial well-being in patients with advanced cancer. *Journal of Psychosocial Oncology, 7*, 105–119.

Litwin, M. S., Hays, R. D., Fink, A., & Ganz, P. A. (1995). Quality-of-life outcomes in men treated for localized prostate cancer. *Journal of the American Medical Association, 273*(2), 129–135.

Maguire, P. (1988). Breast conservation versus mastectomy: Psychological considerations. *Seminars in Surgical Oncology, 5*, 137–144.

Maunsell, E., Brisson, J., & Deschenes, L. (1992). Psychological distress after initial treatment of breast cancer: Assessment of potential risk factors. *Cancer, 70*, 120–125.

McNair, P. M., Lorr, M., & Droppleman, L. (1971). *POMS manual.* San Diego, CA: Educational and Industrial Testing Services.

Meyerowitz, B. E., Watkins, I. K., & Sparks, F. C. (1983). Psychosocial implications of adjuvant chemotherapy: A two-year follow-up study. *Cancer, 52,* 1541–1545.

Morris, T., Greer, H. S., & White, P. (1977). Psychological and social adjustment to mastectomy: A two-year follow-up study. *Cancer, 40*, 2381–2387.

Moyer, A. (1997). Psychosocial outcomes of breast-conserving surgery versus mastectomy: A meta-analytic review. *Health Psychology, 16*, 284–298.

Penman, D., Bloom, J. R., Fotopolis, S., Cook, M., Murowski, B., Gates, C., Holland, J., Ross, R., & Flamer, D. P. (1986–1987, Fall/Winter). The impact of mastectomy on self-concept and social function: A combined cross-sectional and longitudinal study with comparison groups. *Women and Health, 2*(3–4), 99–130.

Rosenberg, M. (1965). *Society and adolescent self image.* Princeton, NJ: Princeton University Press.

Sarna, L. (1993). Women with lung cancer: Impact on quality of life. *Quality of Life Research, 2*(1), 13–22.

Satariano, W. A., Rageb, N. E., Branch, L. G., & Swanson, G. M. (1990). Difficulties in physical function reported by middle aged and elderly women with breast cancer: A case control comparison. *Journal of Gerontology, 45*(1), 3–11.

Schag, C. A. C., Ganz, P. A., Polinksy, M. I., Fred, C., Hirji, K., & Persersen, L. (1993). Characteristics of women at risk for psychosocial distress in the year after breast cancer. *Journal of Clinical Oncology, 11*, 783–793.

Schag, C. A. C., & Heinrich, R. (1989). *CAncer Rehabilitation and Evaluation System manual.* Los Angeles: Cares Consultants.

Schain, W. (1979). *Breast Cancer Problems Checklist.* Unpublished manuscript.

Shover, L. R. (1991). The impact of breast cancer on sexuality, body image and intimate relationships. *CA-A Cancer Journal for Clinicians, 42*(2) 112–120.

Stewart, A. L., & Ware, J. E. (Eds.). (1992). *Measuring function and well-being: The medical outcomes study approach.* Durham, NC: Duke University Press.

Stewart, S. L., Fobair, P., D'Onofrio, C., & Bloom, J. R. (2000). *Body image and sexual problems in young women with breast cancer.* Manuscript in preparation.

Sugarbaker, P. H., Barofsky, I., Rosenberg, S. A., & Gianola, F. J. (1982). Quality of life assessment of patients in extremity sarcoma clinical trials. *Surgery, 91,* 17–23.

Wan, G. J., Counte, M. A., & Cella, D. F. (1997). The influence of personal expectations on cancer patients' reports of health-related quality of life. *Psycho-Oncology, 6,* 1–11.

Ware, J. E. (1984). Conceptualizing disease impact and treatment outcomes. *Cancer, 53,* 2316–2323.

Ware, J. E. (1991). Conceptualizing and measuring generic health outcomes. *Cancer, 64* (Suppl.), 774–779.

Ware, J. E. (1993). *SF-36 Health Survey: Manual and interpretation guide.* Boston: The Health Institute, New England Medical Center.

CHAPTER 4

Quality-of-Life Measurement in Oncology

David Cella

The value of any intervention, including those directed at people with cancer, is determined by judging its impact on quantity and quality of life (QOL). That impact, measured against cost, determines value. Whereas quantity of life is easy to measure, QOL measurement poses challenges and creates debate. Historically, quantity of life (survival time) has been the standard and most comfortable indicator of treatment effectiveness. Recognizing that time without quality is of questionable value, cancer treatment investigators have tended to assume that adding time would add value. Although frequently correct, this is not always true, especially when treatment toxicity, late effects, and second malignancies are taken into account.

Now, with the recent availability of valid and practical QOL questionnaires, we have the opportunity to measure quality alongside quantity of life when evaluating cancer treatment effectiveness. This allows us (a) to confirm the assumption that the time added by therapy is of sufficient value to justify its cost and (b) to examine the value of therapies that do not add time to life but do improve QOL. The critical trade off is not always between toxicity and survival time; sometimes a treatment temporarily palliates tumor-induced symptoms without extending survival. Patients may find this desirable even in the face of competing toxicity. Only a careful evaluation of patient-reported QOL can allow one to evaluate these trade-offs between symptom relief and toxicity.

QOL evaluation entails a multidimensional quantification of health and well-being, as reported by the patient. Many practical and valid questionnaires are available and can be evaluated using standard psychometric criteria (Bohrnstedt, 1983; Campbell & Fiske, 1959). These questionnaires are described in detail and have been compiled for reference elsewhere (Cella & Bonomi, 1995; Kornblith & Holland, 1994). This chapter focuses on the definition and measurement of QOL and provides a brief summary of emerging research issues.

Defining and Measuring QOL

There is wide consensus that QOL is both subjective and multidimensional (Aaronson, 1988; Aaronson et al., 1993; Cella & Cherin, 1988; Schipper et al., 1984;

Stewart, Ware, & Brook, 1981). Cella and Cherin (1988) developed a working definition of QOL that laid a groundwork for measurement: "Quality of life refers to patients' appraisal of and satisfaction with their current level of functioning as compared to what they perceive to be possible or ideal" (p. 70). This earlier definition was modified to explicitly incorporate the multidimensionality of QOL: "Health-related quality of life refers to the extent to which one's usual or expected physical, emotional and social well-being are affected by a medical condition or its treatment" (Cella, 1995, p. 73). This definition provides minimum requirements for QOL measurement: that it obtains the patient's perspective and that it captures physical, mental, and social well-being.

Aggregating Versus Disaggregating Scores

A review of the many available questionnaires revealed that more than 30 names for QOL dimensions were listed by various authors (Kornblith & Holland, 1994). Careful review of the descriptions of these dimensions and available factor analytic studies suggests up to seven distinct dimensions: (a) physical concerns (symptoms; pain), (b) functional ability (activity), (c) family well-being, (d) emotional well-being, (e) treatment satisfaction (including financial concerns), (f) sexuality and intimacy (including body image), and (g) social functioning. There are at least two higher order factors as well: physical well-being and mental well-being (Hays & Stewart, 1990). Finally, summary dimensions can have practical and policy value: a global evaluation of QOL (i.e., a single question rating the patient's global or overall perception of QOL or health status) and a total score (i.e., the sum of dimension scores into an aggregate index of QOL; Cella, 1995; Kornblith & Holland, 1994).

Factor analytic and aggregate index studies have suggested that the physical dimension could be divided into two categories: symptom (i.e., physical experience) and function (i.e., physical abilities and activities; Stewart et al., 1981). Mental well-being assessment should ideally capture both positive and negative mood and symptoms. The social aspects of QOL have been notoriously the most difficult to capture with short measurement approaches. Unfortunately, issues related to cost and burden have meant that brief measurement approaches appear to be required in most contemporary health services research. As a result, the social well-being dimension has tended to be underrepresented. It therefore remains poorly understood, despite growing appreciation of its importance in treatment decision making (Yellen & Cella, 1995), valued life activity (Ditto et al., 1996), and survival from cancer (Helgeson, Cohen, & Fritz, 1998).

QOL is indeed multidimensional, but it does not necessarily follow that reported QOL scores should always remain disaggregated when being reported. There are benefits to reporting QOL data in both disaggregated and aggregated form. Disaggregated dimension scores give one a more detailed and precise estimation of the different areas of patient function and well-being. This is usually preferred by the clinician. Aggregated scores and summary indexes are critical, however, to enable decision makers to meaningfully adjust time for its quality. Summary scores lose some precision, but they are preferred by treatment outcome evaluators such as health economists, health policy reviewers, and some clinicians. A summary of dimension scores is the only way QOL self-report can provide a "bottom line." Nevertheless, QOL dimension scores are more detailed than an aggregated score, and they provide differential sensitivity in some cases. Compared with physically based scales, psychosocial scales are less sensitive to change in a primarily physical rating (e.g., performance status) and less sensitive to differences in groups formed on the basis of physical characteristics (e.g., extent of disease). For example, the emotional functioning scale of the EORTC Quality of Life Questionnaire (EORTC QLQ; Aaronson et al., 1993) was unable to detect change in patient performance status rating (PSR; Aaronson et al., 1993) or in extent of disease (Bergman, Sullivan, & Sorenson, 1992; Osoba et al., 1994). It was also shown to be less sensitive than the physical scales to differences in PSR groups (Aaronson et al., 1993; Bergman et al., 1992; Wisloff et al., 1996). Similar findings have been reported for the Functional Assessment of Cancer Therapy–Breast (FACT–B) Measurement System (Brady et al., 1997; Cella et al., 1993; Cella, Bonomi, et al., 1995). Moreover, the Profile of Mood States (POMS; McNair, Lorr, & Droppleman, 1981), a widely used measure of emotional distress, closely paralleled findings we have reported for the emotional well-being and social well-being scales in breast cancer (Brady et al., 1997). It frequently is difficult to show differences in emotional well-being between people diagnosed with cancer and those without cancer (Andrykowski, Brady, & Hunt, 1993; Cella & Tross, 1986).

Using the Functional Living Index-Cancer (FLIC), Ganz and Coscarelli (1995) found no difference in patient QOL by nodal status, adjuvant chemotherapy, and type of surgery. Ganz and colleagues (1993) also found that the psychological distress scale of the CAncer Rehabilitation Evaluation System (CARES) did not distinguish among clinical disease status groups of HIV-positive patients. Moreover, McHorney, Ware, and Raczek (1993), in their validity studies of the Medical Outcome Study Short Form–36 (MOS SF–36; McHorney, Ware, Lu, & Sherbourne, 1994), presented data demonstrating that measures of mental health are insensitive detectors of change in physical health. Ware and colleagues (1995) also demonstrated that physical and mental health can diverge across time, as in an aging population. If the physical components of mental well-being are extracted from measures of mental well-being, the relationship between the two is modest. A major problem encountered in using earlier measures of psychological distress in the medical population is that these measures are laden with physical symptoms (e.g., appetite, sleep, fatigue).

Notwithstanding the above point supporting separate reporting of QOL dimension scores, there remains strong and justifiable pressure to aggregate dimension scores into a summary index. Ultimate, "bottom-line" decision making depends on having a manageable summary of benefits and problems caused by treatments. We (Brady et al., 1997; Cella et al., 1993; Cella, Bonomi, et al., 1995) and others (Ganz & Coscarelli, 1995; Ganz et al., 1993; McHorney et al., 1993; Ware et al., 1995) have aggregated dimension scores into summary indexes for practical application. This allows for comparing the usefulness of psychometric QOL evaluation with utility assessment to determine patients' preferences or valuations for their current health. We typically recommend using a physical Trial Outcome Index (TOI; Cella, Bonomi, et al., 1995; Brady et al., 1997) as an efficient and precise summary measure of physical and functional well-being in clinical trials (see Brady et al., 1997; Cella, Bonomi, et al., 1995). We recommend this as an analytic strategy for purposes of enhancing measurement sensitivity, reducing data points, and summarizing physical and functional outcomes. It is, however, recommended that the entire multidimensional FACT be administered and evaluated, because the TOI inadequately captures the psychosocial dimensions of QOL, dimensions that contribute significant and unique information (Yellen & Cella, 1995).

Disease-Specific Versus Generic Assessment

Generic and disease-specific instruments have competing advantages and disadvantages. Instruments that strike a balance between these two approaches have tended to become most popular in oncology. Disease-specific and treatment-specific questions are usually of benefit when added to a general measure of QOL. Together, they can provide comparability across diseases (types of cancer, in this context) and sensitivity to specific issues or symptoms relevant to a given disease or treatment. For example, lymphedema is important to women who have had breast surgery, and items related to it should arguably be included in a breast cancer QOL instrument. However, such items are irrelevant to other cancers. The availability of disease-specific questions that need not be asked of all patients is therefore an asset because it allows for the ideal combination of questionnaire length and content coverage.

There is no single best QOL questionnaire for every application. Often, a scale that is good in one setting is inappropriate in another. The frequent absence of a clearly superior questionnaire places the investigator in the uncomfortable position of worrying that important information may be untapped by an insensitive measure. This fear of missing what is most important can lead to a burdening of the patient with a wide array of questions asked as a protection against the investigator's uncertainty. To minimize responder burden and maintain statistical validity, investigators are advised to be judicious in their selection. Typically, the best strategy is to pick the questionnaire that comes closest to asking the most clinically appropriate questions, confirm its reliability and validity, and supplement it with a few additional questions targeted to the disease, condition, or treatment under study.

Emerging Research Issues in QOL Assessment

QOL measurement in oncology has progressed to a point where challenges that have until now been elusive are being overcome by researchers. Some of these challenges include (a) obtaining cross-culturally valid assessment; (b) enhancing interpretability and determining clinical significance; (c) standardizing scores across common instruments; (d) implementing computerized, practical assessment; and (e) combining quality with quantity in the analysis of longitudinal data. These five challenges are somewhat hierarchical inasmuch as the later ones depend on successful accomplishment of the preceding ones.

Cross-Cultural Validity

Culture influences health behavior and perceptions by shaping explanations of sickness, social position, and meaning of life (Harwood & Kleinmann, 1981; Pennebaker & Epstein, 1983). In any multicultural context, people with medical conditions possess attributes that create barriers to standard QOL evaluation, such as different language and low literacy. Most commonly used QOL instruments were developed first only in the English language. Exceptions include the World Health Organization QOL questionnaire (WHOQOL; Sartorius, 1993; WHOQOL group, 1993, 1995), EuroQol (Brooks et al., 1991; Nord & EuroQol., 1991; EuroQol Group, 1990), and the Rotterdam Symptom Checklist (de Haes, van Knippenberg, & Neijt, 1990; Watson et al., 1992).

There is increasing need for multilingual QOL instruments that are acceptable and valid across cultures. Thus, many groups have gone about translating and validating questionnaires originally written in the English language. Translation of an existing single-language document ideally involves an iterative forward–backward–forward sequencing and review of differences on an item-by-item basis. *Decentering*, or selective modification of the source document on the basis of problems encountered in this process, is ideal when possible. The final translated document should be pretested for acceptability and content validity and then implemented in multilingual clinical trials, where the derived data can then be tested statistically for cross-cultural equivalence or bias. Translations are available for the CARES (Ganz & Coscarelli, 1995; Schag, Ganz, & Heinrich, 1991), the EORTC-QLQ-C30 (Aaronson et al., 1993; Osoba et al., 1994), the FACT Measurement System (Bonomi et al., 1996; Cella & Bonomi, 1996; Cella et al., 1993; Cella, Bonomi, et al., 1995), the FLIC (Clinch, 1996; Schipper et al., 1984), the MOS SF–36 (McHorney, Ware, Lu, & Sherbourne, 1994; McHorney et al., 1993; Ware et al., 1995), the Sickness Impact Profile (SIP; Bergner et al., 1981; Chwalow et al., 1992; De Bruin, DeWitte, & Diederiks, 1992), the Nottingham Health Profile (NHP; Hunt et al., 1981; Wiklund, 1990), the McMaster Health Index (Chambers, 1993; Chambers et al., 1982), and the Southwest Oncology Group questionnaire (SWOG; Moinpour, 1994). Information about current status of translations for any questionnaire is best obtained from the scale developer; however, a good review can be found in Spilker (1996).

When an instrument developed in English with primarily Anglo-European patients is adapted to other languages or cultures, it is important to produce a culturally equivalent instrument. This is best understood not as an effort to make different groups of people look the same, but to ensure that different groups of people are evaluated without significant bias. To expect any measure of QOL to be free of cultural influence is unrealistic. However, we must work toward constructing measures on the basis of common cores of items that are not culture biased, neither more attractive nor more offensive to one group or another. Developing item equivalence across cultures does not imply that measures show equivalent QOL levels across different groups of people. Indeed, levels of QOL may differ across cultural or linguistic groups. This is an empirical question that should be addressed without prior assumptions. *Equivalence* in this context refers to the absence of differential item functioning.

The issue of literacy arises in connection with language and culture. It is desirable to justify paraprofessional interview assessment of QOL as an equivalent (or at least equivalent with correction) form of QOL data collection. The demand of cost-efficiency in multicenter clinical trials precludes the administration of a QOL interview to all patients. Self-administered questionnaire is usually the method of choice. However, this carries the risk of excluding or at least confusing low-literacy patients who cannot complete the form. Because low-literacy patients require interviewer administration, and because most high-literacy patients in clinical trials are asked (for reasons of convenience and cost) to complete the questionnaire without assistance, it is important to evaluate the comparability of self- and interviewer administration and of low versus high literacy. This requires a three- (rather than two-) facet psychometric analysis: Patients and QOL items (the usual two facets) are specified and measured, and the interviewers themselves are specified and measured for their influence on the response levels of the patients they assess.

Analyzing for statistical equivalence of measurement is a two-step process (Cella, Lloyd, & Wright, 1996; Chang & Cella, 1997; Gonin, Lloyd, & Cella, 1996). The first step is at the measurement level, where the purpose is to determine whether a given rating scale works in the same manner with different groups of people. This step is crucial when one is interested in detecting systematic measurement bias and a particular rating scale is used with different groups of people (e.g., Hispanic vs. Black non-Hispanic vs. White non-Hispanic culture; Spanish vs. English language; high vs. low literacy) or administered in different ways (e.g., self vs. interviewer). Then the extent to which each QOL item with which the rating scale is used performs similarly across different reference groups is of critical interest when determining which of the QOL items can be used to provide an unbiased basis for comparing groups. We need rating scale categories and QOL items that match across groups on both category step and item "difficulty." The measurement step of equivalence construction and testing provides that reassurance.

The second step after establishing and evaluating equivalence is the analysis level, in which we evaluate scale measure differences across reference groups and test conditions to determine what real differences exist. We are seeking assurance that any detected group difference (as analyzed in the analysis step) is not based on items that are systematically biased in favor of one of the groups.

Enhancing Interpretability and Determining Clinical Significance

It is possible to achieve reliability and validity of measurement yet still be unable to interpret the data collected. In most cases, particularly if QOL measurement experts are successful, the end user of a QOL questionnaire will not be a psychometrician or social scientist; it will be a health care provider making individual treatment decisions, a policy analyst deciding on resource allocation, or a health care payer deciding whether or not to cover a given therapy. For this to work, difference scores must be placed in a context of understandability and credibility, extending beyond statistical significance and even effect size.

A large clinical trial might obtain statistically significant differences between treatment groups, and these differences may reflect measurement of a true effect (i.e., the instrument was valid; it measured what it claimed to measure and detected a real difference). Still, because of the large sample size (and perhaps the small score difference), one might question the clinical meaning of the difference score (Braitman, 1983). Is the difference clinically significant? What is the meaningful pattern of change that deserves clinical attention? Does a significant difference between treatment groups transfer to single-case interpretation? What is the meaning of a 5-, 10-, or 15-point change score? There are few available answers to these and related questions. Some approaches that have been used include the statistical examination of effect size across different thresholds of quality of life (Kraemer, 1992), calibration of change–difference scores to an external criterion (Aaronson et al., 1993; Brady et al., 1997; Cella et al., 1993; Cella, Bonomi, et al., 1995), direct longitudinal assessment of patients (Guyatt, Walter, & Norman, 1987; Jaeschke, Singer, & Guyatt, 1989), determination of population weights or valuations (Torrance, 1986; Torrance & Feeny, 1989), and interviews to derive values or preferences for various health states (e.g., Singer et al., 1991). For 7-point Likert scaling of symptoms, Jaeschke et al. (1989) have suggested that a difference of approximately 0.5 units per item is a minimal clinically important difference. For individual assessment, Jacobson and Truax (1991) recommended a Reliable Change Index that estimates whether a change measured is real or simply a consequence of imprecise measurement. Their suggestions are based on data collected in such a way as to allow calibration of change scores to meaningful criteria.

All of these approaches offer some data about meaningful differences in QOL scores within and across patients over time. It is this area of clinical significance that ultimately determines whether people pay close attention to change in QOL over time and across treatment options. Considerably more research effort must be expended in this area before we have clear and convincing data about clinical significance and value attached to measure change.

Standardizing Scores Across Common Instruments

Many current clinical trials have included QOL as a primary or secondary endpoint. Furthermore, many clinicians would like to integrate knowledge about individual patients' QOL into their daily practice and clinical decision making. Although this increased interest has been encouraging, implementation of QOL measurement in clinical trials and in clinical practice has been hampered by the absence of a "gold standard" instrument. Several QOL instruments have been validated for use with cancer patients, each with its own set of questions and scoring rules. However, even the most ambitious of oncology clinicians can be expected to master only one of these many available instruments. As a result, we are creating a potential Tower of Babel in which we lack a common language (Cella, Gonin, & Lloyd, 1995). An additional concern is that the use of raw scores is problematic because raw scores are not usually equal-interval measures.

To correct these problems, one could demonstrate equivalence of questionnaires and then generate a common, standardized metric ("Q-score") for QOL (Cella, Gonin, & Lloyd, 1995; Chang & Cella, 1997; Gonin et al., 1996). If two instruments are shown to be equivalent, then the Q-score has the same value for any given person, regardless of which questionnaire is administered. The procedure involves five steps:

1. Simultaneously administer two QOL questionnaires.
2. Convert raw scores to (equal interval) logit measures.
3. Assess the agreement (equivalence) of the logit measures.
4. Obtain the functional relationship between the logit measures through orthogonal least-squares regression.
5. Derive universal Q-scores from the logit measures.

With this procedure, one can derive a Q-score conversion table ranging, for example, from 0 to 100 ($M = 50$, $SD = 10$). One can then administer either of the equated instruments and derive an equivalent Q-score, which can evolve to have a standard meaning to the clinician, regardless of questionnaire administered. This same 5-step approach can be applied to any two instruments, including common subscales and higher order factors. Details of possible applications of equating methodology can be found elsewhere (Cella et al., 1996; Chang & Cella, 1997; Gonin et al., 1996).

Implementing Computerized, Practical Assessment

The demand for practical, on-line assessment for outcomes monitoring and management has grown dramatically over the past decade. Health care reimbursement and accreditation agencies are increasingly requiring accountability for medical treatment. Demonstrating improved QOL as a function of therapy is one way to justify treatment.

Whether to show outright improvement or simply to monitor treatment progress for quality improvement purposes, there is now a great need for streamlined, electronic acquisition and scoring of QOL data obtained in the clinical setting over time. One way to do this is to have patients complete forms that can be scanned electronically, scored, and stored with minimal staff effort. Another way is to have patients complete a questionnaire that is administered on the computer itself, eliminating yet another step in the process. A third approach is to create new, "adaptive" tests on a computer at the time of assessment, selecting each next question on the basis of the patient's previous responses. Computerized adaptive testing (CAT) uses an item response theory (IRT) measurement model to characterize the probabilities of responding to an entire series of questions as a function of previous responses, selecting the next question on the basis of which is likely to provide the maximum amount of information.

The response (or *option*) characteristic curve for an item is a measure of item effectiveness at every level of the underlying (latent) variable being measured. This is also referred to as an *item characteristic curve*. In an IRT model, if the probability of responding positively to an item increases as a function of increase in the latent variable measured, then this is a good item, because it discriminates among differences in that latent variable. In addition, the rate of change in the probability of endorsing an item indicates the degree of effectiveness of an item at any point on the latent variable. This capability of IRT approaches to measurement allows the user to select items that have maximum discrimination ability for a given patient being assessed. An item bank, if properly implemented, allows one to conduct CAT, minimizing item length while maximizing measurement sensitivity and precision (McHorney, 1997; Revicki & Cella, 1997).

An added unique feature of IRT measurement models is that they allow one to examine questions for bias or, more appropriately, "differential item functioning" (Angoff, 1993), when applied to one group compared with another. A good, unbiased item is one that has a similar likelihood of endorsement relative to the other items in the scale, across groups. This does not necessarily mean that different groups respond with equal intensity to a given item, but rather that the item shows a similar probability of being endorsed by people from groups that are equal on the underlying trait. Such a demonstration provides added confidence that differences in health status (found between, e.g., men vs. women, Latinos vs. African Americans, or English-speaking vs. French-speaking patients) are based on real differences and not items that are responded to differently across groups. An IRT approach to the Beck Depression Inventory (Ramsay, 1991) recently demonstrated that despite many differences in expression of depression between men and women, the items of the BDI function similarly across gender and can therefore be treated as unbiased (Santor, Ramsay, & Zuroff, 1994).

Risks of Test Brevity

Consumers of QOL data, whether patients, health providers, health planners, payers, or legislators, naturally seek the most efficient questionnaire available to meet their needs (Bice, 1976). To have practical utility, a QOL questionnaire must be as brief as possible without sacrificing precision beyond what is acceptable. Test brevity carries risk that important data for a given group of patients are missed. Properly appreciated, test efficiency minimizes not only item length but also risk of insensitivity, thereby maximizing precision relative to length. IRT models that exploit information about item "difficulty" (likelihood of endorsement), and perhaps also item discrimination, can empirically maximize test efficiency and precision. Item pooling, and subsequent banking and CAT, can allow one to select the best next question given the information obtained from previous questions, thereby minimizing the number of questions asked of any given person without compromising precision.

An *item bank* is a repository consisting of carefully calibrated questions that develop, define, and quantify a common underlying theme or domain (Choppin, 1968). If an item bank is sufficiently deep and complete in its coverage of the domain, it forms an operational definition of the variable being measured, such as physical well-being, mental well-being, social well-being, or general QOL. An item bank is built from the item repository using an IRT measurement model that builds an operational definition of the domain. Measurement precision can be sharpened or dulled within this approach by setting one's tolerance for error up front, depending on one's assessment goal. For example, to describe the QOL of large populations of patients and compare them with reference groups, without the need to discriminate fine differences, one would preset the testing program to a limited number of questions. Conversely, if fine precision were desired, a larger set of questions within the difficulty range of the patient's true QOL ("ability") would be included in the assessment.

Flexible assessment length, within the adaptive testing framework of IRT-based computer assessment, is new to health status assessment. Although unprecedented, it is not impractical. It does require a fairly high level of technological readiness, including available computers for assessment and software for converting item banks into testing programs. Another prerequisite is the availability of large data sets to establish item and response characteristic curves that are used by the CAT program to select item presentation sequence. The technology is within reach, however, and the advantages are potentially profound. For example, form burden to the patient and the investigator are eliminated. Assessment can be tailored to the diverse needs of clinicians and researchers. Assessments become comparable across a variety of contexts. Finally, the use of this technology provides immediate feedback on the quality of data collection and construct validity of the assessment across a variety of patient groups (McHorney, 1997; Revicki & Cella, 1997).

Advantages and Disadvantages of Item Banking

One great advantage of item banking is that it allows for streamlined adaptive testing to take place, minimizing time spent in assessment relative to information obtained.

Use of an item bank can also minimize and even eliminate floor and ceiling effects. Use of an item bank–CAT approach allows the user to specify the degree of precision desired (i.e., longer assessment for individual assessment and brief assessment for large-group classification). This approach also identifies inconsistent response patterns that threaten validity of measurement and allows for determination of bias (*differential item functioning*).

Because item banking works best in conjunction with CAT, a disadvantage of this approach is the requirement of a high degree of technology and patient acceptance of computerized assessment. It also requires extensive preliminary collection of item repositories and derivation of item characteristic curves from which to derive functioning banks. Finally, the approach requires "buy-in" from consumers and continued support of item bank expansion–refinement.

Combining Quality With Quantity in the Analysis of Longitudinal Data

In the evaluation of cancer clinical trials, the final common pathway of all of the above work is the combination of data on QOL with survival time. Life quantity (survival) analyses have emphasized the time-to-event approach, whereas in the past QOL analyses have tended to rely on longitudinal multivariate analysis of variance models. The latter carry insurmountable hurdles with regard to informative censoring and other missing data problems; the former is problematic because it is unclear how to define an "event" in QOL data. This is a problem in part because it is difficult to know what is a significant difference. Furthermore, even if a significant difference score were known, a time-to-event analysis would not readily allow cases back into the analysis, which would be desirable because patients get better and worse over time.

Missing Data

Missing data pose the greatest challenge to the statistician attempting to make sense of a QOL data set from a clinical trial or clinical program database. The first issue to be addressed in an analysis is whether or not the data are missing at random. Data that are missing at random (both "missing completely at random" or "missing at random") can be modeled or imputed with reasonable accuracy using estimation models that draw from available data. Data not missing at random cannot be so easily modeled; in fact, there are no good models for doing so. Patient disability and death, common reasons for missing data over time in a data set, are not random events with regard to the QOL data set. Therefore, unfortunately, nonrandomly missing data always present an analytic challenge. Random reasons for missing data (e.g., staff forgetting) are easier to handle (and obviously are best avoided). Because understanding missing data mechanisms are so important to later analyses, it is recommended that any data collection plan (e.g., in a clinical trial) include a reporting of why patients did not complete specific questions or entire questionnaires. The more detailed information that is available, the greater the investigator's and statistician's ability to determine whether missing data encountered in the data are random or not. For this reason, planning how to report reasons for missing data is best done in consultation with the trial statistician who is doing the analysis.

Despite the problems associated with imputing missing values, imputation of missing data is superior to dropping cases with missing data and analyzing only those with all available data. This leads to greatly distorted conclusions, particularly in data sets that have patient drop out over time as a result of illness, death, or even reasons not clearly random or nonrandom (e.g., lost to follow-up). Therefore, having imputed values for missing data, one must now conduct a QOL analysis when there is no clearly correct approach. Slope analysis is possible when there is a consistent (linear) direction of change and at least two assessments (Korn & O'Fallon, 1990). Area under the curve analysis is another approach that has intuitive appeal in that it is conceptually similar to quality-adjusted time, summing areas under the sequence of trapezoids laid out over time (Cox et al., 1992). Mixed models such as combining repeated measures analysis of variance and growth curve models (Diggle, Liang, & Zeger, 1994) also have promise because they can use all available data, including incomplete cases. Joint mixed effects–survival models (Schluchter, 1992) have appeal because they offer the opportunity to jointly estimate survival and QOL. A recent issue of *Statistics in Medicine* (Bernhard & Gelber, 1998) is devoted to minimizing and handling missing data in longitudinal QOL studies and is highly recommended for more in-depth discussion of this issue.

Utilities, Quality-Adjusted Life-Years, and Quality-Adjusted Time Without Symptoms or Toxicity

Related to the analysis problem is the recognition of the need to combine health status data with utility data in some way. Health status measurement approaches have the strength of descriptive accuracy and measurement sensitivity; utility approaches have the strength of a single index weight for a given period of time, which is anchored to a 0 (*death*) to 1.0 (*perfect health*) scale tied to economic (utility) theory. Perhaps the best of these complementary approaches can be combined into a unified approach that allows for simple, meaningful, and sensitive evaluation of QOL in a clinical trial.

Bush, Chen, and Patrick (1973) described a technique that adjusts survival time downward to a degree proportional to the amount of disability or toxicity endured. Variations on this theme have been called *quality-adjusted life-years* (QALYs; (Weinstein, 1983), *well-years*, (Kaplan & Bush, 1982), and (in the cancer treatment context) *quality-adjusted time without symptoms or toxicity* (Q-TWiST; Gelber & Goldhirsch, 1986; Gelber, Goldhirsch, & Cavalli, 1991). These approaches are most useful in health policy decision making or in cases in which the effectiveness of two or more competing treatments or programs must be evaluated for relative efficacy. The utility approach to health status measurement evolved from a tradition of cost–benefit analysis into cost-effectiveness approaches and, more recently, into cost-utility approaches (Torrance, 1987). The cost-utility approach extends the cost-effectiveness approach conceptually by evaluating the QOL benefit produced by the clinical effects of a treatment, thereby including the (presumed) patient's perspective. To be used this way, QOL must be measured as a utility because, by definition, utilities can be multiplied by time to produce an adjusted time that is less than or equal to actual survival time.

Two general cost-utility methods are the "standard gamble" approach and the time trade-off approach (Torrance, 1986). In the standard gamble approach, people are asked to choose between their current state of health and a gamble in which they have various probabilities for death or perfect health (cure). The time trade-off method involves asking people how much time they would be willing to give up in order to live out their remaining life expectancy in perfect health. All utility approaches share in common the use of a 0–1 scale in which 0 = *death* and 1 = *perfect health*. In practice, most cost-utility analyses use expert estimates of utility weights or, in some cases, weights provided by healthy members of the general public. It is often assumed that these weights are reasonable approximations of patient preferences. However, several studies have demonstrated that utilities obtained from patients are generally higher than those provided by physicians, which are, in turn, higher than utilities for the same health states obtained from healthy individuals (Boyd et al., 1990). There are practical impediments to collection of utilities directly from patients, including the complexity of the concepts involved and the requirement for an interviewer-administered questionnaire (often unfeasible in the cooperative group setting). In addition, utility assessments provide little information on important disease and treatment-specific problems and are probably less sensitive to changes in health status over time than are psychometric data (Tsevat et al., 1993; Canadian Erythropoietin Study Group, 1990). Finally, the few studies that have been done involving simultaneous measurement of utilities and health status have found them at best to be moderately correlated, with measures of mood and depression correlating more highly than other measures with utilities (Tsevat et al., 1991).

A modified utility approach has been developed to evaluate the effectiveness of adjuvant therapy (Gelber & Goldhirsch, 1986; Gelber, Goldhirsch, & Cavalli, 1991). This approach, the Q-TWiST, discounts survival time spent with toxicity or symptoms relative to disease-free survival off therapy. Thresholds for decision making were determined by modeling actual survival data, and judgments were made by the investigators regarding where patient preferences were likely to fall relative to these threshold values. There is no theoretical reason why actual patient preference data could not be used in the Q-TWiST analyses or other studies of quality-adjusted survival. If the relationship between psychometric data and utilities can be established, it will become possible to collect psychometric data and base utility estimates on the reports of patients rather than the best guesses of others. This is a significant area for further research, and many groups of assessment teams are working on it.

Conclusion

In oncology treatment evaluation and planning, QOL assessment has come a long way over the past 10 years. QOL is a multidimensional, subjective, and fluid endpoint, so its measurement must be comprehensive, include the patient's perspective, and be sensitive to meaningful change. Given the challenges and burdens of most cancer treatment systems, QOL measurement must also be brief. There is no gold standard or best QOL measure. It is important to be aware of the strengths and weaknesses of available questionnaires when setting out to study QOL. There are at least five exciting and emerging new areas of research in the development of QOL measurement in oncology: establishing cross-cultural validity; enhancing interpretability of scores; standardizing scores across questionnaire; implementing computerized, practical assessment; and combining quantity of life with QOL in longitudinal data analysis. Social, statistical, and measurement scientists have a tremendous opportunity to contribute meaningfully to the future health and well-being of our society by immersing themselves in these new challenges to measuring and evaluating QOL in people with cancer.

References

Aaronson, N. K. (1988). Quality of life: What is it? How should it be measured? *Oncology*, 2(5), 69–74.

Aaronson, N. K., Ahmedzai, S., Bergman, B., Bullinger, M., Cull, A., Duez, N. J., Filiberti, A., Flechtner, H., Fleischman, S. B., & de Haes, J. C. (1993). The European Organization for the Research and Treatment of Cancer QLQ-C30: A quality of life instrument for use in international clinical trials in oncology. *Journal of the National Cancer Institute*, 85(5), 365–376.

Andrykowski, M. A., Brady, M. J., & Hunt, J. W. (1993). Positive psychosocial adjustment in potential bone marrow transplant recipients: Cancer as a psychosocial transition. *Psycho-Oncology*, 2, 261–276.

Angoff, W. H. (1993). Perspectives on differential item functioning methodology. In P. W. Holland & H. Wainer (Eds.), *Differential item functioning* (pp. 3–23). Hillsdale, NJ: Lawrence Erlbaum Associates.

Bergman, B., Sullivan, M., & Sorenson. S. (1992). Quality of life during chemotherapy for small cell lung cancer. II. A longitudinal study of the EORTC core quality of life questionnaire and comparison with the Sickness Impact Profile. *Acta Oncologica*, 31, 19–28.

Bergner, M., Bobbitt, R. A., Carter, W. B., & Gilson, B. S. (1981). The Sickness Impact Profile: Development and final revision of a health status measure. *Medical Care*, 19, 787–806.

Bernhard, J., & Gelber, R. D. (Eds.). (1998). Workshop on missing data in quality of life research in cancer clinical trials: Practical and methodological issues [Special issue]. *Statistics in Medicine, 17*(5–7).

Bice, T. W. (1976). Comments on health indicators: Methodological perspectives. *International Journal of Health Services, 6,* 509–520.

Bohrnstedt, G. W. (1983). Measurement. In P. H. Rossi, J. D. Wright, & A. B. Anderson (Eds.), *Handbook of survey research* (pp. 70–121). New York: Academic Press.

Bonomi, A. E., Cella, D. F., Bjordal, K., Sperner-Unterweger, B., Gangeri, L., Bergman, B., Willems-Groot, J., Hanquet, P., & Zittoun, R. (1996). Multilingual translation of the Functional Assessment of Cancer Therapy (FACT) quality of life measurement system. *Quality of Life Research, 5*(3), 309–320.

Boyd, N. F., Sutherland, H. J., Heasman, K. Z., Tritchler, D. L., & Commings, B. J. (1990). Whose utilities for decision analysis? *Medical Decision Making, 10,* 58–67.

Brady, M. J., Cella, D. F., Mo, F., Bonomi, A. E., Tulsky, D. S., Lloyd, S. R., Deasy, S., Cobleigh, M., & Shiomoto, G. (1997). Reliability and validity of the Functional Assessment of Cancer Therapy-Breast (FACT-B) quality of life instrument. *Journal of Clinical Oncology, 15*(3), 974–986.

Braitman, L. (1983). Statistical, clinical and experimental evidence in randomized controlled trials. *Annals of Internal Medicine, 98,* 407–408.

Brooks, R., Jendteg, S., Lindgren, B., Perrson, U., & Bjork, S. (1991). EuroQol: Health related quality of life measurement. Results from the Swedish questionnaire exercise. *Health Policy, 18,* 37–48.

Bush, J. W., Chen, M., & Patrick, D. L. (1973). Cost-effectiveness using a health status index: Analysis of the New York State PKU screening program. In R. Berg (Ed.), *Health status indexes* (pp. 172–208). Chicago: Hospital Research and Educational Trust.

Campbell, D. T., & Fiske, D. W. (1959). Convergent and discriminant validation by the multitrait-multimethod matrix. *Psychological Bulletin, 56,* 85–105.

Canadian Erythropoietin Study Group. (1990). Association between recombinant human erythropoietin and quality of life and exercise capacity of patients receiving hemodialysis. *British Medical Journal, 300,* 573–578.

Cella, D. F. (1995). Measuring quality of life in palliative care. *Seminars in Oncology, 22* (2, Suppl. 3), 73–81.

Cella, D. F., & Bonomi, A. E. (1995). Measuring quality of life: 1995 update. *Oncology, 9*(Suppl. 11), 47–60.

Cella, D. F., & Bonomi, A. E. (1996). The Functional Assessment of Cancer Therapy (FACT) and Functional Assessment of HIV Infection (FAHI) quality of life measurement system. In B. Spilker (Ed.), *Quality of life and pharmacoeconomics in clinical trials* (pp. 203–214). New York: Raven Press.

Cella, D. F., Bonomi, A. E., Lloyd, S., Tulsky, D. S., Kaplan, E., & Bonomi, P. (1995). Reliability and validity of the Functional Assessment of Cancer Therapy–Lung (FACT-L) quality of life instrument. *Lung Cancer, 12,* 199–220.

Cella, D. F., & Cherin, E. A. (1988). Quality of life during and after cancer treatment. *Comprehensive Therapy, 4*(5), 69–75.

Cella, D. F., Gonin, R., & Lloyd, S. (1995). The Q-Score: Scaling the Tower of Babel in quality of life (QL) measurement. *Proceedings of the ASCO, 14,* 305 (Abstract #886).

Cella, D. F., Lloyd, S. R., & Wright, B. D. (1996). Cross-cultural instrument equating: Current research and future directions. In B. Spilker (Ed.), *Quality of life and pharmacoeconomics in clinical trials* (pp. 707–715). New York: Raven Press.

Cella, D. F., & Tross, S. (1986). Psychological adjustment to survival from Hodgkin's disease. *Journal of Consulting and Clinical Psychology, 54,* 616–622.

Cella, D. F., Tulsky, D. S., Gray, G., Sarafian, B., Linn, E., Bonomi, A., Silberman, M., Yellen, S. B., Winicour, P., Brannon, J., Eckberg, K., Lloyd, S., Purl, S., Blendowski, C., Goodman, M., Barnicle, M., Stewart, I., McHale, M., Bonomi, P., Kaplan, E., Taylor, S., IV, Thomas, C. R., Jr., & Harris, J. (1993). The functional assessment of cancer therapy scale (FACT): Development and validation of the general measure. *Journal of Clinical Oncology, 11*(3), 570–579.

Chambers, L. W. (1993). The McMaster Health Index Questionnaire: An update. In S. R. Walker & R. M. Rosser (Eds.), *Quality of life assessment: Key issues in the 1990's* (pp. 131–149). London: Kluwer Academic.

Chambers, L. W., Macdonald, L. A., Tugwell, P., Buchanan, W. W., & Kraag, G. (1982). The McMaster Health Index Questionnaire as a measure of quality of life for patients with rheumatoid disease. *Journal of Rheumatology, 9,* 780–784.

Chang, C. H., & Cella, D. (1997). Equating health-related quality of life instruments in applied oncology settings. *Physical Medicine and Rehabilitation: State of the Art Reviews, 11*(2), 397–406.

Choppin, B. (1968). An item bank using sample-free calibration. *Nature, 219,* 870–872.

Chwalow, A. J., Lurie, A., Bean, K., Parent du Chatelet, I., Venot, A., Dusser, D., Duout, Y., & Strauch, G. (1992). A French version of the Sickness Impact Profile (SIP): Stages in the cross validation of a generic quality of life scale. *Fundamental Clinical Pharmacology, 6,* 319–326.

Clinch, J. (1996). The Functional Living Index-Cancer: Ten years later. In B. Spilker (Ed.), *Quality of life and pharmacoeconomics in clinical trials* (pp. 215–226). New York: Raven Press.

Cox, D. R., Fitzpatrick, R., Fletcher, A. I., Gore, S. M., Spiegelhalter, D. J., & Jones, D. R. (1992). Quality of life assessment: Can we keep it simple? (with discussion) *Journal of the Royal Statistical Society, 155,* 353–393.

De Bruin, A. F., De Witte, L. P., & Diederiks, J. P. (1992). Sickness Impact Profile: The state of the art of a generic functional status measure. *Social Science Medicine, 8,* 1003–1014.

de Haes, J. C. J. M., Raatgever, J. W., van der Burg, M. E. L., Hamersma, E., & Neijt, J. P. (1987). Evaluation of the quality of life of patients with advanced ovarian cancer treated with combination chemotherapy. In N. K. Aaronson & J. Beckmann (Eds.), *The quality of life of cancer patients* (p. 215). New York: Raven Press.

de Haes, J. C. J. M., van Knippenberg, F. C. E., & Neijt, J. P. (1990). Measuring psychological and physical distress in cancer patients: Structure and application of the Rotterdam Symptom Checklist. *British Journal of Cancer, 62*, 1034–1038.

Diggle, P. J., Liang, K. Y., & Zeger, S. L. (1994). *Analysis of longitudinal data.* New York: Oxford University Press.

Ditto, P. H., Druley, J. A., Moore, K. A., Danks, J. H., & Smucker, W. D. (1996). Fates worse than death: The role of valued life activities in health-state evaluations. *Health Psychology, 15*, 332–343.

EuroQol Group, the. (1990). EuroQol—A new facility for the measurement of health-related quality of life. *Health Policy, 16*, 199–208.

Ganz, P., & Coscarelli, A. (1995). Quality of life after breast cancer: A decade of research. In J. E. Dimsdale & A. Baum (Eds.), *Quality of life in behavioral medicine research* (pp. 97–113). Hillsdale, NJ: Erlbaum.

Ganz, P., Coscarelli, A., Schag, C. A., Kahn, B., Peterson, L., & Hirji, K. (1993). Describing the health-related quality of life impact of HIV infection: Findings from a study using the HIV Overview of Problems-Evaluation System (HOPES). *Quality of Life Research, 2*, 109–119.

Gelber, R. D., & Goldhirsch, A. (1986). A new endpoint for the assessment of adjuvant therapy in postmenopausal women with operable breast cancer. *Journal of Clinical Oncology, 4*(12), 1772–1779.

Gelber, R. D., Goldhirsch, A., & Cavalli, F. (1991). Quality-of-life adjusted evaluation of adjuvant therapies for operable breast cancer. The International Breast Cancer Study Group. *Annals of Internal Medicine, 114*(8), 621–628.

Gonin, R., Lloyd, S., & Cella, D. F. (1996). Establishing equivalence between scaled measures of quality of life. *Quality of Life Research, 5*, 20–26.

Guyatt, G., Walter, S., & Norman, G. (1987). Measuring change over time: Assessing the usefulness of evaluative instruments. *Journal of Chronic Diseases, 40*, 171.

Harwood, A., & Kleinmann, A. (1981). Ethnicity and clinical care: Selected issues in treating Puerto Rican patients. *Hospital Physician, 17*(9), 113–118.

Hays, R. D., & Stewart, A. L. (1990). The structure of self-reported health in chronic disease patients. *Psychological Assessment: A Journal of Consulting and Clinical Psychology, 2*(1), 22–30.

Helgeson, V. S., Cohen, S., & Fritz, H. L. (1998). Social integration and cancer incidence and mortality. In J. C. Holland (Ed.), *Handbook of psycho-oncology: Vol. 2. Social ties and cancer* (pp. 99–109). New York: Oxford Press.

Hunt, S., McKenna, S. P., McEwen, J., Williams, J., & Papp, E. (1981). The Nottingham Health Profile: Subjective health status and medical consultations. *Social Science and Medicine, 15A*, 221–229.

Jacobson, N. S., & Truax, P. (1991). Clinical significance: A statistical approach to defining meaningful change in psychotherapy research. *Journal of Consulting and Clinical Psychology, 59*, 12–19.

Jaeschke, R., Singer, J., & Guyatt, G. H. (1989). Measurement of health status: Ascertaining the minimal clinically important difference. *Controlled Clinical Trials, 10*, 407–415.

Kaplan, R. M., & Bush, J. W. (1982). Health-related quality of life measurement for evaluation, research and policy analysis. *Health Psychology, 1, 61–80.*

Korn, E. L., & O'Fallon, J. (for the Statistics Working Group). (1990). Statistical considerations. In S. G. Nayfield, B. J. Hailey, & M. McCabe (Eds.), *Quality of life assessment in cancer clinical trials: Report of the workshop on quality of life research in cancer clinical trial.* Bethesda, MD: National Cancer Institute, United States Health and Human Services.

Kornblith, A. B., & Holland, J. C. (1994). *Handbook of measures for psychological, social and physical function in cancer: Vol. 1. Quality of life.* New York: Memorial Sloan-Kettering Cancer Center.

Kraemer, H. (1992). Reporting the size of effects in research studies to facilitate assessments of practical or clinical significance. *Psychoneuroendocrinology, 17, 527–536.*

McHorney, C. A. (1997). Generic health measurement: Past accomplishments and a measurement paradigm for the 21st century. *Annals of Internal Medicine, 127, 743–750.*

McHorney, C. A., Ware, J. E., Lu, J. F. R., & Sherbourne, C. D. (1994). The MOS 36-Item Short Form Health Survey (SF-36). III. Tests of data quality, scaling assumptions and reliability across diverse patient groups. *Medical Care, 32*(1), 40–66.

McHorney, C. A., Ware, J. E., & Raczek, A. E. (1993). The MOS 36-item short-form health survey (SF-36): II. Psychometric and clinical test of validity in measuring physical and mental health constructs. *Medical Care, 31, 247–263.*

McNair, D. M., Lorr, M., & Droppleman, L. F. (1981) *Profile of mood states.* San Diego, CA: Educational and Industrial Testing Service.

Moinpour, C. M. (1994). Quality of life assessment in Southwest Oncology Group clinical trials: Translating and validating a Spanish questionnaire. In J. Orley & W. Kuyken (Eds.), *Quality of life assessment: International perspectives* (pp. 83–97). Berlin, Germany: Springer-Verlag.

Nord, E., & EuroQol. (1991). Health-related quality of life measurement. Valuations of health states by the general public in Norway. *Health Policy, 18, 25–36.*

Osoba, D., Zee, B., Pater, J., Warr, D., Kaizer, L., & Latreille, J. (1994). Psychometric properties and responsiveness of the EORTC quality of life questionnaire (QLQ-30) in patients with breast, ovarian and lung cancer. *Quality of Life Research, 3, 353–364.*

Pennebaker, J. W., & Epstein, D. (1983). Implicit psychophysiology: Effects of common beliefs and idiosyncratic physiological responses on symptom reporting. *Journal of Personality, 51*(3), 468–496.

Ramsay, J. O. (1991). Kernel smoothing approaches to nonparametric item characteristic curve estimation. *Psychometrika, 56, 611-630.*

Revicki, D. A., & Cella, D. (1997). Health status assessment for the twenty-first century: Item response theory, item banking and computer adaptive testing. *Quality of Life Research, 6, 595–600.*

Santor, D. A., Ramsey, J. O., & Zuroff, D. C. (1994). Nonparametric item analysis of the Beck Depression Inventory: Evaluating gender item bias and response option weights. *Psychological Assessment, 6, 255–270.*

Sartorius, N. (1993). WHO's work on the epidemiology of mental disorders. *Social Psychiatry & Psychiatric Epidemiology, 28*(4), 147–155.

Schag, C. A., Ganz, P. A., & Heinrich, R. L. (1991). CAncer Rehabilitation Evaluation System-Short Form (CARES-SF): A cancer specific rehabilitation and quality of life instrument. *Cancer, 68,* 1406–1413.

Schipper, H., Clinch, J., McMurray, A., & Levitt, M. (1984). Measuring the quality of life of cancer patients: The Functional Living Index-Cancer: Development and validation. *Journal of Clinical Oncology, 2*(5), 472–483.

Schluchter, M. D. (1992). Methods for the analysis of informatively censored longitudinal data. *Statistics in Medicine, 11,* 1861–1870.

Singer, P., Tasch, E., Stocking, C., Rubin, S., Siegler, M., & Weichselbaum, R. (1991). Sex or survival: Trade-offs between quality and quantity of life. *Journal of Clinical Oncology, 9,* 328–334.

Spilker, B. (Ed.). (1996). *Quality of life and pharmacoeconomics in clinical trials* (2nd ed.). Philadelphia: Lippincott-Raven.

Stewart, A. L., Ware, J. E., & Brook, R. H. (1981). Advances in the measurement of functional status: Construction of aggregate indexes. *Medical Care, 19,* 473–488.

Torrance, G. (1986). Measurement of health state utilities for economic appraisal. *Journal of Health Economics, 5*(1), 1–30.

Torrance, G. W. (1987). Utility approach to measuring health-related quality of life. *Journal of Chronic Diseases, 40*(6), 593–603.

Torrance, G., & Feeny, D. (1989). Utilities and quality-adjusted life years. *International Journal of Technology Assessment in Health Care, 5*(4), 559–575.

Tsevat, J., Cook, E. F., & Soukup, J. R., Broste, S. K., Dawson, N. V., Matchar, D. B., Harrell, F. E., Phillips, R. S., Bergner, M., Lynn, J., Oye, R. K., & Goldman, L. (1991). Utilities of the seriously ill [Abstract]. *Clinical Research, 39,* 589A.

Tsevat, J., Goldman, L., Soukup, J. R., Lamas, G. A., Connors, K. F., Chapin, C. C., & Lee, T. H. (1993). Stability of time-tradeoff utilities in survivors of myocardial infarction. *Medical Decision Making, 13*(2), 161–165.

Ware, J. E., Kosinski, M. A., Bayliss, M. S., McHorney, C. A., Rogers, W. H., & Raczek, A. (1995). Comparison of methods for scoring and statistical analysis of SF-36 health profile and summary measures: Summary of results from the Medical Outcomes Study. *Medical Care, 33,* AS264–AS279.

Watson, M., Law, M., Maguire, G. P., & Robertson, B. (1992). Further development of a quality of life measure for cancer patients: The Rotterdam Symptom Checklist (Revised). *Psycho-Oncology, 1,* 35–44.

Weinstein, M. C. (1983). Cost-effective priorities for cancer prevention. *Science, 221*(4605), 17–23.

Wiklund, I. (1990). The Nottingham Health Profile—A measure of health-related quality of life. *Scandanavian Journal of Primary Health Care, 1,* 15–18.

Wisloff, F., Eika, S., Hippe, E., Hjorth, M., Holmberg, E., Kaasa, S., Palva, I., & Westin, J. for the Nordic Myeloma Study Group. (1996). Measurement of health-related quality of life in multiple myeloma. *British Journal of Hematology, 92,* 604–613.

World Health Organization. (1993). Study protocol for the World Health Organization project to develop a quality of life assessment instrument (WHOQOL). *Quality of Life Research, 2*(2), 153–159.

World Health Organization. (1995). The World Health Organization quality of life assessment (WHOQOL) [Position paper]. *Social Science & Medicine, 41*(10), 1403–1409.

Yellen, S. B., & Cella, D. (1995). Someone to live for: Social well being, parenthood status and decision-making in oncology. *Journal of Clinical Oncology, 13,* 1255–1264.

CHAPTER 5

Long-Term Adjustment in Cancer Survivors

Integration of Classical-Conditioning and Cognitive-Processing Models

William H. Redd

Katherine N. DuHamel

Suzanne M. Johnson Vickberg

Jamie L. Ostroff

Meredith Y. Smith

Paul B. Jacobsen

Sharon L. Manne

Long-term survival for many cancer patients has markedly increased in the past decade. Unfortunately, life after cancer is often associated with chronic adjustment problems, including anxiety, depression, and concentration difficulties. The purpose of this chapter is to examine the utility of posttraumatic stress disorder (PTSD) to conceptualize long-term psychosocial adjustment difficulties. Of particular interest is the role of classical-conditioning and cognitive-processing models in the development, maintenance, and treatment of adjustment disorders following successful medical treatment for cancer.

We begin the chapter with a brief discussion of aspects of treatment that might contribute to the development of adjustment problems. We then consider research on PTSD in cancer survivors, specifically, research with survivors of breast cancer, lymphoma, and hematological malignancies. We examine the controversy surrounding the inclusion of cancer as a criterion stressor for PTSD in the most recent revision (1994) of the American Psychiatric Association's *Diagnostic and Statistical Manual of Mental Disorders* (*DSM–IV*). Next, we review the possible roles of classical conditioning and cognitive–social processing to the development of long-term adjustment problems. In this chapter we present initial results from our ongoing research with survivors of bone marrow transplantation (BMT), a procedure used in the treatment of leukemia and other cancers.

Distress Associated With Cancer Treatment

The negative sequelae of diagnosis and treatment for cancer are well-known: Surgery can be disfiguring; radiation can cause fatigue, soreness, and long-term cosmetic changes; and chemotherapy often induces nausea, vomiting, hair loss, and weight change. Psychological effects are often no less debilitating. Research has shown that many of these aversive side effects continue after all treatment has ended. Indeed, our preliminary data from breast cancer survivors suggest that more than half experience such symptoms even 3 or more years after the completion of all treatment.

Each phase of breast cancer treatment (diagnosis, surgery, chemotherapy, and radiation) can cause considerable distress (Jacobsen & Holland, 1991). Biopsy is accompanied by the fear of a life-threatening cancer diagnosis, which evokes anxiety and depression (Cassileth et al., 1984; Craig, Comstock, & Geiser, 1974; Hughes, Royle, Buchannan, & Taylor, 1986; Jacobsen & Holland, 1991; Stanton & Snider, 1993; Taylor et al., 1985; Weisman & Worden, 1976). Further distress is experienced if results are positive. In a study comparing women with positive and negative biopsy results, cancer diagnosis was associated with depression, anger, and confusion (Stanton & Snider, 1993). Surgery also engenders psychological distress (Jamison, Wellisch, & Pasnau, 1978; Maguire et al., 1978; Watson, Greer, Blake, & Shrapnell, 1984). Although distress appears to be most pronounced in the immediate postoperative period, such reactions have been shown to linger for months, even years. In one longitudinal study of mastectomy patients, Morris, Greer, and White (1977) found that 46% of patients reported experiencing psychological distress 3 months after surgery, 28% reported such feelings for 12 months, and 25% experienced persistent surgery-related distress for more than 2 years. Research comparing reactions to mastectomy and lumpectomy have found similar levels of postoperative distress (Fallowfield, Baum, & Maguire, 1986; Steinberg, Juliano, & Wise, 1985; Wolberg, Romsaas, Tanner, & Malec, 1989). Kemeny, Wellisch, and Schain (1988) identified one exception in which distress levels in the immediate postoperative period were found to be higher in mastectomy patients than in lumpectomy patients.

Adjuvant chemotherapy and radiotherapy are also associated with psychological distress (Forester, Kornfeld, & Fleiss, 1978; Holland, Rowland, Lebovits, & Rusalem, 1979; Maguire et al., 1978). Holland and her colleagues found that patients experience a significant increase in depression and anger over the course of radiotherapy, in most cases attributed to treatment-induced anorexia, fatigue, and general lack of well-being. In addition to the distress associated with the postchemotherapy side effects (nausea, vomiting, anorexia, hair loss, fatigue, mouth sores, diarrhea, tingling, and numbness), between 25% and 75% of breast cancer patients (depending on the emetogenic potential of the chemotherapeutic agents) developed anticipatory anxiety and nausea, which, for some patients, are as stressful as the disease itself (Redd, 1990; Redd, Silverfarb, Andersen, Andrykowski, & Bovbjerg, 1991). Leventhal and his research team (Leventhal, Easterling, Coons, Luchterhand, & Love, 1986) found that patients' emotional distress was directly related to the number of treatment side effects they experienced.

Several studies of breast cancer survivors (e.g., Northouse, 1988, 1989) have examined distress levels after surgery. Levels of psychological distress were generally as high at 18 months postsurgery as they were earlier in the course of treatment. In another study (Vinokur, Threatt, Vinokur-Kaplan, & Satariano, 1990), patients showed no improvement in mental health or well-being at 4 and 10 months posttreatment. Aside from increased distress levels, specific behavioral symptoms such as conditioned anxiety and nausea have been documented. In our research (Redd, Dadds, Futterman, Taylor, & Bovbjerg, 1993), we found that more than half of breast cancer survivors reported that reminders of treatment still elicited anxiety and nausea 6–24 months after completion of treatment. For some, levels of distress during these "recollection" sessions equaled those experienced during the actual treatment.

In Cella, Pratt, and Holland's (1986) study of survivors of Hodgkin's disease, patients were observed to have "conditioned" responses more than 10 years posttreatment. In addition to conditioned side effects, many cancer patients also experience intrusive thoughts and bouts of anxiety affecting quality of life. Common long-term reactions include anxiety-evoking imagery relating to diagnosis and treatment (Cella, Pratt, & Holland, 1986; Kornblith, Anderson, Cella, Tross, Zuckerman, Cherin, Canellos, et al., 1992; Lesko, 1990); nightmares and flashbacks of treatment (Smith & Lesko, 1988; Woods & Earp, 1978); avoidance of thoughts and feelings associated with cancer (Cella & Tross, 1986; Kornblith, Anderson, Cella, Tross, Zuckerman, Cherin, Weiss, et al., 1992); constricted affect; and feelings of isolation, detachment, and estrangement from others (Baider & Sarell, 1984; Pot-Mees, 1989; Woods & Earp, 1978). These data are consistent with the notion that cancer survivors may experience symptoms of PTSD .

One of the most toxic of cancer treatments is BMT, used in the treatment of leukemia and other hematologic malignancies. Although many cancer survivors who receive BMT appear to adjust well posttreatment (Pelcovitz et al., 1996, Stuber, Nader, Yasuda, Pynoos, & Cohen, 1991), studies have found that a significant number continue to experience psychosocial problems, including depression, anxiety, and sexual and occupational difficulties (Lesko, 1993). BMT is associated with a variety of severe and repeated physical and psychological stressors that can precipitate psychiatric symptoms and long-term psychosocial sequelae (Lesko, 1989; Patenaude, 1990). Stress responses can include anxiety, depression, withdrawal, anger, hostility, survivor guilt, sleep difficulties, anorexia, agitation, suicidal thoughts, and treatment noncompliance (Jenkins, Livingston, & Whittaker, 1991; Lesko, 1993). Clinical research suggests that each phase of BMT can cause considerable psychological distress. Hickman catheter placement can cause anxiety, depression, fear, and negative body image (Lesko, 1993). In response to pre-BMT chemotherapy, patients experience anxiety; severe episodes of vomiting, nausea, and fatigue (Lesko, 1993); and pain from mouth sores that is often severe (Chapko, Syrjala, Schilter, Cummings, & Sullivan, 1989). Although patients undergoing total body irradiation are given nonsedating antiemetics (e.g., Kytril, Zofran), some patients' symptoms break through and are not alleviated with these medications. Jenkins and colleagues (1991) found that 28% of BMT recipients interviewed after treatment was completed reported major depressive episodes during this pre-BMT preparatory phase. Syrjala, Chapko, Vitaliano, Cummings, and Sullivan (1993) found that 27% of the BMT patients interviewed reported depression and 41% reported anxiety. During post-BMT inpatient convalescence, patients often report anxiety, mild depression, sleep disturbance (Ford, 1990), pain, irritability, impaired concentration, and stress reactions (Lesko, Ostroff, Mumma, Mashberg, & Holland, 1992).

In retrospective studies of BMT survivors, psychological symptoms varied considerably. Many survivors appear to return to premorbid psychosocial levels of functioning (Lesko, 1993); however, some survivors continue to experience emotional distress. Wolcott, Wellisch, and Fawzy (1986) conducted a study of survivors of allogeneic BMT 1.5–7.5 years post-BMT and found that 25% reported emotional distress, low self-esteem, decreased life satisfaction, and chronic physical sequelae. Fifteen to 20% had psychological distress requiring intervention. Jenkins and colleagues (1991) found that 3–67 months posttreatment, 40% of survivors suffered from depression with impaired functioning. In comparing acute and chronic leukemia survivors at least 1 year posttreatment with normative samples of physically healthy individuals, Ostroff, Mashberg, and Lesko (1989) observed that BMT survivors reported significantly higher levels of global psychological distress. Vickberg et al. (1996) found that BMT survivors had more PTSD symptoms and higher psychological distress as compared with breast cancer survivors treated with traditional therapies. In a prospective longitudinal study of psychological adjustment to BMT, Syrjala, Chapko, and Cummings (1988) found that 34%–41% of BMT patients suffered from anxiety and depression to a significantly higher degree at pre-BMT baseline (1 standard deviation) than did the general population. Symptoms did not diminish with time. Indeed, pre-BMT depression predicted poorer physical and psychological health following BMT (3 and 12 months post-BMT). More recently, Syrjala and her associates (Syrjala et al., 1993) found that one third of BMT patients experienced increased levels of distress at three assessment points: pre-BMT, 3 months post-BMT, and 12 months post-BMT.

Long-Term Adjustment and PTSD Symptoms

Although a number of investigators have likened posttreatment adjustment difficulties in BMT recipients to PTSD, there is considerable debate concerning the notion that adjustment problems in long-term survivors of cancer represent PTSD (Yehuda

& McFarlane, 1995). The possible relevance of PTSD for cancer is highlighted by recent changes in *DSM–IV* stressor criteria (American Psychiatric Association, 1994). In *DSM–IV*, life-threatening illness, such as cancer, is identified as a traumatic stressor capable of causing PTSD. However, there is little research on PTSD associated with cancer diagnosis and treatment. Only four cancer studies have been published that assessed PTSD in cancer survivors or their family members (Alter et al., 1996; Cordova et al., 1995; Pelcovitz et al., 1996; Stuber et al., 1991). All of the studies had a small sample size (6–55 participants). Considerable variation occurs in the (a) stressor event (e.g., cancer diagnosis, specific treatment procedures, or both); (b) duration of posttreatment follow-up (1–14 years); (c) patient age; (d) cancer site; and (e) treatment type. One of the earliest PTSD studies in oncology examined pediatric patients at post-BMT (Andrykowski, Grady, & Hunt, 1993) and found that survivors had intrusive thoughts concerning the transplant or avoidance of treatment reminders. Cordova and colleagues (1995) found that 5%–10% of the breast cancer survivors surveyed had PTSD, which was negatively associated with quality of life, income, and age. (Cordova et al., 1995). Furthermore, a visit after 1 year revealed a positive correlation between initial symptoms and symptoms at follow-up (Andrykowski, Cordova, McGrath, Sloan, & Kenady, 2000).

Two studies addressing PTSD in survivors and their families were conducted as part of the *DSM–IV* field trials. In the first study (Alter et al., 1996), women who had survived cancer ($n = 27$) for at least 3 years following diagnosis and active treatment were compared with a healthy group of women who were sociodemographically matched and drawn from the same community. Survivors displayed significantly higher levels of re-experiencing (e.g., flashbacks), avoidance, and hyperarousal symptoms than did those in the comparison group. Among the survivors, one patient met criteria for current PTSD (symptoms that persist for at least 1 month and have been present at some point during the previous 6 months), and six met criteria for lifetime PTSD (symptoms that have occurred at least 6 months prior to assessment). Neither current nor lifetime PTSD was diagnosed in members of the comparison group. No differences were found between those meeting criteria for lifetime PTSD and those not meeting criteria (age, cancer diagnosis, type of treatment received, severity of illness, and time since diagnosis or start of treatment).

In the second study, mothers of pediatric cancer survivors were compared with mothers of healthy children ($N = 25$; Pelcovitz et al., 1996). Significant differences were evident in the prevalent PTSD symptoms. Mothers of survivors were more likely to experience intrusive recollections, reliving of the experience and distressing reminders (reexperiencing), diminished interest in activities, feelings of detachment from others, a sense of a foreshortened future (avoidance), sleep disturbances, difficulty concentrating, and hypervigilance (hyperarousal). Overall, 25% of the mothers of cancer survivors met criteria for current PTSD, and 54% met criteria for lifetime PTSD. None in the comparison group were diagnosed with current PTSD, and only 4% met criteria for lifetime PTSD. Illness severity, perceived distress level, and level of social support did not predict onset of either current or lifetime PTSD. The only significant predictor identified was the number of high-magnitude events experienced by the patient in the past. Although they did not study PTSD specifically, Stuber, Christakis, Houskamp, and Kazak (1996) found that 12.5% of the survivors, 39.7% of the mothers, and 33.0% of the fathers reported symptoms consistent with a severe level of posttraumatic stress. Similarly, Kazak and colleagues (1997) studied 130 survivors of pediatric leukemia and their parents and found that 14% of the survivors, 40% of the mothers, and 31% of the fathers had PTSD in the moderate to severe range.

As this review indicates, estimates of PTSD incidence vary appreciably across studies from a low of 4% for current PTSD diagnosed in a cohort of breast cancer survivors (Alter et al., 1996) to a high of 50% for chronic PTSD in a sample of pediatric BMT survivors (Stuber et al., 1991). These figures fall within the range of PTSD prevalence rates reported in studies of at-risk populations but are higher than those reported for general population studies (American Psychiatric Association, 1994). The variability in estimated rates of PTSD may be attributed to differences in the characteristics of the individuals sampled, in their disease and treatment, as well as in the methods used to diagnose PTSD.

BMT may be especially likely to lead to PTSD, as BMT shares some of the qualities of other well-documented traumatic stressors. Our initial data from cancer survivors up to 11 years post-BMT indicated that approximately 13%–14% had symptoms indicating PTSD. For example, one man, 5 years post-BMT, reported flashbacks of various medical procedures. He also had recurrent nightmares of being in the hospital and physical symptoms such as sweating, triggered by treatment reminders. Sixty-nine percent of those individuals not meeting criteria for PTSD diagnosis reported having experienced one or more PTSD symptoms. We have also found that, as compared with BMT survivors who did not report PTSD symptoms, those who did were more likely to also experience existential distress (Vickberg et al., 1996) and to have had a high number of stressful life events experienced within the past year (DuHamel, Ostroff, et al., 2000). High levels of PTSD symptoms were associated with lower quality of life (Smith, Redd, DuHamel, Vickberg, & Ricketts, 1999). BMT survivors may in fact experience greater trauma-related symptoms posttreatment than patients who undergo other methods of cancer treatment. This hypothesis is based on preliminary comparisons of results from our BMT research with findings from our initial research (DuHamel, Vickberg, Smith, & Papadopoulos, 1998) on posttreatment adjustment among breast cancer survivors who had not received BMT. Extensive interviews (using standardized diagnostic questionnaires) of 54 breast cancer survivors who had not received BMT found that none met diagnostic criteria for PTSD. Although this hypothesis must be more fully explored through systematic comparisons, it does suggest that the BMT survivor may experience a unique constellation of adjustment problems after completing treatment.

There is some controversy regarding whether PTSD can be brought about by cancer and its treatment (Yehuda et al., 1995). Although PTSD, by definition, is precipitated by an intensely distressing event that is outside the range of usual human experience (American Psychiatric Association, 1987, 1994), this factor alone is not sufficient to explain the phenomenon of PTSD. Not all people exposed to the same stressful event develop the disorder. Among people exposed to a life-threatening traumatic event, most do not experience a distress response of sufficient magnitude to merit the diagnosis of PTSD, although many experience PTSD symptoms (Foa, Steketee, & Rothbaum, 1989). In prior research, risk factors identified as associated with an increased likelihood of developing PTSD or PTSD symptoms include such patient variables as age, gender, marital status, income, race, and level of education (Frueh, Smith, & Libet, 1996; Kessler, Sonnega, Bromet, Hughes, & Nelson, 1995; Shalev, Bonne, & Eth, 1996). For example, Stuber and colleagues (1996) found that age at cancer diagnosis was positively associated with PTSD symptoms in childhood leukemia survivors. Also identified as risk factors are degrees of social support (Andersen, 1992; Fontana, Schwartz, & Rosenheck, 1997; Perry, Difede, Musngi, Frances, & Jacobsberg, 1992), cognitive processing of the event (Creamer, Burgess, & Pattison, 1990, 1992), personal history of psychological problems (Davidson & Baum, 1986), and recent stressful life events (DuHamel, Smith, Vickberg, Papadopoulos, et al., in press; Yehuda & McFarlane, 1995). For example, in a recent study by Fontana and colleagues (1997), low family support was associated with PTSD in female Vietnam veterans. This study, along with others (Fontana & Rosenheck, 1994; Manne, DuHamel, Gallelli, & Redd, in press; Perry et al., 1992), highlight the role of social support as a moderator of PTSD. Previous research has also found that recent life events (experienced in the time since the trauma) are associated with increased levels of PTSD symptoms (Koopman, Classen, & Spiegel, 1994; Yehuda & McFarlane, 1995). Our cross-sectional study confirms the role of recent stressful life events in the development of PTSD. Although some of these variables (i.e., race, education) were not found to be associated with PTSD or PTSD symptoms (DuHamel, Redd, Smith, Papadopoulos, et al., 1996), our negative results may be related to the homogeneity of our sample (e.g., limited distribution across ethnic groups).

Role of Classical Conditioning, Cognitive–Social Processing, and Dispositional Factors in Posttreatment Distress

There are two empirically investigated theories regarding the etiology of PTSD: Keane's conditioning model (Keane, Fisher, Krinsley, & Niles, 1994; Keane, Zimering, & Caddell, 1985) and Foa's information-processing model (Foa & Kozak, 1986). Both are behavioral. Keane's model maintains that patients come to associate previously neutral stimuli (conditioned stimulus; CS) with the trauma (unconditioned stimulus; UCS), such that re-exposure to the CS elicits a fear or traumatic response (conditioned response; CR). Thus, smells, thoughts, sounds, and visual images (CS) associated with a trauma (e.g., rape, combat, life-threatening disease and treatment; UCS) can elicit anxiety and distress (CR) in individuals even after the trauma has ended (Keane et al., 1985). Clinical research is consistent with this classical-conditioning theory (Keane, Albano, & Blake, 1992); there is a linear relationship between conditioning characteristics of the traumatic event (i.e., frequency, intensity, and duration) and the occurrence of PTSD symptoms. PTSD symptoms are maintained through instrumental learning. That is, avoidance of the feared stimuli is negatively reinforced (through reduction in anxiety) in individuals with PTSD and, as a result, there is no opportunity for extinction to occur. Although PTSD appears to develop through conditioning processes, additional factors may moderate the emergence of the disorder. Risk factors include previous or familial psychopathology (Foy, Resnick, Sipprelle, & Carroll, 1987), high-magnitude trauma history (Pelcovitz et al., 1996), recent stressful life events (DuHamel, Smith, et al., in press; Yehuda et al., 1995), prior psychiatric disorder (e.g., anxiety and depression; Barlow, 1988; J. R. T. Davidson & Fairbank, 1993) weak social support (Barlow, 1988; Green, Grace, Lindy, Gleser, & Leonard, 1990), low income (Cordorva et al., 1995), and poor coping style (Green, Lindy, & Grace, 1985; Schwartz, Lerman, Miller, Daly, & Masny, 1995).

As BMT is associated with a variety of aversive contingencies (e.g., nausea, pain, isolation), we hypothesize that BMT survivors are at risk for PTSD or PTSD symptoms. Our reasoning is consistent with Keane and colleagues' (1985) conditioning model; previously neutral stimuli can become associated with aversive features of BMT (e.g., pain, nausea) such that the BMT survivor experiences a CR (fear, anxiety, etc.) when he or she is reexposed to CSs that were established during the course of BMT. As in the occurrence of PTSD among war veterans and victims of violent crimes, classical conditioning during the course of BMT can occur as a result of a single pairing. Indeed, individuals who had completed BMT treatment 5 years previously reported that they continued to experience anxiety and nausea whenever they returned to the hospital where they had been treated, even when the visit was unrelated to their follow-up care (DuHamel, Ostroff, et al., 2000; Smith et al., 1999). We have observed similar conditioned reactions in survivors of breast cancer (Redd, 1993).

Although conditioning models such as Keane et al.'s (1985) explain the acquisition of fear to previously neutral stimuli and the persistence of avoidance symptoms, they have been criticized on the grounds that they do not account for the occurrence of other types of PTSD symptoms (e.g., pervasive anxiety, increased startle response, emotional numbness) and that they do not incorporate any conceptualization of meaning (Vickberg et al., 1996; Foa et al., 1989). Foa and Kozak (1986) have argued that an information-processing model of fear, derived from previous research (Carver et al., 1993; Lang, 1977), provides a more adequate explanation of the development of PTSD. According to this model, fear is represented in a memory network that includes information regarding (a) the feared stimulus event; (b) possible verbal, physiological, and behavioral responses to the event or situation; and (c) the semantic interpretation of both the event and responses (Foa & Kozak, 1986). This fear network offers the individual a "road map" for escaping or avoiding the traumatic event (Foa & Kozak, 1986). Activation of this fear structure depends on two factors: the individual's subjective appraisal of the event and stressor magnitude. Subjective appraisal includes perception of life threat, perceived potential for physical violence, the experience of extreme fear, attribution of personal helplessness (March, 1990), feeling unprepared (J. R. T. Davidson & Smith, 1990), and perceptions of suffering and of low control (Green et al., 1985). Stressor magnitude includes such aspects as intensity, duration, degree of predictability, and extent of perceived controllability (Foa et al., 1989; Green et al., 1985; Sutker, Uddo-Crane, & Allain, 1991).

As noted by Foa and colleagues (1989), most people who experience a life-threatening traumatic event develop fear and other PTSD symptoms, but for the majority, these symptoms subside (e.g., they do not develop chronic PTSD). On the basis of their fear network theory, Foa and colleagues (Foa & Kozak, 1986; Foa et al., 1989) have proposed that people with chronic PTSD may differ from those whose symptoms are short-lived in the size of their fear structure and their response intensity. Consistent with Foa and colleagues' model, individuals who believed themselves to be safe at the time of the event (or perceive that the event is unpredictable and uncontrollable) should develop larger fear structures than those who do not believe themselves to be safe. Those who perceived the event as placing their lives in greater danger (e.g., have higher perceived threat) should respond more intensely than those who perceived their life to be in less danger, leading in both cases to higher risk for chronic PTSD.

Information-processing models, such as Foa and Kozak's (1986), differ most significantly from conditioning theories in their emphasis on the role of individual perception or "meaning assignment" in determining the traumatogenicity of a given event (Kreitler & Kreitler, 1988). Although some empirical support for both models exists (Blanchard, Kolb, & Gerardi, 1986; Keane et al., 1985; Malloy, Fairbank, & Keane, 1983), neither theory has undergone extensive empirical testing in the context of cancer.

Creamer and his associates (1990, 1992) have proposed a cognitive-processing model to explain the nature and course of psychological reactions in the wake of life trauma. Their model builds on the work of previous cognitive theories (Foa & Kozak, 1986; Foa et al., 1989; Horowitz, 1973, 1982, 1986) and maintains that individuals have mental schemas that contain information about past experience as well as notions regarding personal safety and vulnerability. The occurrence of a traumatic event challenges the person's worldview and creates a fear structure that is stored in active memory, causing emotional reactions and disturbing intrusive thoughts. The size of the fear structure is determined by a number of factors related to the trauma, including the threat to life, the potential for personal suffering, and the intensity of the fear. Pretrauma personality and prior experience also affect fear structure. For recovery to occur, the event must be integrated into the individual's schema, or the schema must be modified. The individual experiences conflict between the desire to avoid the intrusive thoughts and associated distress and the need to make sense of the event. According to Creamer's model, intrusive thoughts are an indication that the fear structure has been activated. Creamer and colleagues proposed that the presence of the intrusive thoughts indicate that cognitive processing is occurring. Successful cognitive processing involves achieving an understanding of the event, either through assimilation or accommodation. Thus, activation and modification of the fear memory network results in immediately high levels of intrusive thoughts and psychological distress but reduced future intrusive thoughts and psychological distress.

Research supports the cognitive-processing model. Appraisal of threat has been associated with higher levels of intrusive thoughts, which in turn were associated with higher levels of avoidance and immediate psychological distress (Creamer et al., 1992; Miller, Rodoletz, Schroeder, Mangan, & Sedlacek, 1996; Schwartz, et al., 1995). A number of studies suggest that cognitive processing is generally associated with subsequent reduced levels of distress (Brewin, Dalgleish, & Joseph, 1996; Creamer et al., 1990, 1992; McIntosh, Silver, & Wortman, 1993).

Two issues that have been highlighted in recent reviews (e.g., Brewin et al., 1996) of cognitive-processing models suggest the necessity of including other types of cognitive processing (in addition to intrusion and avoidance). Although descriptions of cognitive processing have typically emphasized involuntary processes (e.g., intrusive thoughts are involuntary), Brewin and colleagues have suggested that voluntary efforts at processing may also play an important role in the recovery from negative life events (Brewin et al., 1996). Second, descriptions of cognitive processing have assessed "negative" efforts (avoidance) while giving relatively little attention to more positive efforts to cognitively process, such as attempts to reappraise the event in more positive or meaningful ways, accept the situation, or try to process the event in the context of social interaction (Brewin et al., 1996; Baum, Cohen, & Hall, 1993; Greenberg, 1995). As pointed out by Baum and colleagues (1993) and Greenberg (1995), individual differences in processing may be explained more fully if models take these variables into account.

In addition to taking steps to desensitize oneself (either through natural reexposure to the threatening cues or formal systematic desensitization with a behavior therapist; Foa & Kozak, 1986), individuals process events through talking with others. Most individuals confronting a crisis report feeling an overwhelming need to discuss the event and their responses with others (Coates, Wortman, & Abbey, 1979), and most individuals do so (Rimer, Philipport, Boca, & Mesquita, 1992). This desire to talk appears to be prompted by intrusive thoughts or activation of the fear structure (Lepore, Silver, Wortman, & Wayment, 1996; Manne et al., in press). The need to talk about the event typically dissipates over time (Lepore et al., 1996; Manne et al., in press). As outlined by Tait and Silver (1989), talking with others who provide support and empathy may facilitate recovery in a number of ways. First, discussion may allow discharge of emotions (Freud, 1957). Second, it may provide an opportunity for desensitization and learning to tolerate aversive thoughts for longer periods (Horowitz, 1986; Rachman, 1980). Third, talking to others may facilitate provision of emotional support. Fourth, it may serve to prompt cognitive processing and thereby facilitate adjustment (Clark, 1993). Some theorists have proposed that support can function as *coping assistance*, a resource upon which individuals draw in order to deal more effectively with stressors (Thoits, 1986). Significant others may assist individuals in effectively integrating and processing events. Family and friends can also encourage the search for meaning in the event, so that it can be assimilated into the individual's worldview. As such, individuals are aided in changing their points of view so that the event no longer challenges life assumptions (accommodation). They are also assisted in appraising the problem as less threatening. Responses of others can facilitate the process of finding meaning in the negative life event. Emotional support, the reassurance of value and affection, can provide the safe environment in which an individual who is distressed about a traumatic life event can work on his or her cognitive processing of the event. In either case, the intrusive thoughts associated with the negative life event become less distressing and less frequent as the individual develops new ways of thinking about the experience (i.e., he or she has processed the events). Thus, both emotional support and assistance in reframing the events (guidance) can promote cognitive processing.

Significant others may not always respond in ways that facilitate recovery, however. They may be uncomfortable discussing the event and the individual's reactions (Herbert & Dunkel-Schetter, 1992). Comments to mothers of pediatric cancer patients such as "But your child is doing all right now" or "I'm sure he'll be okay" are not uncommon (Lehman, Ellard, & Wortman, 1986). Such "unhelpful" responses may become stronger, and more damaging, when the individual continues to communicate distress after a return to "normal" functioning is considered by others to be appropriate (Coyne, 1976). Individuals who continue to discuss the event and their emotional reactions may encounter difficulties within their social network. Peers may become uncomfortable, change the topic, withdraw, or may even criticize the individual for not "moving on" or coping better. We have documented these reactions to mothers of pediatric cancer survivors (Manne et al., in press) and adult patients (Manne, Taylor, Dougherty, & Kemeny, 1997).

The absence of social processing can serve to maintain or actually increase psychological distress. Most relevant to cognitive-processing theory is the inhibition of thoughts and feelings by others. Such inhibition of thoughts and feelings can impair recovery (Pennebaker, 1989) and lead to increased emotional distress (Lepore et al., 1996). A second effect of the absence of social processing is increased use of avoidance. Results from work with adult cancer patients has indicated that spousal avoidance of or withdrawal from the patient is associated with avoidant coping

(Manne, Pape, Taylor, & Dougherty, 1999). We found that avoidance mediates the association between the spouse's negative responses and psychological distress. However, not everyone needs to talk about the traumatic event with others in order to deal with it successfully. Studies have shown that between 5% (Lepore et al., 1996) and 10% (Rimer et al., 1992) of individuals do not feel the need to talk about events with their peers.

Dispositional Factors and Prior Life History

There is considerable empirical support for the notion that what the individual brings to a negative life event—personality, coping style, psychiatric history, and prior stressful events—affects cognitive processing of the event as well as immediate and long-term adjustment. Each of these factors serves to predispose the individual to react in a characteristic manner. These personality traits influence how individuals appraise, cope with, and respond to life events. Most research in this area has focused on optimism and pessimism (Scheier & Carver, 1992). First, a number of studies have found that pessimists are more likely than optimists to have negative expectations about the outcomes of life events and appraise situations as more threatening (Carver et al., 1993). Second, pessimists cope with negative life events in a characteristic manner (Scheier & Carver, 1992), disengaging from goal-directed efforts and using avoidant ways of coping; optimists are more likely to use acceptance and reframing (Carver et al., 1993). Third, both optimism and pessimism have strong influences on psychological distress. In a longitudinal study of women undergoing surgical treatment of breast cancer, Carver and colleagues (1993) found that optimism (as determined from responses to the Life Orientation Test; Scheier & Carver, 1985) was inversely related to distress. Follow-up assessments also revealed that the distress associated with pessimism persisted beyond the acute treatment phase. Coping strategies have also been shown to mediate the association between optimism and psychological outcomes. In Carver et al.'s (1993) breast cancer research, acceptance coping partially mediated the effect of optimism on long-term psychological distress.

Regarding the role of coping style in the cognitive processing of stressful life events, the research of Miller and colleagues (Miller, Rodoletz, Schroeder, Mangan, & Sedlacek, 1996; Miller, Shoda, & Hurley, 1996) on high-monitoring coping style (characterized by cognitive vigilance to and amplification of threat-related cues) has particular relevance. Working with cancer patients as well as healthy volunteers, Miller and colleagues found that high monitors tend to overestimate the potential severity and unpredictability of aversive events (Lerman, Daly, Masny, & Balshem, 1994; Lepore et al., 1996). Coping through monitoring is also associated with intrusive ideation (Borkovec & Lyonfields, 1993; Meichenbaum, 1992; Muris & van Zuuren, 1992; Muris, van Zuuren, & de Vries, 1994). According to Miller's Monitoring Process Model (MPM; Miller, Shoda, & Hurley, 1996), high monitoring is associated with increased intrusive ideation about the stressor and encoding neutral information as threatening. As a result, high monitors experience greater levels of anxiety following negative life events.

A third construct that has relevance to cognitive processing of negative life events is psychiatric history. There is a large body of research on the role of prior psychopathology in adjustment to negative life events. Foy and colleagues (1987) found that prior psychopathology is associated with increased intrusive and avoidant ideation and with psychological distress. Foy's results are consistent with those of McFarlane (1988) on the role of prior psychopathology in PTSD. Not only are individuals with prior psychopathology more likely to experience persistent distress, they are also more likely to perceive medical events as more threatening than are other individuals (McFarlane, 1988).

Finally, prior stressful life events are predictive of responses to current severe negative life events. Individuals with a greater number of prior stressful life events appraise situations as more threatening. Our preliminary work found that breast cancer survivors who had undergone recent stressful life events perceived their cancer as more life-threatening (Vickberg et al., 1997). A number of researchers (Koopman et al., 1994; Solomon & Flum, 1988; Yehuda et al., 1995) have found that stressful life events before and after a focal negative event are associated with increased intrusive and avoidant ideation regarding the trauma as well as increased psychological distress. These studies suggest that cognitive and social processing, as well as dispositional characteristics and personal history, may play a crucial role in the development and persistence of psychological distress among mothers of children undergoing BMT.

Conclusion

It is clear that a significant number of cancer survivors and their family members experience moderate to severe trauma-related adjustment problems. In many cases, such symptoms continue long after all treatment and follow-ups are complete. These problems appear to relate to classical conditioning, cognitive, and social factors. Although conceptualizing such distress actions in terms of PTSD has clinical and theoretical utility, the question of whether or not such symptoms reliably fulfill criteria of PTSD as set forth in the *DSM–IV* is not the critical question. Rather than debating diagnostic systems, it is more important that we explore mechanisms underlying trauma-related symptoms in cancer survivors. This line of research holds the promise of guiding the development of new interventions and better theories of posttreatment adjustment.

Significant numbers of cancer survivors have intrusive thoughts and other anxiety-related symptoms of distress. A factor in survivors' psychological recovery is resolving overriding anxiety about their treatment and view of their "overall safety" in the world. A critical component of such desensitization is talking with others about their fears and concerns. This "naturally occurring" process of desensitization points out the integration of what appear to be disparate processes: behavioral reexposure and traditional nondirective supportive psychotherapy. This integration may be important to adjustment in many areas and merits careful study.

References

Alter, C. L., Pelcovitz, D., Axelrod, A., Goldenberg, B., Harris, H., Meyers, B., Grobois, B., Mandel, F., Septimus, A., & Kaplan, S. (1996). Identification of PTSD in cancer survivors. *Psychosomatics, 37,* 137–143.

American Psychiatric Association. (1987). *Diagnostic and statistical manual of mental disorders* (3rd ed., rev.). Washington, DC: Author.

American Psychiatric Association. (1994). *Diagnostic and statistical manual of mental disorders* (4th ed.). Washington, DC: Author.

Andersen, B. L. (1992). Psychological interventions for cancer patients to enhance the quality of life. *Journal of Consulting and Clinical Psychology, 60,* 552–568.

Andrykowski, M. A., Cordova, M. J., McGrath, P. C., Sloan, D. A., & Kenady, D. E. (2000). Stability and change in PTSD-like symptoms following breast cancer treatment: A one year follow-up. *Psycho–Oncology, 9*(1), 69–78.

Andrykowski, M. A., Grady, M. J., & Hunt, J. W. (1993). Positive psychosocial adjustment in potential BMT recipients: Cancer as a psychosocial transition. *Psycho–Oncology, 2,* 261–276.

Baider, L., & Sarell, M. (1984). Coping with cancer among Holocaust survivors in Israel. An exploratory study. *Journal of Human Stress, 10,* 121–127.

Barlow, D. (1988). *Anxiety and its disorders.* New York: Guilford Press.

Baum, A., Cohen, L., & Hall, M. (1993). Control and intrusive memories as possible determinants of chronic stress. *Psychosomatic Medicine, 55,* 274–286.

Blanchard, E., Kolb, L., & Gerardi, R. J. (1986). Cardiac response to relevant stimuli as an adjunctive tool for diagnosing post-traumatic stress disorder in Vietnam veterans. *Behavior Therapy, 17,* 596–606.

Borkovec, T. D., & Lyonfields, J. D. (1993). Worry: Thought suppression of emotional processing, In H. W. Krohne (Ed.), *Attention and avoidance: Strategies in coping with aversiveness* (pp. 255–273). Gottingen, Germany: Hogrefe & Huber.

Brewin, C. R., Dalgleish, T., & Joseph, S. (1996). A dual representation theory of posttraumatic stress disorder. *Psychological Review, 103,* 670–686.

Carver, C. S., Pozo, C., Harris, S. D., Noriega, V., Scheier, M. F., Robinson, D. S., Ketcham, A. S., Moffat, F. L. J., & Clark, K. C. (1993). How coping mediates the effect of optimism on distress: A study of women with early stage breast cancer. *Journal of Personality and Social Psychology, 65,* 375–390.

Cassileth, B. R., Lusk, E. J., Strouse, T. B., Miller, D. S., Brown, L. L., Cross, P. A., & Tenaglia, A. N. (1984). Psychosocial status in chronic illness: A comparative analysis of six diagnostic groups. *New England Journal of Medicine, 311,* 506–511.

Cella, D. F., Pratt, A., & Holland, J. C. (1986). Persistent anticipatory nausea, vomiting, and anxiety in cured Hodgkin's disease patients after completion of chemotherapy. *American Journal of Psychiatry, 143,* 641–643.

Cella, D. F., & Tross, S. (1986). Psychological adjustment to survival from Hodgkin's disease. *Journal of Consulting and Clinical Psychology, 54,* 616–622.

Chapko, M. K., Syrjala, K. L., Schilter, L., Cummings, C., & Sullivan, K. M. (1989). Chemoradiotherapy toxicity during bone marrow transplantation: Time course and variation in pain and nausea. *Bone Marrow Transplantation, 4,* 181–186.

Clark, L. F. (1993). Stress and the cognitive-conversational benefits of social interaction. *Journal of Social and Clinical Psychology, 12,* 25–55.

Coates, D., Wortman, C. B., & Abbey, A. (1979). Reactions to victims. In I. H. Frieze, D. Bartal, & J. S. Carroll (Eds.), *New approaches to social problems* (pp. 21–52). San Francisco: Jossey-Bass.

Cordova, M. J., Andrykowski, M. A., Redd, W. H., Kenady, D. E., McGrath, P. C., & Sloan, D. A. (1995). Frequency and correlates of posttraumatic-stress-disorder-like symptoms after treatment for breast cancer. *Journal of Consulting and Clinical Psychology, 63,* 981–986.

Coyne, J. (1976). Toward an interactional description of depression. *Psychiatry, 39,* 38–40.

Craig, T. J., Comstock, G. W., & Geiser, P. B. (1974). The quality of survival in breast cancer: A case control comparison. *Cancer, 33,* 1451–1457.

Creamer, M., Burgess, P., & Pattison, P. (1990). Cognitive processing in post-trauma reactions: Some preliminary findings. *Psychological Medicine, 20,* 597–604.

Creamer, M., Burgess, P., & Pattison, P. (1992). Reaction to trauma: A cognitive processing model. *Journal of Abnormal Psychology, 101,* 452–459.

Davidson, J. R. T., & Fairbank, I. A. (1993). The epidemiology of posttraumatic stress disorder. In J. R. T. Davidson & E. B. Foa (Eds.), *Posttraumatic stress disorder: DSM–IV and beyond* (pp. 147). Washington, DC: American Psychiatric Press.

Davidson, J. R. T., & Smith, R. D. (1990). Traumatic experiences in psychiatric outpatients. *Journal of Traumatic Stress, 3,* 459–474.

Davidson, L. M., & Baum, A. (1986). Chronic stress posttraumatic stress disorders. *Journal of Consulting and Clinical Psychology, 54,* 303–308.

DuHamel, K. N., Ostroff, J. S., Bovbjerg, D. H., Pfeffer, M., Morasco, B. J., Papadopoulos, E., & Redd, W. H. (2000). Trauma-focused intervention after bone marrow transplantation: A case study. *Behavioral Therapy, 31,* 175–186.

DuHamel, K., Redd, W. H., Smith, M., Papadopoulos, E., Rosen, L., & Vickberg, S. (1996). *PTSD in bone marrow transplant survivors.* Paper presented at the Annual Meeting of the Society for Behavioral Medicine, Washington, DC.

DuHamel, K. N., Smith, M. Y., Vickberg, S. M. J., Papadopoulos, E., Ostroff, J., Winkel, G., Manne, S., & Redd, W. H. (in press). Trauma symptoms in bone marrow transplant survivors: The role of non-medical life events. *Journal of Traumatic Stress.*

DuHamel, K. N., Vickberg, S. M. J., Smith, M., & Papadopoulos, E. (1998). *PTSD as a model for understanding adjustment problems in bone marrow transplant survivors.* Paper presented at the annual meeting of the Society for Behavioral Medicine, New Orleans, LA.

Fallowfield, L. I., Baum, M., & Maguire, G. P. (1986). Effects of breast conservation on psychological morbidity associated with diagnosis and treatment of early breast cancer. *British Medicine Journal, 293,* 1331–1334.

Foa, E. B., & Kozak, M. J. (1986). Emotional processing of fear: Exposure to corrective information. *Psychological Bulletin, 99,* 20–35.

Foa, E. B., Steketee, G., & Rothbaum, B. O. (1989). Behavioral/cognitive conceptualizations of post-traumatic stress disorder. *Behavior Therapy, 20,* 155–176.

Fontana, A., & Rosenheck, R. (1994). Posttraumatic stress disorder among Vietnam theater veterans: A causal model of etiology in a community sample. *Journal of Nervous and Mental Disease, 182,* 677–684.

Fontana, A., Schwartz, L. S., & Rosenheck, R. (1997). Posttraumatic stress disorder among female Vietnam veterans: A causal model of etiology. *American Journal of Public Health, 87,* 169–175.

Ford, R. E. (1990). Psychosocial and ethical issues in bone marrow transplantation. In C. A. Kasprisin & E. L. Snyder (Eds.), *Bone marrow transplantation: A nursing perspective* (pp. 129–115). Arlington, VA: American Association of Blood Banks.

Forester, B., Kornfeld, D., & Fleiss, J. (1978). Psychiatric aspects of radiotherapy. *American Journal of Psychiatry, 135,* 960–963.

Foy, D. W., Resnick, H. S., Sipprelle, R. C., & Carroll, E. M. (1987). Premilitary, military and postmilitary factors in the development of combat related posttraumatic stress disorder. *Behavior Therapist, 10,* 3–9.

Freud, S. (1957). Repression. In J. Strachney (Ed.), *The standard edition and the complete psychological works of Sigmund Freud* (pp. 146–158). London: Hogarth Press.

Frueh, B. C., Smith, D. W., & Libet, J. M. (1996). Racial differences on psychological measures in combat veterans seeking treatment for PTSD. *Journal of Personality Assessment, 66,* 41–53.

Green, B. L., Grace, M. C., Lindy, J. D., Gleser, G. C., & Leonard, A. (1990). Risk factors for PTSD and other diagnoses in a general sample of Vietnam veterans. *American Journal of Psychiatry, 147,* 729–733.

Green, B. L., Lindy, J. D., & Grace, M. C. (1985). Posttraumatic stress disorder—Toward DSM–IV. *Journal of Nervous and Mental Disease, 173,* 406–411.

Greenberg, M. A. (1995). Cognitive processing of traumas: The role of intrusive thoughts and reappraisals. *Journal of Applied Social Psychology, 25,* 1262–1296.

Herbert, T. B., & Dunkel-Schetter, C. (1992). Negative social reactions to victims: An overview of responses and their determinants. In L. Montada, S. H. Filipp, & M. J. Lerner (Eds.), *Life crises and experiences of loss in adulthood* (pp. 497–518). Hillsdale, NJ: Erlbaum.

Holland, J. C., Rowland, J., Lebovits, A., & Rusalem, R. (1979). Reactions to cancer treatment: Assessment of emotional response to adjuvant radiotherapy as a guide to planned intervention. *Psychiatric Clinics of North America, 2,* 347–358.

Horowitz, M. J. (1973). Phase orientated treatment of stress response syndromes. *American Journal of Psychotherapy, 27,* 506–515.

Horowitz, M. J. (1982). Stress response syndromes and their treatment. In H. Goldbert (Ed.), *Handbook of stress* (p. 711). New York: Free Press.

Horowitz, M. J. (1986). *Stress response syndromes* (2nd ed). Northvale, NJ: Jason Aronson Press.

Hughes, J. E., Royle, G. T., Buchannan, R., & Taylor, I. (1986). Depression and social stress among patients awaiting breast biopsy. *Journal of Psychosomatic Research, 32,* 173–180.

Jacobsen, P. B., & Holland, J. C. (1991). The stress of cancer: Psychological responses to diagnosis and treatment. In C. Cooper & M. Watson (Eds.), *Coping and stress: Psychological, biological, and coping studies* (pp. 147–169). New York: Wiley.

Jamison, K. R., Wellisch, D. K., & Pasnau, R. O. (1978). Psychosocial aspects of mastectomy. I. The woman's perspective. *American Journal of Psychiatry, 135,* 432–436.

Jenkins, P. L., Livingston, A., & Whittaker, I. A. (1991). A retrospective study of psychosocial morbidity in bone marrow transplant recipients. *Psychosomatics, 32,* 65–71.

Kazak, A. E., Meeske, K., Penati, B., Barakat, L. P., Christakis, D., Meadows, A. T., Casey, R., Penati, B., & Stuber, M. L. (1997). Posttraumatic stress, family functioning, and social support in survivors of childhood leukemia and their mothers and fathers. *Journal of Consulting and Clinical Psychology, 65,* 120–129.

Keane, T. M., Albano, A. M., & Blake, D. D. (1992). Current trends in the treatment of post-traumatic stress symptoms. In M. Basoglu (Ed.), *Torture and its current treatment approaches* (pp. 363–401). London: Cambridge University Press.

Keane, T. M., Fisher, L. M., Krinsley, K. E., & Niles, B. L. (1994). Post-traumatic stress disorder. In R. T. Amerman & M. Hersen (Eds.), *Handbook of prescriptive treatments for adults* (pp. 237–260). New York: Plenum Press.

Keane, T. M., Zimering, R. T., & Caddell, J. M. (1985). A behavioral formulation of posttraumatic stress disorder in Vietnam veterans. *Behavior Therapist, 8,* 9–12.

Kemeny, M., Wellisch, D. K., & Schain, W. S. (1988). Psychosocial outcome in a randomized surgical trial for treatment of primary breast cancer. *Cancer, 62,* 1231–1237.

Kessler, R. C., Sonnega, A., Bromet, E., Hughes, M., & Nelson, C. B. (1995). Posttraumatic stress disorder in the National Comorbidity Survey. *Archives of General Psychiatry, 52,* 1048–1060.

Koopman, C., Classen, C., & Spiegel, D. (1994). Predictors of posttraumatic stress symptoms among survivors of the Oakland/Berkeley, Calif., firestorm. *American Journal of Psychiatry, 151,* 888–894.

Kornblith, A. B., Anderson, I., Cella, D. F., Tross, S., Zuckerman, E., Cherin, E., Canellos, G. P., Kosty, M. P., & Cooper, M. R. (1992). Comparison of psychosocial adaptation and sexual function of survivors of advanced Hodgkin disease treated by MOPP, ABVD, or MOPP alternating with ABVD. *Cancer, 70,* 2508–2516.

Kornblith, A. B., Anderson, I., Cella, D. F., Tross, S., Zuckerman, E., Cherin, E., Weiss, R. B., Cooper, M. R., Silver, R. T., & The Cancer and Leukemia Group. (1992). Hodgkin disease survivors at increased risk for problems in psychosocial adaptation. *Cancer, 70,* 2214–2224.

Kreitler, S., & Kreitler, J. (1988). Trauma and anxiety: The cognitive approach. *Journal of Traumatic Stress, 1*, 35–56.

Lang, P. J. (1977). Imagery in therapy: An information processing analysis of fear. *Behavior Therapy, 8*, 495–510.

Lehman, D. R., Ellard, I. H., & Wortman, C. B. (1986). Social support for the bereaved: Recipients' and providers' perspectives on what is helpful. *Journal of Consulting and Clinical Psychology, 54*, 438–446.

Lepore, S. J., Silver, R. C., Wortman, C. B., & Wayment, H. A. (1996). Social constraints, intrusive thoughts, and depressive symptoms among bereaved mothers. *Journal of Personality and Social Psychology, 70*, 271–282.

Lerman, C., Daly, M., Masny, A., & Balshem, A. M. (1994). Attitudes about genetic testing for breast–ovarian cancer susceptibility. *Journal of Clinical Oncology, 12*, 843–850.

Lesko, L. M. (1989). Bone marrow transplantation. In J. C. Holland & J. H. Rowland (Eds.), *Handbook of psycho-oncology: Psychological care of the patient with cancer* (pp. 163–173). New York: Oxford University Press.

Lesko, L. M. (1990). Surviving hematological malignancies. Stress responses and predicting psychological adjustment. *Progress in Clinical and Biological Research, 352*, 423–437.

Lesko, L. M. (1993). Psychiatric aspects of bone marrow transplantation: Part II: Life beyond transplant. *Psycho–Oncology, 2*, 185–193.

Lesko, L. M., Ostroff, J. S., Mumma, G. H., Mashberg, D. E., & Holland, J. C. (1992). Long-term psychological adjustment of acute leukemia survivors: Impact of bone marrow transplantation versus conventional chemotherapy. *Psychosomatic Medicine, 54*, 30–47.

Leventhal, H., Easterling, F., Coons, H. L., Luchterhand, C. M., & Love, R. R. (1986). Adaptation to chemotherapy treatments. In B. L. Andersen (Ed.), *Women with cancer. Psychological perspectives* (pp. 172–103). New York: Springer-Verlag.

Maguire, G. P., Lee, E. G., Bevington, D. J., Kuchemann, C. S., Crabtree, R. J., & Cornell, C. E. (1978). Psychiatric problems in the first year after mastectomy. *British Medical Journal, 1*, 963–965.

Malloy, P., Fairbank, J., & Keane, T. (1983). Validation of a multi-method assessment of post-traumatic stress disorders in Vietnam veterans. *Journal of Consulting and Clinical Psychology, 51*, 488–494.

Manne, S., DuHamel, K., Gallelli, K., & Redd, W. H. (in press). Association of psychological vulnerability factors to post-traumatic stress symptomatology in parents of pediatric cancer survivors. *Psycho-Oncology.*

Manne, S., Pape, S., Taylor, K., & Dougherty, J. (1999). Spouse support, coping, and mood among individuals with cancer. *Annals of Behavioral Medicine, 21*, 111–121.

Manne, S., Taylor, K., Dougherty, J., & Kemeny, N. (1997). Social support and negative responses in the marital relationship: Their association with psychological adjustment among individuals with cancer. *Journal of Behavioral Medicine, 20*, 101–125.

March, J. S. (1990). The nosology of posttraumatic stress disorder. *Journal of Anxiety Disorders, 4*, 61–82.

McFarlane, A. C. (1988). The aetiology of post-traumatic stress disorders following a natural disaster. *British Journal of Psychiatry, 152,* 116–121.

McIntosh, D. N., Silver, R. C., & Wortman, C. B. (1993). Religion's role in adjustment to a negative life event: Coping with the loss of a child. *Journal of Personality and Social Psychology, 65,* 812–821.

Meichenbaum, D. (1992). Stress inoculation training: A twenty year update. In R. L. Woolfolk & P. H. Lehrer (Eds.), *Principles and practice of stress management* (pp. 373–406). New York: Guilford Press.

Miller, S. M., Rodoletz, M., Schroeder, C. M., Mangan, C. E., & Sedlacek, T. V. (1996). Applications of the monitoring process model to coping with severe long-term medical threats. *Health Psychology, 15,* 216–225.

Miller, S. M., Shoda, Y., & Hurley, K. (1996). Applying cognitive–social theory to health-protective behavior: Breast self-examination in cancer screening. *Psychological Bulletin, 119,* 70–94.

Morris, T., Greer, H. S., & White, P. (1977). Psychological and social adjustment to mastectomy: A two year follow-up. *Cancer, 40,* 2381–2387.

Muris, P., & van Zuuren, F. (1992). Monitoring, medical fears, and physical symptoms. *British Journal of Clinical Psychology, 31,* 360–362.

Muris, P., van Zuuren, F. J., & de Vries, S. (1994). Monitoring, blunting, and situational anxiety: A laboratory study on coping with a quasi-medical stressor. *Personality and Individual Differences, 16,* 365–372.

Northouse, L. L. (1988). Social support in patients' and husbands' adjustment to breast cancer. *Nursing Research, 37,* 91–95.

Northouse, L. L. (1989). A longitudinal study of the adjustment of patients and husbands to breast cancer. *Oncology Nursing Forum, 16,* 511–516.

Ostroff, J., Mashberg, D., & Lesko, L. (1989). *Stress responses among bone marrow transplantation survivors* [Abstract]. American Psychosomatic Medicine Annual Meeting, San Francisco, CA.

Patenaude, A. F. (1990). Psychological impact of bone marrow transplantation: Current perspectives. *Yale Journal of Biology and Medicine, 63,* 515–519.

Pelcovitz, D., Goldenberg, B., Kaplan, S., Weinblatt, M., Mandel, F., Meyers, B., & Vinciguerra, V. (1996). Post-traumatic stress disorder in mothers of pediatric cancer survivors. *Psychosomatics, 37,* 116–126.

Pennebaker, J. W. (1989). Confession, inhibition, and disease. In L. Berkowitz (Ed.), *Advances in experimental social psychology* (pp. 211–244). Orlando, FL: Academic Press.

Perry, S. P., Difede, J., Musngi, G., Frances, A. J., & Jacobsberg, L. (1992). Predictors of posttraumatic stress disorder after burn injury. *American Journal of Psychiatry, 147,* 69–75.

Pot-Mees, C. (1989). *The psychosocial effects of bone marrow transplantation in children.* Delft, Netherlands: Eburon.

Rachman, S. (1980). Emotional processing. *Behaviour Research and Therapy, 18,* 51–60.

Redd, W. H. (1990). Management of anticipatory nausea and vomiting with cancer chemotherapy. In K. M. Foley, J. J. Bonica, & V. Ventafridda (Eds.), *Advances in pain research and therapy: Second International Congress on Cancer Pain* (pp. 345–357). New York: Raven Press.

Redd, W. H., Dadds, M. R., Futterman, A. D., Taylor, K. L., & Bovbjerg, D. H. (1993). Nausea induced by mental images of chemotherapy. *Cancer, 72,* 629–636.

Redd, W. H., Silverfarb, P. M., Andersen, B. L., Andrykowski, M. A., & Bovbjerg, D. H. (1991). Physiologic and psychobehavioral research in oncology. *Cancer, 67,* 813–822.

Rimer, B., Philipport, T., Boca, S., & Mesquita, B. (1992). Long-lasting cognitive and social consequences of emotion: Social sharing and rumination. *European Review of Social Psychology, 3,* 225–258.

Scheier, M. F., & Carver, C. S. (1985). Optimism, coping and health: Assessment and implications of generalized outcome expectancies. *Health Psychology, 4,* 219–247.

Scheier, M. F., & Carver, C. S. (1992). Effects of optimism on psychological and physical well-being: Theoretical overview and empirical update. *Cognitive Therapy and Research, 16,* 201–228.

Schwartz, M. D., Lerman, C., Miller, S. M., Daly, M., & Masny, A. (1995). Coping disposition, perceived risk, and psychological distress among women at increased risk for ovarian cancer. *Health Psychology, 14,* 232–235.

Shalev, A. Y., Bonne, O., & Eth, S. (1996). Treatment of posttraumatic stress disorder: A review. *Psychosomatic Medicine, 58,* 165–182.

Smith, K., & Lesko, L. M. (1988). Psychosocial problems in cancer survivors. *Oncology, 2,* 33–44.

Smith, M. Y., Redd, W. H., DuHamel, K. N., Vickberg, S. M. J., & Ricketts, P. (1999). Validation of the Posttraumatic Stress Disorder Checklist–Civilian in survivors of bone marrow transplantation. *Journal of Traumatic Stress, 12,* 485–499.

Solomon, Z., & Flum, H. (1988). Life events, combat stress reaction and post-traumatic stress disorder. *Social Science & Medicine, 3,* 319–325.

Stanton, A., & Snider, P. (1993). Coping with a breast cancer diagnosis: A prospective study. *Health Psychology, 12,* 16–23.

Steinberg, M. D., Juliano, M. A., & Wise, L. (1985). Psychological outcome of lumpectomy versus mastectomy in the treatment of breast cancer. *American Journal of Psychiatry, 142,* 34–39.

Stuber, M. L., Christakis, D. A., Houskamp, B., & Kazak, A. E. (1996). Posttrauma symptoms in childhood leukemia survivors and their parents. *Psychosomatics, 37,* 254–261.

Stuber, M. L., Nader, K., Yasuda, P., Pynoos, R. S., & Cohen, S. (1991). Stress responses after pediatric bone marrow transplantation: Preliminary results of a prospective longitudinal study. *Journal of the American Academy of Child and Adolescent Psychiatry, 30,* 952–957.

Sutker, P. B., Uddo-Crane, M., & Allain, A. N. (1991). Clinical and research assessment of posttraumatic stress disorder: A conceptual overview. *Psychological Assessment, 3,* 520–530.

Syrjala, K. L., Chapko, M. K., & Cummings, C. (1988). Physical and psychological functioning in the first year after bone marrow transplantation: A prospective study [Abstract]. *The Society of Behavioral Medicine Scientific Sessions.*

Syrjala, K. L., Chapko, M. K., Vitaliano, P. P., Cummings, C., & Sullivan, K. M. (1993). Recovery after allogeneic marrow transplantation: Prospective study of predictors of long-term physical and psychosocial functioning. *Bone Marrow Transplantation, 11,* 319–327.

Tait, R., & Silver, R. C. (1989). Coming to terms with major negative life events. In J. S. Uleman & J. A. Bargh (Eds.), *Unintended thought* (pp. 351–382). New York: Guilford Press.

Taylor, S. E., Lichtmann, R. R., Wood, J. V., Bluming, A. Z., Dosik, G. M., & Leibowitz, R. L. (1985). Illness-related and treatment-related factors in psychological adjustment to breast cancer. *Cancer, 55,* 2506–2513.

Thoits, P. (1986). Social support as coping assistance. *Journal of Consulting and Clinical Psychology, 54,* 416–423.

Vickberg, S. M. J., Redd, W. H., Ricketts, P., DuHamel, K. N., Bovbjerg, D., Schrimshaw, E. W., Steinmayer, K., & Currie, V. (1997). *Perceptions of breast cancer: Examining the "cancer as trauma" assumption.* Poster presented at the Annual Meeting of the American Psychological Association, Chicago.

Vickberg, S., Redd, W. H., Smith, M., DuHamel, K., Papadopoulous, E., & Rosen, L. (1996, May). *PTSD and existential life attitudes in bone marrow transplant survivors.* Poster presented at the American Psychiatric Annual Meeting, New York.

Vinokur, A. D., Threatt, B. A., Vinokur-Kaplan, D., & Satariano, W. A. (1990). The process of recovery from breast cancer for younger and older patients. Changes during the first year. *Cancer, 65,* 1242–1254.

Watson, M., Greer, S., Blake, S., & Shrapnell, K. (1984). Reaction to a diagnosis of breast cancer: Relationship between denial. *Cancer, 53,* 2008–2012.

Weisman, A., & Worden, J. (1976). The existential plight in cancer: Significance of the first 100 days. *International Journal of Psychiatry in Medicine, 7,* 1–15.

Wolberg, W. H., Romsaas, E. P., Tanner, M. A., & Malec, I. F. (1989). Psychosexual adaptation to breast cancer surgery. *Cancer, 63,* 1645–1655.

Wolcott, D. L., Wellisch, D. K., & Fawzy, F. I. (1986). Adaptation of adult bone marrow transplant recipient long term survivors. *Transplantation, 41,* 478–483.

Woods, N. F., & Earp, J. L. (1978). Women with cured breast cancer. A study of mastectomy patients in North Carolina. *Nursing Research, 27,* 279–285.

Yehuda, R., & McFarlane, A. C. (1995). Conflict between current knowledge about posttraumatic stress disorder and its original conceptual basis. *American Journal of Psychiatry, 152,* 1705–1713.

Yehuda, R., Kahana, B., Schneidler, J., Southwick, S. M., Wilson, S., & Giller, E. L. (1995). Impact of cumulative lifetime trauma and recent stress on current posttraumatic stress disorder symptoms in Holocaust survivors. *American Journal of Psychiatry, 152,* 1815–1818.

CHAPTER 6

A Social–Cognitive Processing Model of Emotional Adjustment to Cancer

Stephen J. Lepore

Cancer diagnosis and treatments can profoundly and, sometimes, irrevocably alter people's lives. The specter of death looms large at diagnosis, and the threat of recurrence can evoke lasting concerns and distress. Cancer treatments are invasive, painful, and often create long-term negative side effects. Yet despite the dread, discomfort, and dysfunction associated with this disease, some individuals are able to maintain or quickly reestablish their precancer emotional equilibrium. Understanding this adjustment process is a primary goal of psychologists and health care providers who conduct psychosocial interventions with cancer patients (Andersen, 1992). By examining natural processes and predictors of adjustment in cancer patients, we can find clues to designing effective interventions.

A primary predictor of emotional adjustment in people who have cancer is the quality of their interpersonal relationships in the recovery period. In particular, the availability of social support from close family and friends is associated with better adjustment (Glanz & Lerman, 1992; Helgeson & Cohen, 1996; Rowland, 1989), whereas strained relationships are associated with poorer adjustment (de Ruiter, de Haes, & Tempelaar, 1993; Lepore, 1997a; Lepore & Helgeson, 1998; Lepore & Ituarte, 1999; Manne, 1999; Manne & Glassman, 2000; Manne, Taylor, Dougherty, & Kemeny, 1997). This chapter applies a social–cognitive processing theory of adjustment to stressors to explain how the social context of recovery influences emotional adjustment to cancer. The theory also is applied to understanding who benefits from psychosocial interventions for cancer and why.

Cognitive Processing

Because cancer is a life-threatening illness, it can be classified as a traumatic life event (American Psychiatric Association, 1994). Like other traumas, it can dissolve

The research reported in this chapter was partly supported by National Institute of Mental Health Grants 1-54217, 1-49432, CA-68354, and CA-61303.

people's everyday assumptions about life. It can cause people to question core beliefs they hold about themselves, their relationships with others, and their future—beliefs that help people to maintain a sense of self-worth, predictability, coherence, and control in the world (Janoff-Bulman, 1992). By challenging individuals' preexisting mental models of themselves and the world, cancer can take a major psychological toll. According to cognitive-processing theories, emotional distress associated with traumas is largely due to the discrepancy between people's mental models of themselves or the world and the meaning inherent in a trauma (Epstein, 1991). Confronting, contemplating, and reevaluating aversive, trauma-related stimuli may facilitate emotional adaptation by helping people to integrate novel, trauma-related information into preexisting mental models (Horowitz, 1986; Janoff-Bulman, 1992; McCann & Pearlman, 1990; Parkes, 1971; Rachman, 1980; van der Kolk & van der Hart, 1991).

Cognitive integration could occur through mental processes of assimilation (i.e., reappraising events to fit preconceptions) or accommodation (i.e., changing mental models to fit information inherent in a traumatic event). Through assimilation and accommodation processes, people with cancer can interpret their illness in personally meaningful terms, integrate threatening and confusing aspects of the disease into a coherent conceptual framework, and achieve intellectual or emotional resolution. For instance, to preserve a sense of control, cancer patients could attribute their disease to a smoking habit rather than to random or unknown causes. Or, instead of an assimilation process, patients might mentally accommodate the disease by changing their views about control over health outcomes. In addition to facilitating integration, repeated mental exposure to cancer-related stimuli could foster healthy adaptation through habituation or desensitization to cancer-related thoughts and stimuli. If the cognitive processing occurs in a supportive or benign social context, associations between the traumatic stimuli and negative emotional responses may be weakened or supplanted by positive emotional responses.

Horowitz (1986) has argued that cognitive processing of traumatic events is characterized by alternating cycles of intrusion (i.e., unbidden thoughts and images of the event intrude into consciousness) and avoidance (i.e., attempting not to think about the event). In cancer survivors, these trauma symptoms are common and may be experienced years after diagnosis (Alter et al., 1996; Cella & Tross, 1986; Cordova et al., 1995; Epping-Jordan, Compas, & Howell, 1994; Horowitz, 1982; Lepore & Helgeson, 1998). In theory, intrusive thoughts emerge from individuals' need to integrate trauma-related information into their mental models—a process that Horowitz (1986) referred to as the *completion tendency*. Thus, intrusive thoughts are a marker of incomplete cognitive processing, and they may stimulate cognitive processing by bringing aspects of a trauma into consciousness. Although intrusions may be functionally adaptive, they are also emotionally disturbing. For this reason, people may adopt avoidant coping strategies, which can prevent them from becoming emotionally overwhelmed when they think of or are reminded of their trauma.

However, if avoidance is excessive, it can interfere with cognitive processing (Horo-witz, 1986).

Theorists recently have called for more research on individual and situational factors that can modulate cognitive processing (Brewin, Dalgleish, & Joseph, 1996; Greenberg, 1995; Jones & Barlow, 1990; Litz, 1992; Tait & Silver, 1989). Such research is necessary to explain failures in cognitive processing. For example, such research might reveal why intrusive thoughts become fixated in some people (Baum, Cohen, & Hall, 1993; Lehman, Wortman, & Williams, 1987), why some people perpetually search for meaning after a trauma (R. L. Silver, Boon, & Stones, 1983), or why some people are fixated on avoiding thinking or talking about a trauma. Such research also can point to avenues of intervention to facilitate emotional adaptation to cancer. According to a social–cognitive processing model that my colleagues and I have been developing, social–contextual variables, such as social support and social constraints on disclosure, can account for much of the variance in cognitive-processing success.

Social Modulation of Cognitive Processing

In numerous interview studies with trauma survivors, including cancer patients, the majority of respondents report that they have talked about their trauma with others (Pennebaker & Harber, 1993; Rime, 1995). This social sharing normally occurs shortly after a negative event (Rime, 1995) and, in some cases, continues for years after an event (Lehman et al., 1987). Talking with others may facilitate cognitive processing of traumatic experiences. As noted above, such experiences can challenge core assumptions that people hold in order to maintain a sense of coherence, predictability, control, and self-worth. One way that people may reduce the disso-nance created by traumatic events is to initiate communication (Festinger, Riecken, & Schachter, 1956). However, despite the strong urge and tendency for people to talk about traumatic events, there is actually little empirical evidence that talking per se boosts emotional adjustment (Rime, 1995). To account for these unexpected findings, my colleagues and I have argued that the emotional benefits of talking are moderated by the social response of others (e.g., Lepore, Silver, Wortman, & Way-ment, 1996). Benefits should be accrued if talking is met with supportive, receptive, or noncritical social responses, but not if talking is met with unsupportive, unre-ceptive, or critical social responses.

A positive, or supportive, social environment should enhance cognitive process-ing by enabling people to contemplate and discuss trauma-related thoughts and feelings (Albrecht, Burleson, & Goldsmith, 1994; Clark, 1993; Pennebaker, 1993; R. L. Silver & Wortman, 1980). Supportive, or empathic, social networks help people to maintain or reestablish a positive self-concept, because such responses validate people's experiences and affirm that they are loved and esteemed (Albrecht

& Adelman, 1987). Discussing traumas with supportive others might help people to maintain or reestablish a coherent worldview (Janoff-Bulman, 1992). Supportive others can suggest new and positive perspectives on a traumatic experience, provide information on how to cope, or encourage individuals to accept their situation (Clark, 1993; Lepore et al., 1996; R. L. Silver et al., 1983). Positive social responses also may facilitate consolidation of traumatic memories, thereby reducing the need for further processing (e.g., searching for meaning, rumination; see Lepore, Ragan, & Jones, 2000). A final benefit is this: When people are able to talk about traumatic thoughts in a benign social context, they may be able to increase control over negative emotional responses or supplant negative emotional responses to intrusive thoughts with neutral or positive ones.

In contrast, an unsupportive or critical social network should impede cognitive processing and adjustment. When individuals disclose stressful experiences in a negative social context, or one in which network members are not fully supportive, it can result in increased psychological distress (Major et al., 1990; Major, Zubeck, Cooper, Cozzarelli, & Richards, 1997). My colleagues and I have argued that unexpected or negative social responses to disclosures about traumas could impede cognitive processing if individuals counter-respond by trying not to think or talk about traumas (Kliewer, Lepore, Oskin, & Johnson, 1998; Lepore, 1997b, 1997c; Lepore & Helgeson, 1998; Lepore et al., 1996). Active attempts at thought suppression can prolong intrusive thoughts (Wegner, 1994). Inhibition of talking and thinking about traumas also can interfere with cognitive processing in other ways, including limiting individuals' access to new information and alternative perspectives, which may be critical for cognitive integration of trauma-related information (Janoff-Bulman, 1992; Pennebaker, 1989, 1993; Tait & Silver, 1989). People who are constrained in talking about traumas also might engage in a perpetual search for meaning, because they are unable to accept or understand their traumatic experience. Inhibition also can diminish the chance to habituate to trauma-related stimuli: Not thinking or talking about a trauma reduces opportunities to form new, nonthreatening associations with trauma-related stimuli (Bootzin, 1997; Coates & Winston, 1983; Creamer, Burgess, & Pattison, 1990; Keane, Zimmering, & Caddell, 1985; Lepore, 1997a; Stiles, 1987). Thus, constraints on disclosure can undermine individuals' ability to gain control over negative emotions (Lepore & Greenberg, in press).

Empirical Studies on the Social–Cognitive Processing Model of Adjustment

Evidence from a growing number of studies is consistent with the social–cognitive processing model of adjustment. In a cross-sectional study of good-prognosis prostate cancer survivors, Lepore and Helgeson (1998) found that a subset of men reported constraints in talking with significant others about their cancer (e.g., others avoided talking about the cancer, acted uncomfortable when they visited, or expressed difficulties talking about cancer). These men, when compared with their peers who had relatively few constraints in talking, reported more cancer-related intrusive thoughts and were more likely to avoid thinking and talking about their cancer. Moreover, constraints in talking with others potentiated the positive association between intrusive thoughts and poor mental health. As shown in Figure 6.1, there were stronger negative associations between intrusive thoughts and mental health in men who had high constraints in talking with their spouse (panel A) or family and friends (panel B) than in men who had relatively few constraints in talking with these network members.

A more rigorous test of the model was provided in a longitudinal study on the emotional adaptation of women who had been treated for localized breast or colon cancer (Lepore, 1997b). Data were collected from approximately 100 women 3 months (T1) and 11 months (T2) after their diagnosis. Regression analyses were used to examine whether T1 social constraints moderated the association between T1 intrusive thoughts and T2 negative affect, after statistically controlling for T1 negative affect. The social-constraints measure was similar to the one used in the prostate cancer study. It tapped women's perceptions of how family and friends reacted when they attempted to talk about their cancer (e.g., did not understand your situation, changed the subject when you tried to discuss your cancer, minimized your problems, gave you the idea they did not want to hear about it). The intrusive thoughts measure assessed how frequently women had intrusive thoughts about cancer. Negative affect was measured using the Positive and Negative Affect Scales, or PANAS (Watson, Clark, & Tellegen, 1988).

There was a significant interaction between social constraints and intrusive thoughts, which replicated the findings from the prostate cancer study. Again, social constraints appeared to moderate the association between intrusive thoughts and emotional adjustment. As shown in Figure 6.2, level of intrusive thoughts was associated with an increase in negative affect in women who had high social constraints, but it was unrelated to negative affect in women with relatively few social constraints. Other analyses suggested that social constraints also moderated the frequency of talking about cancer-related intrusive thoughts. As shown in Figure 6.3, higher intrusive thoughts were associated with increases in talking over time in women low in social constraints but not in women with relatively high social constraints. Furthermore, social constraints moderated the association between intrusive thoughts and frequency of breast self-examinations. Over time, higher intrusive thoughts were associated with more frequent monthly breast self-examinations (for recurrence) in women low in social constraints than in women high in social constraints. These latter findings are consistent with the notion that social constraints lead to increases in avoidant coping, which could account for failures in cognitive processing.

FIGURE 6.1

Slopes of the relation between intrusive thoughts about prostate cancer and mental health as a function of social constraints from spouse (panel A) and family/friends (panel B). Low constraints are represented with squares, and high constraints are represented with triangles. Low intrusive thoughts = − 1 standard deviation, and high intrusive thoughts = + 1 standard deviation. Higher scores indicate better mental health. From "Social Constraints, Intrusive Thoughts, and Mental Health in Prostate Cancer Survivors," by S. J. Lepore & V. Helgeson, 1998, Journal of Social and Clinical Psychology, 17, p. 99. Copyright 1998 by The Guilford Press. Reprinted with permission.

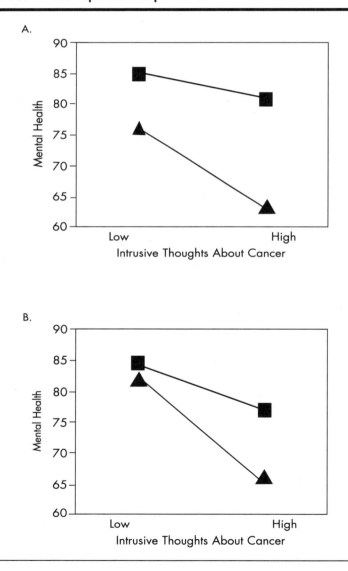

FIGURE 6.2

Slopes of the relation between intrusive thoughts about cancer and residualized negative affect as a function of social constraints from family and friends. Low constraints are represented with squares, and high constraints are represented with triangles. Low intrusive thoughts = − 1 standard deviation, and high intrusive thoughts = + 1 standard deviation. Higher scores indicate more negative affect. These findings were originally presented in Social Constraints, Intrusive Thoughts, and Negative Affect in Women With Cancer, by S. J. Lepore, April 1997, paper presented at the Society of Behavioral Medicine in San Francisco, CA.

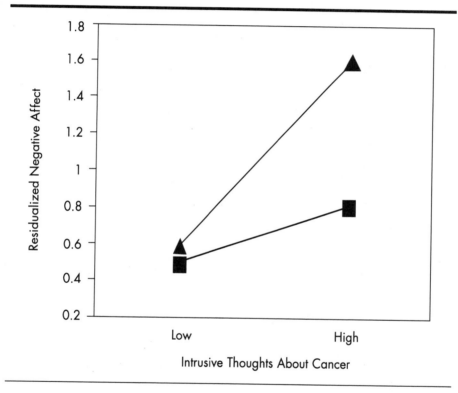

Manne (1999) examined the social moderation of the emotional effects of intrusive thoughts in a sample of patients with breast, lung, or colorectal cancer. Manne focused on the effects of critical and avoidant responses from the patients' spouse. Patients in active treatment for cancer completed measures of cancer-specific critical and avoidant responses by their spouses, intrusive thoughts about cancer, and psychological distress at two time points spaced 3 months apart. Presumably, critical and avoidant responses from a spouse would constrain social sharing. Psychological distress at T2 was predicted by T1 intrusions, criticism by spouse, avoidance by spouse, Intrusions × Criticism interaction, and Avoidance × Criticism interac-

FIGURE 6.3

Slopes of the relation between intrusive thoughts about cancer and residualized amount of talking about cancer as a function of social constraints from family and friends. Low constraints are represented with squares, and high constraints are represented with triangles. Low intrusive thoughts = − 1 standard deviation, and high intrusive thoughts = + 1 standard deviation. Higher scores indicate more negative affect. These findings were originally presented in Social Constraints, Intrusive Thoughts, and Negative Affect in Women With Cancer, by S. J. Lepore, April 1997, paper presented at the Society of Behavioral Medicine in San Francisco, CA.

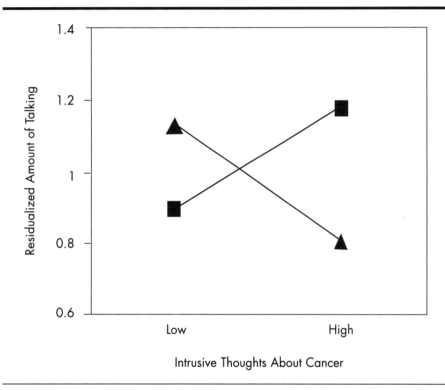

Intrusive Thoughts About Cancer

tion, controlling for T1 psychological distress. Criticism interacted with intrusions. Intrusive thoughts were associated with increases in distress at T2 in patients with high spouse criticism, but not in patients with relatively low spouse criticism and avoidance. There was a marginal ($p < .06$) interaction between avoidance and intrusions. The directional of this effect was similar to the interaction between criticism and intrusions. These findings suggest that critical responses might be more detrimental than avoidant responses.

In a study of gynecological cancer patients, Lutgendorf, Anderson, Larsen, Buller, and Sorosky (1999) found interactive effects of social support seeking and intrusive thoughts on symptoms of anxiety and depression. Data were collected during interviews conducted at two time points: after diagnosis but before surgery (T1) and again 6 months later (T2). Regression analyses were used to examine whether T2 social support seeking moderated the association between T2 intrusive thoughts and T2 symptoms, controlling for symptoms at T1. There was a significant interaction for both outcomes. Plots of the interactions indicated that the positive association between intrusive thoughts and symptoms was stronger in women who tended not to seek emotional support than in women who did use this coping method. Although support seeking is somewhat different from the social variables that Lepore and colleagues used (i.e., negative social reactions to disclosure, inadequate support), it is probable that patients' willingness to seek support is inversely related to the quality of the support that they have available to them (Lepore, 1997c).

Evidence from studies with other trauma populations also reveals the powerful effects of the social environment on cognitive–emotional processes of adaptation. In a study of bereaved mothers, level of intrusive thoughts at 3 weeks postloss was associated with increases in depressive symptoms if mothers felt constrained in talking about the loss but not if they felt relatively unconstrained (Lepore et al., 1996). In a study of women who had had an abortion, intrusive thoughts of the abortion 2 years later were more strongly associated with distress in women who had talked relatively little about their emotions with others than in women who had talked to a greater extent (Major & Gramzow, 1999). In a study on children exposed to inner-city violence, results showed that violence exposure was associated with higher levels of internalizing symptoms in children (Kliewer et al., 1998). The highest risk group for internalizing symptoms consisted of children with a high level of violence-related intrusive thoughts combined with a low level of social support or a high level of social constraints. Finally, in a study of people left homeless by a fire disaster, investigators found a synergistic effect of conflicted social relationships and intrusive thoughts on psychological distress symptoms (R. C. Silver & Holman, 1994). Psychological distress symptoms, intrusive thoughts, and social conflict with network members were measured shortly after the fire disaster and were used to predict psychological distress symptoms 1 year later. Controlling for initial level of distress symptoms, level of intrusive thoughts was positively associated with subsequent distress symptoms in individuals who had a high level of social conflict but not in those who had a low level of social conflict.

In summary, the quality of interpersonal relationships appears to influence cognitive–emotional processes of adaptation to cancer, as well as other major life stressors. Data from several studies reveal that the quality of cancer survivors' interpersonal relationships is related to the frequency and impact of intrusive thoughts about cancer, as well as how people cope with cancer-related thoughts and stimuli. Poorer social relationships are correlated with more inhibitory behaviors, such as avoidance of thinking and talking about cancer, or monitoring for recurrence. Furthermore, individuals who have unsupportive and critical social ties tend to be more psychologically distressed by cancer-related intrusive thoughts than are individuals with relatively supportive and uncritical social ties. The inhibitory behaviors of cancer patients with unsupportive social networks may account for the greater emotional distress that they experience relative to their peers with more supportive social networks. However, the mechanisms explaining the interactive effects of unsupportive social interactions and intrusive thoughts on distress have yet to be clearly demonstrated. Nonetheless, the social modulation of coping and emotional responses to intrusive thoughts appears to be a robust phenomenon, because it has been observed in a variety of trauma populations, including bereaved mothers, people in a fire disaster, women having an abortion, and children exposed to inner-city violence. In the remainder of this chapter, I consider the implications of these basic research findings for psychosocial interventions with cancer patients.

Implications for Psychosocial Interventions

In a recent review article, Helgeson and Cohen (1996) found mixed effects of social support groups on adjustment to cancer. One possible explanation for these unexpected findings is that individual differences determine who benefits from attending support groups. On the basis of the social–cognitive processing model described above, it would appear that only individuals with inadequate social coping resources would benefit from participating in a support group. People with adequate social coping resources should be able to maintain or quickly reestablish their emotional equilibrium after being diagnosed with cancer (cf. Andersen, 1992). Most support groups provide both education and sharing of experiences with peers. For cancer survivors who have inadequate support resources from their social network, education and sharing of experiences could help them to develop adaptive mental models of their situation. For instance, cancer patients who participate in a support group can develop greater feelings of control, or self-efficacy, as a result of learning coping strategies through direct education or social sharing with peers. They also should be less distressed by cancer-related intrusive thoughts as a result of having their thoughts and feelings validated by peers.

A colleague, Vicki Helgeson, and I tested some of these ideas in a study of men who had been treated for localized prostate cancer (Lepore & Helgeson, 1999). Shortly after their cancer treatment, men were randomly assigned to a control group or an intervention group. All men were interviewed 2 weeks before (T1) and 2 weeks after (T2) the intervention period. The median length of time from diagnosis to the initial interview was 142 days; from treatment to the initial interview it was 41 days. The primary treatment for most men was surgery (83%), although some received radiation or a combination of surgery and radiation (21%).

The intervention group consisted of 6 weekly lectures and facilitated discussion with peers. The lectures covered topics representing central concerns for this population: (a) overview of prostate cancer and its causes, (b) the role of nutrition and exercise in cancer, (c) management of the physical side effects of treatments, (d) relaxation and stress management, (e) communication with family and friends and intimacy with spouse, and (e) follow-up care and health promotion. During the discussion component of the intervention, men and their wives convened in separate rooms. A psychologist facilitated the men's discussions, and an oncology nurse facilitated the wives' discussions. The facilitators emphasized sharing of experiences, with the goal of validating and normalizing experiences. They also ensured that there was a nonjudgmental atmosphere, where individuals could feel comfortable sharing or listening. Finally, facilitators kept the discussion focused on the topic of the night and controlled any misinformation that would arise in the discussions. The control group did not receive any intervention.

Relative to the men in the control group, men who participated in the intervention had greater improvements in mental health, as measured by the mental health index of the Medical Outcome Study, Short Form 36 (Stewart, Hays, & Ware, 1988). From T1 to T2, the intervention group also reported significantly fewer interpersonal conflicts, larger increases in perceived control over their health and functioning, and lower distress associated with cancer-related intrusive thoughts. Men in the intervention groups also reported less avoidance of cancer-related thoughts over time, but this effect was marginal. Frequency of intrusive thoughts was unaffected by the intervention.

The most interesting finding came from analyses of individual differences. As predicted, there were interactive effects of group (control, intervention) and social coping resources (low, high) on changes in mental health. These effects showed that the intervention was especially beneficial to men with inadequate social resources. As shown in Figure 6.4, a low level of social support from family and friends was associated with poorer mental health in the control group, but not in the intervention group. Men with a high level of social support from family and friends had relatively good mental health in both the control and intervention group. Amount of social support from the wife did not interact with group. However, satisfaction with wife support did. As shown in Figure 6.5, a low level of satisfaction with support from the wife was associated with poorer mental health in the control group but not in the intervention group. Men with a high level of satisfaction with wife support had relatively good mental health in both the control and intervention group.

In summary, preliminary evidence suggests that support groups that emphasize education and sharing of experiences may be beneficial for cancer patients with inadequate support from family and friends. Men who have adequate social support from family and friends might not benefit emotionally from support groups. However, the presence of this subset of well-adjusted men may have positively influenced the well-being of men with inadequate support. Thus, I would not recommend conducting a support group consisting entirely of patients with poor mental health and inadequate social support. The intervention also influenced mental models in a positive way (i.e., increased perceived control) and reduced distress associated

FIGURE 6.4

Slope of the relation between support received from family and friends and residualized mental health as a function of experimental group. The intervention group is represented with a square, and the control group is represented with a triangle. Low intrusive thoughts = −1 standard deviation, and high intrusive thoughts = +1 standard deviation. Higher scores indicate better mental health. From "Psychoeducational Support Group Enhances Quality of Life After Prostate Cancer," by S. J. Lepore & V. S. Helgeson, 1999, Cancer Research, Therapy and Control, 8, p. 89. Copyright 1999 by Harwood Academic Publishers. Reprinted with permission.

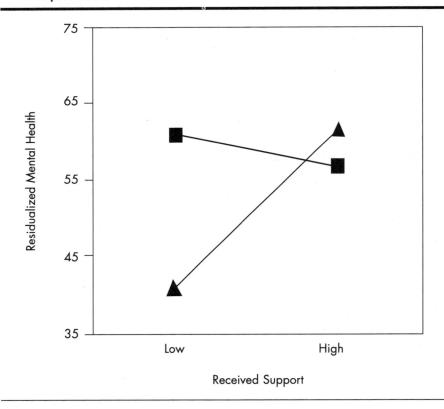

with cancer-related intrusive thoughts. These latter findings suggest that cognitive processing and desensitization to intrusive thoughts may be important mediators of the benefits of social support groups.

General Conclusions and Future Directions

The studies discussed in this chapter indicate that supportive and uncritical social relationships buffer people from the negative emotional effects of trauma-related

FIGURE 6.5

Slope of the relation between satisfaction with spouse support and residualized mental health as a function of experimental group. The intervention group is represented with a square, and the control group is represented with a triangle. Low intrusive thoughts = − 1 standard deviation, and high intrusive thoughts = + 1 standard deviation. Higher scores indicate better mental health. From "Psychoeducational Support Group Enhances Quality of Life After Prostate Cancer," by S. J. Lepore & V. S. Helgeson, 1999, Cancer Research, Therapy and Control, 8, p. 89. Copyright 1999 by Harwood Academic Publishers. Reprinted with permission.

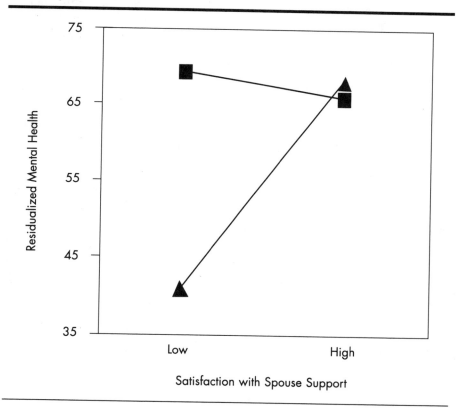

intrusive thoughts. The exact mechanisms underlying these buffering effects are not yet established and present many research opportunities.

Supportive social environments might reduce distress by facilitating cognitive processing and integration of traumatic experiences. Some of the studies reviewed in the chapter have produced effects consistent with this notion. For instance, supportive social responses to the disclosures of prostate cancer patients (Lepore & Helgeson, 1998) and bereaved mothers (Lepore et al., 1996) facilitated talking and reduced avoidant thinking and behaviors. By talking and thinking about their traumas, individuals may be able to restore their basic assumptions about themselves and the world.

Additional research is needed to uncover the exact mechanisms involved in emotional adaptation. One mechanism that has been suggested in this chapter could be labeled the *completion hypothesis*. According to this explanation, talking with supportive and uncritical others helps to restore basic beliefs about the self and the world that people use to maintain a sense of coherence, predictability, and self-worth. The prostate cancer intervention study revealed that patients who participated in a support group were more likely to gain a sense of control over their illness. Much more evidence of this sort is needed before we can take stock in the completion hypothesis.

An alternative to the completion hypothesis is the *desensitization hypothesis*. As noted above, people who confront trauma-related thoughts and stimuli in a benign social context may be able to supplant negative emotional responses to traumatic stimuli with neutral or positive responses. Such a process would clearly account for the Intrusion × Social Environment interactions described in this chapter. The desensitization hypothesis could also explain why participation in the prostate cancer support group reduced the emotional impact of intrusive thoughts but not the frequency of intrusive thoughts. If social support facilitates "completion," or reduces the discrepancy between individuals' mental models and information inherent in a trauma, then in theory it also should dispel intrusive thoughts. From the desensitization perspective, one would not necessarily predict a reduction in the frequency of intrusive thoughts. It is of course also possible that in time men in the intervention group would experience a more rapid decline in intrusive thoughts than would men in the control group. Because the follow-up measures were taken just a couple of weeks after the intervention, thoughts about prostate cancer were probably still fresh for those men who participated in the support group. It is also possible that both completion and desensitization processes are operating. Because thoughts about cancer, or other traumas, are less distressing to people with adequate rather than inadequate social outlets, they may be in a better position to achieve intellectual and emotional resolution.

A final and important challenge for future research is to untangle the effects of different components of social support groups (Redd, 1995). In the prostate cancer intervention study, there was an education and peer discussion arm. The group was run in this manner because we assumed that talking with supportive others and receiving information about an illness and how to cope with its side effects should enhance self-concept (through validation, affirmation, and normalization) and help people to make sense of an illness. We also assumed that the educational topics would provide a focus for the discussions. Recent findings with breast cancer patients indicate that discussion with peers does not necessarily enhance the psychological well-being of cancer patients (Helgeson, Cohen, Schulz, & Yasko, 1999). Therefore, we must be careful in assuming that the social sharing that took place between men in the prostate cancer support group is responsible for the improvements in their mental health. In an ongoing, large-scale clinical trial, we are examining how education versus education combined with peer discussion affects the quality of life of men with prostate cancer.

References

Albrecht, T. L., & Adelman, M. B. (1987). *Communicating social support.* Newbury Park, CA: Sage.

Albrecht, T. L., Burleson, B. R., & Goldsmith, D. (1994). Supportive communication. In M. L. Knapp & G. R. Miller (Eds.), *Handbook of interpersonal communication* (2nd ed., pp. 419–449). Thousand Oaks, CA: Sage.

Alter, C. L., Pelcovitz, D., Axelrod, A., Godenberg, B., Harris, H., Meyers, B., Grobois, B., Mandel, F., Septimus, A., & Kaplan, S. (1996). Identification of PTSD in cancer survivors. *Psychosomatics, 37,* 137–143.

American Psychiatric Association. (1994). *Diagnostic and statistical manual of mental disorders* (4th ed.). Washington, DC: Author.

Andersen, B. L. (1992). Psychological interventions for cancer patients to enhance quality of life. *Journal of Consulting and Clinical Psychology, 60,* 552–568.

Baum, A., Cohen, L., & Hall, M. (1993). Control and intrusive memories as possible determinants of chronic stress. *Psychosomatic Medicine, 55,* 274–286.

Bootzin, R. R. (1997). Examining the theory and clinical utility of writing about emotional experiences. *Psychological Science, 8,* 167–169.

Brewin, C., Dalgleish, R., & Joseph, S. (1996). A dual representation theory of posttraumatic stress disorder. *Psychological Bulletin, 103,* 670–686.

Cella, D., & Tross, S. (1986). Psychological adjustment to survival from Hodgkin's disease. *Journal of Consulting and Clinical Psychology, 54,* 616–622.

Clark, L. F. (1993). Stress and the cognitive-conversational benefits of social interaction. *Journal of Social and Clinical Psychology, 12,* 25–55.

Coates, D., & Winston, T. (1983). Counteracting the deviance of depression: Peer support groups for victims. *Journal of Social Issues, 39,* 169–194.

Cordova, M. J., Andrykowski, M. A., Kenady, D. E., McGrath, P. C., Sloan, D. A., & Redd, W. H. (1995). Frequency and correlates of posttraumatic-stress-disorder-like symptoms after treatment for breast cancer. *Journal of Consulting and Clinical Psychology, 63,* 981–986.

Creamer, M., Burgess, P., & Pattison, P. (1990). Cognitive processing of post-trauma reactions: Some preliminary findings. *Psychological Medicine, 58,* 597–604.

de Ruiter, J., de Haes, J., & Tempelaar, R. (1993). Cancer patients and their network: The meaning of the social network and social interactions for quality of life. *Supportive Care in Cancer, 1,* 152–155.

Epping-Jordan, J. E., Compas, B., & Howell, D. C. (1994). Predictors of cancer progression in young adult men and women: Avoidance, intrusive thoughts, and psychological symptoms. *Health Psychology, 13,* 539–547.

Epstein, S. (1991). The self-concept, the traumatic neurosis and the structure of personality. In D. Ozer, J. N. Healy, & A. J. Stewart (Eds.), *Perspectives on personality* (pp. 80–95). Greenwich, CT: JAI Press.

Festinger, L., Riecken, H. W., & Schachter, S. (1956). *When prophecy fails.* Minneapolis: University of Minnesota Press.

Glanz, K., & Lerman, C. (1992). Psychosocial impact of breast cancer: A critical review. *Annals of Behavioral Medicine, 14,* 204–212.

Greenberg, M. (1995). Cognitive processing of traumas: The role of intrusive thoughts and reappraisals. *Journal of Applied Social Psychology, 25,* 1262–1296.

Helgeson, V. S., & Cohen, S. (1996). Social support and adjustment to cancer: Reconciling descriptive, correlational, and intervention research. *Health Psychology, 15,* 135–148.

Helgeson, V. S., Cohen, S., Schulz, R., & Yasko, J. (1999). Effects of education and peer discussion group interventions on 6-month adjustment to stage I and II breast cancer. *Archives of General Psychiatry, 56,* 340–347.

Horowitz, M. (Ed.). (1982). *Stress response syndromes and their treatment.* New York: Free Press.

Horowitz, M. J. (1986). *Stress response syndromes* (2nd ed.). New York: Jason Aronson.

Janoff-Bulman, R. (1992). *Shattered assumptions: Toward a new psychology of trauma.* New York: Free Press.

Jones, J. C., & Barlow, D. H. (1990). The etiology of posttraumatic stress disorder. *Clinical Psychology Review, 10,* 299–328.

Keane, T. M., Zimmering, R. T., & Caddell, J. M. (1985). A behavioral formulation of posttraumatic stress disorder in Vietnam veterans. *The Behavior Therapist, 8,* 9–12.

Kliewer, W. L., Lepore, S. J., Oskin, D., & Johnson, P. D. (1998). The role of social and cognitive processes in children's adjustment to community violence. *Journal of Consulting and Clinical Psychology, 66,* 199–209.

Lehman, D. R., Wortman, C. B., & Williams, A. F. (1987). Long-term effects of losing a spouse or child in a motor vehicle death. *Journal of Personality and Social Psychology, 52,* 218–231.

Lepore, S. J. (1997a). Expressive writing moderates the relation between intrusive thoughts and depressive symptoms. *Journal of Personality and Social Psychology, 73,* 1030–1037.

Lepore, S. J. (1997b, April). *Social constraints, intrusive thoughts, and negative affect in women with cancer.* Paper presented at the meeting of the Society of Behavioral Medicine, San Francisco, CA.

Lepore, S. J. (1997c). Social–environmental influences on the chronic stress process. In B. Gottlieb (Ed.), *Coping with chronic stressors* (pp. 133–160). New York: Plenum.

Lepore, S. J., & Greenberg, M. A. (in press). Mending broken hearts: Effects of expressive writing on mood, cognitive processing, social adjustment, and health following a relationship breakup. *Psychology & Health.*

Lepore, S. J., & Helgeson, V. (1998). Social constraints, intrusive thoughts, and mental health in prostate cancer survivors. *Journal of Social and Clinical Psychology, 17,* 89–106.

Lepore, S. J., & Helgeson, V. S. (1999). Psychoeducational support group enhances quality of life after prostate cancer. *Cancer Research, Therapy and Control, 8,* 81–91.

Lepore, S. J., & Ituarte, P. H. G. (1999). Optimism about cancer enhances mood by reducing negative social interactions. *Cancer Research, Therapy and Control, 8,* 165–174.

Lepore, S. J., Ragan, J. D., & Jones, S. (2000). Talking facilitates cognitive–emotional processes of adaptation to an acute stressor. *Journal of Personality and Social Psychology, 78,* 499–508.

Lepore, S. J., Silver, R. C., Wortman, C. B., & Wayment, H. A. (1996). Social constraints, intrusive thoughts, and depressive symptoms among bereaved mothers. *Journal of Personality and Social Psychology, 70,* 271–282.

Litz, B. T. (1992). Emotional numbing in combat-related post-traumatic stress disorder: A critical review and reformulation. *Clinical Psychology Review, 12,* 417–432.

Lutgendorf, S., Anderson, B., Larsen, K., Buller, R. E., & Sorosky, J. I. (1999). Cognitive processing, social support coping, and distress in gynecological cancer patients. *Cancer Research, Therapy, and Control, 8,* 9–19.

Major, B., Cozzarelli, C., Sciacchitano, A. M., Cooper, M. L., Testa, M., & Mueller, P. M. (1990). Perceived social support, self-efficacy, and adjustment to abortion. *Journal of Personality and Social Psychology, 59,* 452–463.

Major, B., & Gramzow, R. H. (1999). Abortion as stigma: Cognitive and emotional implications of concealment. *Journal of Personality and Social Psychology, 77,* 735–745.

Major, B., Zubeck, J. M., Cooper, M. R., Cozzarelli, C., & Richards, C. (1997). Mixed messages: Implications of social conflict and social support within close relationships for adjustment to a stressful life event. *Journal of Personality and Social Psychology, 72,* 1349–1363.

Manne, S. L. (1999). Intrusive thoughts and psychological distress among cancer patients: The role of spouse avoidance and criticism. *Journal of Consulting and Clinical Psychology, 67,* 539–546.

Manne, S. L., & Glassman, M. (2000). Perceived control, coping efficacy, and avoidance coping as mediators between spouses' unsupportive behaviors and cancer patients' psychological distress. *Health Psychology, 19,* 155–164.

Manne, S. L., Taylor, K. L., Dougherty, J., & Kemeny, N. (1997). Social support and negative responses in the marital relationship: Their association with psychological adjustment among individuals with cancer. *Journal of Behavioral Medicine, 20,* 101–125.

McCann, I. L., & Pearlman, L. A. (1990). *Psychological trauma and the adult survivor: Theory, therapy, and transformation.* New York: Brunner/Mazel.

Parkes, C. M. (1971). Psycho-social transitions: A field study. *Social Science and Medicine, 5,* 101–115.

Pennebaker, J. W. (1989). Confession, inhibition, and disease. In L. Berkowitz (Ed.), *Advances in experimental social psychology* (Vol. 22, pp. 211–244). Orlando, FL: Academic Press.

Pennebaker, J. W. (1993). Putting stress into words: Health, linguistic, and therapeutic implications. *Behaviour Research and Therapy, 31,* 539–548.

Pennebaker, J. W., & Harber, K. (1993). A social stage model of collective coping: The Loma Prieta earthquake and the Persian Gulf war. *Journal of Social Issues, 49*, 125–146.

Rachman, S. (1980). Emotional processing. *Behaviour Research and Therapy, 18*, 51–60.

Redd, W. H. (1995). Behavioral research in cancer as a model for health psychology. *Health Psychology, 14*, 99–100.

Rime, B. (1995). Mental rumination, social sharing, and the recovery from emotional exposure. In J. W. Pennebaker (Ed.), *Emotion, disclosure, & health* (pp. 271–292). Washington, DC: American Psychological Association.

Rowland, J. H. (1989). Developmental stage and adaptation: Adult model. In J. C. Holland & J. H. Rowland (Eds.), *Handbook of psychooncology: Psychological care of the patient with cancer* (pp. 25–43). New York: Oxford University Press.

Silver, R. C., & Holman, E. A. (1994, June). *Social responses to disclosure following traumatic life events.* Paper presented at the International Conference on Emotion, Disclosure, and Health, Taos, NM.

Silver, R. L., Boon, C., & Stones, M. H. (1983). Searching for meaning in misfortune: Making sense of incest. *Journal of Social Issues, 39*, 81–102.

Silver, R. L., & Wortman, C. B. (1980). Coping with undesirable life events. In J. Garber & M. E. P. Seligman (Eds.), *Human helplessness: Theory and applications* (pp. 279–340). New York: Academic Press.

Stewart, A. L., Hays, R. D., & Ware, J. E. (1988). The MOS Short-Form General Health Survey. *Medical Care, 26*, 724–735.

Stiles, W. B. (1987). "I have to talk to somebody": A fever model of self disclosure. In V. J. Derlega & J. H. Berg (Eds.), *Self-disclosure: Theory, research, and therapy* (pp. 257–282). New York: Plenum.

Tait, R., & Silver, R. C. (1989). Coming to terms with major negative life events. In J. S. Uleman & J. A. Bargh (Eds.), *Unintended thought* (pp. 351–382). New York: Guilford Press.

van der Kolk, B. A., & van der Hart, O. (1991). The intrusive past: The flexibility of memory and the engraving of trauma. *American Imago, 48*, 425–454.

Watson, D., Clark, L. A., & Tellegen, A. (1988). Development and validation of brief measures of positive and negative affect: The PANAS scales. *Journal of Personality and Social Psychology, 54*, 1063–1070.

Wegner, D. M. (1994). Ironic processes of mental control. *Psychological Review, 101*, 34–52.

PART 2

Bases of Intervention: Targets and Processes

CHAPTER 7

A Biobehavioral Model for Psychological Interventions

Barbara L. Andersen

The psychological–behavioral aspects of cancer, sometimes termed *issues of quality of life* (QOL), are ones of great importance for those with cancer. Although this seems obvious enough, these issues are often forgotten when dealing with other, seemingly more pressing concerns. Every year millions of federal dollars are made available for research to fight the disease, either directly, as with treatment trials, or indirectly, with research on genetic and biologic factors. This occurs because the numbers of cancer patients are staggering: Each year more than 1.4 million individuals in the United States are diagnosed and another half million people—one person every 90 seconds—die of the disease (Greenlee, Murray, Bolden, & Wingo, 2000). Unfortunately, the attention (and the funding) often stops there, with little translation into proportionately substantive initiatives in cancer control. What are cancer control studies about? Too few have been about the individuals dying from the disease every 90 seconds (Spiegel et al., 1989). The majority have been about the newly diagnosed (Spiker, Trijsburg, & Duivenvoorden, 1997) and, more recently, about the process of surviving cancer (Gotay & Muraoka, 1998).

Who are the cancer survivors? Survivor groups can be determined by considering data on disease incidence and trends in cancer death rates. In combination, the data provide an indication of how many cancer survivors of what disease type there will be, given current incidence and trends in death rates. The data suggest that among women, the survivors will largely come from the breast, colorectal, and gynecologic cancer groups. There will be proportionately smaller numbers of bladder and leukemia survivors because of the lower incidence of these diseases. In the case of breast cancer (about 24% of the total survivor group), women will be there largely because

This research was supported by U.S. Army Medical Research Acquisition Activity Grant DAMD17-96-1-6294, National Institutes of Mental Health Grant R01 MH51487, and the Walther Cancer Foundation.

of the disproportionately large numbers diagnosed each year, rather than because of any improvements in survival rates. Considering other prevalent disease sites, 25% of women will have had colorectal or gynecologic cancer, but they will be more highly represented among the survivor group because of the improvements in therapy cure rates.

For men, the largest numbers of survivors will come from the ranks of prostate, colorectal, and bladder cancer patients. There will be smaller numbers of oral, leukemia, and stomach cancer survivors because of the lower incidence of these diseases. As in the case of breast cancer, men with prostate cancer will be in the survivor group because of the large numbers of men diagnosed each year (about 12% of the total survivor group), rather than because of any improvements in survival rates. Also similar to the women, the men with colorectal and bladder cancer will be more highly represented among the survivor group because of the improvements in therapy cure rates. Finally, the survivor group will be predominantly female (75%); breast (24%), colorectal (15%), and prostate (12%) cancers together will account for more than half of the people living with cancer (Stat Bite, 1998).

What are the important QOL issues for individuals with cancer? Preventing or reducing psychosocial morbidity is the focus of intervention efforts. Stress and poor QOL may also have implications for biological processes or health conditions, such as disease progression and spread. We have offered a biobehavioral model (Andersen, Kiecolt-Glaser, & Glaser, 1994) for considering the psychological and QOL stresses of cancer, and we propose mechanisms by which psychological–behavioral responses may influence biological processes and, perhaps, health outcomes. In this chapter I consider the biobehavioral model and evidence for it, but I frame the discussion in the context of the role of psychological interventions for cancer patients and their potential importance for health outcomes. I also illustrate the utility of the model with data from an ongoing clinical trial, the Stress and Immunity Breast Cancer Project.

Psychological Interventions for Cancer Patients: Asking the Right Questions

> What treatment, by whom, is most effective for this individual, with that specific problem, under which set of circumstances, and how does it come about? (Paul, 1969)

This quotation came from a chapter entitled "Behavior Modification Research: Design and Tactics" (p. 44), which was written by Gordon Paul and appeared in Cyril Franks's book, *Behavior Therapy: Appraisal and Status,* published in 1969. This timeless, insightful perspective on a difficult question, namely, "Is psychotherapy effective?" became an important theoretical and research rallying point for investigators conducting treatment comparison investigations, discussing psychotherapy change processes, studying individual differences, and others topics—virtually any arena where the role or effects of a psychological intervention was considered. I bring this familiar and important perspective into the discussion of the biobehavioral model of cancer and interventions for cancer patients. To answer the question regarding the effectiveness of psychosocial interventions with cancer patients, I address important issues in the conceptualization, design, conduct, and outcomes of psychological interventions with cancer patients.

What Treatment, by Whom, Is Most Effective?

Several models of interventions for cancer patients have been developed. These have included, for example, Spiegel's supportive-expressive group therapy (Spiegel & Yalom, 1978; see Spiegel & Diamond, this volume, chapter 12), psychoeducational interventions, such as that used by Fawzy (see Fawzy, Fawzy, & Canada, this volume, chapter 13), and multicomponent efforts. The research literature of the recent decades has focused largely on demonstrating effectiveness of multicomponent interventions rather than making treatment comparisons, although such efforts have appeared in the past (Telch & Telch, 1986) and may well be more prominent in the coming decade (e.g., see Helgesen, Cohen, Schulz, & Yasko, this volume, chapter 14). As the multicomponent effort has been the standard, the research literature indicates that effective therapy components have included the following (Andersen, 1992; Meyer & Mark, 1995):

- relaxation training or related strategies (e.g., guided imagery) to lower "arousal,"
- information about the disease and treatment,
- an emotionally supportive context to address fears and anxieties about the disease,
- behavioral and cognitive coping strategies,
- focused interventions for disease-specific problems, and
- social support.

Even though we do not yet know which components are critical in producing change, preliminary evidence can be obtained from current clinical trials. For example, if assessment modules are included for each therapy component, patient process data on the use of specific intervention components can be related to change on the outcome variables. Data from this "bootstrapping" methodology can subsequently be used to design treatment comparison studies experimentally manipulating the most effective treatment components that have emerged from the bootstrapping data.

Which Individuals Receive Treatment? Do Individual Differences Exist in Risk for Psychosocial/QOL Morbidity?

How are individual differences among cancer patients construed? Types of psychological variables that have been offered have included information-processing models (e.g., Suzanne Miller's monitor-blunter conceptualization; see chapter 18, this volume), consideration of socioeconomic differences as moderators (e.g., Meyerowitz, Richardson, Hudson, & Leedham, 1998), social–cognitive processing (see Lepore, this volume, chapter 6), and others. Alternatively, some have suggested that some cancer treatment experiences are more traumatic than others and result in heightened risk for distress (Cordova, Andrykowski, & Kenady, 1995; see Redd et al., this volume, chapter 5), in contrast to individual differences in response to the treatments.

In considering this issue, it is useful to note important considerations for future research. First, as indicated above, there are different domains of individual differences that could be examined. These can include, for example, disease- and treatment-relevant psychological, behavioral, and physiological (e.g., individuals with chronically "low" vs. "high" immune responses) differences. Research has largely focused on psychological ones (as indicated by the examples above) and approximations of medical ones (e.g., contrasting QOL outcomes for patients who differ in stage of disease). Second, researchers might consider the "fit" of the individual difference to the to-be-predicted outcome. Stated simply, specific individual differences are likely to be better predictors for particular outcomes rather than others (or all outcomes). An example of an individual difference measure to predict risk for a specific type of morbidity will be used for illustration.

Sexual functioning represents an important area of psychosocial morbidity following cancer, and I have tested a model for predicting risk for decrements in sexual behavior and sexual dysfunction (Andersen, 1994). The model was used to operationalize the magnitude of disease and treatment as well as posttreatment health changes affecting sexuality. However, even after considering these important risk factors for sexual morbidity, we found that a sexually relevant individual difference variable—sexual self-schema—could be used to predict significant decrements in sexual behavior and reductions in sexual responsiveness. The predictive value of the model and the outcome-relevant individual-difference variable was reported initially for women with gynecologic cancer (Andersen, Woods, & Copeland, 1997) and replicated with women with breast cancer (Yurek, Farrar, & Andersen, 2000). The sexual self-schema construct was designed as an individual-difference variable for sexual and romantic domains and predicts sexual behavior, responses, and cognitions (Andersen & Cyranowski, 1994; Andersen, Cyranowski, & Espindle, 1999). For my purposes here, however, it serves as an example of tailoring the test of the individual-difference variable to the relevant outcome to maximize predictive power.

What Are the Problems to Treat? What Are the Targets for Change or Outcomes of Cancer Control Psychological Interventions?

Outcomes from psychological interventions generally include, in order of frequency, emotional adjustment, social adjustment, and health outcomes. In contrast, health behaviors and compliance have rarely been an intervention target, although data suggest that such a broadened approach would be important. For example, certain health behaviors, such as dietary intake of fiber or fat, have been related to breast cancer risk (Ballard-Barbash, Forman, & Kipnis, 1999). Problems with compliance cut across many diseases and illnesses. So, too, in cancer, noncompliance with treatment can literally have life-threatening consequences. Depending on the nature of the behavior, it can affect local or distant control of the disease. Noncompliance with radiotherapy can, for example, limit control of the disease at the tumor site or the nodal site, where the risk for metastases is high. Lower levels of compliance with chemotherapy raise the risk of distant metastases and reduce survival time or rate (e.g., Budman et al., 1998).

Psychological interventions can produce improvements in mood, lowered emotional distress, and, typically, more adaptive and fewer maladaptive coping strategies. Improvements in other social or behavioral aspects are inconsistent. However, that we can reliably enhance QOL for cancer patients provides the necessary conditions to move forward and examine biologic mechanisms of change and test for health effects. In the main, measures of disease signs, symptoms, or cancer endpoints have not been included, although there is increasing interest in doing so, as evidenced by the work in such areas as menopausal sequelae following chemotherapy (Carpenter et al., 1998) and fatigue (Andrykowski, Curran, & Lightner, 1998). Studies that have included disease endpoints have, in general, reported lower rates of recurrence or longer survival times (e.g., Fawzy et al., 1993; Spiegel et al., 1989); however, the mechanisms for these effects have been unclear.

How Does Change Occur? What Mechanisms Exist for Biobehavioral Change With Psychological Interventions?

We have viewed stress, QOL, health behaviors, and compliance as the major psychological and behavioral factors in a conceptual model of adjustment to the cancer stressor (Andersen, Kiecolt-Glaser, & Glaser, 1994). Also part of the model are the physiological systems—the endocrine and the immune systems—which may be important for moderating the effects of stress on disease progression. Use of specific endocrine and immune parameters, operationalized with such assays as that for cortisol or natural killer (NK) cell function, respectively, are relevant to the physiologic effects of stress (in the case of the cortisol as an endocrine measure) and risk for disease progression (as in the case of NK cell lysis for immunity); however, these are only examples of possible appropriate measures. Carefully chosen measures of each physiologic system may provide important "windows" on the process of the mind effecting the body in the context of cancer. Few studies have measured endocrine and immune responses, instead relying on psychological or behavioral measures. An exception to this is the research by Fawzy and colleagues (Fawzy,

Cousins, et al., 1990; Fawzy, Kemeny, et al., 1990), who conducted a randomized investigation to reduce stress for newly diagnosed and surgically treated melanoma patients. They reported lower levels of mood disturbance and enhanced immune function (e.g., NK cell lysis) for the psychoeducational intervention group.

To test the direct and indirect effects of psychological and behavioral interventions on biologic and disease processes, it is important to consider the basic research in cancer immunology, cell biology, and tumor immunology (see Finn, this volume, chapter 10; and Triozzi, this volume, chapter 11). These areas are not typically familiar ground for psychologists in general and psychoneuroimmunology (PNI) researchers in particular. However, we cannot ignore the decades of effort and discoveries in these areas and studies of the body's own immunologic fight against cancer. While two decades of research in PNI has brought many advances, the participants in the studies have primarily been healthy individuals undergoing stressful life circumstances or acute stressors (Herbert & Cohen, 1993a, 1993b). The salient exception to this paradigm are studies of individuals with HIV (e.g., Bower, Kemeny, Fahey, & Taylor, 1998).

Psychosocial researchers using immunology measures to examine questions of biobehavioral mechanisms should attend to contextual aspects of cancer, which may covary with immune outcomes and which differ in significant ways from the paradigms used in previous PNI research, including that (a) cancer patients are often ill (or at least recovering) from medical events, such as surgery, chemotherapy, or invasive procedures, which have immunologic consequences; (b) cancer therapies produce immunologic perturbations of varying magnitudes and varying durations, and many of these effects are not yet well documented; and (c) rigorous experimental control is difficult to achieve, and potentially important confounding differences between groups to be compared must be addressed with other strategies (e.g., selection of a homogeneous sample; stratification for a more heterogeneous sample). Taken together, these circumstances challenge investigators interested in biobehavioral responses to move along with the rapid developments in immunology and cell biology and incorporate these exciting new methods (e.g., studies of gene expression) into intervention trials.

Summary

Are interventions for cancer patients effective? The simple answer is an unqualified "yes." Multicomponent treatments achieve broadband improvement—reductions in stress, improved moods, improved social outcomes and, perhaps, reductions in physical symptoms. Moreover, there are positive suggestions that such changes could also be linked to improved biological responses or health outcomes; however, in the coming decade we will require additional data to document the breadth and reliability of such effects and possibilities. Research on individual differences is at the earliest of stages; we are currently at the point of demonstrating the effects of the differences rather than manipulating them or using them to identify individuals for preventive efforts. Finally, investigators attempting to understand the mechanisms for linking psychological–behavioral responses to disease outcomes come to the field at an exciting time with the expanding methods and discoveries in genetics, cell biology, and immunology. This offers great opportunities and challenges for behavioral scientists to merge basic and behavioral sciences research in contemporary cancer control research.

An Experiment With the Biobehavioral Model: The Stress and Immunity Breast Cancer Project

The biobehavioral model is being tested with an experiment, the Stress and Immunity Breast Cancer Project, a randomized clinical trial with women with Stage II or III breast cancer. This group was specifically selected because of their difficult struggle: Current cancer survival data predict that 40% of women with Stage II disease and 60% of women with Stage III disease will experience a recurrence within a 5-year interval. Taken together, the study sample participants have, on average, a 50–50 chance that within 5 years they will experience a recurrence of disease, and at least half of that sample may also die of their disease.

Our hypothesis is that women being treated with the psychological intervention will show lowered stress, increased QOL, more positive health behaviors and fewer negative ones, and greater compliance and, perhaps, reduction in stress hormone (endocrine) responses and an enhancement of immune responses; these events will lead, in turn, to a significant reduction in the frequency of recurrence or to an extension of the disease-free interval. Women enter the trial within days of their breast surgery and prior to beginning any additional radiation, chemotherapy, or hormonal therapy. Assignment to an intervention plus assessment group versus an assessment only group is stratified by prognostic and psychological factors.

The intervention arm of the study is derived from the biobehavioral model. Constructs of the model—stress, quality of life, health behavior, compliance—have been translated to specific intervention components to reduce stress, enhance quality of life, ensure compliance and treatment adherence, and promote health behavior change. For example, the stress reduction component includes a general adaptation syndrome conceptualization of stress and our body's response to it as well as training in progressive muscle relaxation. Our approach differs from previous interventions in that a significant portion of the intervention (approximately 40%) is focused on behavioral factors—progressive relaxation, compliance, and positive health behaviors. Preliminary data from the project suggests that these strategies may be particularly important for the reduction of physiologic aspects of stress because they represent active, behavioral coping efforts.

When the project began we were first interested in testing the relationship between stress and immunity as the women entered the trial, which was following surgery and prior to beginning adjuvant therapy (Andersen et al., 1998). Regression analyses tested a model to predict NK cell lysis—a functional measure of the workings of a relevant immune response—in vitro killing of cells. Three variables chosen for control—age, disease stage, and days since surgery—were entered as Step 1. Step 2 consisted of the percentage of cells (lymphocytes) that were NK and therefore available to lyse (kill), because the percentage of NK cells would obviously contribute to the total amount of the lysis. This factor was indeed important as it accounted for 15% of the variance in the total lysis. Finally, in Step 3, stress (as measured by the Impact of Event Scale; Horowitz, Wilner, & Alvarez, 1979) accounted for significant, additional variance, with the entire model accounting for 21% of the variance.

We also examined the reliability of the effect. Indeed, the same negative stress effect was there across all of the effector:target cell (E:T) ratios for NK cell lysis. Moreover, the same negative effect of stress was found for the poorer response of the NK cells to recombinant gamma interferon, a biological response modifier used to enhance NK cell activity. That is, stress contributed to the NK cells being less responsive to gamma interferon, again across all E:T ratios.

We also tested T-cell responsiveness to stress. The first simple test was to predict the numbers of T cells, and stress could predict both T-cell counts and percentages. More important was to test for down regulation of T-cell functional responses. We conducted assays in which a monoclonal antibody to the T-cell receptor was added to stimulate the peripheral blood leukocytes, and we then measured proliferation (cell division). Again it was found that stress lowered the level of responsiveness of the T lymphocytes. Another way to study the same process is to stimulate the T cells with a mitogen and measure proliferation (i.e., rate of cell division). The reliability of this phenomenon was tested with two mitogens, Concanavalin A and phytohemagglutinin (PHA), and then tested across three concentrations each. Again, the same negative stress effect was found, replicated across different mitogens and concentrations of each mitogen.

In summary, these analyses controlled for factors expected to exert long- or short-term effects on these immune responses. In all cases, the models tested were significant, and the contribution of stress was significant and in the correct (inhibitory) direction, both between and within assays. All models accounted for 15% to 30% of the variance. Stress assessed following diagnosis and definitive surgical treatment was reliably related to impairment of the functional responses of NK cells and T lymphocytes. These findings suggest that if an individual with cancer is significantly stressed, and nothing is done to alleviate it, then stress may negatively influence his or her immune response.

The focus of the trial is to experimentally determine whether an intervention designed to reduce cancer-related stress and enhance mood could also influence biologic responses, that is, to down-regulate (lower) endocrine stress responses and up-regulate (enhance) immune responses. Prior to beginning standard adjuvant therapy, all patients complete a psychological, behavioral, biological, and health assessment. Women are randomized to one of two arms: intervention and assessment or assessment only. The 12-month psychological–behavioral intervention consists of an intensive phase with weekly sessions for 4 months and then a maintenance phase with monthly sessions for 8 months. Monitoring of all patients is repeated at 4, 8, and 12 months. The data will provide the opportunity to examine psychological and biological mechanisms.

Conclusion

The results from psychological intervention studies are encouraging. The psychological and behavioral effects are essential, and our hope is to make them as robust as possible to enhance the women's lives and be able to test the questions regarding health effects and examination of endocrine and immune mechanisms. Our assessment strategy, at all levels and within all domains, is one of converging operations. The experiment is extraordinarily simple (contrasting something with nothing), but it is simple by design, because the mechanisms and the outcomes of the adjustment to the cancer stressor are complex and poorly understood. In characterizing immunity, some textbooks refer to an *immune cascade*, meaning that any specific immune response can involve a complex cascade of events that extends over many days. Furthermore, we know now that direct and peripheral products of stress can play many roles in regulating this cascade, and so the effects of stress will be variable as well. Thus far, data suggest that the interventions are capable of producing positive psychological effects, and perhaps biological effects as well. We await further results regarding the disease implications of these findings.

References

Andersen, B. L. (1992). Psychological interventions for cancer patients to enhance the quality of life. *Journal of Consulting and Clinical Psychology, 60,* 552–568.

Andersen, B. L. (1994). Surviving cancer. *Cancer, 74,* 1484–1495.

Andersen, B. L., & Cyranowski, J. C. (1994). Women's sexual self schema. *Journal of Personality and Social Psychology, 67,* 1079–1100.

Andersen, B. L., & Cyranowski, J. C., & Espindle, D. (1999). Men's sexual self schema. *Journal of Personality and Social Psychology, 76,* 645–661.

Andersen, B. L., Farrar, W. B., Golden-Kreutz, D., Kutz, L. A., MacCallum, R., Courtney, M. E., & Glaser, R. (1998). Stress and immune responses following surgical treatment of regional breast cancer. *Journal of the National Cancer Institute, 90*(1), 30–36.

Andersen, B. L., Kiecolt-Glaser, J. K., & Glaser, R. (1994). A biobehavioral model of cancer stress and disease course. *American Psychologist, 49,* 389–404.

Andersen, B. L., Woods, X. A., & Copeland, L. J. (1997). Sexual self schema and sexual morbidity among gynecologic cancer survivors. *Journal of Consulting and Clinical Psychology, 65,* 221–229.

Andrykowski, M. A., Curran, S. L., & Lightner, R. (1998). Off-treatment fatigue in breast cancer survivors: A controlled comparison. *Journal of Behavioral Medicine, 21,* 1–18.

Ballard-Barbash, R., Forman, M. R., & Kipnis, V. (1999). Dietary fat, serum estrogen levels, and breast cancer risk: A multifaceted story. *Journal of the National Cancer Institute, 91,* 492–534.

Bower, J. E., Kemeny, M. E., Fahey, J. L., & Taylor, S. E. (1998). Cognitive processing, discovery of meaning, CD4 decline, and AIDS related mortality among bereaved HIV-seropositive men. *Journal of Consulting and Clinical Psychology, 66,* 979–986.

Budman, D. R., Berry, D. A., Cirrincione, C. T., Henderson, I. C., Wood, W. C., Weiss, R. B., Ferree, C. R., Muss, H. B., Green, M. R., Norton, L., & Frei, E., III. (1998). Dose and dose intensity as determinants of outcome in the adjuvant treatment of breast cancer. *Journal of the National Cancer Institute, 90,* 1205–1211.

Carpenter, J. S., Andrykowski, M. A., Cordova, M., Cunningham, L., Studts, J., McGrath, P., Kenady, D., Sloan, D., & Mussen, R. (1998). Hot flashes in postmenopausal women treated for breast carcinoma. *Cancer, 82,* 1682–1691.

Ciborowski, P., Hiltbold, E. M., Barratt-Boyes, S., & Finn, O. J. (1999). MUC1 mucin as a tumor antigen in breast cancer. In A. M. Bowcock (Ed.), *Breast cancer: Molecular genetics, pathogenesis and therapeutics* (pp. 453–468). Totowa, NJ: Humana Press.

Cordova, M. J., Andrykowski, M. A., & Kenady, D. E. (1995). Frequency and correlates of posttraumatic stress disorder-like symptoms after treatment for breast cancer. *Journal of Consulting and Clinical Psychology, 63,* 981–986.

Dhabhar, F. S., Miller, A. H., McEwen, B. S., & Spencer, R. L. (1995). Effects of stress on immune cell distribution: Dynamics and hormonal mechanisms. *Journal of Immunology, 154,* 5511–5527.

Fawzy, F. I., Cousins, N., Fawzy, N. W., Kemeny, M. E., Elashoff, R., & Morton, D. (1990). Structured psychiatric intervention for cancer patients: I. Changes over time in methods of coping and affective disturbance. *Archives of General Psychiatry, 47,* 720–725.

Fawzy, F. I., Fawzy, N. W., Hyun, C. S., Gutherie, D., Fahey, J. L., & Morton, D. (1993). Malignant melanoma: Effects of a early structured psychiatric intervention, coping, and affective state on recurrence and survival six years later. *Archives of General Psychiatry, 50,* 681–689.

Fawzy, F. I., Kemeny, M. E., Fawzy, N. W., Elashoff, R., Morton, D., Cousins, N., & Fahey, J. L. (1990). A structured psychiatric intervention for cancer patients: II. Changes over time in immunological measures. *Archives of General Psychiatry, 47,* 729–735.

Gotay, C. C., & Muraoka, M. Y. (1998). Quality of life in long-term survivors of adult-onset cancers. *Journal of the National Cancer Institute, 90,* 656–667.

Greenlee, R. T., Murray, T., Bolden, S., & Wingo, P. A. (2000). Cancer statistics, 2000. *CA-A Cancer Journal for Clinicians, 50,* 7–33.

Henderson, R. A., & Finn, O. J. (1996). Human tumor antigens are ready to fly. *Advanced Immunology, 62,* 217–256.

Herbert, T. B., & Cohen, S. (1993a). Depression and immunity: A meta-analytic review. *Psychological Bulletin, 113*, 472–486.

Herbert, T. B., & Cohen, S. (1993b). Stress and immunity in humans: A meta-analytic review. *Psychosomatic Medicine, 55*, 364–379.

Horowitz, M., Wilner, N., & Alvarez, W. (1979). Impact of Event Scale: A measure of subjective stress. *Psychosomatic Medicine, 41*(3), 209–218.

Jerome, K. R., Lomenech, N., & Finn, O. J. (1996). Tumor-specific cytotoxic T cell clones from patients with breast and pancreatic adenocarcinoma recognize EBV-immortalized B cells transfected with polymorphic epithelial mucin complementary DNA. *Journal of Immunology, 151*, 1654–1657.

Meyer, T. J., & Mark, M. M. (1995). Effects of psychosocial interventions with adult cancer patients: A meta-analysis of randomized experiments. *Health Psychology, 14*, 101–108.

Meyerowitz, B. E., Richardson, J., Hudson, S., & Leedham, B. (1998). Ethnicity and cancer outcomes: Behavioral and psychosocial considerations. *Psychological Bulletin, 123*, 47–70.

Paul, G. L. (1969). Behavior modification research: Design and tactics. In C. M. Franks (Ed.), *Behavior therapy: Appraisal and status* (pp. 29–62). New York: McGraw-Hill.

Spiegel, D., Bloom, J. R., Kraemer, H. C., & Gottheil, E. (1989). Effect of psychosocial treatment on survival of patients with metastatic breast cancer. *Lancet, 2*, 888–891.

Spiegel, D., & Yalom, I. D. (1978). A support group for dying patients. *International Journal of Group Psychotherapy, 28*, 233–245.

Spiker, A. V., Trijsburg, R. W., & Duivenvoorden, H. J. (1997). Psychological sequelae of cancer diagnosis: A meta-analytical review of 58 studies after 1980. *Psychosomatic Medicine, 59*, 280–293.

Stat bite: Persons living with major cancers in the United States, 1998. (1998). *Journal of the National Cancer Institute, 90*(8), 565.

Telch, C. F., & Telch, M. J. (1986). Group coping skills instruction and supportive group therapy for cancer patients: A comparison of strategies. *Journal of Consulting and Clinical Psychology, 54*, 802–808.

Wyllie, A. H. (1980). Glucocorticoid-induced thymocyte apoptosis is associated with endogenous endonuclease activation. *Nature, 284*, 555–556.

Yurek, D., Farrar, W., & Andersen, B. L. (2000). Breast cancer surgery: Comparing surgical groups and determining individual differences in post operative sexuality and body change stress. *Journal of Consulting and Clinical Psychology, 68*, 697–709.

CHAPTER 8

Group Processes in Therapeutic Support Groups

Paul B. Paulus

For many years I have been interested in the relationship of group factors such as crowding and social interaction to the health and well-being of individuals in a wide range of contexts (e.g., Paulus & Nagar, 1987). I examined a limited number of issues related to group dynamics, such as the stress-inducing impact of uncontrolled interactions in crowded prisons and the potentially positive impact of social interaction for Army families living near Army posts (Paulus, 1987; Paulus, Nagar, Larey, & Camacho, 1996). My knowledge of group dynamics and of health psychology has remained mostly in discrete unrelated cognitive categories. Recently, however, I have come to realize the many ways in which principles of group dynamics can be related to the ways in which individuals cope with cancer and other serious health problems. The focus of my research in the last few years has been on group creativity and teamwork (Paulus, Brown, & Ortega, 1999; Paulus, Larey, & Dzindolet, 2000). In particular, we have been interested in understanding the social and cognitive processes related to the idea-generation and sharing process. The principles that underlie the performance of idea-generating groups may have implications for the effectiveness of the sharing process in the therapeutic support groups.

In this chapter I discuss briefly the exciting potential of connections between the group dynamics literature and research on social factors in health. Research on groups has a long and distinguished history and has focused on many problems of practical interest, such as conflict resolution, bargaining, decision making, and social influence (cf. Hare, Blumberg, Davies, & Kent, 1994; Paulus, 1980, 1989). Much of the theoretically oriented research has been done in laboratory settings, but there is also much interesting research on family interaction, therapy groups, and teamwork (Cohen & Bailey, 1997; Levine & Moreland, 1990). I focus primarily on the implica-

This chapter was written while the author was a visiting scholar at the University of Pittsburgh and Carnegie Mellon University.

tions of general group processes for coping with serious health problems, and especially on the dynamics of structured support groups that involve sharing of feelings and information.

The Sharing Process

One of the most fundamental aspects of group interaction is the opportunity it provides for development of a shared reality (Levine, Resnick, & Higgins, 1993). In groups we can compare our abilities, attitudes, and feelings with those of others (Festinger, 1954). This facilitates the development of our self-concept and sense of uniqueness (Suls & Wills, 1991). However, in many domains of our life there is a high level of uncertainty about how one should construe reality in that there are no objective standards. For example, how important is freedom of speech versus the sensitivity of certain segments of society? This uncertainty often characterizes our response to the diagnosis of a serious illness. What does it mean, and what is likely to happen? Should I tell my friends? What should my friends and family do to help me deal with it? Given this level of uncertainty, it is quite likely that there will be a strong desire for social comparison. Individuals tend to seek out those who are similar to themselves when they seek to understand social reality (Festinger, 1954). Thus, those who have been diagnosed with a particular form of cancer should tend to seek out those with a similar type of cancer to discuss feelings, strategies, and hopes.

Not all individuals are equally likely to seek out such social comparison opportunities. Some individuals are loners or are uncomfortable in groups. Social interaction anxiety (Leary & Kowalski, 1993), introversion (Barry & Stewart, 1997), and sociability (Bouchard, 1969) are just some of the characteristics related to desire to interact with others and the reactions to group interactions. It is likely that group interventions such as social support groups are most effective for those individuals who are socially inclined. It is even possible that group interactions may hinder adjustment of individuals who are low in social inclinations. Social loners may find individual-coping strategies such as cognitive reevaluation and exercise and individual-based programs such as education and individual counseling most helpful. Group interventions are sometimes quite successful (see also Spiegel & Diamond, this volume, chapter 12) and at other times produce negative reactions (see also Helgeson, Cohen, Schulz, & Yasko, this volume, chapter 14). The social characteristics of the group members could be partly responsible for these disparate outcomes. One would expect that the typical group would have a mixture of high- and low-sociable individuals. This could be optimum in that the high-sociable members may prime the sharing pump because they are outgoing and talkative and may in turn encourage participation of low-sociable members. For example, Barry and Stewart (1997) found that groups with 20% to 40% extroverts outperformed groups with a higher or lower percentage of extroverts on creativity problem-solving tasks. It is interesting that group members rated openness of the communication within the group as not related to the percentage of extroverts. Thus, it is likely that introverts and extroverts have equal interest in sharing their thoughts and feelings, and supportive or well-facilitated group interactions should elicit meaningful sharing by all group members.

One factor that is likely to be critical in the extent to which group members (in particular introverted ones) openly share their feelings in a group is the degree to which the group context is nonevaluative or supportive. This has been emphasized in the group creativity and team innovation literatures (Osborn, 1957; West & Anderson, 1996). Osborn (1957, 1963) felt strongly that it is important to defer judgment of shared ideas or feelings during the sharing process to insure that all pertinent perspectives are shared. West and Anderson (1996) found that support for innovation in the organization was a critical factor in determining the extent to which top management teams developed innovations. In support groups there are several factors that may inhibit openness among group members. There may be a high level of evaluation apprehension in newly formed groups (Paulus & Murdoch, 1971). Group members may have a strong desire to gain approval and be concerned about the reactions of group members to their feelings. If group members have not shared their feelings before in a group setting, there may be a strong uncertainty about the appropriateness of their thoughts and feelings. There often is a desire for consensus in groups (Janis, 1982). Thus, when conflicting perspectives are shared in the group, there may be a tendency of group members to be more supportive of certain perspectives than others. To avoid further conflict, group members may inhibit sharing of thoughts and feelings inconsistent with the dominant group perspective.

Alternatively, therapeutic goals may involve reinforcing the types of thoughts and feelings presumed to be consistent with effective coping or adjustment (e.g., optimism vs. pessimism). However, if an open sharing process involving all group members is desired, group members should feel free to share all of their thoughts and feelings. This will increase the likelihood that individuals will be exposed to conflicting perspectives, which in turn may stimulate a careful reassessment of the validity of their own thoughts and feelings (Levine & Thompson, 1996). If the group members become concerned about persuading others about the validity of their own perspectives, resulting group conflicts may be a source of additional tension and stress.

Support groups are likely to go through a series of stages or phases (Levine & Moreland, 1994). In the initial phases of group sharing, there may be a focus on the negative aspects of the present life dilemma. Because groups tend to polarize or become more extreme when there is an apparent consensus for a particular point of view (cf. Myers, 1982), the group exchange of negative feelings may further increase the negative affect experienced by group members. Lepore (this volume, chapter 6) presents some evidence that those who focus on negatives have more impact on the group than those who focus on positives. However, it is also possible that these negative effects are restricted to the initial group interactions. Once there has been a purging of negative emotions, group members may focus on ways to develop a more positive perspective. Conflicts in the group may be resolved and may even stimulate the group members to develop clearer and more cognitively consistent perspectives (Levine et al., 1993; Nemeth, 1995). Thus, the initial focus on expressing negative feelings may shift to a focus on dealing with these feelings, effective coping strategies, and the positive aspects of one's dilemma.

One factor that could shift the group in a positive direction is a tendency toward downward comparison. In order to feel better about one's health status, individuals may compare themselves with those who are less fortunate (Taylor, 1989). For example, married women diagnosed with breast cancer may compare themselves favorably with those who are not married. Those with Stage 1 cancer may find comfort in comparing themselves with those with Stage 2 or 3. However, upward comparison processes may also become more prevalent in later sessions as group members may begin to focus on survivors or those who have dealt successfully with the emotional consequences of a cancer diagnosis.

The Positive Perspective on Group Sharing

One interesting phenomenon is that group members may have very positive perceptions of their effectiveness. For example, members of groups involved in idea generation rate their performance more favorably than those who perform in isolation even though performance of the group members is inferior (Paulus, Dzindolet, Poletes, & Camacho, 1993). Groups also appear to enjoy their experience more than do solitary performers. Thus, self-ratings may be poor indicators of actual effectiveness of group activities and should not be used as sole indicators of effectiveness of group interventions. One very positive feature of many of the studies presented in this volume is that they use objective physiological measures of intervention outcomes. These studies can thus determine to what extent participant perceptions and objective physiological outcomes are consistent. These two indicators clearly may not be independent. Participant perceptions or feelings about the psychosocial intervention may play an important role in determining its actual effect on health.

There appears to be a general presumption that the sharing process in social support groups is eventually beneficial. However, even after overcoming initial conflicts and negativity, how can we be sure that such groups begin focusing on the most appropriate domains or topics and develop a shared reality that is helpful in coping with cancer? Those with a naive belief in the wisdom of groups might believe that groups inevitably discover the most useful strategies or reality for their group members. This type of positive image of groups is shared by those who have been promoting teamwork in organizations (Tjosvold, 1991). Organizations are increasingly turning to teamwork as part of a strategy of redesigning the work process to increase worker motivation and effective use of talent. Many case studies have strongly supported the efficacy of teamwork, and members of self-managing teams rate their effectiveness more favorably than do those in traditional teams. However, the data comparing the actual effectiveness of self-managing teams are often mixed (Cohen & Bailey, 1997; Cotton, 1993). Only teams that are self-managed seem to be related to positive outcomes (Cohen & Bailey, 1997). These teams have a lot of autonomy in making decisions about the work process. Presumably, these types of teams lead to higher levels of motivation, better use of talent, and better adjustment to changing external factors (Goodman, Devadas, & Hughson, 1988). However, autonomous teams require much training in order to function effectively (Stevens & Campion, 1994).

What are the implications of the teamwork literature for support groups? It suggests that these groups should be given a great degree of autonomy so that they can discover the most effective means of functioning for their particular group. Too much control by the facilitator may limit member motivation and the ability of the group to reach its unique therapeutic potential. However, groups should be trained in effective group dynamics so that they function effectively without strong outside control or intervention by a facilitator.

The Negative Perspective on Group Sharing

Although teamwork is popular, one often encounters negative stories about group effectiveness. That is, groups on their own may drift, get into nonproductive discussions, and do a poor job of tapping their potential. There is often a great disparity in the contributions of group members (Bonita & Hollingshead, 1997). Some members tend to dominate the discussions or group interactions (Bales, 1970). Other members may not be highly motivated to contribute to the group discussion. Group research has documented a variety of instances of reduced motivation in groups, such as social loafing or free riding (Shepperd, 1993). Problems of group effectiveness are clearly evident in studies of idea sharing in groups. These studies have often used Osborn's (1957) brainstorming rules to encourage the sharing of ideas. These rules encourage individuals to share all thoughts that come to mind, to be accepting of all ideas as they are presented, and to try to generate as many ideas as possible. Even with the use of these rules, groups generate many fewer ideas than comparable numbers of individual idea generators. This may reflect the reduced motivation of group members, a concern about how others might react to one's ideas, or the inability to fully share one's ideas in groups when one is competing with other group members for time (Diehl & Stroebe, 1987). Group members also tend to match their idea generation rate to that of other group members, particularly the low-performing ones (Camacho & Paulus, 1995; Paulus & Dzindolet, 1993).

Another problem with groups that is evident from the group decision and idea generation literature is that groups share only a very limited amount of the information or ideas relevant to a particular issue (Connolly, Routhieaux, & Schneider,

1993; Gettys, Pliske, Manning, & Casey, 1987). This is reflected in observations of groupthink in which groups tend to limit expression of ideas inconsistent with the dominant group perspective (Janis, 1982). Groups also are more likely to focus on information or ideas that they have in common rather than unshared perspectives (Stewart & Stasser, 1995). That is, there is a bias to reinforce those ideas that are expressed in the group. This commonality bias may limit the extent to which individuals express their unique perspectives (Gigone & Hastie, 1993). Ironically, these perspectives may be most important because they may stimulate much group discussion or reflection. However, it is exactly these unique perspectives that may lead to lack of support and a negative experience in groups.

Improving the Group Sharing Process

The perspective from group idea generation studies is that groups may actually inhibit one's ability to fully share one's feelings and ideas. However, there are a number of ways to counteract this problem. Groups may be provided with sufficient time for all members to share their perspectives. Yet even under such conditions, group members generate fewer ideas than do solitary individuals (Diehl & Stroebe, 1991). A promising alternative is for group leaders to help groups function in a more productive manner or to train groups to function effectively (Offner, Kramer, & Winter, 1996; Oxley, Dzindolet, & Paulus, 1996). Another possibility is to combine individual sharing with group sharing. Writing about past traumas can be quite therapeutic (Lepore, 1997; Pennebaker, 1993). Writing out one's thoughts and feelings prior to a group session may ensure that each individual taps into the full range of relevant issues prior to the group discussion. During group discussion, the group may tend to focus on a very limited set of issues. Prior solitary idea generation may make more salient other areas that the group needs to explore. With appropriate facilitation, these diverse issues may be more easily elicited if groups have prior individual focusing sessions. Alternatively, group members may benefit from working through some of the issues raised in the group discussion right after the group session. Even though this may occur naturally in the course of the subsequent days, the many competing events of one's life may inhibit a full working through mentally of these issues. Furthermore, an individual follow-up session may allow for rehearsal of key issues and further development of their relevance for the individual and specific ways that the individual might want to act on some of the shared ideas. This incubation or concretization period may be very useful in ensuring the successful application of insights gained from the group discussion (Csikszentmihalyi & Sawyer, 1995).

It would also be possible to use information gained from individualistic writing sessions to compose groups with similar mental models or concerns. This might increase the likelihood that groups would provide reinforcement and support and would help in the developing of a shared reality. Alternatively, it might be necessary to "prime" groups to consider certain perspectives or issues. The prewriting experience may provide information about areas of denial or avoidance. The groups can then be led to consider these issues or other important issues by a facilitator. This presumes a strong knowledge base for determining the types of issues that should be considered by groups. This may vary with the type of group or population and type of problem.

The way the problem is structured in the group may also be quite important. Groups have a higher overall rate of performance or idea sharing when their session is divided into smaller time periods or segments than when there is just one overall session (Kelly & Karau, 1993). Time segmentation seems to affect the overall pacing of the group activity. One way to approach time segmentation is to ask the group to discuss different aspects of a problem in sequential periods of time rather than having the group consider all aspects simultaneously (Coskun, Paulus, Brown, & Sherwood, in press; Dennis, Valacich, Connolly, & Wynne, 1996). The sequential approach seems to lead to a more extensive tapping of the cognitive content related to an issue or problem than a simultaneous approach.

The studies of psychosocial interventions with cancer patients have involved the use of a wide variety of interventions—social support groups, educational information, and telephone counseling. These different types of modalities vary in the extent to which they involve face-to-face contact with others. Face-to-face contact may be important in situations where there is sharing of feelings. Access to many pertinent nonverbal cues may facilitate the effectiveness of the emotional sharing process. For example, studies comparing face-to-face and computer based interaction have found that group decision making is facilitated in face-to-face contexts (McGrath & Hollingshead, 1994). However, electronic groups help avoid the type of blocking often experienced in verbal sharing groups (Gallupe, Bastianutti, & Cooper, 1991).

All of the social support group studies presented in this volume have involved face-to-face groups. It would be of interest to determine the effectiveness of other modalities of interaction. It may be difficult for participants to attend support groups on a regular basis. Electronic support groups could be compared with face-to-face groups to determine their relative effectiveness. The electronic groups could be designed to interact simultaneously, or the group could access a designated chat room at regular times. Clearly, however, electronic or written exchange of feelings may have less impact and result in much less commitment to the sharing process than occurs in face-to-face groups. However, even if that is the case, some combination of modalities may be optimal. There may be some initial reticence to share one's personal feelings with other strangers in a face-to-face format. An initial period of sharing using some anonymous procedure (either writing or electronic) may help reduce this type of inhibition. Studies of self-disclosure have demonstrated that people respond to written or oral personal self-disclosures with their own intimate disclosures (Davis, 1976). I have used a writing self-disclosure exercise several times as a class demonstration. Very personal feelings are shared after a short period of self-disclosure exchanges among pairs of students. At the end of the exercise there is often a strong desire to continue exchanging self-disclosures with the partner. Electronic support groups may be particularly useful as a means of continuing group contact after the actual sessions have been completed. Access to such electronically based interactions can allow one to assess the nature of these interactions and how they are related to individual and group adjustment.

One positive feature of some of the studies presented in this volume is their ability to use random assignment to treatments. Random assignment is not common in the study of groups outside laboratory settings. In many real world contexts this is either not feasible or it is not possible to get the cooperation of the organization. For example, no study compares traditional and self-managed teams in which team members are randomly assigned (Cohen & Ledford, 1994). It is likely that there are important differences in participant characteristics that determine whether they end up as a self-managing or a traditional team. In some of the psychosocial interventions, volunteers may refuse random assignment but are still included in the study. With sufficient samples, these studies have an interesting opportunity to examine differences in outcomes between those who are randomly assigned and those who are not.

In summary, there is much potential benefit from a more careful integration of the literature on group dynamics with the use of support groups in health care. The groups literature suggests a number of interesting avenues for research and application in the area of social interventions and health. The study of support groups and health outcomes provide an exciting new arena for the study of group processes.

References

Bales, B. F. (1970). *Personality and interpersonal behavior*. New York: Holt Rinehart, & Winston.

Barry, B., & Stewart, G. L. (1997). Composition, process, and performance in self-managed groups: The role of personality. *Journal of Applied Psychology, 82*, 62–78.

Bonito, J. A., & Hollingshead, A. B. (1997). Participation in small groups. In B. R. Burleson, A.W. Kunkel, et al. (Eds.), *Communication yearbook 20* (pp. 227–261). Thousand Oaks, CA: Sage.

Bouchard, T. J. (1969). Personality, problem-solving procedure, and performance in small groups. *Journal of Applied Psychology Monographs, 53*, 1–28.

Camacho, L. M., & Paulus, P. B. (1995). The role of social anxiousness in group brainstorming. *Journal of Personality and Social Psychology, 68*, 1071–1080.

Cohen, S. G., & Bailey, D. E. (1997). What makes teams work: Group effectiveness research from the shop floor to the executive suite. *Journal of Management, 23*, 239–290.

Cohen, S. G., & Ledford, G. E. (1994). The effectiveness of self-managing teams: A quasi-experiment. *Human Relations, 47*, 13–43.

Connolly, T., Routhieaux, R. L., & Schneider, S. K. (1993). On the effectiveness of group brainstorming: Test of one underlying cognitive mechanism. *Small Group Research*, 24, 490–503.

Coskun, H., Paulus, P. B., Brown, V., & Sherwood, J. J. (in press). Cognitive stimulation and problem presentation in idea generating groups. *Group Dynamics: Theory, Research, and Practice.*

Cotton, J. L. (1993). *Employee involvement.* Newbury Park, CA: Sage.

Csikszentmihalyi, M., & Sawyer, K. (1995). Creative insight: The social dimension of a solitary moment. In R. J. Sternberg & J. E. Davidson (Eds.), *The nature of insight* (pp. 329–363). Cambridge, MA: MIT Press.

Davis, J. D. (1976). Self-disclosure in an acquaintance exercise: Responsibility for level of intimacy. *Journal of Personality and Social Psychology, 33,* 787–792.

Dennis, A. R., Valacich, J. S., Connolly, T., & Wynne, B. E. (1996). Process structuring in electronic brainstorming. *Information Systems Research, 7,* 268–277.

Diehl, M., & Stroebe, W. (1987). Productivity loss in brainstorming groups: Toward the solution of a riddle. *Journal of Personality and Social Psychology, 53,* 497–509.

Diehl, M., & Stroebe, W. (1991). Productivity loss in idea-generating groups: Tracking down the blocking effect. *Journal of Personality and Social Psychology, 61,* 392–403.

Festinger, L. (1954). A theory of social comparison processes. *Human Relations, 7,* 117–140.

Gallupe, R. B., Bastianutti, L. M., & Cooper, W. H. (1991). Unblocking brainstorms. *Journal of Applied Psychology, 76,* 137–142.

Gettys, C. F., Pliske, R. M., Manning, C., & Casey, J. T. (1987). An evaluation of human act generation performance. *Organizational Behavior and Human Decision Processes, 39,* 23–31.

Gigone, D., & Hastie, R. (1993). The common knowledge effect: Information sharing and group judgment. *Journal of Personality and Social Psychology, 65,* 959–974.

Goodman, P. S., Devadas, R., & Hughson, T. L. G. (1988). Groups and productivity: Analyzing the effectiveness of self-managing teams. In J. P. Campbell & R. J. Campbell (Eds.), *Productivity in organizations* (pp. 295–327). San Francisco: Jossey-Bass.

Hare, A. P., Blumberg, H. H., Davies, M. F., & Kent, M. V. (1994). *Small group research: A handbook.* Norwood, NJ: Ablex.

Janis, I. L. (1982). *Groupthink* (2nd ed.). Boston: Houghton-Mifflin.

Kelly, J. R., & Karau, S. J. (1993). Entrainment in small groups. *Small Group Research,* 24, 179–198.

Leary, M. R., & Kowalski, R. (1993). The Interaction Anxiousness Scale: Construct and criterion-related validity. *Journal of Personality Assessment, 61,* 136–146.

Lepore, S. J. (1997). Expressive writing moderates the relation between intrusive thoughts and depressive symptoms. *Journal of Personality and Social Psychology, 73,* 1030–1037.

Levine, J. M., & Moreland, R. L. (1990). Progress in small groups research. *Annual Review of Psychology, 41,* 585–634.

Levine, J. M., & Moreland, R. L. (1994). Group socialization: Theory and research. In W. Stroebe & M. Hewstone (Eds.), *The European review of social psychology* (Vol. 5, pp. 305–336). Chichester, England: Wiley.

Levine, J. M., Resnick, L. B., & Higgins, E. T. (1993). Social foundations of cognition. *Annual Review of Psychology, 44,* 585–612.

Levine, J. M., & Thompson, L. (1996). Conflict in groups. In E. T. Higgins & A. W. Kruglanski (Eds.), *Social psychology: Handbook of basic principles* (pp. 745–776). New York: Guilford Press.

McGrath, J. E., & Hollingshead, A. B. (1994). *Groups interacting with technology.* Thousand Oaks, CA: Sage.

Myers, D. G. (1982). Polarizing effects of group interaction. In H. Brandstatter, J. H. Davis, & G. Stocker-Kreichgauer (Eds.), *Group decision making* (pp. 125–161). New York: Academic Press.

Nemeth, C. J. (1995). Dissent as driving cognition, attitudes, and judgements. *Social Cognition, 13,* 273–291.

Offner, A. K., Kramer, T. J., & Winter, J. P. (1996). The effects of facilitation, recording, and pauses on group brainstorming. *Small Group Research, 27,* 283–298.

Osborn, A. F. (1957). *Applied imagination.* New York: Scribner.

Osborn, A. F. (1963). *Applied imagination* (2nd ed.). New York: Scribner.

Oxley, N. L., Dzindolet, M. T., & Paulus, P. B. (1996). The effects of facilitators on the performance of brainstorming groups. *Journal of Social Behavior and Personality, 11,* 633–646.

Paulus, P. B. (Ed.). (1980). *Psychology of group influence.* Hillsdale, NJ: Erlbaum.

Paulus, P. B. (1987). *Prison crowding: A psychological perspective.* New York: Springer-Verlag.

Paulus, P. B. (Ed.). (1989). *Psychology of group influence* (2nd ed.). Hillsdale, NJ: Erlbaum.

Paulus, P. B., Brown, V., & Ortega, A. H. (1999). Group creativity. In R. E. Purser & A. Montuori (Eds.), *Social creativity* (Vol. 2, pp. 151–176). Cresskill, NJ: Hampton.

Paulus, P. B., & Dzindolet, M. T. (1993). Social influence processes in group brainstorming. *Journal of Personality and Social Psychology, 64,* 575–586.

Paulus, P. B., Dzindolet, M. T., Poletes, G., & Camacho, L. M. (1993). Perception of performance in group brainstorming: The illusion of group productivity. *Personality and Social Psychology Bulletin, 19,* 78–89.

Paulus, P. B., Larey, T. S., & Dzindolet, M. T. (2000). Creativity in groups and teams. In M. Turner (Ed.), *Groups at work: Advances in theory and research* (pp. 319–338). Mahwah, NJ: Erlbaum.

Paulus, P. B., & Murdoch, P. (1971). Anticipated evaluation and audience presence in the enhancement of dominant responses. *Journal of Experimental Social Psychology, 7,* 280–291.

Paulus, P. B., & Nagar, D. (1987). Environmental influences on social interaction and group development. In C. Hendrick (Ed.), *Review of personality and social psychology* (Vol. 9, pp. 68–90). Beverly Hills, CA: Sage.

Paulus, P. B., Nagar, D., Larey, T. S., & Camacho, L. M. (1996). Environmental, lifestyle, and psychological factors in the health and well-being of military families. *Journal of Applied Social Psychology, 26,* 2053–2075.

Pennebaker, J. W. (1993). Putting stress into words: Health, linguistic, and therapeutic implications. *Behavioral Research and Therapy, 31,* 539–548.

Shepperd, J. A. (1993). Productivity loss in performance groups: A motivation analysis. *Psychological Bulletin, 113,* 67–81.

Stevens, M. J., & Campion, M. A. (1994). The knowledge, skill, and ability requirements for teamwork: Implications for human resource management. *Journal of Management, 20,* 503–530.

Stewart, D. D., & Stasser, G. (1995). Expert role assignment and information sampling during collective recall and decision–making. *Journal of Personality and Social Psychology, 69,* 619–628.

Suls, J. M., & Wills, T. A. (Eds.). (1991). *Social comparison: Contemporary theory and research.* Hillsdale, NJ: Erlbaum.

Taylor, S. E. (1989). *Positive illusions.* New York: Basic Books.

Tjosvold, D. (1991). *Team organization: An enduring competitive advantage.* New York: Wiley.

West, M. A., & Anderson, N. R. (1996). Innovation in top management teams. *Journal of Applied Psychology, 81,* 680–693.

Traumatic Stress as a Target for Intervention With Cancer Patients

Andrew Baum

Donna M. Posluszny

A major theme in behavioral medicine, health psychology, and related disciplines has been the role of stress, emotions, thoughts, and behaviors in the etiology of disease. These factors appear to affect vulnerability to infection, pathogenic processes that contribute to disease, and a variety of other conditions associated with ill health. However, behavioral and psychological processes are also important after diseases have developed and been diagnosed. Regardless of their causes, diseases like cancer and heart disease are stressful and expose people to a broad range of threats, burdens, and potential losses. They often pose sudden and intense life threat, introducing the possibility of psychological trauma, and many aspects of their treatment are stressful as well. Disruption of one's everyday routine and of family and work relationships can compound these treatment effects. At the same time, diseases disturb homeostasis and strain the physiological systems that regulate mood, behavior, and resistance to disease. The specific effects of a disease, the body's reactions to these changes, psychological trauma when life threat is involved, and the often potent effects of treatment can produce considerable dysfunction and distress. We focus in this chapter on the stressful aspects of serious illness, specifically on psychological trauma associated with life threat and associated challenges to one's fundamental outlook on life.

Cancer appears to be unusually stressful regardless of whether one has it or not. Many people grow up fearing cancer, and the prospect of cancer appears to be upsetting and associated with worry (e.g., Berman & Wandersman, 1990). Those who know they are at elevated risk appear to experience additional worry and chronic stress (e.g., Kash, Holland, Halper, & Miller, 1992; Lerman et al., 1995; Lerman, Kash, & Stefanek, 1994; Valdimarsdottir et al., 1995). Because cancer can cause severe pain, typically involves surgery and aversive adjuvant therapy, and too often has a poor prognosis, the possibility or reality of having cancer is very threatening. Once cancer is diagnosed and is being treated, stressors may include life threat, side effects of cancer treatment, and the need to engage in close surveillance after treatment. Similarly, the social stigma associated with having cancer, occupational discrimination often encountered by patients and survivors, and disease- or treatment-related changes in one's body or functional status also appear to be stressful. These sources of stress are important because they pose a challenge and burden for even the most resilient people, but they also suggest ways to reduce the impact of stress. Interventions to support or enhance adjustment to these stressors are associated with better quality of life and longer survival in some cases (e.g., Fawzy, Fawzy, Arndt, & Pasnau, 1995; Helgeson & Cohen, 1996; Spiegel, Bloom, Kraemer, & Gottheil, 1989).

Many of these stressors are addressed in psychosocial interventions designed to enhance the well-being of cancer patients. Most interventions concentrate on a particular stage of treatment, ranging from presurgical stress reduction to coping with the completion of treatment. Some interventions focus on coping with chemotherapy and radiation therapy, and others may be primarily concerned with survival or posttreatment surveillance or palliation. This approach acknowledges that patient needs and sources of stress change as one progresses through different stages of treatment. That each intervention may have a different focus underscores the complexity of the disease and the observation that having cancer is stressful for many reasons. Many of the most stressful aspects of the disease are discrete, time-limited stressors that may occur sequentially. Simply stated, learning that one has cancer triggers a series of other stressors that occur because one has cancer or is being treated for it.

However, it is likely that the diagnosis of cancer has important effects on people independent of the stressors described above. A recent meta-analysis confirmed that the social disruption, treatment side effects, and other stressors that confront cancer patients are disturbing and stressful but that these stressors do not explain all patient distress (Meyer & Mark, 1995). Less well-studied are the lasting effects of the cancer diagnosis itself, the existential sources of stress introduced by acute and chronic life threat, and the lingering psychological effects of the shock to the system associated with one's cancer diagnosis. Learning that one has cancer is bad news, regardless of one's prognosis or style of coping. This life threat is experienced in the context of ongoing burdens and supports and should play a major role in adjustment and well-being.

This suggests that a cancer diagnosis is a psychological blow that can produce cognitive and emotional crises and persistent distress. It also indicates that this turmoil and stress create a broader context in which stressors associated with surgery, chemotherapy, and other upsetting aspects of having cancer are experienced. Learning that one has cancer challenges one's beliefs about the world and about one's sense of safety. It also may force reconsideration of life priorities, expectations, and aspirations. The sudden and intense life peril introduced by such a diagnosis and the considerable fear most people experience when they think about having cancer set the stage for catastrophic thoughts or other reactions to the reality of cancer.

These effects of trauma associated with diagnosis likely persist as the discrete stressors associated with treatment are superimposed on them. In such cases, persistent stress may affect response to discrete disease-related stressors. As it does, it is in turn transformed, and this changing nature of traumatic stress may make it difficult to identify or to track. We consider these possibilities in some detail and suggest that traumatic stress can undermine adjustment to cancer treatment, quality of life, and survival and should be a target of psychotherapeutic interventions.

A Model of Cancer and Traumatic Stress

We propose that serious illnesses like cancer are complex stressors composed of several interrelated stressors triggered by the identification of the disease. When diseases like cancer are initially diagnosed, serious life threat is introduced and psychological trauma is likely. As the process of treating or living with the disease unfolds, additional, discrete stressors are encountered and dealt with, often one or two at a time. Social stigmatization, occupational discrimination, and other enduring social problems may also characterize this experience. We propose that these sources of stress combine to determine the experience of people with cancer and affect a range of outcomes, including disease course, quality of life, and response to treatment.

Traumatic and Nontraumatic Stress

The model we propose is based on two assumptions, the first of which is that traumatic stress is different from stress or even from extreme stress. Some theorists have defined *traumatic stress* as an extreme point on a stress continuum ranging roughly from the irritation or impatience associated with daily hassles and minor stressors to the more severe responses associated with cataclysmic events. Traumatic stress in this system is exaggerated or extremely severe stress; it differs from other instances of stress only in degree and not quality. However, common experiences with extreme stress suggest that the relationships among points on such a continuum are geometric rather than arithmetic and that there are qualitative differences in how stressors of different magnitude or "threat capacity" are experienced. Clearly, the severity of a threat or loss contributes to the magnitude of stress that is experienced, but other factors appear to be important as well (Davidson & Baum, 1986).

Traumatic stressors also appear to be more personally disruptive than extreme stressors that do not convey life threat. Some manifestations of traumatic stress are symptoms of arousal that resemble most stress reactions, but other aspects of traumatic stress response are more unusual. Emotional numbing, persistent unwanted and intrusive thoughts about the stressor, and temporal distortions or dissociation are much more pronounced and reliably related to psychological trauma than during or after most stressors. There also appear to be differences in the biological manifestations of regular stress and traumatic stress, including differences in resting hormonal profiles and rhythms (e.g., Mason, Giller, Kosten, Ostroff, & Harkness, 1986; Yehuda, Resnick, Kahana, & Giller, 1993). This suggests that experiences associated with traumatic or cataclysmic events are different from those associated with other sources of stress and that these differences appear to be more than just differences in magnitude of response.

Cancer can be discovered suddenly and without warning or as a result of a slowly unfolding series of tests and concerns. The increasingly stressful nature of information about cancer as it is gradually introduced should have different effects depending on whether this slower unfolding of events is desensitizing and leaves people more prepared (and less disturbed by the diagnosis) or is sensitizing and additive and generates steadily increasing fear and threat. However, for most people, whether anticipated or not, the diagnosis represents a sudden interruption and a severe life threat. It is hypothesized that this causes people to question basic social and existential assumptions and to re-evaluate their priorities and goals. The extent to which the suddenness of the diagnosis affects response is not clear, but either way, the impact of the diagnosis can be overwhelming, dominating people's thoughts and feelings and changing them forever. This is not typical of most stressors but is rather like a cataclysmic or traumatic event. One should not expect people to experience a cancer diagnosis as "just another major stressor."

Stressors Associated With Cancer

Another key assumption of this model is the characterization of cancer treatment as a series of discrete major sources of demand or stress. Adjustment to cancer is a process of coping with a number of sequential and overlapping stressors characterizing treatment or one's social environment (see Figure 9.1). To a large extent these stressors must be dealt with while one is also coping with the impact of the diagnosis; soon after the diagnosis, most patients must undergo surgery that may be disfiguring, affect incontinence, alter sexual activity, or affect fertility. Surgery may also cause considerable pain, discomfort, and body image concerns and threaten self-esteem. In addition, many patients face adjuvant treatment soon after surgery, frequently characterized by aversive side effects and a variety of social problems or problems of daily living. As we have noted, these stressors are generally time-limited and may "engulf the field," drawing attention away from other issues and focusing attention on the sources of threat associated with them. As one focuses attention on coping with side effects of chemotherapy, for example, issues related to psychological trauma may be ignored or repressed. To the extent that social and treatment-related stressors draw attention away from resolution of unresolved distress related to life threat, they may push trauma to the background and interfere with ongoing coping. These stressors also interact with underlying trauma, and it is possible that subsequent

FIGURE 9.1

Stress associated with cancer as sequential overlapping clusters associated with premorbid risk and fear, diagnosis, treatment, and survival.

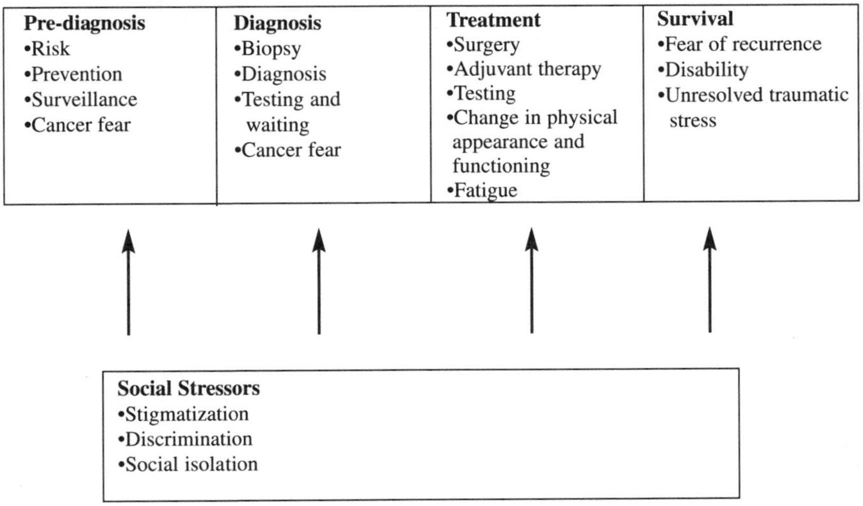

Pre-diagnosis	Diagnosis	Treatment	Survival
•Risk	•Biopsy	•Surgery	•Fear of recurrence
•Prevention	•Diagnosis	•Adjuvant therapy	•Disability
•Surveillance	•Testing and	•Testing	•Unresolved traumatic
•Cancer fear	waiting	•Change in physical	stress
	•Cancer fear	appearance and	
		functioning	
		•Fatigue	

Social Stressors
•Stigmatization
•Discrimination
•Social isolation

stressors and the process of coping with them also affect manifestations of traumatic stress. In effect, adjustment to cancer involves coping with a series of stressors associated with cancer treatment that are superimposed on the psychological effects of having cancer.

To the extent that the psychological crises that arise from the diagnosis of cancer can be resolved or accommodated, their effects may be short-lived or delayed. However, if some adaptation and resolution of these sources of threat cannot be readily achieved, this underlying distress may affect adjustment to subsequent stressors occurring as a result of cancer treatment (see Figure 9.2). Traumatic stress has an array of negative sequelae, but the extent to which ongoing, unresolved traumatic stress may affect more acute, discrete events is not known. There is evidence of persistent stress responding among trauma victims (e.g., Baum & Fleming, 1993; Delahanty et al., 1996; Mason et al., 1986; Yehuda et al., 1993), but it is not clear how ongoing traumatic stress affects an individual's experience of a new stressor or trauma. The limited literature on the effects of chronic stress on acute reactivity to new, acute stressors suggests that the magnitude and duration of acute response are affected (e.g., Gump & Matthews, 1999).

The majority of studies suggest that chronic stress is associated with a slower recovery to prestress resting levels of response (e.g., Fleming, Baum, Davidson, Rectanus, & McArdle, 1987). This could entail effects of chronic stress on feedback

FIGURE 9.2

The superimposition of treatment-related and social stressors associated with cancer on traumatic stress related to the diagnosis. As a result of this superimposition, responses may be transformed or altered to both kinds of stressor.

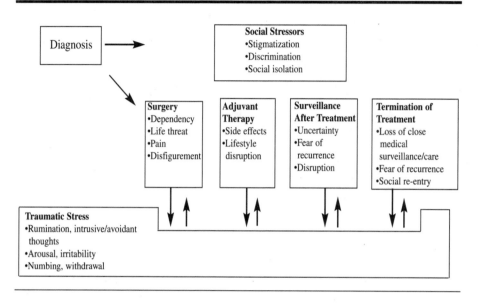

systems or other mechanisms of recovery after stress. Some studies suggest that chronic stress suppresses reactivity to subsequent acute stressors, and others indicate potentiation of response (Gump & Matthews, 1999). An even more limited literature addresses the effects of traumatic stressors on newly experienced stressful events. Several studies indicate that prior trauma is associated with greater distress when subsequent stressors are experienced (e.g., King, King, & Foy, 1996; Koopman, Classen, & Spiegel, 1994; Resnick, Yehuda, Pitman, & Foy, 1995; Ullman & Siegel, 1994; Yehuda, McFarlane, & Shalev, 1998). One particularly relevant study found that cancer patients who survived the Holocaust experienced more distress than those without such a history of trauma (Peretz, Baider, Ever-Hadani, & De-Nour, 1994).

A growing literature on adjustment to cancer and a smaller literature on cancer as a trauma suggest that there are gaps in our knowledge of how people experience cancer diagnosis. Clinical manifestations of traumatic stress, including posttraumatic stress disorder (PTSD), are not typical among cancer patients even though their rates of morbidity are higher than the general population (Alter et al., 1996). However, most of these studies considered patients long after their diagnosis. Later in this chapter, we review definitions of traumatic stressors and models of trauma and its consequences. Research on trauma, particularly medical trauma, is also reviewed. Studies that have examined cancer and trauma and more traditional research and theory on adjustment to cancer are described in later sections.

Psychological Trauma

Several conceptualizations of psychological trauma have been proposed. Some have been broader treatments of the concept of trauma, but many are primarily concerned with understanding the etiology and maintenance of PTSD. Regardless of their breadth, all of these models include description of initiating events, responses, and sequelae. The occurrence of a traumatic event is generally depicted as the precipitating factor of a syndrome of persistent distress. However, these precipitating events are characterized in varying ways.

Traumatic events are broadly defined as events that threaten or actually harm one's life or physical integrity (American Psychiatric Association, 1994). Earlier versions of the *Diagnostic and Statistical Manual of Mental Disorders* (e.g., the third edition, *DSM–III*, American Psychiatric Association, 1980, and the third revised edition, *DSM–III–R*; American Psychiatric Association, 1987) included definitions of traumatic events as unusual or beyond the realm of normal human experience. Unlike most stressors, traumatic events pose severe life threat. Traumatic events are cataclysmic, often overwhelming one's perceptual field and dominating conscious and unconscious thoughts (Baum, 1987). Regardless of whether one focuses on qualitative differences between extreme and traumatic stressors or ignores the differences in sources of threat and disruption, it is clear that trauma is associated with stress responses that can become persistent and disruptive and with coping designed in part to integrate the trauma into existing assumptions about the world. Disasters, war, serious motor vehicle accidents, abuse, rape, and injury are all considered to be traumatic.

Although traumatic events are associated with acute distress for most people affected by them, people's reactions differ, and not everyone exposed to a traumatic event experiences unusual or persistent distress (e.g., Keane, Zimmering, & Caddell, 1985). Traumatic events are probably more universal in causing distress than are less severe stressors, but reactions to events are dependent in part on how they are appraised (e.g., Lazarus, 1966; Lazarus & Folkman, 1984). For example, some people may surf the large waves at the beach as a hurricane approaches, whereas most people might evacuate the area. If the event is not perceived as life-threatening or if people think they can deal with a threatening event and emerge unscathed, they may not experience stress or show stress-related effects. However, traumatic events are usually considered sufficiently "out of the ordinary" and convey sufficient life threat to minimize variability in people's appraisal of the event (Janoff-Bulman, 1992).

According to some formulations, traumatic stress is produced by reactions to an event or situation that is completely different from the commonplace or what one could reasonably expect to encounter. Confrontation with threatening events that are beyond the realm of normal experience is thought to be unusually stressful, shaking people's assumptions and beliefs about the world and themselves (Janoff-Bulman, 1992). The experience is particularly problematic when available information is at odds with what victims previously believed or experienced (e.g., Janoff-Bulman & Frieze, 1983). Others have described trauma similarly as the experience of intense loss, anger, betrayal, helplessness, and denial and avoidance of these feelings following extraordinary threat or harm (Horowitz, 1976). The impact of a traumatic stressor is painful because it conflicts with elements of the psyche. Others view trauma as a state associated with difficulty in encoding or understanding a novel, extremely threatening experience (Foa, Steketee, Rothbaum, 1989). These theories share the premise that traumatic events are perceived as novel and highly threatening and the resulting experience is upsetting and highly emotional. Taken together, these theories suggest that *traumatic stress* can be defined as an intense negative, emotional experience characterized by challenge to one's fundamental beliefs of safety and meaning in the world and by intrusive or ruminative thoughts, avoidance, helplessness, fear, and horror.

The reaction to a traumatic event is complex. These events constitute a special case of chronic stress that is caused by an acute event that can greatly outlive its precipitating conditions (Baum, O'Keeffe, & Davidson, 1990). One mechanism underlying this unusual persistence is the experience of intrusive thoughts about the stressor (Baum, Cohen, & Hall, 1993). Traumatic events also introduce new, related stressors that persist beyond the initiating event (e.g., Baum & Fleming, 1993). In some cases a traumatic event initiates a cascade of other events that are related but distinct. For example, being involved in a serious motor vehicle accident can be a highly threatening and traumatic event itself, even if there are no further complications. However, in many instances, the aftermath of the accident can involve a series of related events, including hassles and pain associated with rehabilitation and physical therapy, financial difficulties, inconvenience caused by possible loss of license or insurance, lost work time, and arrangements for child care (Baum et al., 1990). These events are secondary to the traumatic event (accident) and likely occur in the context of ongoing traumatic stress resulting from the severe threats associated with the accident. Each of these secondary stressors has the potential to affect mood and behavior, but it does so in the context of ongoing reactions to traumatic aspects of the initial stressor. These secondary stressors may affect the quality of one's long-term response to the traumatic event, extending or exacerbating stress responses after the initial event has ended (Baum et al., 1990).

Models of Psychological Trauma and PTSD

Several models of traumatic response have been proposed, and serious mental health outcomes of trauma have been conceptualized as PTSD. These models include information-processing theories that focus on how we incorporate new, threatening information in our environment or on how reexperiencing of the traumatic event is critical to one's adaptation (Horowitz, 1976). Other models are derived from learning theory and describe how people form associations during the traumatic event and how those associations are maintained through conditioning (e.g., Foa et al., 1989; Keane et al., 1985). Disruption of people's basic beliefs about meaning and order in the world are central to the assumptive world model (Janoff-Bulman, 1988/1995, 1992). Finally, biological models emphasize the impact of trauma on physiological functioning over time that may influence psychological adaptation (e.g., van der Kolk, 1988).

Information-processing models address how individuals perceive, selectively attend to, and retrieve information from memory. These models suggest that experiences are organized in memory in the form of schemas, or networks, of information. These schemas allow us to quickly process and react to new information by mapping the new information onto what we already know and using the schema as a template. Once a particular schema is activated, we quickly direct attention to schema-relevant, information in the environment (Williams, Watts, MacLeod, & Mathews, 1988). Reactions can include cognitive, behavioral, and physiological changes and may be particularly strong for personally meaningful material (Pillemer, 1984).

This perspective is related to research on fear networks (e.g., Lang, 1985), an information-processing theory of fear and anxiety that maintains that fear-relevant stimuli are encoded in highly organized networks in memory. A person with an anxiety disorder has a schema of fear that is easily activated for the specific feared stimulus and then for related stimuli as the fear generalizes. Extending this to traumatic stress, one can see that the networks that organize trauma may be particularly large and easily activated because of their emotional content (Foa et al., 1989). When a trauma network is activated, the resulting emotional response may prevent people from attending to other information or may link the new information in the environment to the trauma network. Although it is not known how multiple traumatic events may affect information processing of future traumatic events, it has been proposed that a history of trauma may make activating or forming new traumatic schemas easier (Hyer and Associates, 1994).

Learning theory has also been used to explain how traumatic experiences occur and become perpetuated in PTSD-like syndromes. According to this model, any stimulus associated with a traumatic event can come to elicit a conditioned response similar to that associated with the original event. Stimulus generalization can occur, and stimuli that are more peripheral to the trauma come to elicit a conditioned response similar to the original reaction to the original stimulus. This increases opportunities for the conditioned response to occur over time. Avoidance behaviors can also develop and be reinforced by decreasing distress. Avoidance behaviors include keeping away from reminders, decreasing awareness and distress through drugs or alcohol, and using dissociation to keep unpleasant experiences from conscious awareness (van der Kolk & Ducey, 1989). These behaviors can perpetuate the problem and prevent people from recognizing that traumatic memories are aversive but not life-threatening. Moreover, people may become highly vigilant for trauma-related stimuli, increasing the likelihood that reminiscent stimuli are recognized. Conditioning may also explain how responses can continue after the stressor or threat is gone.

Horowitz (1976) proposed an information-processing model incorporating some psychodynamic constructs first advanced by Freud. Freud (1920/1955) coined the term *traumatic neurosis* to describe a condition that may occur after severe shock from threat to life, as in an accident. He noted that those who suffered from traumatic neurosis had continuing dreams about the situation of extreme threat and would awaken with "renewed terror." Horowitz (1976, 1997) suggested that adjustment to a traumatic event requires incorporation of the event into existing schemas. Alternatively, people can develop new schemas, but this would presumably require more work and might still require some degree of integration of the disturbing information. Until this process is complete, the trauma remains in active memory and is out of conscious awareness. Denial and emotional numbing are used to keep from becoming aware of and overwhelmed by threatening information. Intrusions and avoidance may even coexist; an individual may experience both denial about one aspect of a traumatic event and intrusive repetitions about another aspect of the same event (Fairbank & Nicholson, 1987). However, motivation to integrate the trauma or to overcome and resolve the underlying anxiety allows intrusive thoughts and images about the trauma to intrude into awareness (Horowitz, 1973, 1997). Because these intrusions are uncontrollable, unwarranted, and often upsetting, denial and numbing are used to minimize them. This cycle of avoidance and intrusion allows people to process a little more information, and with each cycle the trauma is closer to being fully integrated. PTSD results when one cannot integrate the trauma, possibly because of directing most effort toward denial or avoidance and perpetuating the cycles of intrusions and avoidance.

Reexperiences of traumatic stressors are usually vivid and are described as though they were going on in the present (van der Kolk & Fisler, 1995). Part of the normal memory process results in altered memories over time; specific details are forgotten or no longer have the same emotional experience as when the event occurred. However, some traumatic memories do not appear to habituate like this. In one longitudinal study of men who had participated in World War II, those who recalled the horrific combat experience in more benign terms (compared with when they had initially described and recounted it in comparable detail 45 years earlier) were less likely to have PTSD than men who did not modify their story (Lee, Vaillant, Torrey, & Elder, 1995). Men with PTSD described their experiences in the same emotionally laden terms as they had years before.

Basic beliefs about meaning and order in the world form the basis of the assumptive world model (Janoff-Bulman, 1988/1995, 1992; Taylor, 1983). These basic beliefs reflect assumptions we make that define our personalities and guide our behavior. These include safety or the belief that one is safe in many contexts, beliefs about people generally being good or bad, assumptions derived from religion, and beliefs about whether the world is random or orderly. Most people, prior to any serious victimization, feel relatively invulnerable to negative events (Janoff-Bulman & Frieze, 1983; Weinstein, 1988). Victims experience a lost sense of safety whether they are victims of crime (e.g., Krupnick & Horowitz, 1981), disease (e.g., Taylor, 1983; Wortman & Dunkel-Schetter, 1979), or disasters (e.g., Green, 1994). It has been proposed that people seem to operate on the beliefs that the world is a good place where events are meaningful and the self is good (Janoff-Bulman, 1992). This set of assumptions about the world provides people with a sense of stability and invulnerability and helps them to make sense of what is happening around them. For most people, these assumptions go relatively unchallenged, until they are faced with an event that does not easily fit into existing assumptive worlds or schemas. When this occurs, people try to integrate the event into their assumptions in order to minimize psychological distress. If they cannot make sense of the event, their integrated distress persists (Janoff-Bulman, 1992; Janoff-Bulman & Wortman, 1977; Taylor, 1983).

Biological models of trauma focus on stress symptoms associated with physiological reactions and interactions with genetic predispositions. Hyperarousal of the sympathetic nervous system, disregulation of the hypothalamic–pituitary–adrenocortical axis, and abnormalities of the endogenous opioid system and sleep have been associated with trauma and PTSD (e.g., Friedman, 1991; Kolb, 1987; Yehuda et al., 1993). For example, urinary free-cortisol levels are lower among PTSD patients than in patients with most other psychiatric disorders (Mason et al., 1986). One model (e.g., van der Kolk, 1988) is based on neurohormonal disruption at the time of a traumatic event, which affects how memories are consolidated and stored. Subsequent symptoms of PTSD, such as exaggerated startle responses that are resistant to habituation, are thought to be related to chronic autonomic overarousal and extreme autonomic responses to trauma-relevant stimuli.

The hyperarousal pattern associated with trauma-related stimuli can be characterized as a conditioned emotional response (Kolb, 1987). Frequent reliving of a traumatic event in flashbacks or nightmares causes a release of stress hormones, which further strengthens the memory. Another aspect of this theory suggests that excessive stimulation of the central nervous system at the time of the trauma may result in permanent neuronal changes that have a negative effect on learning, habituation, and stimulus discrimination (Kolb, 1987). Symptoms of PTSD also may develop from a complex interaction of genetically determined biological and psychological predispositions to respond to stress with chronic autonomic overarousal and a tendency toward distorted processing of information along with extremely negative affect (Jones & Barlow, 1990).

These models of PTSD suggest that traumatic stress is more intense and over-whelming and that it is supported by larger networks of fear and anxiety-producing information than is more routine stress. Stress following trauma also appears to involve more rumination, possibly because of the need for cognitive reorganization and acceptance of discordant information. Traumatic stress appears to involve chal-lenges to basic assumptions about the world, including beliefs about its randomness, benign qualities, safety, and predictability. These challenges can be painful and distressing and may be processed in an alternative sequence of intrusions and avoidance until adaptation is achieved. Traumatic stress appears to outlast the event or events that precipitated it. Temporal distortions and dissociation may be more likely in cases where threat is very severe.

Adjustment to Trauma

One of the great truths about human response to stressors, no matter how large or small they may be, is that reactions are variable and often hard to predict. Many sources of variability are tied up with appraisal, coping, resources, and resiliency, but the strength or stability of threat appears to be inversely related to variability in the short term. Acute reactions to traumatic events appear to be more stereotypic than reactions to more common stressors (e.g., Green, 1990; Horowitz, 1973; Shalev, Bonne, & Eth, 1996). During and immediately after a traumatic event, people tend to experience shock and disbelief, often blocking out all or most of the threat. At this point some form of time disturbance or dissociation can occur, presumably to help to distance oneself from the threat. Depersonalization, numbing or absence of emotional responsiveness, and dissociative amnesia are possible in the face of an overwhelming stressor (Shalev, 1992). This distancing can be adaptive because it helps to prevent becoming overwhelmed with intense feelings of horror or helpless-ness. Memory for the event is also affected by temporal distortions, and the "unreal" quality of some traumatic stressors may reinforce their capacity to threaten people.

After the event has passed and the individual begins to regain some sense of safety and control, responses become more variable. Many show steady improvement in mood and well-being, but others exhibit continued or even heightened distress long after the initial event is experienced. More persistent stress responses are associated with reexperiencing the event through thoughts, images, or dreams. This repeated replaying of upsetting memories is thought to serve the function of modify-ing or reducing the intensity of the emotions associated with the trauma in order to create tolerance for the content of the memories (Horowitz & Reidbord, 1992). However, some people do not adapt and continue to reexperience the event, often with the same intensity as when it originally occurred (Baum et al., 1993). They may also experience symptoms of heightened arousal, such as difficulty sleeping, poor concentration, exaggerated startle response, and hypervigilance. However, some investigators have suggested that what characterizes traumatic stress and PTSD is the alternation between intrusive reexperiencing of the trauma and denial or numbing of emotional responsiveness (e.g., Foa, Zinbarg, & Rothbaum, 1992).

Data bear this out. Whether or not people develop PTSD or become seriously impaired, they are likely to experience intrusive thoughts about the event (Creamer, Burgess, & Pattison, 1992; McFarlane, 1992; Shalev, 1992). For example, about half of a sample of individuals involved in motor vehicle accidents reported moderate levels of intrusive thoughts and avoidance, and about a third reported higher levels of intrusive thoughts and avoidance within 2 weeks of the accident (Bryant & Harvey, 1996). In other studies of individuals involved in motor vehicle accidents, a third or more of the samples met threshold or subthreshold criteria for PTSD when assessed within 1–4 months of their accident (Blanchard et al., 1996; Delahanty et al., 1997; Ursano, Fullerton, Vance, & Kao, 1999). Major natural and technological disasters are also associated with persistent intrusive and avoidant ideation (e.g., Baum, Cohen, & Hall, 1993; Davidson & Baum, 1986; Ironson et al., 1997; McFarlane, 1988, 1992).

The immediate response following a traumatic stressor is typically more extreme and consistent than is later response as symptoms of traumatic stress typically change over time. For example, Rothbaum and Foa (1992) described PTSD symptoms in 94% of rape victims 1 week after the trauma, 53% two months later, and 47% nine months later. Similarly, symptoms related to traumatic stressors declined in the majority of individuals involved in motor vehicle accidents (e.g., Delahanty et al., 1997; Dougall, Craig, & Baum, 1999). Some people who are victimized by threatening, powerful events clearly do not adapt as readily as others exhibiting substantial chronic stress burdens. Whether this is associated with changes in physiological arousal and in specific stress-related systems or with differences in coping, resources, vigilance, and other intervening variables, this suggests that for a substantial number of cancer patients dealing with treatment or survivorship stressors, the disruption and trauma associated with the diagnosis persist well beyond it.

Cancer, Stress, and Trauma

The findings and theories described in the preceding sections also suggest that cancer or its diagnosis has the potential to be traumatic. Cancer diagnosis introduces immediate life threat; it challenges assumptions and expectations about safety, the world, and how long one has in it. For many, the diagnosis is an overwhelming and "paralyzing" stressor. Although most of the data suggest that many psychological issues associated with cancer diagnosis and treatment are readily resolved and short-lived, these data may not provide direct tests of hypotheses characterizing the traumatic nature of cancer and may underestimate the impact of this event.

We have argued that cancer can be considered both traumatic and stressful. Although medical research and clinical care have progressed to the point that many people diagnosed with cancer can be treated and survive, cancer remains a highly feared disease and many people still believe that it is inevitably fatal (Berman & Wandersman, 1990). Its treatment is also highly aversive and disruptive to one's life, and research has documented stressful aspects of cancer such as adjustment to chemotherapy and radiation treatment (e.g., Christman, 1990; Holland, Rowland, Lebovits, & Rusalem, 1979; Jacobsen, Bovbjerg, & Redd, 1993; Meyerowitz, 1980). Less work has been directed toward investigating the possibility that underlying trauma may be characteristic of cancer. As noted, hearing that one has cancer may challenge one's beliefs about safety and what one expects for himself or herself. Existing beliefs about oneself as a healthy person may be transformed into beliefs about one's vulnerability to harm or recurrence. Assumptions regarding personal safety and the just nature of the world, evaluations of self-worth, perceived control, one's relationship with family, and beliefs about the spiritual world may all be called into question. The ensuing cognitive turmoil and reorganization may lead to emotional sequelae of trauma, including PTSD.

We have proposed that cancer is a complex stressor, composed of interacting but partially independent threats, harm, or loss. When people learn that they have cancer, a series of treatment-related stressors is initiated and a number of social stressors are triggered as well. Major, treatment-related stressors include surgery, adjuvant chemotherapy, radiotherapy, and immunotherapy; the approaching end of treatment; follow-up surveillance; and pain. These stressors are linked to one another as aspects of treatment but are generally sequential and can occur independently of one another. Persistent social stressors are also likely, and the disruption of normal routines may increase one's experience with daily hassles. All of these stressors occur in the context of often sudden and immediate life threat and the psychological trauma that can be associated with such threat (see Figure 9.3). The potential for traumatic stress and its interactions with these other stressors define the experience of cancer and offer suggestions for enhancing patient care. The slowly growing literature addressing these issues is generally consistent with the depiction of cancer as a complex stressor.

Trauma

The broader PTSD inclusion criteria in the 4th edition of the *DSM* (*DSM–IV*; American Psychiatric Association, 1994) have led to more thorough investigations of trauma and PTSD in medical patients, particularly in women with breast cancer (Alter et al., 1996; Andrykowski, Cordova, Studts, & Miller, 1998; Cordova et al., 1995; Green et al., 1998). In addition, PTSD symptoms have also been examined in life-threatening medical conditions such as myocardial infarction (Doerfler, Pbert, & DeCosimo, 1994) and severe burn injuries (Patterson, Carrigan, Questad, & Robinson, 1990; Perry, Difede, Musngi, Frances, & Jacobsberg, 1992; Roca, Spence, & Munster, 1992). This research has focused on describing the psychological

FIGURE 9.3

Cancer-related stressors occur in the context of often sudden and immediate life threat and the psychological trauma that can be associated with such threat. PTSD = posttraumatic stress disorder.

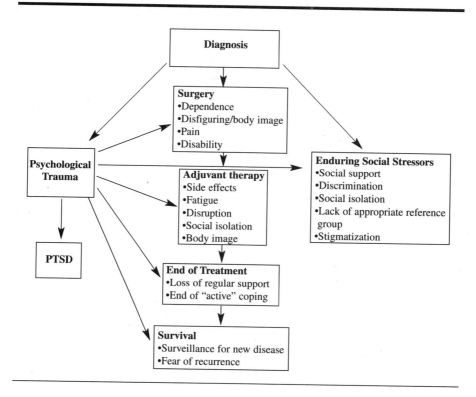

sequelae of these medical events, determining the incidence of clinical syndromes, and understanding the factors that affect clinical symptoms or syndromes.

Findings from these studies have been reassuring in that they indicate less debilitating distress than might be expected. Sudden onset of a myocardial infarction or undergoing coronary bypass surgery can be traumatic, but patients with these conditions, as a group, experience relatively low levels of distress (Doerfler et al., 1994). About 8% of these patients met *DSM–III–R* (American Psychiatric Association, 1987) criteria for PTSD related to their medical event 6–12 months after it occurred, and an additional 8% met criteria for major depressive disorder. Studies of burn patients also indicate that the majority of patients did not develop PTSD but that a subgroup did not appear to adapt very well and experienced more extensive distress (e.g., Perry et al., 1992; Roca et al., 1992).

Evidence of traumatic stress and PTSD in cancer patients is similar. The life-threatening nature of the diagnosis and its profound impact on one's day-to-day functioning make adjustment to this illness difficult. Investigations have found that cancer patients and survivors report more symptoms of reexperiencing, avoidance, and arousal than do healthy control patients (e.g., Alter et al., 1996). When patients were asked about their reactions to diagnosis, many reported similar themes of trying to understand why it occurred, changing their outlook on life, and looking for sources of hope (O'Connor, Wicker, & Germino, 1990). Others described it as the worst experience they had ever had (Alter et al., 1996). Data suggest that the diagnosis of cancer is very stressful and, although less common than once feared, some mental health problems occur in its wake (e.g., Cordova et al., 1995; Devlen, Maguire, Phillips, & Crowther, 1987a, 1987b; Maguire et al., 1978; Manuel, Roth, Keefe, & Brantley, 1987; Stanton & Snider, 1993). Taken together, these findings suggest that the distress and cognitive turmoil described by Horowitz (1976) and Janoff-Bulman (1992) are relevant to cancer and that its diagnosis can be traumatic.

Women at higher risk for breast cancer express more worry and distress about breast cancer than do women who are at lower risk (e.g., Lerman et al., 1995). Consistent with earlier assertions, data suggest that people are generally worried about cancer and are distressed even by precancerous conditions that are highly treatable. One week after testing, women who had received results indicating presence of cervical intra-epithelial neoplasia (CIN; a precursor to invasive cervical cancer) reported more intrusive thoughts about cancer than did women who had received negative results (Palmer, Tucker, Warren, & Adams, 1993). Three to 6 weeks later, despite having completed treatment, women with a positive indication of CIN still reported more intrusive thoughts. Reasons for persistent stress were probably related to the lasting impact of life threat; women reported that they feared recurrence and the progression of CIN to cancer (Palmer et al., 1993).

In studies of major stress reactions and PTSD among cancer patients and survivors, fairly low rates of impairment have been reported. Typically this research has considered people with relatively good prognoses, studying them several years after diagnosis and treatment of the disease (e.g., Alter et al., 1996). Cordova et al. (1995) examined women with early stage breast cancer 6–60 months after treatment (M = 31 months). About half reported repeated disturbing thoughts about their cancer, mostly focused on side effects of surgery and fear of recurrence. About a third reported experiencing nausea, heart palpitations, and panic when something reminded them of their cancer treatment or other aspects of their illness. Only 3 of the 55 women (5.5%) met criteria for concurrent cancer-related PTSD. Using an alternate scoring method of looking at the pattern of responses, 6 out of 55 women (11%) were judged likely to meet criteria for a diagnosis of cancer-related PTSD.

Although a substantial percentage of affected patients reported troublesome intrusive thoughts and distress related to their cancer, relatively few could be diagnosed with PTSD. This may have been related to participants' generally good prognoses (they were all diagnosed with early stage cancer). In addition, assessment of PTSD symptoms was made long after discovery and treatment of the cancer, in some cases as much as 5 years later. Several studies suggest that posttraumatic stress syndromes gradually diminish and remit after 1 year or so (e.g., McFarlane, 1988; Rothbaum & Foa, 1992; Ursano, Fullerton, Kao, & Bhartiya, 1995).

A related cross-sectional study incorporating these 55 women with 27 additional patients bears on these possibilities (Andrykowski et al., 1998). The 82 participants were early stage breast cancer patients and were studied an average of 37 months posttreatment. Rates of PTSD were again low, with only 5 women (6%) exhibiting current cancer-related PTSD and 3 more (4%) showing lifetime cancer-related PTSD. However, the length of time since treatment was negatively correlated with levels of PTSD symptoms, suggesting that the long time frames in those studies may be one reason for low rates of PTSD. Those women who had been diagnosed more recently reported more symptoms (Andrykowski & Cordova, 1998). The data also suggested that low rates of observed PTSD were partly due to the good prognosis of early stage breast cancer. More advanced disease at diagnosis was associated with more severe cancer-related PTSD symptoms.

These studies suggest that some women with early stage breast cancer experienced symptoms of PTSD years after diagnosis and treatment. They also suggest that stage of disease is associated with more extreme symptoms and that PTSD is more prevalent among advanced or recurrent cancer survivors (Andrykowski & Cordova, 1998). Few have looked at symptoms of traumatic stress soon after diagnosis or treatment. In one major study, researchers (Green et al., 1998) looked at PTSD closer to the diagnosis of cancer and assessed PTSD in 160 women with early stage (i.e., Stage I or II) breast cancer 4–12 months after cancer diagnosis and treatment. All women rated their diagnosis as the most stressful experience related to their cancer, more than 33% of the sample had experienced at least one symptom of intrusion since diagnosis, and 20% were still experiencing symptoms at the time of assessment. However, only 5 (3%) of the women met criteria for lifetime cancer-related PTSD. Another study of early stage breast cancer patients estimated that about 12% met criteria for PTSD 1 year after surgery (Tjemsland, Soreide, & Malt, 1998).

Most of these studies were conducted with breast cancer survivors. There are some exceptions. For example, Cella and Tross (1986) compared male Hodgkins lymphoma survivors with an age-matched sample of healthy men. Survivors were defined by extended disease-free survival (range = 6–140 months). Intrusive thoughts, distress, and sexual problems were measured in both groups. Patients with advanced disease and those who were diagnosed within 2 years of the study reported nearly twice as many intrusive thoughts as did control patients. Patients who were diagnosed more than 30 months earlier reported the same levels of intrusive thoughts as the control group, suggesting a decline in intrusive thoughts over time. However, the cross-sectional nature of this study limits the conclusions that can be drawn. As a group, cancer survivors showed significantly more sexual problems, distress, and more illness-related concerns than did healthy control patients. Not surprisingly, advanced stage patients who were more recently diagnosed reported the greatest levels of distress (Cella & Tross, 1986).

Although research in this area is not extensive, it provides some evidence of traumatic stress as a major component of adjustment to cancer. Had studies been initiated sooner or with more severely affected patients, observed distress and PTSD might have been more substantial. It is interesting to note, however, that although symptoms of traumatic stress are relatively common among cancer patients, relatively few classifiable mental health problems or cases of PTSD are typically observed. Research has found substantial emotional disturbance among cancer patients, but even when rates are as high as 44%, patients with DSM–III (American Psychiatric Association, 1980) clinical syndromes were primarily diagnosed with adjustment disorders, and only a small minority were diagnosed with major anxiety or depression (Derogatis et al., 1983). This is consistent with other studies of mental health among cancer patients (e.g., Dean, 1987) and is likely influenced by disease stage and site as well as social support, quality of medical care, and mental health history. Reasons for the relatively low rates of major mental health problems in cancer patients remain an important area of investigation.

Stress

One explanation for lower than expected rates of PTSD is that the trauma associated with cancer diagnoses is quickly buried by more immediate stressors associated with treatment or other aspects of life as a cancer patient. To recapitulate earlier discussions, these stressors are discrete, are usually managed within a finite time frame, and are superimposed on the underlying life threat and associated reevaluation of one's assumptions and beliefs. As new and highly feared stressors are layered on top of traumatic stress associated with the diagnosis, symptoms of that trauma may be masked, and psychological work on resolving threats to one's worldview may temporarily cease while the individual copes actively with more immediate treatment-related stressors. For example, a woman learning that she has breast cancer may experience shock and stress upon diagnosis but must almost immediately consider, anticipate, and experience surgery. After recovery from surgery, she typically must cope with radiation or chemotherapy (or both) and their side effects. All the while, she is coping with profound social disruption, stigmatization from dependency, and other issues. The result of this cascade of stressors may be suspension of active coping with the traumatic elements of cancer as attention is drawn to other issues.

The preexistence of traumatic stress does not diminish the importance or impact of these discrete, often treatment-related stressors. Uncertainty appears to be a major source of stress and may explain the aversiveness of waiting for results of tests or treatments, anticipating surgery, or thinking about possible recurrence (e.g., Green et al., 1998). Dependence issues and more immediate threats associated with surgery contribute to stress, as do the aversive side effects of chemotherapy, radiotherapy, and other adjuvant therapies. These side effects can evoke fear, cause disruption and social stigmatization, and otherwise threaten or inhibit coping behavior. Concerns about body image and social and occupational difficulties as a result of having cancer are also stressful (e.g., Andersen, 1989; Meyerowitz, 1980; Taylor et al., 1985). Many cancer patients experience significant distress immediately after diagnosis and throughout treatment (e.g., Dean, 1987; Devlen, Maguire, Phillips, & Crowther, 1987a; Maguire et al., 1978; Manuel, Roth, Keefe, & Brantley, 1987; Stanton & Snider, 1993). Stanton and Snider measured mood among 117 women before breast biopsy, after diagnosis, and after surgery among those who had cancer. Not surprisingly, cancer patients reported more negative mood after diagnosis than did benign patients, with prebiopsy distress controlled. However, cancer patients' mood returned to prebiopsy levels after surgery. The investigators speculated that the rapid recovery of mood might have been due to the relief of having taken a concrete action against the disease and having completed surgery successfully and safely.

Adjuvant chemotherapy, radiotherapy, and immunotherapy also appear to be stressful and often follow quickly after surgery. In one study, breast cancer and malignant lymphoma patients were interviewed five times during the course of chemotherapy (Love, Leventhal, Easterling, & Nerenz, 1988). Most reported experiencing nausea, hair loss, and fatigue. Toward the end of chemotherapy, almost half reported that they had thought of quitting treatment and that this was related to extent of distress and difficulty tolerating treatment. Patient ratings of treatment difficulty increased over time and were related to the number and severity of side effects experienced. A study of lung, breast, and head and neck cancer patients that measured distress before the start of radiation therapy and again shortly after the end of treatment suggested that distress was greatest shortly after completion of treatment (Eakes, Rakfal, Keel, & Gaiser, 1996). Furthermore, effects of adjuvant treatment may linger after treatment ends (Meyerowitz, 1983). Women who received chemotherapy for breast cancer reported that they were still experiencing physical problems from the treatment more than 2 years after completing it. Physical problems included persistent weight changes, a loss of energy, and cessation or interruption of menstruation. Patients reported that it took more than 6 months after chemotherapy to return to their normal level of functioning, and about one third reported that they were still very fearful of recurrence (Meyerowitz, 1983).

Stress and the End of Treatment

The finding that lung, breast, and head and neck cancer patients experienced more distress at the end of adjuvant therapy (Eakes et al., 1996) could reflect several processes. It may suggest that adjuvant therapy is aversive, but it also raises the possibility that completion of treatment may constitute another discrete stressor. The time immediately after treatment ends can be filled with mixed feelings of relief, sadness related to perceived loss of regular contact with medical staff, and fear of recurrence. Among women with breast cancer studied before radiation therapy, during the 2nd week of treatment and at the end of treatment, depression and anger were greatest at the end of treatment (Holland et al., 1979). After active treatment, such as chemotherapy or radiation therapy, cancer patients may have difficulty knowing what to do to further combat their disease or to prevent recurrence, and these feelings of helplessness could contribute to depression (Maguire, 1988). In another study, about one third of women completing adjuvant treatment reported that the termination of treatment was upsetting (Ward, Viergutz, Tormey, deMuth, & Paulen, 1992). Those who were most upset by termination of treatment had been more depressed since the onset of treatment, tended to view their illness as chronic, and had more side effects during their last cycle of chemotherapy (Ward et al., 1992).

Although research suggests that mental health problems and major psychological disorders are not characteristic of cancer patients, data suggest that having cancer and adjusting to its treatment are stressful (Hughes, 1982). Prospective studies of patient adjustment studying patients before surgery and 3 months and 12 months after surgery have found greater distress among patients than in a control group of women randomly selected from the community (Dean, 1987).

Prospective studies of stress also suggest that coping with cancer may be best viewed as dealing with a succession of major treatment-related stressors experienced in the context of ongoing distress caused by the impact of life threat and uncertainty. For example, in Hughes's (1982) study of early stage breast cancer patients, 80% reported a period of significant, persistent emotional distress related to breast cancer, with severe distress or depression present in 18% of patients. By the end of the year, distress levels had subsided, but more than half of the women expressed continuing worries about their diagnosis of cancer and feared recurrence. The notion that more immediate treatment-related stressors may mask symptoms of traumatic stress related to cancer diagnosis provides some explanations for curiosities in the data on stress and cancer. There are data consistent with cognitive and emotional aspects of trauma, and there is evidence of persistent distress among cancer patients. Furthermore, the apparently stressful nature of the end of treatment may be a function of the reemergence of traumatic stress as most discrete treatment-related stressors abate.

Stress and Disease Severity

As noted above, the low observed rates of PTSD and other major mental health problems among cancer patient populations may be artifactual and attributable to the time frames and narrow range of disease severity typically studied. Most research on PTSD and cancer has been conducted in early stage cancer patients assessed several years after their diagnosis and treatment. Many of these patients had excellent prognoses, and 90% or more expected to survive the disease, so its severity or experience as a life threat may have been diminished. The seriousness of the disease or magnitude of life threat associated with later stage or more advanced cancers could be related to greater distress and PTSD risk. Distress also appears to decrease over time for most patients, suggesting that studies following 5-year survivors may not find much evidence of distress. Although studies have not directly addressed these issues using mental health outcomes, the pattern of data makes these conclusions very likely.

For example, a study of ovarian cancer patients, most with advanced stage disease, compared responses a week after surgery, a week after completing chemotherapy, and every 3 months for a year (Kornblith et al., 1995). More than a third of the patients reported moderate to severe anxiety and depression immediately after surgery, and those patients who reported the most distress reported significantly more physical symptoms and poorer physical functioning. In general, patients maintained stable levels of distress over the year, although those patients who died during the year had exhibited increasing levels of distress up until the time of their death. In contrast, Andersen, Anderson, and deProsse (1989a) found that women with gynecological cancer exhibited anxiety and depression after diagnosis but that distress declined over time. Four months later, no differences were found for distress between cancer patients and a control group. The cancer patients in this study were in the earlier stages of the disease, with better prognoses than the patients in the Kornblith et al. (1995) study, and this may have produced these inconsistent findings.

Studies of lymphoma patients across stage of disease (or better or poorer prognosis) also support the notion that more severe or advanced cancers might produce more significant distress. More distress was observed when cancer was advanced or when patients did not respond to treatment (Pettingale, Burgess, & Greer, 1988). In a different study, survivors of advanced stage Hodgkins disease exhibited continuing distress 6½ years after completing treatment (Kornblith et al., 1992). The severity or aversiveness of treatment also affects lasting response: 12–19% of women with breast cancer who had more serious treatment with bone marrow transplants met criteria for PTSD (Jacobsen et al., 1998). Research has also identified components of posttraumatic stress among some patients and survivors. People confronting a diagnosis or recurrence of cancer also reported high levels of cancer-related intrusions and avoidance (Cella et al., 1990; Cella & Tross, 1986; Palmer et al., 1993), similar in range to other individuals who had recently experienced traumatic events (e.g., Baum et al., 1993; Cella & Tross, 1986; Ironson et al., 1997; Zilberg, Weiss, & Horowitz, 1982). Many cancer patients reported moderate levels of cancer-related intrusions and avoidance several years after diagnosis (Alter et al., 1986; Cordova et al., 1995). A smaller number met *DSM–IV* (American Psychiatric Association, 1994) criteria for cancer-related PTSD years after diagnosis (Alter et al., 1996; Andrykowski et al., 1998).

Traumatic Stress

The literature suggests that reactions to cancer diagnoses may be traumatic, and some cases of PTSD may be related to this experience. As is the case for many psychiatric disorders, the prevalence of PTSD is relatively low in cancer patients but cannot be readily compared with other traumatic events because of different time frames and measures. Research has described sources of threat associated with cancer diagnosis that suggest it is a traumatic event. Patients confronting initial diagnoses or news of recurrence often have existential concerns and seek to determine the cause or reason for their illness (e.g., McCorkle & Quint-Benoliel, 1983; O'Connor et al., 1990; Taylor et al., 1985). Challenges to assumptions about one's life expectancy and the justness of the world and attempts to find meaning or grow from the experience are common themes in studies of cancer patients and survivors (e.g., Carver et al., 1993). There is also some evidence of continued stress and remote PTSD in cancer survivor populations, suggesting that some aspects of survival are stressful, that unresolved traumatic stress and cognitive disorganization are still active (and unmasked), or both. The conclusion that stress associated with discrete, disease-related stressors can be affected by an underlying traumatic stress has a number of implications.

Effects of Traumatic Stress on Subsequent Stressors

It was suggested earlier that persistent stress associated with psychological trauma may affect the ways in which treatment-related stressors are perceived or the ways people cope with them. Adjustment to subsequent stressors may be compromised for those patients who continue to experience stress as a result of cancer diagnosis, and resulting coping and adaptation may be more tenuous. Findings from studies of the effects of chronic stress on response to acute stressors are mixed. Some studies show potentiated responses, but others show suppression of response. A more consistent observation is that chronic stress inhibits recovery from new stressors (e.g., Gump & Matthews, 1999). An ongoing stressor or history of trauma may affect reactions and adjustment to discrete situational stressors or classes of stressors such as surgery or side effects of treatment. Those patients who experience trauma as a result of cancer diagnosis and for whom the reaction persists may have greater difficulty adjusting over time and continue to experience unresolved distress.

There are two studies that suggest that an earlier trauma or previous diagnosis of cancer affects subsequent reactions to cancer. Cancer patients who had survived the Holocaust experienced greater distress after diagnosis of cancer than did those who had not experienced the Holocaust (Peretz et al., 1994). Similarly, research on the impact of recurrent malignancies of mixed cancer sites also showed evidence of heightened distress (Cella, Mahon, & Donovan, 1990). In this study, all patients had been disease free for 1–10 years, had been diagnosed in the last month with recurrence, and were undergoing adjuvant therapy. In general, patients reported that their adjustment to recurrence was more difficult than their adjustment to the initial diagnosis and that intrusions and avoidant thoughts were frequent and disturbing. Almost all patients reported that they were less hopeful after this recurrence than when they were initially diagnosed, and half expressed concerns that their physician would decide not to treat the recurrent disease. Twenty percent felt their family would be less supportive of them than during the initial diagnosis, and most reported that the medical staff was providing less treatment information and attention to them than during the first bout with cancer (Cella et al., 1990).

PTSD

If traumatic stress is so clearly linked to the diagnosis of cancer, why is it not manifest as PTSD or more readily detected in cancer populations? There are several possibilities. First, most patients probably cope effectively and may resolve threats associated with cancer diagnoses quickly, making PTSD less likely. Another possibility is that PTSD or the effects of traumatic stress among cancer patients may not appear exactly as they do in most instances of severe stress or victimization. Traumatic stress may be manifest in different ways when major stressors such as those associated with surgery are quickly superimposed on it, and the influences of each major but time-limited treatment stressor may transform PTSD symptoms as well. For example, people who are exposed to a traumatic stressor and then are quickly faced with a succession of major stressors may not experience intrusive or ruminative thoughts about the initial event but may instead experience unwanted or uncontrollable thoughts about existential concerns, more generalized apprehensiveness, or reactivity to a range of stimuli. Alternately, they may focus on more controllable mundane aspects of the cascade of stressors following diagnosis, and hence the content of their concerns and intrusions may change as these stressors change.

In most cases of PTSD, intrusive thoughts and reminiscences are related to the traumatic event, but with the intervening stressors associated with having cancer and being treated for it, these symptoms of PTSD may be transformed and may be manifest as a different set of symptoms. If one is seeking to make a PTSD diagnosis and asks about reexperiencing symptoms, patients' answers may be misleading. In most cases diagnostic criteria have included stressor-related stimuli and intrusive thoughts that were often related to soldiers' combat experiences in Vietnam, the events or experiences associated with disasters and serious accidents, and other aspects of traumatic events (e.g., Blanchard et al., 1996; Delahanty et al., 1996; Keane et al., 1995). In cases in which new stressors supplant attention to trauma, such as cancer, intrusive thoughts after treatment may no longer reflect rumination about cancer but could reflect worries about safety, control, and uncertainty that might have appeared secondary to the trauma. The ongoing nature of the sources of trauma and the continuing threat associated with cancer are different from most of these traumatic events, and we should expect that manifestations of traumatic stress would be different as well. In addition, changes in social support or other interpersonal losses subsequent to cancer and cancer treatment may affect how symptoms are expressed. Generalized worry about the future, diminished confidence in one's ability to predict or control future events, and an intrusive sense of mortality may form the basis for continued distress and symptom expression.

Conclusion

The studies described in this chapter offer ample evidence that having and being treated for cancer are stressful experiences and that some of this stress may linger beyond active and successful treatment of the disease. Patients experience distress at the time of diagnosis and during or immediately after adjuvant treatment (Eakes et al., 1996; Holland et al., 1979; Love et al., 1988; Stanton & Snider, 1993). Distress associated with the experience of treatment may affect adherence (Gilbar & De-Nour, 1989), and side effects of chemotherapy can continue after the cessation of treatment (Kornblith et al., 1992; Meyerowitz, 1983). Stress may decrease over time after diagnosis or after completion of stressful procedures, although completion of treatment may be stressful for some patients (e.g., Andersen et al., 1989b; Dean, 1987; Holland et al., 1979; Hughes, 1982). Patients with advanced disease may be more likely to continue to experience stress and adjustment problems than patients with early stage disease (e.g., Kornblith et al., 1995; Pettingale et al., 1988). Evidence of traumatic stress associated with a cancer diagnosis or of its continued effects on coping and well-being is incomplete, and research is needed in several areas.

Adjustment to cancer is a dynamic, complex process that may contribute to the variability of disease course and response to treatment. Much remains unknown regarding the manner in which people cope with cancer. Future research should address the issue of whether observed rates of psychiatric disorders among cancer patients are due to this notion of symptom transformation, to the tendency to study early stage patients with relatively good prognoses, to the long intervals between cancer diagnosis and measurement of PTSD characteristic of some studies, or whether PTSD simply does not occur in this population as often as in other traumatized groups. The roles of uncertainty, denial or acceptance, appraisal, and life threat in response to the diagnosis also need to be studied to provide a clearer picture of how persistent traumatic stress is manifest in this population. Finally, the opportunities to address trauma-related stressors early in the process of coping with cancer may have a broad effect and lessen distress and adjustment problems across the entire process. Research should also address whether interventions designed to facilitate adjustment of cancer patients (and enhance quality of life) should target the traumatic aspects of cancer or anticipate the dual impact of life threat and discrete treatment or social stressors on patient coping and well-being. The potential that continued treatment of cancer patients with chemoprevention agents like tamoxifen may have for reducing or exacerbating distress should also be explored and addressed in these interventions. Systematic consideration of these and related issues should provide important insights into the nature of stress and adjustment to cancer and improve the overall quality of care and management of this serious illness.

References

Alter, C., Pelcovitz, D., Axelrod, A., Goldenberg, B., Harris, H., Meyers, B., Grobois, B., Mandel, F., Septimus, A., & Kaplan, S. (1996). Identification of PTSD in cancer survivors. *Psychosomatics, 37,* 137–143.

American Psychiatric Association. (1980). *Diagnostic and statistical manual of mental disorders* (3rd ed.). Washington, DC: Author.

American Psychiatric Association. (1987). *Diagnostic and statistical manual of mental disorders* (3rd ed., rev.). Washington, DC: Author.

American Psychiatric Association. (1994). *Diagnostic and statistical manual of mental disorders* (4th ed.). Washington, DC: Author.

Andersen, B. (1989). Health psychology's contribution to addressing the cancer problem: Update on accomplishments. *Health Psychology, 8,* 683–703.

Andersen, B., Anderson, B., & deProsse, C. (1989a). Controlled prospective longitudinal study of women with cancer: I. Sexual functioning outcomes. *Journal of Consulting and Clinical Psychology, 57,* 683–691.

Andersen, B., Anderson, B., & deProsse, C. (1989b). Controlled prospective longitudinal study of women with cancer: II. Psychological outcomes. *Journal of Consulting and Clinical Psychology, 57,* 692–697.

Andrykowski, M., & Cordova, M. (1998). Factors associated with PTSD symptoms following treatment for breast cancer: Test of the Andersen model. *Journal of Traumatic Stress, 11,* 189–203.

Andrykowski, M., Cordova, M., Studts, J., & Miller, T. (1998). Posttraumatic stress disorder after treatment for breast cancer: Prevalence of diagnosis and use of the PTSD Checklist–Civilian Version (PLC–C) as a screening instrument. *Journal of Consulting and Clinical Psychology, 66,* 586–590.

Baum, A. (1987). Toxins, technology, and natural disasters. In G. R. VandenBos, B. K. Bryant, et al. (Eds.), *Cataclysims, crises, and catastrophes: Psychology in action.* The master lectures, Vol. 6. (pp. 5–53). Washington, DC: American Psychological Association.

Baum, A., Cohen, L., & Hall, M. (1993). Control and intrusive memories as possible determinants of chronic stress. *Psychosomatic Medicine, 55,* 274–286.

Baum, A., & Fleming, I. (1993). Implications of psychological research on stress and technological accidents. *American Psychologist, 48,* 665–672.

Baum, A., O'Keeffe, M., & Davidson, L. (1990). Acute stressors and chronic response: The case of traumatic stress. *Journal of Applied Social Psychology, 20,* 1643–1654.

Berman, S., & Wandersman, A. (1990). Fear of cancer and knowledge of cancer: A review and proposed relevance to hazardous waste sites. *Social Science and Medicine, 31*, 81–90.

Blanchard, E., Hickling, E., Taylor, A., Loos, W., Forneris, C., & Jaccard, J. (1996). Who develops PTSD from motor vehicle accidents? *Behavior Research and Therapy, 34*, 1–10.

Bryant, R., & Harvey, A. (1996). Initial posttraumatic stress responses following motor vehicle accidents. *Journal of Traumatic Stress, 9*, 223–234.

Carver, C., Pozo, C., Harris, S., Noriega, V., Scheier, M., Robinson, D., Ketcham, A., Moffat, F., & Clark, K. (1993). How coping mediates the effect of optimism on distress: A study of women with early stage breast cancer. *Journal of Personality and Social Psychology, 65*, 375–390.

Cella, D. F., Mahon, S. M., & Donovan, M. I. (1990). Cancer recurrence as a traumatic event. *Behavioral Medicine, 16*(1), 15–22.

Cella, D., & Tross, S. (1986). Psychological adjustment to survival from Hodgkin's disease. *Journal of Consulting and Clinical Psychology, 54*, 616–622.

Christman, N. (1990). Uncertainty and adjustment during radiotherapy. *Nursing Research, 39*, 17–20.

Cordova, M., Andrykowski, M., Kenady, D., McGrath, P., Sloan, D., & Redd, W. (1995). Frequency and correlates of posttraumatic-stress-disorder-like symptoms after treatment for breast cancer. *Journal of Consulting and Clinical Psychology, 63*, 981–986.

Creamer, M., Burgess, P., & Pattison, P. (1992). Reaction to trauma: A cognitive model. *Journal of Abnormal Psychology, 101*, 452–459.

Davidson, L., & Baum, A. (1986). Chronic stress and posttraumatic stress disorders. *Journal of Consulting and Clinical Psychology, 54*, 303–308.

Dean, C. (1987). Psychiatric morbidity following mastectomy preoperative predictors and types of illness. *Journal of Psychosomatic Research, 31*, 385–392.

Delahanty, D. L., Dougall, A. L., Schmitz, J. B., Hawken, L., Trakowski, J. H., Jenkins, F. J., & Baum, A. (1996). Time course of natural killer cell activity and lymphocyte proliferation in response to two acute stressors in healthy men. *Health Psychology, 15*(1), 48–55.

Delahanty, D., Herberman, H., Craig, K., Hayward, M., Fullerton, C., Ursano, R., & Baum, A. (1997). Acute and chronic distress and posttraumatic stress disorder as a function of responsibility for serious motor vehicle accidents. *Journal of Consulting and Clinical Psychology, 65*, 560–567.

Derogatis, L., Morrow, G., Fetting, J., Penman, D., Piasetsky, S., Schmale, A., Heinrichs, M., & Carnicke, C. (1983). The prevalence of psychiatric disorders among cancer patients. *Journal of the American Medical Association, 249*, 751–757.

Devlen, J., Maguire, P., Phillips, P., & Crowther, D. (1987a). Psychological problems associated with the diagnosis and treatment of lymphomas: II. Prospective study. *British Medical Journal, 295*, 955–957.

Devlen, J., Maguire, P., Phillips, P., Crowther, D., & Chambers, H. (1987b). Psychological problems associated with the diagnosis and treatment of lymphomas: II. Retrospective study. *British Medical Journal, 295*, 953–954.

Doerfler, L., Pbert, L., & DeCosimo, D. (1994). Symptoms of posttraumatic stress disorder following myocardial infarction and coronary artery bypass surgery. *General Hospital Psychiatry, 16*, 193–199.

Dougall, A. L., Craig, K. J., & Baum, A. (1999). Assessment of characteristics of intrusive thoughts and their impact on distress among victims of traumatic events. *Psychosomatic Medicine, 61*(1), 38–48.

Eakes, G., Rakfal, S., Keel, E., & Gaiser, J. (1996). The cancer experience: Responses of patients receiving outpatient radiotherapy. *Journal of Psychosocial Oncology, 14*, 19–30.

Fairbank, J. A., & Nicholson, R. A. (1987). Theoretical and empirical issues in the treatment of post-traumatic stress disorder in Vietnam veterans. *Journal of Clinical Psychology, 43*(1), 44–55.

Fawzy, F., Fawzy, N., Arndt, L., & Pasnau, R. (1995). Critical review of psychosocial interventions in cancer care. *Archives of General Psychiatry, 52*, 100–113.

Fleming, I., Baum, A., Davidson, L. M., Rectanus, E., & McArdle, S. (1987). Chronic stress as a factor in physiologic reactivity to challenge. *Health Psychology, 6*(3), 221–237.

Foa, E., Steketee, G., & Rothbaum, B. (1989). Behavior/cognitive conceptualization of post-traumatic stress disorder. *Behavior Therapy, 20*, 155–176.

Foa, E. B., Zinbarg, R., & Rothbaum, B. O. (1992). Uncontrollability and unpredictability in post-traumatic stress disorder: An animal model. *Psychological Bulletin, 112*, 218–238.

Freud, S. (1955). Beyond the pleasure principle. In J. Strachey (Ed. and Trans.), *The standard edition of the complete psychological works of Sigmund Freud* (Vol. 18, pp. 3–64). London: Hogarth Press. (Original work published 1920)

Friedman, M. (1991). Biological approaches to the diagnosis and treatment of post-traumatic stress disorder. *Journal of Traumatic Stress, 4*, 67–91.

Gilbar, O., & De-Nour, A. (1989). Adjustment to illness and dropout of chemotherapy. *Journal of Psychosomatic Research, 33*, 1–5.

Green, B. (1990). Defining trauma: Terminology and generic stressor dimension. *Journal of Applied Social Psychology, 20*, 1632–1642.

Green, B. (1994). Psychosocial research in traumatic stress: An update. *Journal of Traumatic Stress, 7*, 341–362.

Green, B., Rowland, J. H., Krupnick, J. L., Epstein, S. A., Stockton, P., Stern, N. M., Spertus, I. L., & Steakley, C. (1998). Prevalence of post-traumatic stress disorder in women with breast cancer. *Psychosomatics, 39*(2), 102–111.

Gump, B., & Matthews, K. (1999). Do background stressors influence reactivity to and recovery from acute stressors? *Journal of Applied Social Psychology, 29*(3), 469–494.

Helgeson, V., & Cohen, S. (1996). Social support and adjustment to cancer: Reconciling descriptive, correlational, and intervention research. *Health Psychology, 15*, 135–148.

Holland, J., Rowland, J., Lebovits, A., & Rusalem, R. (1979). Reactions to cancer treatment. *Psychiatric Clinics of North America, 2*, 347–358.

Horowitz, M. (1973). Phase oriented treatment of stress response syndromes. *American Journal of Psychotherapy, 27*, 506–515.

Horowitz, M. (1976). *Stress response syndromes*. New York: Jason Aronson.

Horowitz, M. (1997). *Stress response syndromes: PTSD, grief, & adjustment disorders*. New York: Jason Aronson.

Horowitz, M., & Reidbord, S. (1992). Memory, emotion, and response to trauma. In S. Christianson (Ed.), *The handbook of emotion and memory: Research and theory* (pp. 343–357). Hillsdale, NJ: Erlbaum.

Hughes, J. (1982). Emotional reactions to the diagnosis and treatment of early breast cancer. *Journal of Psychosomatic Research, 26*, 277–283.

Hyer, L., and Associates. (1994). *Trauma victim: Theoretical and practical suggestions*. Muncie, IN: Accelerated Development.

Ironson, G., Wynings, C., Schneiderman, N., Baum, A., Rodriguez, M., Greenwood, D., Benight, C., Antoni, M., LaPerriere, A., Huang, H., Klimas, N., & Fletcher, M. (1997). Posttraumatic stress symptoms, intrusive thoughts, loss, and immune function after Hurricane Andrew. *Psychosomatic Medicine, 59*, 128–141.

Jacobsen, P., Bovbjerg, D., & Redd, W. (1993). Anticipatory anxiety in women receiving chemotherapy for breast cancer. *Health Psychology, 12*, 469–475.

Jacobsen, P. B., Widows, M. R., Hanna, D. M., Andrykowski, M. A., Kronish, L. E., & Fields, K. K. (1998). Post-traumatic stress disorder symptoms after bone marrow transplantation for breast cancer. *Psychosomatic Medicine, 60*, 366–371.

Janoff-Bulman, R. (1992). *Shattered assumptions: Towards a new psychology of trauma*. New York: Free Press.

Janoff-Bulman, R. (1995). Victims of violence. In G. Everly & J. Lating (Eds.), *Psychotraumatology* (pp. 73–86). New York: Plenum. (Original work published 1988)

Janoff-Bulman, R., & Frieze, I. (1983). Theoretical perspective for understanding reactions to victimization. *Journal of Social Issues, 39*, 1–17.

Janoff-Bulman, R., & Wortman, C. (1977). Attributions of blame and coping in the "real world": Severe accident victims react to their lot. *Journal of Personality and Social Psychology, 35*, 351–363.

Jones, J. C., & Barlow, D. H. (1990). The etiology of posttraumatic stress disorder. *Clinical Psychology Review, 10*(3), 299–328.

Kash, K. M., Holland, J. C., Halper, M. S., & Miller, D. G. (1992). Psychological distress and surveillance behaviors of women with a family history of breast cancer. *Journal of the National Cancer Institute, 84*, 24–30.

Keane, T., Zimmering, R., & Caddell, J. (1995). A behavioral formulation of posttraumatic stress disorder in Vietnam veterans. *The Behavior Therapist, 8*, 9–12.

King, D. W., King, L. A., & Foy, D. W. (1996). Prewar factors in combat-related posttraumatic stress disorder: Structural equation modeling with a national sample of female and male Vietnam veterans. *Journal of Consulting and Clinical Psychology, 64*(3), 520–531.

Kolb, L. (1987). A neuropsychological hypothesis explaining post traumatic stress disorders. *The American Journal of Psychiatry, 144,* 989–995.

Koopman, C., Classen, C., & Spiegel, D. (1994). Predictors of posttraumatic stress symptoms survivors of the Oakland/Berkeley, Calif., firestorm. *American Journal of Psychiatry, 151,* 888–894.

Kornblith, A., Anderson, J., Cella, D., Tross, S., Zuckerman, E., Cherin, E., Hendersen, E., Weiss, R., Cooper, R., Silver, R., Leone, L., Canellos, G., Gottlieg, A., & Holland, J. (1992). Hodgkin disease survivors at increased risk for problems in psychosocial adaptation. *Cancer, 70,* 2214–2224.

Kornblith, A., Thaler, H., Wong, G., Vlamis, V., Lepore, J., Loseth, D., Hakes, T., Hoskins, W., & Portenoy, R. (1995). Quality of life of women with ovarian cancer. *Gynecologic Oncology, 59,* 231–242.

Krupnick, J., & Horowitz, M. (1981). Stress response syndromes: Recurrent themes. *Archives of General Psychiatry, 38,* 428–435.

Lang, P. (1985). The cognitive psychophysiology of emotion: Fear and anxiety. In A. Tuma & J. Maser (Eds.), *Anxiety and the anxiety disorders* (pp. 131–170). Hillsdale, NJ: Erlbaum.

Lazarus, R. (1966). *Psychological stress and the coping process.* New York: McGraw Hill.

Lazarus, R., & Folkman, S. (1984). *Stress, appraisal and coping.* New York: Springer.

Lee, K., Vaillant, G., Torrey, W., & Elder, G. (1995). A 50-year old prospective study of psychological sequelae of World War II combat. *American Journal of Psychiatry, 152,* 516–522.

Lerman, C., Kash, K., & Stefanek, M. (1994). Younger women at increased risk for breast cancer: Perceived risk, psychological well-being, and surveillance behavior. *Journal of the National Cancer Institute Monographs, 16,* 171–176.

Lerman, C., Lustbader, E., Rimer, B., Daly, M., Miller, S., Sands, C., & Balshem, A. (1995). Effects of individualized breast cancer risk counseling: A randomized trial. *Journal of the National Cancer Institute, 87,* 286–292.

Love, R., Leventhal, H., Easterling, D., & Nerenz, D. (1988). Side effects and emotional distress during cancer chemotherapy. *Cancer, 63,* 604–612.

Maguire, G. P. (1988). Psychological morbidity among cancer patients—who needs help? *Oncology (Huntington), 2*(6), 55–59, 62–64.

Maguire, G., Lee, E., Bevingtom, D., Kuchemann, S., Crabtree, R., & Cornell, C. (1978). Psychiatric problems in the first year after mastectomy. *British Medical Journal, 1,* 963–965.

Manuel, G., Roth, S., Keefe, F., & Brantley, B. (1987). Coping with cancer. *Journal of Human Stress, 13*(4), 149–158.

Mason, J., Giller, E., Kosten, T., Ostroff, R., & Harkness, L. (1986). Urinary free-cortisol in post-traumatic stress disorder. *Journal of Nervous and Mental Diseases, 174,* 145–149.

McCorkel, R., & Quint-Benoliel, J. (1983). Symptom distress, current concerns and mood disturbance after diagnosis of life-threatening disease. *Social Science and Medicine, 17,* 431–438.

McFarlane, A. (1988). The phenomenology of posttraumatic stress disorders following a natural disaster. *The Journal of Nervous and Mental Disease, 176,* 22–29.

McFarlane, A. (1992). Avoidance and intrusion in posttraumatic stress disorder. *Journal of Nervous and Mental Disease, 180,* 439–445.

Meyer, T., & Mark, M. (1995). Effects of psychosocial interventions with adult cancer patients: A meta-analysis of randomized experiments. *Health Psychology, 14,* 101–108.

Meyerowitz, B. (1980). Psychosocial correlates of breast cancer and its treatment. *Psychological Bulletin, 87,* 108–131.

Meyerowitz, B. (1983). Postmastectomy coping strategies and quality of life. *Health Psychology, 2*(2), 117–132.

O'Connor, A., Wicker, C., & Germino, B. (1990). Understanding the cancer patient's search for meaning. *Cancer Nursing, 13,* 165–175.

Palmer, A. G., Tucker, S., Warren, R., & Adams, M. (1993). Understanding women's responses to treatment for cervical intra-epithelial neoplasia. *British Journal of Clinical Psychology, 32,* 101–112.

Patterson, D. R., Carrgian, L., Questad, K. A., & Robinson, R. (1990). Posttraumatic stress disorder in hospitalized patients with burn injuries. *Journal of Burn Care & Rehabilitation, 11*(3), 181–184.

Peretz, T., Baider, L., Ever-Hadani, P., & De-Nour, A. (1994). Psychological distress in female cancer patients with Holocaust experience. *General Hospital Psychiatry, 16,* 413–418.

Perry, S., Difede, J., Musngi, G., Frances, A., & Jacobsberg, L. (1992). Predictors of posttraumatic stress disorder after burn injury. *American Journal of Psychiatry, 149,* 931–935.

Pettingale, K. W., Burgess, C., & Greer, S. (1988). Psychological response to cancer diagnosis— I. Correlations with prognostic variables. *Journal of Psychosomatic Research, 32*(3), 255–261.

Pillemer, D. (1984). Flashbulb memories of the assassination attempt on President Reagan. *Cognition, 16,* 63–80.

Resnick, H., Yehuda, R., Pitman, R., & Foy, D. (1995). Effect of previous trauma on acute plasma cortisol level following rape. *American Journal of Psychiatry, 152,* 1675–1677.

Roca, R., Spence, R., & Munster, A. (1992). Posttraumatic adaptation and distress among adult burn survivors. *American Journal of Psychiatry, 149,* 1234–1238.

Rothbaum, B., & Foa, E. (1992). Subtypes of posttraumatic stress disorder and duration of symptoms. In J. Davidson & E. Foa (Eds.), *Posttraumatic stress disorder: DSM–IV and beyond* (pp. 23–35). Washington, DC: American Psychiatric Press.

Shalev, A. (1992). Posttraumatic stress disorder among injured survivors of a terrorist attack: Predictive value of early intrusion and avoidance symptoms. *Journal of Nervous and Mental Disease, 180,* 505–509.

Shalev, A., Bonne, O., & Eth, S. (1996). Treatment of posttraumatic stress disorder: A review. *Psychosomatic Medicine, 58,* 165–182.

Spiegel, D., Bloom, H., Kraemer, J., & Gottheil, E. (1989). Effect of psychosocial treatment on survival of patients with metastatic breast cancer. *Lancet, 1,* 888–901.

Stanton, A., & Snider, P. (1993). Coping with a breast cancer diagnosis: A prospective study. *Health Psychology, 12,* 16–23.

Taylor, S. (1983). Adjustment to threatening events: A theory of cognitive adaptation. *American Psychologist, 38*(11), 1161–1173.

Taylor, S., Lichtman, R., Wood, J., Bluming, A., Dosik, G., & Leibowitz, R. (1985). Illness-related and treatment-related factors in psychological adjustment to breast cancer. *Cancer, 55,* 2506–2513.

Tjemsland, L., Soreide, J. A., & Malt, U. F. (1998). Post-traumatic distress symptoms in operable breast cancer: III. Status one year after surgery. *Breast Cancer Research & Treatment, 47*(2), 141–151.

Ullman, S., & Siegel, J. (1994). Predictors of exposure to traumatic events and posttraumatic stress sequelae. *Journal of Community Psychology, 22,* 328–338.

Ursano, R. J., Fullerton, C. S., Kao, T. C., & Bhartiya, V. R. (1995). Longitudinal assessment of posttraumatic stress disorder and depression after exposure to traumatic death. *Journal of Nervous and Mental Disease, 183*(1), 36–42.

Ursano, R. J., Fullerton, C. S., Vance, K., & Kao, T. C. (1999). Posttraumatic stress disorder and identification in disaster workers. *American Journal of Psychiatry, 156,* 353–359.

Valdimarsdottir, H., Bovbjerg, D., Kash, K., Holland, J., Osborne, M., & Miller, D. (1995). Psychological distress in women with a familial risk of breast cancer. *Psychooncology, 4,* 133–141.

van der Kolk, B. (1988). The trauma spectrum: The interaction of biological and social events in the genesis of the trauma response. *Journal of Traumatic Stress, 1,* 273–290.

van der Kolk, B., & Ducey, C. (1989). The psychological processing of traumatic experience: Rorschach patterns in PTSD. *Journal of Traumatic Stress, 2,* 259–274.

van der Kolk, B., & Fisler, R. (1995). Dissociation and the fragmentary nature of traumatic memories: Overview and exploratory study. *Journal of Traumatic Stress, 8,* 505–525.

Ward, S., Viergutz, G., Tormey, D., deMuth, J., & Paulen, A. (1992). Patients' reactions to completion of adjuvant breast cancer therapy. *Nursing Research, 41,* 362–366.

Weinstein, N. D. (1988). The precaution adoption hypothesis. *Health Psychology, 7,* 355–386.

Williams, J. M. G., Watts, F. N., MacLeod, C., & Mathews, A. (Eds.). (1988). *Cognitive psychology and emotional disorders.* Chichester, England: John Wiley & Sons.

Wortman, C., & Dunkel-Schetter, C. (1979). Interpersonal relationships and cancer: A theoretical analysis. *Journal of Social Issues, 35,* 120–155.

Yehuda, R., McFarlane, A. C., & Shalev, A. Y. (1998). Predicting the development of posttraumatic stress disorder from the acute response to a traumatic event. *Biological Psychiatry, 44*(12), 1305–1313.

Yehuda, R., Resnick, H., Kahana, B., & Giller, E. (1993). Long-lasting hormonal alterations to extreme stress in humans: Normative or maladaptive? *Psychosomatic Medicine, 55,* 287–297.

Zilberg, N., Weiss, D., & Horowitz, M. (1982). Impact of Event Scale: A cross-validation study and some empirical evidence supporting a conceptual model of stress response syndromes. *Journal of Consulting and Clinical Psychology, 50,* 407–414.

CHAPTER 10

Assessing the Important Effector Mechanisms in the Immune Response Against Cancer

Olivera J. Finn

E ffective treatment for cancer must remove every cancer cell while sparing normal tissue. Even the best chemotherapy, surgery, or radiation cannot fulfill that requirement. The only hope of achieving this goal is by harnessing the immune system. The effective function of the immune system depends on many factors, including age and physical and mental health. Each of these factors alone or in concert may determine whether the immune system recognizes the presence of a tumor (priming of the immune response), responds appropriately (amplification of the immune response), and destroys the tumor (effector phase of the immune response). I review specific cells and molecules that are involved at each step and could be affected by interventions designed to control factors that control the immune response.

Tumor-Specific Immunity

How is tumor-specific immunity elicited? To answer this question one must use as a blueprint well-studied immune responses to viral and bacterial pathogens. Most microorganisms that are encountered frequently do not cause perceptible disease in humans even when they penetrate skin or epithelial barriers. That is because they are quickly eliminated by preformed effector mechanisms of innate immunity, notably macrophages (cells that surround and devour foreign particles or altered

I am indebted to all of my former and current graduate students and fellows who have contributed data that have shaped my ideas. Special thanks go to John McKolanis and Elisabeth Hiltbold from the University of Pittsburgh and to Augusto Ochoa from Tulane Medical School for illustrations in this chapter.

cells) and natural killer (NK) cells (large granular lymphocytes that can kill almost any kind of microinvader). These cells can be activated to eliminate extracellular microorganisms, kill cells invaded by pathogens, and produce cytokines and other inflammatory mediators (Fearon & Locksley, 1996). They also recruit additional phagocytic cells and NK cells to the site of infection and produce additional cytokines or other inflammatory agents and create an inflammation site. If the inflammatory process does not result in complete removal of the infectious agent, it serves to provide support for activation of a second, antigen-specific set of responses known as *adaptive immunity* (Paul & Seder, 1994). While the elements of innate immunity are battling an invading microorganism or altered cell, the antigen is transported to the lymph nodes either as intact microorganisms or within macrophages that serve as antigen-presenting cells (APC). Together with dendritic cells, they take up and process antigen particles and stimulate small numbers of naive helper T cells and cytotoxic T cells that have not been previously exposed to antigen. Soluble particles are bound by naive B cells, which also undergo activation. The rich cytokine soup draining into the lymph node from the inflammation site and new cytokines secreted by specifically activated T and B cells provide just the right environment for these cells to reproduce and proliferate as activated, mature effector cells. This process releases into the periphery antigen-specific helper T cells and cytotoxic T cells, as well as large amounts of antibodies produced by activated B cells that have matured into plasma cells. They can now travel to the original site of inflammation, where the innate immunity is still at work keeping the pathogen in check, or to other sites to which the pathogen may have spread (MacLennan, 1994, Springer, 1994). These specific mechanisms with their varied armamentarium of cytokines can completely eliminate the pathogen. The antigen-specific effector cells and antibodies continue to circulate for some time during which they provide immediate protective immunity to reinfection. Once all antigen is cleared, a subset of these cells further differentiates to provide immunological memory (Sprent, 1994). Memory T and B cells are able to undergo quick expansion and transition into activated effector cells should the same pathogen appear any time in the future, clearing the pathogen before any evidence of disease.

If this blueprint for a successful immune response is applied to the case of a slowly growing spontaneous tumor, certain requirements are not met. Malignant cells, being mostly body tissue ("self"), with only a few tumor-specific mutations, do not generally activate the mechanisms of innate immunity. As a result, there typically is no initial formation of an inflammation site. Knowing the importance of these early events for assuring a more robust course of the later events, one must assume that this is where tumor-specific immunity is first compromised. NK cells have been shown in vitro to be able to kill tumor cells without prior activation (Reyburn et al., 1997), but it is not clear whether this function is significant in vivo or whether it results in NK cell activation at the tumor site, which could mimic in part the early innate response to pathogens. Macrophages have also been shown in vitro to be able to kill tumor cells when activated by certain cytokines, and it is possible that they too may migrate into the tumor and contribute some inflammatory cytokines. However, it is not clear what signals attract them to the tumor site. It is more likely in the case of tumor immunity that the entire process is reversed: Tumors elicit adaptive immunity first, and only later the specific effector T cells and specific antibodies that migrate to the tumor site may provide signals for the nonspecific, innate immunity players to participate in tumor destruction. Consequently, the most important players in eliciting tumor-specific immunity may not be NK cells or macrophages, but rather antigen-specific T cells and B cells of the adaptive immune response. As naive cells in the tumor-draining lymph node, they recognize the existence of tumor antigens processed and presented by APC. This initial activation is followed by proliferation of activated effector cells. Tumor-specific helper and cytotoxic T cells enter circulation and migrate to all sites of the tumor and initiate its destruction. Tumor-specific B cells mature into plasma cells and produce tumor-specific antibodies that bind tumor cells in circulation, marking them for destruction by complement or for elimination by phagocytic cells. Antibodies also accumulate at the sites of tumor where they bind, complement, and activate the innate immune response. Once all the tumor is gone, a subset of the effector cells differentiates into memory cells to provide long-lasting protection against tumor recurrence.

This "reversed order" of events, adaptive immunity elicited before innate immunity, may account for tumor-specific immune responses being quantitatively different (lower numbers of effector cells) as well as qualitatively different (different cytokines produced by the effector cells) from antiviral or antibacterial responses. The quantitative difference is the result of a weaker amplification of effector cells in the absence of the rich cytokine mixture that is produced when inflammation occurs first. The qualitative difference resides in the cytokines produced by mature effector cells. Naive helper T cells can be activated to develop into type 1 or type 2 cells depending on the cytokines they produce (Seder & Paul, 1994). A typical type 1 cytokine is interferon gamma, and a typical type 2 cytokine is interleukin-4 (IL-4). Type 1 cells primarily support development of cytotoxic T cells. These can also mature into type 1 cytolytic T lymphocytes (CTL) that make interferon gamma and other type 1 cytokines, or type 2, CTL that make IL-4 or other type 2 cytokines (Croft, Carter, Swain, & Dutton, 1996). Type 2 helper T cells help differentiation of antibody-producing cells. During early inflammatory responses carried out by the innate immune mechanisms, the abundance of many different cytokines provides a balanced environment in which both type 1 and type 2 cells can develop. When these early responses are missing, the direction of helper T cell development can be easily skewed depending on the most abundant cytokine present at that particular time at the tumor site. If this happens to be a type 2 cytokine, the predominant tumor-specific response that develops may be an antibody response. Whereas antibodies play a role in rounding out the antitumor immune response, it is clear from numerous animal studies that CTL are the effector mechanism primarily responsible for tumor destruction. Thus, biasing the immune response toward a single effector mechanism, such as antibody in the absence of CTL, may further compromise its effectiveness.

Despite these suboptimal conditions, both humoral and cellular immune responses to cancer do develop and have been used to define tumor-specific antigens that have already been explored as possible cancer vaccines. These immune responses are likely to be protective under normal circumstances but may be easier to defeat if a person is threatened with cancer at a time of some strongly immunocompromising episode, such as in the course of treatment for another disease with immunosuppressive drugs or during a prolonged period of stress. The cancer might then grow unimpeded even in the face of existing tumor-specific immunity. The increasing tumor burden can further add to continuous immunosuppression through soluble products secreted by the tumor. Even if the tumor is discovered and removed very early, the chemotherapy treatment that is prescribed in many cases further suppresses the immune system, giving few surviving tumor cells advantage precisely at the time when they would be most susceptible to immune attack. Alternatively, and much more important for the subject of this book, simply facing a diagnosis of a life-threatening disease can alter the patient's mental state in the direction of creating an immunosuppressive environment that favors tumor recurrence.

If we fully understand the processes and the mechanisms involved, it might be possible to control many of the suspected adverse influences that weaken the tumor-specific immune response. This can be accomplished by asking very specific questions regarding the function of the critical immune effector mechanisms and by finding out which ones are either positively or negatively affected by a specific treatment.

Critical Effector Mechanisms in Tumor-Specific Immune Responses

Inasmuch as there is no effective treatment against metastatic disease, the first question asked after surgery should be how to best use the immune response to prevent tumor recurrence. The obvious choices are to strengthen it through vaccination in tumors for which candidate vaccines are becoming available; or to create the most supportive, least immunosuppressive environment in which the immune system can optimally function. This includes (but is not limited to) interventions to eliminate stress as an important immunosuppressor. Ideally, multiple interventions are ultimately combined such that, for example, patients would be vaccinated at the time when their stress levels are judged to be low.

In order for this approach to become an accepted practice, data must be accumulated to show where the immune response has failed and to prove that specific interventions can restore its function. The critical players in tumor-specific immune responses are tumor-specific antigens, antigen-presenting cells, helper T cells, cyto-toxic T cells, and antibodies produced by B cells (Schreiber, 1993). Thus the impor-tant questions to ask are the following:

- Is the tumor recognized by the immune system (does it have tumor-specific antigens)?
- Are the APC, dendritic cells, and macrophages functional (can they process and present tumor antigens)?
- Are tumor-specific helper T cells activated? If so, are they type 1 or type 2?
- Are tumor-specific CTL activated? If so, are they type 1 or type 2?
- Are tumor-specific antibodies produced. If so, what are the isotypes?

The first question has received a lot of attention in the past. The conclusive answer has come as a result of relatively recent advances in our understanding of the nature of antigens in general, how they are processed and presented to T cells, and how they are recognized by T and B cells. It is clear that tumors do not need to contain or express on their surface completely new proteins not expressed by normal cells. Any mutation in a normal protein, even one that does not change the structure or function of that protein, can create a small tumor-specific peptide that can be recognized by the immune system as a tumor-specific antigen. Many such antigens have been defined using T cells derived from cancer patients that recognize tumor cells but not normal cells of the same individual (Henderson & Finn, 1996). The most convenient antigens for vaccine purposes are those that are shared by many tumors. So, generally, the answer to the first question (regarding whether the immune system recognizes tumors) is "yes" and is the one constant in antitumor responses least likely to be subject to influences such as different treatments, age, or mental state. The answers to all the other questions vary from patient to patient and tumor to tumor. The final picture that emerges when these answers are compiled outlines the full extent of immune deviation from what is possible (*immunological outcome*) to what is actually functional in the cancer patient (*disease outcome*). The goal of any intervention designed to improve the immune response against cancer should be geared toward decreasing the magnitude of difference between these two outcomes.

There are very compelling reasons to ask the above questions rather than perform the now standard assays of NK cell function, mitogen stimulation, or cytokine production. The primary reason is that not enough data are currently available to show that changes that are measured in nonspecific immune responses are paralleled by changes in specific immune responses. For example, the disease outcome may show that activation of tumor-specific helper T cells has not occurred, which has led to low frequency of tumor-specific CTL and no tumor-specific antibody produc-tion. At the same time, NK cell function may be perfectly normal, all other T cells (not tumor-specific) may respond to mitogens, and they all may make cytokines.

Similarly, the NK cell function may start low and improve with intervention, giving hope that the disease outcome may change. However, if there are still no tumor-specific CTL or antibodies, the relevant disease outcome will not improve. The attraction of the nonspecific assays has been that they are relatively easy to perform. Although the use of specific assays is not as easy, their use is still recommended. They have been well worked out and are performed routinely in many immunology laboratories (Coligan, 1991; Weir, 1996).

Immunological Versus Disease Outcome in Response to a Breast Cancer Antigen MUC1

To best illustrate how a disease outcome may be measured and then manipulated to a possible and desirable immunological outcome, I use the example of a breast cancer antigen we have studied for many years in hope of using it as a target of a tumor rejection response (Finn et al., 1995). MUC1 is a cell surface protein expressed in low levels on normal epithelial cells. Epithelial adenocarcinomas, such as breast cancer, express very high levels of this protein, which leads to its aberrant processing and subsequent recognition as a tumor-specific antigen by the immune system. When APC, dendritic cells, and macrophages from healthy individuals are grown in vitro and given purified MUC1 protein, they process it efficiently and present it to naive T cells generating potent helper and cytotoxic T cell responses. We contrast that with MUC1-specific responses in advanced breast cancer patients: MUC1-specific CTL can be found, but they are neither potent nor numerous. Helper T cells are not found, leading to the assumption that there is either no processing and presentation of this tumor antigen or (more likely) that the cytokine environment in the tumor-draining lymph node is not supportive of helper T cell activation. Because there are no helper T cells, very few B cells are activated, and the antibody made is primarily Immunoglobulin (Ig) M. The situation is somewhat different in early breast cancer. The frequency of CTL is higher, but it diminishes with tumor progression. Other isotypes of antibody (IgG, IgA) are present, indicating that helper cell activity, even though low, was present to support antibody isotype switch from IgM to IgG, but it also diminished with tumor progression.

In Phase I clinical trials using various forms of MUC1 to formulate several types of vaccines, even in advanced cancer patients some of the disease outcomes have been influenced and brought closer to the desired immunological outcomes. In some patients, the frequency of MUC1-specific CTL was raised above the prevaccination levels (Goydos, Elder, Whiteside, Finn, & Lotze, 1996); in some patients helper T cell activity was elicited together with MUC1-specific IgG (Karanikas et al., 1997). These results were obtained in patients with advanced disease whose disease had not responded to all other forms of therapy. They give hope that similar manipulations of anti-MUC1 immunity early in disease and in combination with other treatments, such as psychosocial intervention to reduce stress, would reproducibly generate the same and better results in most patients.

Measuring Tumor-Specific Immune Responses in Patients Undergoing Intervention

Several trials of psychosocial intervention in breast cancer patients are reported elsewhere in this book. They are a result of the excitement generated in some of the early trials that showed a clear benefit of this form of intervention on disease-free survival and overall survival (Kogon, Biswas, Pearl, Carlson, & Spiegel, 1997; Spiegel, Bloom, Kraemer, & Gottheil, 1989). One of the many hypotheses of the mechanisms underlying the effect of psychosocial intervention on disease-free survival is that reducing stress is beneficial to the function of the immune system and that it is the immune response that keeps the tumor in check. This is a very attractive hypothesis that has yet to be proven. One of the best ways to prove this hypothesis is to evaluate at various times during and following a specific intervention, either tumor-specific immune responses, when specific tumor antigens are available, or appropriate surrogates of tumor-specific responses in cases in which no specific antigens have been identified.

There are several human tumor types for which tumor-specific antigens have been identified and shown in animal models to be targets for tumor rejection (Henderson & Finn, 1996). These include glycoprotein 100 (gp100); tyrosinase; melanoma antigen (MART-1/MelanA) recognized by T cells and several ganglioside antigens for melanomas; a series of melanoma antigens (MAGE) found also in breast tumors and gliomas; growth factor receptor HER-2/neu for breast and ovarian cancer; epithelial MUC1 for breast, pancreas, colon, prostate, lung, and ovarian tumors; carcinoembryonic antigen (CEA) primarily for colon cancer; prostate-specific antigen (PSA) and prostatic acidic phosphatase (PAP) for prostate cancer; oncogene products such as Ras and p53 for a variety of tumors; BCR-ABL for chronic myeloid leukemia; and human papiloma virus (HPV) type 16 antigens E6 and E7 for cervical carcinoma. They provide a wealth of reagents, both proteins and DNA, with which to follow the fate of tumor-specific immune responses before, during, and after intervention and compare those responses between the intervention and the assessment groups.

Using MUC1 as an example, the following are the tests whose results could be very informative. They require drawing blood at specified intervals and separating peripheral blood leukocytes (PBL) and plasma for testing. Plasma can be stored in a $-20°C$ freezer and used in assays for the presence of tumor-specific antibodies. PBL must be frozen at $-70°C$ under controlled conditions to maintain viability of lymphocytes. The samples obtained and stored at various intervals should be tested at the same time to reduce the error caused by experimental variability.

MUC1-Specific Antibodies

There are numerous assays for measuring antibodies, and most are based on the same principle: purified antigen (in this case MUC1) reacts with several dilutions of plasma or serum to allow specific antibodies, if present, to bind the antigen. Unbound material is washed away, and bound antibodies detected by specific, commercially available reagents developed to detect human antibodies. These reagents may detect all antibody isotypes or be specific for IgM, IgG, or IgA. Positive reactivity is detected either by counting radioactivity or by reading optical density. An example of the data obtained at different time intervals on two patients is shown in Figure 10.1. In the case of Patient 1, the data show that antibody levels started high at the time of tumor diagnosis but became much lower when measured 8 months later. In the case of Patient 2, there was an encouraging increase in MUC1-specific antibody over the same period of time. The goal of an intervention would be to either maintain the antibody levels found at the beginning or to raise them. The result seen in Patient 2 would predict a good outcome of the intervention. Disappearance of MUC1-specific antibody would be interpreted as a sign of bad prognosis.

FIGURE 10.1

Measurements of tumor-specific antibodies in plasma of two cancer patients at two different time points from diagnosis using the Enzyme Linked Immunosorbent Assay (ELISA). Optical density (OD) correlates with antibody concentration.

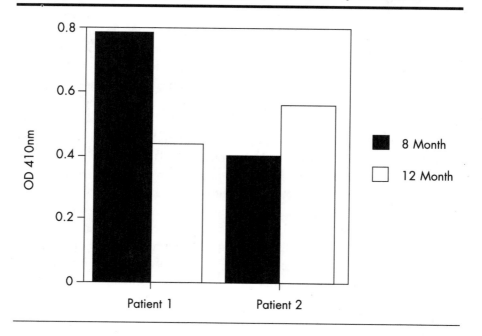

MUC1-Specific CTL

Tumor-specific CTL that circulate in the peripheral blood require a short in vitro culture period in the presence of the tumor antigen to exhibit their cytotoxic function. Previously frozen PBL are cocultured with MUC1$^+$ target cells for up to 7 days. Multiple microcultures are set up at each cell concentration, starting with high numbers and ending with very low numbers of PBL. All these cultures are then tested for the ability to kill a MUC1$^+$ target cell. The target cells are labeled with radioactive tracers, which they release on being lysed. Released radioactivity is a measure of T-cell cytotoxicity. Using a statistical program in combination with a dilution of lymphocytes at which there is no more cytotoxicity, it is possible to determine the frequency of MUC1-specific CTL. An example of data obtained in this type of assay with PBL of three different cancer patients can be seen in Figure 10.2. These patients were entered into a Phase I trial of MUC1 vaccine (Goydos et al., 1996). All three showed an increase in the CTL frequency after vaccination.

FIGURE 10.2

Measurements of tumor-specific cytolytic T lymphocytes frequency in peripheral blood leukocytes of three patients before and after vaccination with a tumor-specific antigen MUC1.

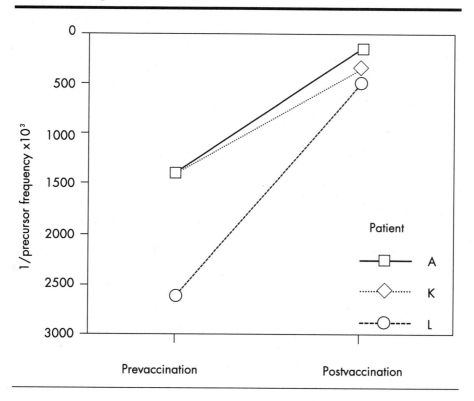

Inasmuch as the goal of this intervention was to increase the CTL numbers, this is an encouraging result. A decrease in their frequency or a total disappearance of the CTL would be seen as a bad sign. Results of other interventions could also be evaluated by the ability to maintain or increase tumor-specific CTL frequency.

MUC1-Specific Helper T Cells

Like the CTL, MUC1-specific helper T cells also require a short-term in vitro culture to exhibit antigen-specific function. Soluble antigen (in this case, purified MUC1 protein or synthetic peptide) is added to small cultures of previously frozen PBL. The APC in the culture process and present the antigen to helper T cells, which get activated and begin to proliferate. Proliferation can be measured simply by counting cells, or more conveniently for large number of samples, by adding radioactive thymidine to the cultures. Thymidine is incorporated into DNA during DNA synthesis. By measuring thymidine incorporation, one can determine the extent of specific helper T cell proliferation. An example of the data obtained is shown in Figure 10.3. Helper cells from two patients are exposed to different forms and different concentrations of the MUC1 tumor antigen. One T-cell population is much more responsive than the other. As before, the goal of an intervention would be to maintain and increase helper T-cell activity. The helper T-cell function should correlate well with antibody levels as well as antibody isotypes. In other words, an increase in helper T-cell function would also be reflected in increasing antibody titers as well as broadening of antibody isotypes.

Measuring Cytokine Production

More important than whether cytokines are produced is a question of what cells produce what cytokines. For example, interferon gamma is a very important cytokine and a hallmark of a type 1 response known to be tumor protective. When a nonspecific stimulus is given to a culture of PBL resulting in interferon gamma detected in the supernatant, a conclusion might be made that this is an indication of a normal type 1 helper cell function. However, NK cells as well as macrophages produce interferon. Thus, interferon can be found in the culture supernatants even if the type 1 cells are completely absent. This is potentially a problem with many cytokines, including IL-4, the hallmark of type 2 responses. In order for the cytokine data to be informative, more refined assays must be used, and they are now available. One of the best is intracellular cytokine staining, which uses the power of the Fluorescence Activated Cell Sorter (FACS) instrument (Becton-Dickinson, San Jose, CA) and a technique that traps the cytokine inside the cell that produces it. The PBL are stimulated with antigen (e.g., MUC1[+] cells, purified MUC-1 protein, MUC1 synthetic peptide), and when activated they are labeled by specific antibodies that can distinguish T cells from other cells and helper T cells from CTL. The next step serves to make the cells permeable and allow access inside the cells to the antibodies detecting specific cytokines. When these multiply-labeled cells are analyzed by FACS, one can precisely determine which cell population (T cells vs. non-T cells, Th vs. CTL)

FIGURE 10.3

Measurements of helper T-cell proliferation in two individuals in response to different concentrations of a tumor-specific antigen, MUC1. Different forms of MUC1 were used: a synthetic peptide (100-mer), a recombinant product (underglycosylated MUC1), or purified protein from the tumor (ascites MUC1). Proliferation of helper T cells in the absence of antigen (No Ag) provided the baseline response. Proliferation was measured by incorporation of radioactive thymidine (^{3}H). CPM indicates counts per minute.

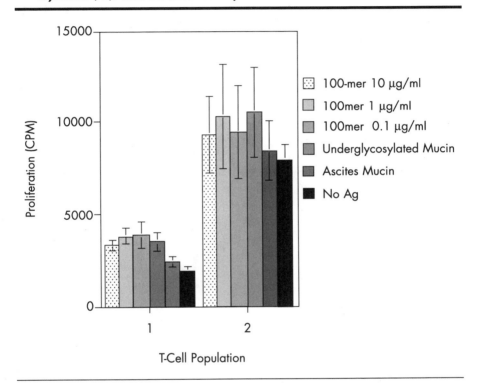

makes what cytokine in response to the antigen (see Figure 10.4). For example, pretreatment samples might indicate that helper T cells are activated, but the only cytokines produced are type 2. This would be a good indication that something has severely biased the tumor-specific immune response toward mostly antibody production, which in turn may explain the failure to control tumor growth. The intervention, in this case, if successful, might be expected to change this situation toward a more balanced response by changing the conditions in favor of the type 1 response. Samples harvested during and after intervention should be examined for evidence that T helper cells are beginning to make type 1 cytokines.

All the experiments described above to test tumor-specific responses using MUC1 antigen can be performed using other tumor antigens more appropriate to specific patient populations under study.

FIGURE 10.4

Fluorescence activated cell sorter analysis of intracellular cytokine production. Quadrant 4 contains cytolytic T lymphocytes (CTL) that carry the CD8 marker (colored in green by an antibody conjugated to a green fluorescent dye, fluoroisothyocyanate, FITC). The X axis indicates amount of green fluorescence. A shift to the right indicates increase in fluorescence, which indicates higher level of expression of the CD8 marker. Quadrant 1 contains helper T lymphocytes that do not carry the CD8 marker and thus are not fluorescent. Stimulation with antigen causes both helper T lymphocytes as well as CTL to produce cytokines. Quadrants 2 and 3 contain cells that make interferon (IFN) gamma (upper panels) or Interleukin-4 (IL-4; lower panels). Cells making cytokines are detected by staining with specific antibodies conjugated to a red fluorescent dye, phycoerythrin (PE). The Y axis indicates amount of red fluorescence. Increase in fluorescence indicates higher level of production of a specific cytokine.

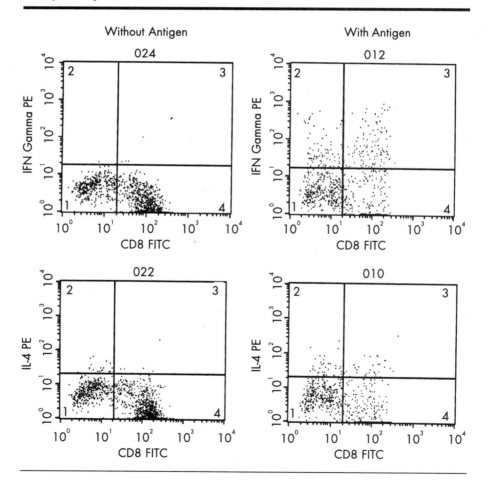

When Can Measurements of Nonspecific Immune Responses Be Informative?

There are circumstances when, even if reagents are available for measuring tumor-specific immune responses, it may still be informative to measure in addition the capacity of all T cells to respond to nonspecific mitogenic stimuli or the ability of NK cells to lyse target cells and make cytokines. Recent work, primarily in patients with advanced cancer and with relatively large tumor burdens, has shown profound deficiencies in T cells, NK cells, and antigen-presenting cells to transmit and interpret activation signals (Finke et al., 1993; Lai et al., 1996; Nagacomi et al., 1993; Zea et al., 1995). The molecular basis for this general form of immune suppression appears to be a drastic reduction in expression of specific phosphotyrosine kinases that participate in signal transduction (Alberola-Ila, Takaki, Kerner, & Perlmutter, 1997). This deficiency is seen in all T cells, not only in tumor-specific cells, and simultaneously in NK cells and APC. The most striking consequence is the inability of these cells to proliferate following activation (the responses to phytohemagglutinin [PHA] are low) or to make cytokines (total cytokine production is low). Activation signals are usually transmitted from the cell surface to the nucleus in order to turn on production of transcription factors, which activate specific genes. Figure 10.5 compares data from three patients with advanced cancer with a healthy individual and shows that cancer patients who suffer from this general immunosuppression lack the ability to make transcription factors necessary to turn on the gamma interferon gene. Only one of three has T cells that can make transcription factors following activation.

The two most intriguing findings in this very recent area of research are that this effect is both nonspecific (all immune cells are affected) and reversible. When patient's lymphocytes are cultured in vitro for a period of 24–48 hours, their normal signaling functions return. It is not clear how early in tumor development this suppression occurs, nor have there been any insights into the cause for the generality of this effect. The most plausible idea is an elaboration either by the tumor or by the immune system (and perhaps even the neuroendocrine system) of a soluble factor or factors that can have this general effect on all cells. The candidate factors have not been proposed and are now only the focus of speculation.

Speculation on the Effect of Stress and Stress Reduction on Tumor-Specific Immune Effector Mechanisms

It has been clear for some time that the immune response is under the influence of neuroendocrine mediators, and the reverse appears to be true. The immune system and the neuroendocrine system provide an integrated mechanism necessary for maintenance of a proper defense function. Lymphocytes, as the key effectors of this

FIGURE 10.5

Molecular analysis of the presence or absence of transcription factors necessary for interferon (IFN) gamma production. Peripheral blood T cells from three cancer patients (P1, P2, and P3) and one healthy individual (N) were purified and their nuclei isolated. The nuclei were disrupted to release nuclear proteins containing transcription factors that bind to interferon gamma gene promoter region and initiate gene transcription. To detect these factors, a radioactive DNA probe was made corresponding to the sequence of the IFN-gamma promoter. The probe was mixed with the nuclear proteins and analyzed by gel electrophoresis and exposure to film. The small DNA probe travels fast through the gel and can be found as a black smear at the bottom of each lane. If the nuclear extract contains IFN-gamma specific transcription factors, they bind to the radioactive probe and create a much bigger complex that travels much slower. We can see that four distinct proteins (indicated by arrows) bind to the probe in the sample from a healthy individual (N). These factors are also present in the sample from P2 but are completely absent from P1 and P3. This suggests that T cells from P1 and P3 would be unable to make IFN-gamma.

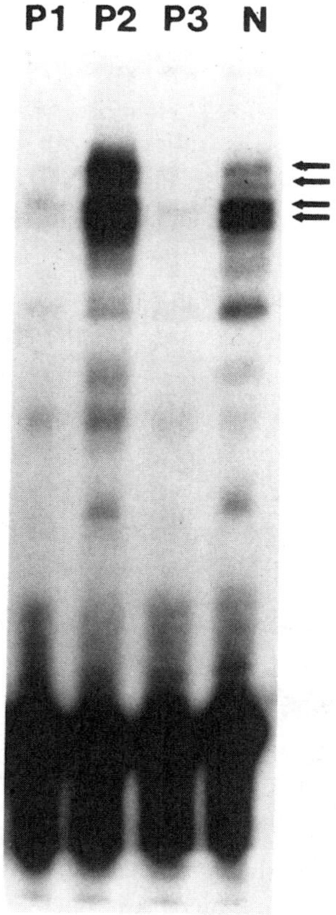

function, have receptors for neuroendocrine peptides and hormones, as well as the ability to produce them. They also make cytokines that in turn can regulate the production of various hormones by the neuroendocrine system. For the purposes of speculation, we can limit discussion to two classes of neuroendocrine mediators, the 31 amino acid opioid peptide β-endorphin (BE) and glucocorticoids. In vivo studies involving administration of exogenous opiates have consistently shown that they have a suppressive effect on specific immune effector mechanisms (Panerai & Sacerdote, 1997). Studies have also been done to show increased levels of BE after experimental stress. In the environment characterized by high levels of BE, NK cell function is inhibited, as is mitogen-induced proliferation of T cells. Most important, the response that remains is biased toward type 2, type 1 being severely suppressed. Under increased BE concentrations, skin allografts are less likely to be rejected, which is one objective test of a real life consequence of the observations made by in vitro assays. Under these same conditions it is highly unlikely that the immune system could stop the growth of the tumor either. No one has yet addressed the molecular bases of the BE effect, but the signal transducing molecules may be a reasonable place to start. These observations beg this question: How can psychosocial or pharmacological interventions be designed to lower the BE levels, recover the balance to the immune response, and ultimately help it reject the tumor?

Corticosteroids are another family of neuroendocrine mediators that can regulate immune responses (Wilckens & De Rijk, 1997). They also show stress-related increase to levels that can be strongly immunosuppressive. One of the mechanisms is by induction of transforming growth factor β (TGF-β), which is a potent inhibitor of T cells, NK cells, and other effector cells of the immune system. The other mechanism clearly can be by interrupting normal signal transduction. Like BE, corticosteroids can influence the type 1–type 2 balance in favor of the type 2 response. Considering that most of these effects appear to be reversible, interventions to balance levels of corticosteroids by reducing stress could be directly responsible for reconstituting a tumor-rejection response. The tools for evaluating this potential at a molecular level are now available, and closer interactions between psychiatrists, psychologists, and immunologists could rapidly advance this important area of investigation.

References

Alberola-Ila, J., Takaki, S., Kerner, J. D., & Perlmutter, R. (1997). Differential signaling by lymphocyte antigen receptors. *Annual Review of Immunology, 15,* 125–154.

Coligan, J. E. (1991). *Current protocols in immunology* (Vol. 1). New York: Greene & Wiley Interscience.

Croft, M., Carter, L., Swain, S. L., & Dutton, R. W. (1996). Generation of polarized antigen-specific CD8 effector populations: Reciprocal action of interleukin-4 and IL-12 in promoting type 2 versus type 1 cytokine profiles. *Journal of Experimental Medicine, 180,* 1715–1728.

Fearon, D. T., & Locksley, R. M. (1996). The instinctive role of innate immunity in the acquired immune response. *Science, 272,* 50–53.

Finke, J. H., Zea, A. H., Stanley, J., Longo, D. L., Mizoguchi, H., Tubbs, R. R., Wiltrout, R. H., O'Shea, J. J., Kudoh, S., Klein, E., Bukowski, R. M., & Ochoa, A. C. (1993). Loss of T-cell receptor zeta chain and p56^{lck} in T-cells infiltrating human renal cell carcinoma. *Cancer Research, 53,* 5613–5616.

Finn, O. J., Jerome, K. R., Henderson, R. A., Pecher, G., Domenech, N., Magarian-Blander, J., & Barratt-Boyes, S. M. (1995). MUC-1 epithelial tumor mucin-based immunity and cancer vaccines. *Immunological Reviews, 145,* 61–89.

Goydos, J. S., Elder, E., Whiteside, T. L., Finn, O. J., & Lotze, M. T. (1996). A phase I trial of a synthetic mucin peptide vaccine. *Journal of Surgical Research, 63,* 298–304.

Henderson, R. A., & Finn, O. J. (1996). Human tumor antigens are ready to fly. *Advances in Immunology, 62,* 217–256.

Karanikas, V., Hwang, L. A., Pearson, J., Ong, C. S., Apostolopoulos, V., Vaughan, H., Xing, P. X., Jamieson, G., Pietersaz, G., Tait, B., Broadbent, R., Thynne, G., & McKenzie, I. F. C. (1997). Antibody and T cell responses of patients with adenocarcinoma immunized with mannan-MUC-1 fusion protein. *Journal of Clinical Investigation, 100,* 2783–2792.

Kogon, M. M., Biswas, A., Pearl, D., Carlson, R. W., & Spiegel, D. (1997). Effects of medical and psychotherapeutic treatment on the survival of women with breast carcinoma. *Cancer, 80,* 225–230.

Lai, P., Rabinowich, H., Crowley-Nowick, P. A., Bell, M. C., Mantovani, G., & Whiteside, T. L. (1996). Alterations in expression and function of signal-transducing proteins in tumor-associated T and natural killer cells in patients with ovarian carcinoma. *Clinical Cancer Research, 2,* 161–173.

MacLennan, I. C. M. (1994). Germinal centers. *Annual Review of Immunology, 12,* 117–139.

Nagacomi, H., Petersson, M., Magnusson, I., Juhlin, C., Matsuda, M., Mellstedt, H., Taupin, J.-L., & Kiessling, R. (1993). Decreased expression of the signal-transducing zeta chain in tumor-infiltrating T-cells, and NK cells of patients with colorectal carcinoma. *Cancer Research, 53,* 5610–5612.

Panerai, A. E., & Sacerdote, P. (1997). β-endorphin in the immune system: A role at last? *Immunology Today, 18,* 317–319.

Paul, W. E., & Seder, R. A. (1994). Lymphocyte responses and cytokines. *Cell, 76,* 241–251.

Reyburn, H., Mandelboim, O., Vales-Gomez, M., Sheu, E. G., Pazmany, L., Davis, D. M., & Strominger, J. L. (1997). Human NK cells: Their ligands, receptors and functions. *Immunological Reviews, 155,* 119–126.

Schreiber, H. (1993). Tumor immunology. In W. E. Paul (Ed.), *Fundamental immunology* (pp. 1143–1178). New York: Raven Press.

Seder, R. A., & Paul, W. E. (1994). Acquisition of lymphokine producing phenotype by CD4$^+$ cells. *Annual Review of Immunology, 12,* 635–673.

Spiegel, D., Bloom, J. R., Kraemer, H. C., & Gottheil, E. (1989). Effect of psychosocial treatment on survival of patients with metastatic breast cancer. *The Lancet, 2*, 888–891.

Sprent, J. (1994). T and B memory cells. *Cell, 76*, 315–322.

Springer, T. A. (1994). Traffic signals for lymphocyte recirculation and leukocyte emigration: The multi-step paradigm. *Cell, 76*, 301–304.

Weir, D. (Ed.). (1996). *The handbook of experimental immunology* (Vol. 1, 5th ed.). Oxford, England: Blackwell.

Wilckens, T., & De Rijk, R. (1997). Glucocorticoids and immune function: Unknown dimensions and new frontiers. *Immunology Today, 9*, 418–424.

Zea, A. H., Curti, B. D., Longo, D. L., Alvord, W. G., Strobl, S. L., Mizoguchi, H., Creekmore, S. P., Powers, G. C., Urba, W. J., & Ochoa, A. C. (1995). Alterations in T cell receptor and signal transduction molecules in melanoma patients. *Clinical Cancer Research, 1*, 1327–1335.

11

Immune System Versus Tumor

Pierre L. Triozzi

Psychosocial interventions can modulate immune responses. How to best evaluate and exploit this phenomenon in cancer patients has to be considered within the context of the many recent advances that have been made in tumor immunology. The immune system can respond to tumors with a variety of cells and their soluble products. Natural killer (NK) cells, macrophages, cytolytic T lymphocytes (CTL), and antibody-secreting plasma cells are the major antitumor "effectors." Dendritic cells, macrophages, and B cells serve as the major *affectors*, cells responsible for presenting tumor-derived antigens to T helper (T_H) lymphocytes and initiating immune responses. The activities of these cells are mediated through the secretion of a variety of cytokines and through complicated interactions between cells. Many more cells are involved. T suppressor (T_s) lymphocytes, neutrophils, and eosinophils may also be important, and cells not considered to be primarily immune in function, such as endothelial cells, can secrete cytokines with significant effects on local immune responses. In addition to antibodies and cytokines, immune cells can secrete lytic enzymes and other factors that can modulate host–tumor interactions, including growth and angiogenic factors. The immune system does not stand alone. Interactions with the neuropsychiatric and endocrine system are well established; so too is the influence of diet, exercise, age, and environment. In cancer patients, the effects of surgery, chemotherapy, and radiation therapy can be profound.

Modulating the immune response in cancer patients generally has been an attractive and aggressively pursued approach and (more specifically) an endpoint of many studies of psychosocial interventions. It is clear that a variety of psychosocial interventions can have a significant impact on immune parameters (Besedovsky, Herberman, Temoshok, & Sendo, 1996). Many recent advances have been made that have allowed for a more rational and mechanistic approach to this phenomenon. At the same time, however, these advances have underscored the enormous complexity of host–tumor immune interactions and, to some extent, have contributed to controversies concerning not only optimal immunologic targets but also the central question of whether or not immune surveillance of cancer even exists. The effects of any intervention, psychosocial or otherwise, has to be considered within the context of the recent advances that have been made in tumor immunology. In this chapter, I review some of these advances and ongoing debates in our understanding of host–tumor interactions and their modulation.

Innate Versus Adaptive Immunity

Innate immunity is the host defense present from birth that does not depend on specific antigen recognition or on immunologic "memory." It is designed to protect the host from invading organisms with which it has not had previous contact and includes a variety of physical barriers (e.g., skin, mucous membranes) and soluble factors (e.g., complement, lysozyme in tears). NK cells and macrophages are the primary cellular effectors of innate immunity.

NK cells are predominantly large granular lymphocytes, the majority of which express CD16 and CD56. NK cells are able to selectively lyse tumor cells and virally infected cells without prior sensitization. The factors that mediate this selectivity are not known. Lysis is mediated in the absence of the expression of a specific antigen in the context of major histocompatibility (MHC) molecules on the target cell. There is actually an inverse relationship with cells expressing MHC class I demonstrating resistance. Newly identified receptors, including NKR-P1 and p58, may be important (Moretta et al., 1997; Ryan & Seaman, 1997). NK cells also express Fc receptors, which bind antibodies; tumor destruction can occur, however, in the absence of specific antibodies.

NK cells have been extensively studied in the setting of cancer. Most studies of psychosocial interventions have measured NK activity as an endpoint. The role of NK cells has been clearly established in animal models. Animals with low levels of NK cell activity have been shown to develop increased numbers of spontaneous and experimental tumors. Animals with augmented NK cell activity have displayed increased resistance. Despite convincing evidence from animal studies, however, the role of NK cells in human cancer is poorly defined. Cells with NK markers or function are not a prominent feature of leukocytic infiltrates in solid tumors and, when present, do not appear to correlate with other prognostic variables. Some studies have found that patients with low NK activity have an increased rate of developing cancers; other studies have not (Pross, Sterns, & MacGillis, 1984). Because NK cells are found primarily in the peripheral blood, it has been postulated that they play a role in preventing blood-borne metastases. Some studies show that reduced NK cell function is associated with increases in metastases and death; others show no relationship, and still others show an inverse relationship (Brittenden, Heys, Ross, & Eremin, 1996).

Macrophages, which derive from peripheral blood monocytes and which are CD14+, represent a major component of the cellular infiltrates of tumors. As with NK cells, activated macrophages engage and lyse transformed cells in preference to normal cells. Again, the recognition structures are not known, and although macrophages do express Fc receptor, selective lysis of tumors can be mediated in the absence of antibodies. Although the results obtained in vitro and in some animal models suggest that macrophages do have the potential to eliminate at least small numbers of tumor cells, there is actually little evidence of antitumor activity in most animal models. Macrophages have not been extensively studied in human cancer patients, and data are conflicting (Mantovani, Bottazzi, Colotta, Sozzani, & Ruco, 1992).

Although potentially lethal, tumors are not truly "invading organisms." More and more tumor immunologists have been focusing on the adaptive immune response, the host defense that does depend on the recognition of specific antigens and that does establish immunologic memory. Antibody-secreting plasma cells, which derive from B cells, and T cells are the primary effectors of adaptive immune responses. B cells recognize antigens in their unprocessed form by engaging the antigen through their receptors, which are the membrane-bound forms of the antibodies they will later secrete. There is very little evidence from animal studies (and virtually no clinical data) that adaptive humoral responses play a significant role in the tumor destruction. Although antibody-secreting plasma cells are not a major component of tumor-infiltrating cells, antibodies that react with a patient's tumor are frequently found in the sera of cancer patients (Old, 1981). Antibodies recognizing tumor-associated determinants such as p75 in patients with melanoma (Vijayasaradhi & Houghton, 1991); p53 in patients with lung, breast, colon, and ovarian cancers (Angelopoulou, Diamandis, Sutherland, Kellen, & Bunting, 1994); and HER-2/neu in patients with breast cancer have been recently identified (Disis et al., 1994). The prognostic significance of tumor-reactive antibodies is not known; their presence may actually confer a worse prognosis (Vlock et al., 1993).

There is more evidence supporting a role for adaptive T-cell responses. T-cell recognition is mediated through T-cell receptors (TCRs). Gene rearrangements during early T-cell development generate a vast repertoire of TCRs specific for potential antigens. In contrast to antibodies, which recognize antigens in their native conformation, the TCR recognizes antigens as a complex of a short peptide bound to an MHC molecule on the surface of the cell presenting the antigen (Germain, 1994). Class I MHC molecules, which in humans include the HLA-A, HLA-B, and HLA-C molecules, are expressed on all cells and are recognized by CD8+ cells. CTL are usually CD8+. Class I MHC molecules normally present endogenous antigens, antigens derived from the cell cytoplasm. Class II MHC, which include HLA-DP, HLA-DQ, and HLA-DR molecules, are expressed on macrophages, dendritic cells, B cells, and occasionally on other cells, including tumor cells. Class II MHC molecules are recognized by CD4+ cells; T_H cells are usually CD4+. Class II MHC molecules normally present exogenous antigens (i.e., antigens taken up from the extracellular space). The extensive polymorphism of MHC molecules means that different individuals will express many different molecules. The peptides that bind and that are presented by individual MHC molecules show distinct structural motifs. Thus, the HLA molecules expressed by an individual play a crucial role in determining the nature of the epitope that is presented. Peptides derived from a tumor may or may not be presented depending on its structure and the HLA haplotype present.

In animal models tumor destruction mediated by T-cell mechanisms appears to be more potent than that mediated by NK cells and also provides the possibility of long-lasting memory. T-cell responses have not been as well studied in humans as NK activity. Assays of T-cell function are technically more difficult than NK assays. T cells that recognize autologous tumors have been identified in the peripheral blood, tumor-draining lymphocytes, and tumors of many melanoma patients. T cells from patients with melanoma have been shown to recognize tumor-associated determinants, such as antigens of the MAGE/GAGE/BAGE family (Boon et al., 1992). Although it has been somewhat more difficult to identify antitumor T cells in other human cancers, T-cell responses have been detected against autologous tumors in patients with colorectal, lung, and breast cancers and against common tumor-associated determinants such as *ras*, p53, bcr/c-abl, and HER-2/neu (Chen, Peace, Rovira, You, & Cheever, 1992; Houbiers et al., 1993; Ioannides et al., 1993; Jung & Schluesener, 1991). The prognostic significance of these T-cell responses, however, is not yet known.

Whether innate or adaptive immune responses are more important in antitumor immunity has not been established; nor do we know whether psychosocial or pharmacological factors should be the focus of intervention. The clinical experience to date provides very little supporting evidence for one or the other. Interleukin-2 (IL-2) therapy routinely enhances NK activity; tumor responses are rarely observed. Interferon-γ is the prototypical macrophage activator; it has not demonstrated antitumor activity in clinical trials. Although responses with CTL derived from tumor-infiltrating lymphocytes and with monoclonal antibodies have been observed, they too are far less frequent than would be predicted from preclinical studies. One's position in the innate versus adaptive debate essentially hinges at present on the weight given to the extensive data generated regarding NK activity in cancer patients, and data are conflicting. Psychosocial interventions have been shown to enhance NK activity in cancer patients. Whether this enhancement has clinical significance is not known. Although the focus of recent studies has been on T-cell-mediated adaptive responses, there is, at present, very little clinical data supporting its role. It is important to note that adaptive immune responses do not occur independently of innate immune responses, and vice versa. It is likely that both innate and adaptive effector mechanisms play roles in the control of tumor growth and that both can be exploited, but a particular mechanism may be more or less important, depending on the tumor and the host.

"Effector" Versus "Affector" Mechanisms

Antitumor immune responses have been primarily considered in terms of effector mechanisms, and much has been learned. As noted, recognition structures are being better characterized. Cell killing is also being better characterized. The basic cytolytic mechanisms of NK and CTL appear to be similar. Both destroy tumors by releasing cytoplasmic granules that contain serine proteases, known as *granzymes*, and a pore-forming protein, known as *perforin*. Both can also destroy tumors by activating a cell surface molecule, the fas ligand, which binds the fas receptor on target cells triggering apoptosis of the target. Both can secrete cytokines with antitumor activity. Antibodies can yield tumor regression by a variety of mechanisms, including comple-ment-mediated and antibody dependent cellular cytotoxicity (ADCC). Antitumor antibodies can also directly modulate the growth and differentiation of tumor cells and induce apoptosis (Trauth et al., 1989). Several mechanisms may also be involved in macrophage tumor cell cytotoxicity, including superoxide production, release of lysosomal products, neutral protease, and secretion of cytokines such as tumor necrosis factor.

Although much has also been learned regarding immune effector mechanisms, as the focus has turned from innate to adaptive immunity, the recent focus has turned from the effector arm to the affector arm and the generation of tumor-antigen-specific T-cell responses. The activation of T cells is controlled at several levels. Two signals are required. The first is the immunostimulatory signal that is induced when the TCR engages the MHC-antigen complex on the antigen-presenting cell (APC). CD4 and CD8 function as coreceptors on the surface of the T cells to assist this binding. The second signal is the "costimulatory" signal provided by molecules, such as B7, on the cell presenting the antigen mediated through costimulatory receptors, which include CD28, on the responding T cell. If both are present, the T cell is activated and proliferates. If the costimulatory molecule is not present on the cell presenting the MHC-antigen complex, the T cell becomes tolerant and undergoes apoptosis. A variety of other cell surface molecules also function to optimize T-cell activation, including a variety of adhesion molecules, such as LFA-1 (CD11a/CD18) on the T cell and ICAM-1 on the cell presenting the antigen. Through poorly described mechanisms, some of the activated cells revert to the resting state to become memory T cells capable of persisting until a subsequent encounter with cells presenting the antigen occurs, which usually elicits a more vigorous response. All cells, including tumor cells, by nature of the capacity to express MHC molecules, can present antigen to T cells. Tumor cells are not, however, "professional" APCs. They do not express MHC class II in conjunction with costimu-latory and other accessory molecules necessary to activate T_H cells. Macrophages, dendritic cells, and B cells do and are "professional" APCs.

Macrophages take up exogenous antigen for MHC class II presentation by a variety of mechanisms, including phagocytosis and Fc receptor uptake of antigen bound to antibodies. Exogenous antigen is broken down into peptide fragments in macrophage lysosomes. The MHC class II molecules present in the endoplasmic reticulum are associated with the invariant chain (Ii) so as to prevent it from binding endogenous peptides. The exogenous peptides and the MHC class II molecules are translocated to an endosomal compartment, where Ii dissociates from the class II molecule and is replaced by the exogenous peptides. The resultant peptide-MHC class II complex is then translocated onto the cell surface. Endogenous peptide fragments for MHC class I presentation are generated in the proteasome. These peptides are then shuttled into the endoplasmic reticulum by transporters associated with antigen processing (TAPs), where they assemble with MCH class I chains and β_2 microglobulin. This trimeric MCH class I complex then reaches the cell surface via the Golgi complex. Some exogenous and endogenous antigens that have been broken down into peptides may leak from the macrophage in a soluble form to be taken up by other APCs. Although the MHC class I pathway generally presents endogenous peptides of cytoplasmic origin, exogenous antigens that are chaperoned by a heat shock protein (HSP) can gain access to the class I processing pathway of certain cells, including macrophages. HSPs derived from tumor cells have been shown to elicit CTL and productive immune responses in animals (Srivastava & Udono, 1994). Macrophages are the primary APC for primed lymphocytes but are not efficient stimulators of naïve T cells.

Much recent attention has focused on dendritic cells, potent APCs that are characterized by their morphology and that are widely dispersed in nonlymphoid tissues (e.g., skin Langerhan cells) and lymphoid tissues (e.g., interdigitating cells). Dendritic cells lack a unique cell surface marker. They do express CD1a and CD83, and although they share a common hematopoietic precursor, they are not thought to be macrophages, because they lack CD14 and nonspecific esterase and have low phagocytic activity. In peripheral tissue "immature" dendritic cells internalize and process antigens. How antigen is taken up is not entirely clear. Dendritic cells do express Fc receptors and are efficient at pinocytosis and endocytosis. After antigen uptake dendritic cells migrate via the afferent lymph to lymphoid organs, where they "mature" and obtain antigen presentation function. As with macrophages, antigens can be presented on class II and class I MHC molecules. In contrast to macrophages, dendritic cells are very effective at stimulating resting naïve T cells (T cells that have not been sensitized to antigens). The reasons for their potent immunostimulatory activity are also not clear. Dendritic cells normally play an important role in contact allergic reactions, atopic disease, and graft rejection. Their role in tumor immunity is not entirely clear. Some data show an altered number of morphology of dendritic cells in the vicinity of epithelial malignancies. Some studies have also shown a positive correlation between the number of tumor-infiltrating dendritic cells and clinical prognosis (Becker, 1992).

In addition to secreting antitumor antibodies, B cells with antitumor surface immunoglobulin may play a role in binding, processing, and presenting tumor antigens to T cells. The current view is that antigens bound to surface immunoglobulin is internalized in endosomes, which then fuse with vesicles containing MHC class II molecules with their invariant chain. The processing of the protein antigen then occurs as described above, and the resultant peptide is then brought to the surface in association with the class II molecules. The unique idiotypic structure of the variable region of antibody can also serve as an antigen that can elicit anti-idiotypic humoral and cellular responses. This idiotypic network may play a role in the regulation of immune responses in conjunction with regulatory T cells.

Effector mechanisms have been easier to study. A variety of assays are available, including the widely applied lymphocyte cytotoxicity assays, but also limiting dilution analysis, delayed type hypersensitivity (DTH) skin testing, TCR usage, and circulating antibodies. Antigen processing and presentation is more difficult to study. Although information can be obtained from DTH testing, lymphoproliferative assays, mixed lymphocyte reactions, measurement of cytokine production, and evaluating TCR signal transduction pathways, assays that specifically and directly assess the multiple steps in antigen processing and presentation that are clinically applicable are not widely available.

Effector and affector mechanisms obviously go hand in hand. The presentation of an antigen to CD4+ T_H cells, however, is the central process in any specific immune response, including the specific response to a tumor, upon which all the other processes depend. A focus on affector mechanisms does not necessarily concede the innate versus adaptive debate to antibody and CTLs and away from macrophages and NK cells. Macrophages are obviously important affectors, and NK cells, by virtue of their capacity to secrete a variety of cytokines, may play an important regulatory role in this process. Study of the interaction of professional APCs (and especially dendritic cells) with T cells is currently a very important area of research in tumor immunology. Whether psychosocial interventions can modulate this key step is not known.

T_H1 Versus T_H2

The antitumor immune response is often considered in terms of cellular and humoral components. For the most part, the cellular versus humoral debate has been reformulated as T_H1 versus T_H2. Animal studies suggest that there are two functional types of T_H activity that are provided. T_H1 is mediated through the secretion of cytokines such as interferon-γ, IL-2, and IL-12 and promotes the cellular immune response mediated by CTL, macrophages, and NK cells. T_H2 is mediated by factors such as IL-4, IL-5, and IL-10 and promotes the humoral response and also eosinophilic inflammation. It has been difficult to demonstrate cells with discrete T_H1/T_H2 function in humans. There appears to be considerable plasticity in the types of cytokines human lymphocytes can secrete. Depending on the dose and timing and on the responding cell, T_H1-type cytokines can promote T_H2-type responses and vice versa. In addition, T_H1 and T_H2 cytokines can be produced by a variety of cells not classically considered to be T_H cells, including CTL, NK cells, and macrophages. The T_H1/T_H2 model, however, has been useful for understanding the immunologic mechanisms involved in several conditions in humans, including infectious diseases, organ transplantation, atopic allergy, and pregnancy. T_H2-associated cytokines (e.g., IL-10) are widely regarded as suppressor factors for T_H1-associated CTL responses. A switch from a T_H1- to a T_H2-type response would be deleterious in conditions in which CTL responses are important, such as HIV-1 infection; likewise a T_H2 to T_H1 switch would be deleterious in conditions in which humoral and eosinophilic inflammation are important, such as leishmaniasis.

Whether the T_H1/T_H2 paradigm will be helpful in understanding the immunology of tumors has not been established. Several lines of evidence do suggest that a cellular response (i.e., T_H1) is more important than a humoral response (i.e., T_H2) in the control of neoplasia. The cytokine profiles observed in several human tumors are consistent with a T_H1 to T_H2 switch, which, in light of the importance of cellular responses in tumor destruction, could explain the progression of tumors in the face of an immune response (Huang et al., 1995). The preeminence of T_H1 over T_H2 in antitumor immune responses is, however, controversial. Humoral responses certainly have the capacity to mediate tumor regressions. Although several lines of evidence support a role for CTL and a T_H1-type response in the control of neoplasia, T_H2-associated cytokines, such as IL-4 and IL-5, have been shown to mediate antitumor activity in murine modules (Hillman et al., 1995; Nakashima, Mita, Takatsu, & Ogawa, 1993). IL-5 is a potent inducer of the accumulation and activation or eosinophils, and some data suggest that the presence of eosinophils in tumors may confer a more favorable prognosis (Fisher et al., 1989; McGinnis et al., 1989). Thus, the functional importance of T_H2 cells in antitumor immune responses requires further investigation.

The cellular versus humoral and T_H1 versus T_H2 debates also extend to how to best identify tumor antigens. Most tumor antigens were initially characterized by their capacity to induce and to be recognized by antibodies. Many were identified by immunizing mice with human tumors and isolating the tumor antigens and then using hybridoma technology to develop monoclonal antitumor antibodies. Tumor-reactive antibodies have been detected in the serum of cancer patients. Most of the antibodies that have been identified have been shown to bind not only the patient's own tumor cells but also tumors of the same histologic type from other donors. Most of the antibodies that have been identified have also been shown to bind to normal tissues. Finally, most of the tumor antigens identified with antibodies are soluble antigens, antigens that are released by the tumor cell into the circulation (Old, 1981).

The emergence of the central role of T cells and the development of new assay systems has now led to the identification of tumor antigens by their capacity to be recognized by lymphocytes. For the most part, these antigens have been identified by reacting proteins expressed by tumors, peptides isolated from tumors, or peptides derived from peptide libraries with T cells derived from cancer patients. Genes for many tumor antigens have been subsequently isolated by expression DNA cloning. Tumor-associated antigens identified by these methods include oncogenes, oncofetal antigens, idiotypic epitopes, viral antigens, mucin molecules, and gangliosides. As with antibody-defined antigens, most T-cell-defined antigens are not tumor-specific and are expressed to various degrees on normal tissue (Boon et al., 1992).

Many antigenic peptides have been identified for melanoma by using clones of T cells isolated from patients (Boon et al., 1992). Melanoma antigens isolated to date have been shown to be nonmutated cellular protein with restricted distribution in normal tissue. Antigens of the MAGE/BAGE/GAGE family are not expressed in any healthy adults with the exception of the testes, and are possibly developmental or oncofetal antigens reexpressed during the process of tumorigenesis. MAGE-1 expression has been found in a variety of tumor types. Other melanoma antigens, tyrosinase, MART-1, and gp100, are present in normal and retinal melanocytes and are differentiation antigens specific to the melanocyte lineage. Immunologic recognition of MAGE-1, MAGE-2, and MAGE-3 is restricted by HLA-A1, whereas recognition of tyrosinase, MART-1, and gp100 is restricted by HLA-A2. As the HLA-A1 haplotype is expressed by approximately 25% of White people and MAGE-1 is detected on 40% of melanomas, only approximately 10% of White patients with melanoma have the ability to respond functionally to MAGE-1. Similarly, HLA-A2 is expressed by 45% of White patients and MART-1 is found in 80% of melanoma, which suggests that some 36% of White patients with melanoma might be able to develop an immune response to MART-1.

The relative merits of targeting tumor antigens identified with antibodies or with T cells cannot be concluded. It should be noted that once tumor antigens are identified as a target for immune therapy, a variety of manipulations can be undertaken to harness both humoral and cellular effector mechanisms, whether or not the target was initially identified with antibodies or with T cells. Although cellular responses appear to play a central role in antitumor immune responses and although the recent focus has been on T-cell-defined antigens, T-cell-defined antigens do have the limitation of HLA restriction. Antibody-defined antigens do not. In addition, because antibodies can recognize proteins in their native configuration, antibody-defined antigens can exploit the capacity of antibodies to bind and directly modulate cellular biology by, for example, binding to an oncogenic growth factor receptor.

Attempts to measure the T_H1/T_H2 cytokine profile in cancer patients in several settings, including in the setting of psychosocial interventions, currently are under way. There are strong biases among tumor immunologists regarding the relative merits of the cellular and humoral, T_H1 and T_H2, and antibody-defined and T-cell-defined tumor antigens, with most favoring the cellular, T_H1, T-cell-defined positions. Again, there really is no direct evidence supporting one over the other at present. As with adaptive versus innate immune responses, it is likely that both play roles, but a particular mechanism or type of antigen may be more or less important, depending on the tumor and the host.

"Self-Nonself" Versus "Danger"

Responses may be innate, adaptive, humoral, or cellular immune. Why aren't tumors eliminated? There are a number of models to account for the intervention of the immune response. The essential role of the immune system is to recognize and specifically respond to foreign agents and not to self components. It is thought that during embryonic development or early life the immune system undergoes negative selection processes to tolerate the body's own tissues, retaining ability to eliminate infectious agents. The immune system learns to distinguish "self" from "nonself." Lymphocyte clones that recognize self are eliminated in the thymus. In the self–nonself model, clones capable of responding with antigens that are expressed by growing tumors may have been previously deleted because they are in that individual self antigen. Thus, there may be "holes" in the repertoire of immune recognition when it comes to tumors. As noted, tumors are not professional APCs. They do not express costimulatory molecules and usually do not express MHC class II. Thus, even if a potentially unique tumor antigen is expressed by the tumor in the context of the MHC complex, the T cell that engages the tumor will not receive the second costimulatory signal and, thus, would be predicted to become tolerant to the antigen.

In the "danger" model the immune system learns what is dangerous (i.e., anything that causes cell stress or lytic cell death) rather than to distinguish self from nonself (Matzinger, 1994). Three signals, not just two, are needed to activate the immune system, and dendritic cells are key. Two of the required signals are the same ones needed to trigger T cells: the first, when a specific antigen presented by d ..idritic cells is recognized by the TCR, and the second, when the costimulatory signal is provided. The key third signal is the "alarm signal" that is delivered only after the dendritic cell has been activated by stressed, damaged, or lysed necrotic cells. In the danger model, the immune system fails to fight tumors because, coming from the perspective of the immune system, small tumors do not induce a significant alarm signal and are not deemed dangerous. The immune system learns to tolerate it. Thus, when cancer is considered in the context of the danger model, "stress" is beneficial.

Tumor cells are not sitting ducks. Because of inherent genetic instability, cells making up tumors are heterogeneous. Heterogeneity of tumor antigen expression, let alone heterogeneity of MHC expression, among the tumor cell population is extensive. Only a fraction of the cells present is likely to express a specific antigenic determinant. In theory, an immune response directed to tumor cells expressing a specific antigen results in the growth of antigen-negative cells. The importance of MHC class I molecules in the presenting of tumor-associated antigens to CD8 + CTL has several implications. It is now well-recognized that the cell surface expression of MHC class I antigens is reduced or lost in a variety of human tumors. Human tumors are frequently characterized by deficiencies in proteasome, TAP, or β2 microglobulin function (Ruiz-Cabello et al., 1991). Again, without MHC expression, there is no T-cell recognition.

Tumors can express cell surface molecules or release factors that can suppress the activity of cytolytic effectors. Tumors themselves have been shown to express fas ligand, and engagement of fas ligand on the tumor with the fas receptor on activated lymphocytes can lead to apoptosis of the lymphocytes (Hahne et al., 1996). Tumor cells can also release factors that affect dendritic cell maturation that could lead to inadequate presentation of tumor antigens (Gabrilovich et al., 1996). Furthermore, tumors can release antigen that can engage effector molecules in the periphery, and, in effect, it is the tumor that is establishing "decoys." The process of tumor neovascularization results in abnormal vessel architecture that leads to increased interstitial pressure that acts to prevent the influx of cells and factors from the vasculature into the tumor (Boucher & Jain, 1992).

The self–nonself model focuses on T cell activation at the level of individual TCRs and their interactions with tumor antigens. The danger model focuses on how to maintain dendritic cell activation and consequently T-cell activation to generate an antitumor immune response. Whether the self–nonself model or the danger model ultimately proves to be an accurate representation of antitumor immune responses is not known. Both models focus tumor immunology on escape phenomena, both focus on affector mechanisms, and both suggest strategies for interventions. The models, however, do suggest significant hurdles that may not be easily overcome by any intervention, psychosocial or otherwise.

Immune Surveillance Versus Immune Facilitation

What is the evidence that an antitumor immune response is actually important? The first argument that is usually made to support the existence of the immune surveillance of tumors is that patients with congenital and acquired immune deficiencies develop an excess of some forms of cancer. The counterargument is that most of the cancers that do develop are cancers of the immune system, such as lymphomas, which can be explained by direct dysregulation of the growth and differentiation of immune cells induced by the growth factors, viruses, or mutations that characterize these conditions. In acquired immune deficiencies that occur iatrogenically in the setting of organ transplant or that occur as a result of chronic viral infections, it may be the constant immune stimulation and not the immune suppression that leads to lymphoreticular malignancies. Non-immune-system cancers can be accounted for by the presence of codeterminants in the people at risk, for example, the use of mutagenic immunosuppressives. It should be noted that immunodeficient nude or SCID mice as well as NK-cell-deficient beige mice do not develop tumors at a markedly increased rate.

A second argument often made is that spontaneous regressions of tumors are the result of immune surveillance. These tumors, however, may be virus-associated, and the immune response may be to viral and not specifically to tumor determinants. What of the immune cells infiltrating tumors and the specific antitumor T-cell and humoral responses that have been identified? The counterargument to this is that the cancer is still there and the responses represent an epiphenomenon. Finally, a variety of immunotherapeutics have been applied in cancer patients, and tumor regressions have been observed. The counterargument can be made that the mechanisms of these tumor regressions have not been clearly established. Immunotherapeutics can modulate a number of other potential factors (e.g., steroid hormone levels) that affect tumor growth independent of the modulation of classic immune effect mechanisms.

There is evidence that the immune response can be deleterious and actually facilitate tumor growth. Some cancers that are characterized by intense immune cell infiltration, such as inflammatory breast cancer, are very refractory to treatment. Macrophages and tumors appear to have a particularly complex relationship (Mantovani et al., 1992). Macrophages are important APCs and play a role in the innate immune responses. On the other hand, macrophages and tumors demonstrate a "symbiotic" relationship, with both secreting a variety of cytokines that can maintain each other's growth. Macrophage-derived factors have tumor-promoting potential and appear to play a central role in tumor vascularization, growth rate, and stroma formation. Macrophages can secrete factors that may help tumors invade and establish in tissues, including proteases, elastase, and collagenase. Macrophages can also down-regulate the immune response by secreting inhibitory cytokines, such as IL-1-receptor antagonist and transforming growth factor (TGF) β (Christ et al., 1994).

Although antibodies can mediate tumor regressions, there is evidence that antibodies can permit progressive tumor growth by accumulating on tumor cells, protecting them from attack by cytotoxic lymphocytes (Manson, 1991). That circulating antigen-antibody complexes can inhibit T-cell function is well recognized. In some studies, the identification of circulating immune complexes in cancer patients has been associated with a poorer prognosis (Vlock et al., 1993). Some data indicate that cytokines produced by the immune cells promote tumor growth. Cytokines appear to be involved in tumors such as Kaposi's sarcoma, which may be initially a paracrine T-cell-cytokine-mediated disease with later autocrine production of these cytokines (Ensoli, Barillari, & Gallo, 1992).

Macrophages and NK cells infiltrate preneoplastic tumors in mice that spontaneously develop breast cancer. Retrovirus-associated breast cancers in mice can be promoted by immune mechanisms, and stimulation of NK cells has been shown to enhance tumor progression in some mouse models of mammary cancer (Callahan, Weeks, Ohuchi, & Schlom, 1989). Some data show that immunosuppression with neonatal thymectomy or anti-lymphocyte/NK antibodies can decrease tumor incidents in mice (Wei, Gill, & Wang, 1993). If women, likewise, have an immune promotion of breast cancer, the incidence of breast cancer in patients receiving therapeutic immunosuppression should be lower than that in a comparable cohort of nonimmunosuppressed patients. In fact, the incidence of breast cancers arising in women receiving immunosuppressive therapy after kidney or heart transplantation has recently been shown to be lower, supporting the possibility of immune facilitation (Stewart, Tsai, Grayson, Henderson, & Opetz, 1995). For all other major cancers, however, the incidence was higher in the immunosuppressed women. Interestingly, the drugs that are effective in causing regressions of metastatic breast cancer in a dose-dependent fashion also cause a dose-dependent reduction of cytokines produced by the immune system (Stewart, Retsky, Tsai, & Verma, 1994).

Although there really is no direct evidence that immune surveillance does play a role in protecting against human cancer, several arguments can be made that immune responses, both innate and adaptive, both humoral and cellular, are important. There are counterarguments, but the predominance of evidence does support a role for immune responses. At the same time, however, there is good evidence that tumors can subvert this response and use it to their advantage. Although intuitively appealing, exploiting the immune system to mediate tumor regression, whether one is considering a pharmacological or nonpharmacological approach, is a formidable task.

Nonspecific Versus Specific Immunotherapy

There are two general strategies of modulating host–tumor interactions: In nonspecific immunotherapy, the goal is to stimulate immune function in general and to elicit tumor destruction as a byproduct of this stimulation. This approach primarily exploits innate immune responses but can also involve CTL and antibodies. In specific immunotherapy, a specific tumor antigen is targeted, and specific effector mechanisms, namely CTL and antibodies, are exploited. Nonspecific and specific immunotherapy can either be active, in which an agent is administered to the host to stimulate host immune responses, or passive, in which immune effector cells or factors are infused or "adoptively transferred" into the host.

Psychosocial interventions are essentially nonspecific immunotherapeutics. Nonspecific immunotherapeutics, namely levamisole, interferon-α, IL-2, and BCG, have made their way into the clinic. These agents have a variety of effects in addition to their immunostimulatory activities, and it is not clear that immune effector mechanisms are actually operational in their antitumor activity. Nonspecific immunotherapeutics have been primarily successful in the treatment of patients with melanoma and renal cell carcinoma, two cancers considered to be immunogenic. Results in other cancers have been very disappointing. The immune system is highly regulated to prevent deleterious autoimmune reactions. It is difficult to nonspecifically stimulate or manipulate one aspect without having effects on other aspects that will have a homeostatic effect. For example, IL-2 can activate NK cells and CTL. At the same time, through the activation of T_S cells and macrophages, factors can be released that down-regulate the activities of the killer cells. Although many nonspecific approaches have been abandoned, novel agents and cytokines, such as the T$_H$1-enhancing IL-12, are generating interest and are being studied in clinical trials. It should be noted that active nonspecific immunotherapy can be effective when administered by local injection. Intravesicular administration of BCG is very effective in treating localized bladder cancers.

With the identification of the lymphokine activated killer (LAK) cell phenomenon, there was considerable interest in adoptive nonspecific immunotherapy using LAK cells generated ex vivo from patients. Cells with LAK activity can lyse a wide variety of tumor and virally infected targets resistant to NK lysis in a non-MHC restricted manner. Although T cells can mediate LAK activity, most LAK activity appears to be due to the activation of NK cells. Results of a number of clinical trials using LAK cells infusion were disappointing, and randomized studies suggested that the addition of LAK cells to IL-2 did not substantially modulate the response rate of IL-2 therapy alone (Rosenberg et al., 1993).

There is much more research focusing on active specific approaches, that is, tumor "vaccines." As most tumor antigens that have been identified are expressed to some degree on normal tissues, it may seem that targeting these antigens would be risky, because of the potential for generating autoimmunity. In some instances, the tissue from which the tumor arises may be dispensable. For example, patients with melanoma are willing to accept the risk of vitiligo in their normal skin that may result in programs that produce antimelanin immune responses. Autoimmunity has not been a limiting problem in clinical trials to date. Normal tissue counterpart of many tumors may express low levels of MHC class I, thus rendering them less sensitive to CTL attack.

Purified or synthetic tumor antigens can be administered with a variety of immunologic adjuvant treatments, such as bacterial products and saponins, to activate T-cell help. Antigens can also be conjugated to carriers such as keynote limpet hemocyanin. Cytokines such as granulocyte-macrophage, colony stimulating factor (GM-CSF), and IL-12 have been administered with defined tumor antigens. Because viral infections can elicit lifelong immunity, vectors such as poxviruses, adenoviruses, retroviruses, and herpes viruses have been developed to express tumor antigens in tissues. The administration of antigen-pulsed dendritic cells has also demonstrated significant clinical promise (Hsu et al., 1996). The ability of the idiotype to function as an antigen can be exploited, and antibodies can be used as an active specific immunotherapy. Another approach under evaluation is to increase the immunogenicity of tumors and let the immune system decide which antigen to attack. This approach does not require knowledge about either the specific T-cell epitope or MHC haplotypes. Weakly immunogenic tumors can provoke effective anticancer response if transfected with costimulatory molecules such as B7 and cytokines such as IL-12 and GM-CSF (Roth & Cristiano, 1997). The identification of specific T-cell antigens has also resulted in the development of adoptive specific therapies using either antigen-specific CTL and/or T$_H$ cells generated ex vivo (Triozzi, 1993).

The development of antitumor monoclonal antibodies led to numerous clinical studies of passive specific immunotherapy. The selectivity for tumors and the lack of associated toxicity make these "magic bullets" very attractive agents. Their ability to destroy common solid tumors, however, has been minimal unless aided by other mechanisms, and a variety of radionuclides, drugs, and toxins have been conjugated to monoclonal antibodies to increase their antitumor activity. Many problems have been identified. Relatively low amounts of the total antibodies injected actually bind the tumor. Very few antibodies appear to diffuse through large tumor masses in particular. A number of the tumor antigens are released from the tumor cell. Thus, monoclonal antibodies can be engaged in the peripheral circulation and never engage the tumor. Most monoclonal antibodies produced by hybridoma technology contain mouse components, which induced human antimouse antibody (HAMA) when injected into patients, which may abrogate the effectiveness of therapy. Recombinant chimeric antibodies that use human constant regions have reduced the production of HAMA. However, idiotypic responses against the variable region of the antibodies are still induced, which may also abrogate their effectiveness (Dillman, 1994).

Antibody-based therapies have shown promising results in the treatment of hematologic malignancies, where some distribution issues noted above are less problematic. For example, a genetically engineered chimeric anti-CD20 antibody, which consists of human constant region and mouse variable regions, has shown considerable promise in patients with relapsed or refractory low-grade B-cell lymphoma. This antibody has been shown to lyse B cells in vitro via complement and ADCC lysis, but, again, whether classic immune effector mechanisms are actually operational in vivo is not clear, as this antibody may directly modulate cell growth and function (Maloney et al., 1994). The mouse monoclonal antibody 17-1A, which recognized a cell surface component of tumor and of normal epithelial cells, has been shown to reduce recurrence rates and improve survival in patients with colorectal cancer. This effect appears to be due to the capacity of the murine monoclonal antibodies to function as a vaccine and induce idiotypic humoral and cellular responses (Fagerberg, Steinitz, Wigzell, Askelof, & Mellstedt, 1995).

Both nonspecific and specific immunotherapeutic approaches have demonstrated clinical antitumor activity, but only in a few cancers and only in a minority of cancer patients with these cancers. There is a considerable discrepancy between the results obtained in preclinical studies and the results obtained clinically. Part of the problem is that our understanding of the immune response is still very superficial. There are other issues, however. For example, many agents have only been tested in the setting of advanced disease where it is unlikely to be of benefit and our capacity to monitor immune therapies clinically is limited. Psychosocial interventions appear to be a reproducible nonspecific immunomodulator whose therapeutic value is not yet known. At any rate, both nonspecific and specific immunomodulators are clinical realities, and the precedent has been set for future development.

Summary

Many advances have been made in our understanding of the complex immune response to tumors, and tumor immunity can no longer be considered a "black box" when one evaluates any intervention, be it psychosocial or pharmacological. Mechanisms of effector function are better understood. Important progress has been made in understanding affector mechanisms, including the processing pathways for presentation of peptide antigens in association with MHC molecules. New insights have been made regarding regulatory mechanisms and the mechanisms by which tumor cells can grow and subvert an intact immune response. Even with these advances, however, the answers to central questions, such as whether or not the immune system plays a role in tumor surveillance, are not known. There is virtually no direct evidence, and data from animal and from human studies are either limited or conflicting.

There are many explanations for the areas of controversy. First of all, the immune response is a very complex biologic phenomenon, and the study of complex biologic phenomena is always characterized by debates. Second, not only is the immune response heterogeneous, there is also considerable heterogeneity among human tumors. Third, our assay systems are not adequate. The animal models and human studies are biased to assess only one aspect. Although our capacity to study immune responses is vastly improved and has moved considerably beyond standard lymphocyte cytotoxicity and circulating antibody assays, very important steps are very difficult to study, particularly in the cancer patient population.

It is not really necessary to clearly establish whether or not innate or adaptive immune responses are more important, whether or not cellular or humoral responses predominate, and whether or not tumor immune surveillance exists in order to exploit the selectivity and power of the immune response. Most would conclude that the immune system can still be modulated to mediate beneficial antitumor activity. Psychosocial interventions can modulate the immune response. How to best exploit this phenomenon has to now be considered within the context of the advances that have been made in tumor immunology. Progress has been great, and in the future more and more host–immune system versus tumor interactions should be settled in favor of the host.

References

Angelopoulou, K., Diamandis, E. P., Sutherland, D. J., Kellen, J. A., & Bunting, P. S. (1994). Prevalence of serum antibodies against the p53 tumor suppressor gene protein in various cancers. *International Journal of Cancer, 58*, 480–487.

Becker, Y. (1992). Anticancer role of dendritic cells (DC) in human and experimental cancers— A review. *Anticancer Research, 12*, 511–520.

Besedovsky, H. O., Herberman, R. B., Temoshok, L. R., & Sendo, F. (1996). Psychoneuroimmunology and cancer: Fifteenth Sapporo Cancer Seminar. *Cancer Research, 56,* 4278–4281.

Boon, T., De Plaen, E., Lurquin, C., Van Den Eynde, B., Van Der Bruggen, P., Traversari, C., Amar-Costesec, A., & Van Pel, A. (1992). Identification of tumour rejection antigens recognised by T lymphocytes. *Cancer Surveys, 13,* 23–38.

Boucher, Y., & Jain, R. K. (1992). Microvascular pressure is the principal driving force for interstitial hypertension in solid tumors: Implications for vascular collapse. *Cancer Research, 52,* 5110–5114.

Brittenden, J., Heys, S. D., Ross, J., & Eremin, O. (1996). Natural killer cells and cancer. *Cancer, 77,* 1226–1243.

Callahan, R., Weeks, M. O., Ohuchi, N., & Schlom, J. (1989). Retroviral-related genes, proto-oncogenes, and breast cancer. *Immunology Series, 43,* 623–642.

Chen, W., Peace, D. J., Rovira, D. K., You, S. G., & Cheever, M. A. (1992). T-cell immunity to the joining region of p210[bcr-abl] protein. *Proceedings of the National Academy of Sciences of the United States of America, 89,* 1468–1472.

Christ, M., McCartney-Francis, N. L., Kulkarni, A. B., Ward, J. M., Mizel, D. E., Mackall, C. L., Gress, R. E., Hines, K. L., Tian, H., Karlsson, S., & Wahl, S. M. (1994). Immune dysregulation in TGF-beta 1-deficient mice. *Journal of Immunology, 153,* 1936–1946.

Dillman, R. O. (1994). Antibodies as cytotoxic therapy. *Journal of Clinical Oncology, 12,* 1497–1515.

Disis, M. L., Calenoff, E., McLaughlin, G., Murphy, A. E., Chen, W., Groner, B., Jeschke, M., Lydon, N., McGlynn, E., Livingston, R. B., Moe, R., & Cheever, M. A. (1994). Existent T-cell and antibody immunity to HER-2/neu protein in patients with breast cancer. *Cancer Research, 54,* 16–20.

Ensoli, B., Barillari, G., & Gallo, R. C. (1992). Cytokines and growth factors in the pathogenesis of AIDS-associated Kaposi's sarcoma. *Immunological Review, 127,* 147–155.

Fagerberg, J., Steinitz, M., Wigzell, H., Askelof, P., & Mellstedt, H. (1995). Human anti-idiotypic antibodies induced a humoral and cellular immune response against a colorectal carcinoma-associated antigen in patients. *Proceedings of the National Academy of Sciences of the United States of America, 92,* 4773–4777.

Fisher, E. R., Paik, S. M., Rockette, H., Jones, J., Caplan, R., & Fisher, B. (1989). Prognostic significance of eosinophils and mast cells in rectal cancer: Findings from the National Surgical Adjuvant Breast and Bowel Project. *Human Pathology, 20,* 159–163.

Gabrilovich, D. I., Chen, H. L., Girgis, K. R., Cunningham, H. T., Meny, G. M., Nadaf, S., Kavanaugh, D., & Carbone, D. P. (1996). Production of vascular endothelial growth factor by human tumors inhibits the functional maturation of dendritic cells. *Nature Medicine, 2,* 1096–1103.

Germain, R. N. (1994). MHC-dependent antigen processing and peptide presentation: Providing ligands for T lymphocyte activation. *Cell, 76,* 287–299.

Hahne, M., Rimoldi, D., Schroter, M., Romero, P., Schreier, M., French, L. E., Schneider, P., Bornand, T., Fontana, A., Lienard, D., Cerottini, J. C., & Tschopp, J. (1996). Melanoma cell expression of Fas(Apo-1/CD95) ligand: Implications for tumor immune escape. *Science, 274,* 1363–1366.

Hillman, G. G., Younes, E., Visscher, D., Ali, E., Lam, J. S., Montecillo, E., Pontes, J. E., Haas, G. P., & Puri, R. K. (1995). Systemic treatment with interleukin-4 induces regression of pulmonary metastases in a murine renal cell carcinoma mode. *Cell Immunology*, *160*, 257–263.

Houbiers, J. G., Nijman, H. W., van der Berg, S. H., Drijfhout, J. W., Kenemans, P., van de Velde, C. J., Brand, A., Momberg, F., Kast, W. M., & Melief, C. J. (1993). In vitro induction of human cytotoxic T lymphocyte responses against peptides of mutant and wild-type p53. *European Journal of Immunology*, *23*, 2072–2077.

Hsu, F. J., Benike, C., Fagnoni, F., Liles, T. M., Czerwinski, D., Taidi, B., Engleman, E. G., & Levy, R. (1996). Vaccination of patients with B-cell lymphoma using autologous antigen-pulsed dendritic cells. *Nature Medicine*, *2*, 52–58.

Huang, M., Wang, J., Lee, P., Sharma, S., Mao, J. T., Meissner H., Uyemura, K., Modlin, R., Wollman, J., & Dubinett, S. M. (1995). Human non-small cell lung cancer cells express a type 2 cytokine pattern. *Cancer Research*, *55*, 3847–3853.

Ioannides, C. G., Fisk, B., Fan, D., Biddison, W. E., Wharton, J. T., & O'Brian, C. A. (1993). Cytotoxic T cells isolated from ovarian malignant ascites recognize a peptide derived from the HER-2/neu proto-oncogene. *Cell Immunology*, *151*, 225–234.

Jung, S., & Schluesener, H. J. (1991). Human T lymphocytes recognize a peptide of single point-mutated, oncogenic ras protein. *Journal of Experimental Medicine*, *173*, 273–276.

Maloney, D. G., Liles, T. M., Czerwinski, D. K., Waldichuk, C., Rosenberg, J., Grillo-Lopez, A., & Levy, R. (1994). Phase I clinical trial using escalating single-dose infusion of chimeric anti-CD20 monoclonal antibody (IDEC-C2B8) in patients with recurrent B-cell lymphoma. *Blood*, *84*, 2457–2466

Manson, L. A. (1991). Does antibody-dependent epitope masking permit progressive tumour growth in the face of cell-mediated cytotoxicity? *Immunology Today*, *12*, 352–355.

Mantovani, A., Bottazzi, B., Colotta, F., Sozzani, S., & Ruco, L. (1992). The origin and function of tumor-associated macrophages. *Immunology Today*, *13*, 265–270.

Matzinger, P. (1994). Tolerance, danger, and the extended family. *Annual Review of Immunology*, *12*, 991–1045.

McGinnis, M. C., Bradley, E. L., Pretlow, T. P., Ortiz-Reyes, R., Bowden, C. J., Stellato, T. A., & Pretlow, T. G. (1989). Correlation of stromal cells by morphometric analysis metastatic behavior of human colonic carcinoma. *Cancer Research*, *49*, 5989–5993.

Moretta, A., Biassoni, R., Bottino, C., Pende, D., Vitale, M., Poggi, A., Mingari, M.C., & Moretta, L. (1997). Major histocompatibility complex class I specific receptors on human natural killer and T lymphocytes. *Immunological Review*, *155*, 105–117.

Nakashima, Y., Mita, S., Takatsu, K., & Ogawa, M. (1993). Interleukin-5 induces tumor suppression by peritoneal exudate cells in mice. *Cancer Immunology, Immunotherapy*, *37*, 227–232.

Old, L. J. (1981). Cancer immunology; the search for specificity—G.H.A. Clowes Memorial Lecture. *Cancer Research*, *41*, 361–375.

Pross, H. F., Sterns, E., & MacGillis, D. R. (1984). Natural killer cell activity in women at "high risk" for breast cancer, with and without benign breast syndrome. *International Journal of Cancer*, *34*, 303–308.

Rosenberg, S. A., Lotze, M. T., Yang, J. C., Topalian, S. L., Chang, A. E., Schwartzentruber, D. J., Aebersold, P., Leitman, S., Linehan , W. M., Seipp, C. A., White, D. E., & Steinberg, S. M. (1993). Prospective randomized trial of high-dose interleukin-2 alone or in conjunction with lymphokine-activated killer cells for the treatment of patients with advanced cancer. *Journal of the National Cancer Institute, 85,* 622–632.

Roth, J. A., & Cristiano, R. J. (1997). Gene therapy for cancer—What have we done and where are we going? *Journal of the National Cancer Institute, 89,* 12–39.

Ruiz-Cabello, F., Perez-Ayala, M., Gomez, O., Redondo, M., Concha, A., Cabrera, T., & Garrido, F. (1991). Molecular analysis of MHC-class-I alterations in human tumour cell lines. *International Journal of Cancer, 6*(Suppl), 123–130.

Ryan, J. C., & Seaman, W. E. (1997). Divergent functions of lectin-like receptors on NK cells. *Immunological Review, 155,* 79–89.

Srivastava, P. K., & Udono, H. (1994). Heat shock protein-peptide complexes in cancer immunotherapy. *Current Opinion in Immunology, 6,* 728–732.

Stewart, T. H., Retsky, M. W., Tsai, S. C., & Verma, S. (1994). Dose response in the treatment of breast cancer. *Lancet, 343,* 402–404.

Stewart, T., Tsai, S. C., Grayson, H., Henderson, R., & Opetz, G. (1995). Incidence of de-novo breast cancer in women chronically immunosuppressed after organ transplantation. *Lancet, 346,* 796–798.

Trauth, B. C., Klas, C., Peters, A. M. G., Matzky, S., Moller, P., Falk, W., Debatin, K. M., & Krammer, P. H. (1989). Monoclonal antibody mediated tumor regression by induction of apoptosis. *Science, 245,* 301–304.

Triozzi, P. L. (1993). Identification and activation of tumor-reactive cells for adoptive cellular immunotherapy. *Stem Cells, 11,* 204–211

Vijayasaradhi, S., & Houghton, A. N. (1991). Purification of an autoantigenic 75-kDa human melanosomal glycoprotein. *International Journal of Cancer, 47,* 298–303.

Vlock, D. R., Schantz, S. P., Fisher, S. G., Savage, H. E., Carey, T. E., & Wolf, G. T. (1993). Clinical correlates of circulating immune complexes and antibody reactivity in squamous cell carcinoma of the head and neck. *Journal of Clinical Oncology, 11,* 2427–2433.

Wei, W. Z., Gill, R. F., & Wang, H. (1993). Mouse mammary tumor virus associated antigens and super antigens-immuno-molecular correlates of neoplastic progression. *Seminars in Cancer Biology, 4,* 205–213.

PART 3

Prevention and Intervention

CHAPTER 12

Psychosocial Interventions in Cancer

Group Therapy Techniques

David Spiegel
Susan Diamond

Advances in cancer medical treatment are primarily extending the lives of patients, converting the disease from a terminal to a chronic illness. Although remarkable cures have been obtained for some rarer forms of cancer, the disease remains the second leading killer of Americans, after heart disease. This means that the importance of helping people live with a chronic life threat; the side effects of arduous treatments; and the personal, social, and vocational consequences of disease-related disability is growing. At the same time, the line between psychosocial and biomedical intervention is blurring as evidence accumulates that medical treatment profoundly affects quality of life, and psychosocial stress and support may affect the quantity of life. In this chapter we review the rationale for psychotherapeutic intervention for cancer patients, examine underlying themes, compare treatment techniques, and review evidence regarding both psychosocial and biomedical outcome.

The Need for Intervention: Psychosocial Problems Among Cancer Patients

Psychological sequelae to a cancer diagnosis are understandably common. Thoughts of death and dying loom following diagnosis, often out of proportion to actual mortality risk. Other psychosocial consequences of a cancer diagnosis can include fears of recurrence, social isolation, marked energy reduction, alterations in body image, loss of previous identity, unanticipated demands on time because of treatment appointments, adherence to treatments that are repugnant and arduous, and financial burden. Although any of these stressors in and of themselves can be unwieldy, their confluence can often be experienced as overwhelming by the already beleaguered cancer patient. Few patients are optimally prepared to tackle all of these problems at once.

A cancer diagnosis is an unequivocally stressful life event that precipitates an increase in subjective levels of distress in the population it affects. For example, approximately 80% of women with breast cancer report substantial distress levels during initial diagnosis and treatments, including anxiety about recurrence, difficulties in sexual functioning, death anxiety, and vocational difficulties. Treatment itself, particularly chemotherapy, provokes recurrent anxiety, which can involve anticipatory nausea and vomiting and a reduction in compliance. Some early studies have demonstrated that 20–30% of patients suffer severe distress for 2 or more years after surgical intervention. A study by Irvine, Brown, Crooks, Roberts, and Browne (1991) showed that women with breast cancer suffered 12% more sexual difficulties than women with benign breast disease and that 46% experienced significant psychological distress. In a study of 99 breast cancer patients, Omne-Ponten, Holmberg, and Sjoden (1994) found that 45% continued to experience significant anxiety and depression 1 year after diagnosis. Ten percent of patients continued to experience severe maladjustment to diagnosis and treatment even at the 6-year follow-up, and breast-conserving surgery was not a factor in mediating psychological distress. A significant minority of breast cancer patients present with continued emotional distress and disturbance that is related to their fear and anxiety regarding disease progression and recurrence.

In a study of 274 breast cancer patients, Vinokur, Threatt, Caplan, and Zimmerman (1989) found persistent mental health problems during the year after diagnosis, including anxiety, depression, and somatic preoccupation. One of the strongest predictors of compromised mental health at 1-year follow-up was appraisal of threat, more so than at initial disease stage. This suggests that subjective threat appraisal is an impressive determinant of adjustment to breast cancer, even more so than initial prognostic variables such as staging. The use of medical treatments not involving disruptive side effects associated with traditional chemotherapy was also found to have an anti-anxiety effect of decreasing threat appraisal.

Depression and anxiety have been found to be particularly prevalent in cancer patients in general in various studies, pain status notwithstanding. Factors associated with increased levels of depression included a higher level of physical disability and more severe illness. As disease progresses, the proportion of patients who are clinically depressed increases. Twenty percent of terminally ill patients are depressed, and this number increases to 60% among those requesting physician-assisted suicide (Chochinov et al., 1995). Derogatis et al. (1983) found that among 215 oncology inpatients, 47% suffered from clinically apparent psychiatric disorders, including major affective disorders (6%), adjustment disorders with depressed mood (12%), and adjustment disorders with mixed emotional features (13%). Approximately 90% of observable psychiatric syndromes were evaluated as responses to or manifestations of disease or treatment. Mermelstein and Lesko (1992) undertook a study that suggested a fourfold increase in the rate of depressive disorders among oncology patients as compared with the general population. Increased incidence of mood disturbance was observed throughout disease course, from undiagnosed breast masses to recurrence. Other studies have demonstrated a 14% incidence of anxiety disorders in women with breast cancer, although only 1.5% of this sample met criteria for a depressive disorder. Moreover, distressed high utilizers (Von Korff, Ormel, Katon, & Lin, 1992) of medical care are very likely to be suffering from psychiatric disorders, which can include major depression, generalized anxiety disorder, and substance abuse. These patients also cost far more to treat (Browne, Arpin, Corey, Fitch, & Gafni, 1990).

Patients' patterns of coping with a cancer diagnosis and their specific types of psychosocial problems and needs remain fairly constant after initial diagnosis. The most pressing concerns of cancer patients involve emotional stress, worries about family members, and acquiring additional information. Patients at increased risk for poor coping and adjustment include those who suffer from social isolation, have a history of recent losses or multiple obligations, or use rigid and inflexible coping strategies. Holland and Rowland (1990) found that breast cancer patients who use more direct and confrontational coping strategies are less distressed than those who use avoidance and denial. Emotional distress is common across the board in cancer patients at all levels of diagnosis and treatment. Particular coping strategies facilitate adjustment to a cancer diagnosis and suggest that psychosocial support should be a potent factor in mediating emotional distress and improving outcome. Furthermore, recent data suggest an inverse relationship between efforts to repress emotion and distress (Classen, Koopman, Angell, & Spiegel, 1996). That is, efforts to suppress dysphoria seem, if anything, to increase it. This suggests that psychotherapeutic techniques designed to facilitate emotional expression might provide relief of distress and better prepare cancer patients to manage future stressors, which are inevitable in the course of the disease and its treatment.

Psychotherapeutic Intervention Methods

Psychosocial support has long been demonstrated to be a critical factor in moderating the effects of difficult life stressors. The literature on psychotherapeutic treatment of cancer patients suggests that emotional suppression and avoidance are associated with poorer coping and offers ample evidence of improvements in mood, coping, and adjustment as a result of psychotherapeutic intervention (Koopman, Hermanson, Diamond, Angell, & Spiegel, 1998). Both group and individual psychotherapies can provide a forum that facilitates expression of feelings appropriate to the disease (Greer, 1991; Greer, Morris, & Pettingale, 1979; Spiegel, 1994, 1995; Spiegel, Bloom, & Yalom, 1981). In so doing, patients are less likely to use repressive coping strategies, and the result is an increased expression of both positive and negative emotions. Emotional suppression negatively affects intimacy in families and hinders opportunities for open expression of affection and concern between patients and their loved ones (Classen et al., 1996). This review emphasizes the role of exploration of affect in psychotherapy, an area that has received relatively less attention than cognitive–behavioral approaches, which focus on social learning, knowledge acquisition, and behavior change.

Psychotherapeutic intervention offers a safe context in which to manage the intrusion of painful and frightening affect. Fears of death and dying, for example, can be overwhelming when the patient has little or no opportunity to fully express them. These normal, yet terrifying, feelings can be better negotiated by patients who have a specific time and place to express and deal with them. In addition, when the patient feels isolated or somehow singled out in his or her experience of anxiety, loss, and fear related to the cancer, the disease-related dysphoria is considerably more intense. Fear and anxiety about death and dying are exacerbated by isolation, because of our frequent conceptualization of death as the ultimate separation from loved ones. Feeling alone in the heat of intense emotions can make the patient feel already a little bit dead, which further aggravates death anxiety. This can be countered (with impressive results) by psychotherapeutic techniques that specifically attend to these kinds of concerns. Group therapy, for example, provides a setting where others experience and share similar distress, which serves to normalize these feelings, rendering them less toxic, alien, and overwhelming (I. D. Yalom, 1995; I. D. Yalom & Greaves, 1977). Patients who questioned their responses to their diagnosis discover that they have, in fact, reacted normally to an abnormal situation. This, in turn, engenders more of a sense of control as patients find that they are able to sustain themselves in the face of adversity.

Many group and individual psychotherapy programs teach specific coping skills, such as how to seek needed medical information, improve communication with physicians and other health care staff, and mobilize family and other social support. Moreover, many effective programs teach specific self-regulation techniques such as self-hypnosis, meditation, biofeedback, and progressive muscle relaxation. These can be extremely effective in reducing such symptoms as pain and anxiety.

These interventions often offer a purely educational component. Both newly diagnosed patients as well as those with advanced disease need and want to know more about the course, prognosis, and treatments for their disease. Knowledge acquisition is an essential element of effective treatment. It is important in making decisions regarding treatment alternatives, informing friends and family about likely outcomes, planning for the future, and feeling more in control of the situation. However, it is critical that the educational aspects of psychotherapeutic interventions do not replace direct medical advice from treating physicians.

Group Therapeutic Factors

Group therapy has been found to provide distinct advantages as a psychotherapeutic intervention for cancer patients.

Social Support

Members of support groups can frequently find a comradeship that they experience nowhere else. They can relate to each other in certain ways that buffer the social isolation often experienced after a diagnosis of cancer. Group psychotherapy offers a new and important social connection at a time when others may withdraw out of fear or awkwardness. The very thing that may hamper other social relationships is, in fact, the "ticket of admission" to such groups and lends itself to an unusual intensity of caring among group members from the start. Being part of a group allows cancer patients to experience a crucial sense of community that is essential for successful coping; moreover, it provides opportunities to learn from each other (Spiegel, 1993a). Social isolation has been demonstrated to be as closely related to age-adjusted mortality as serum cholesterol levels or smoking (House, Landis, & Umberson, 1988). Goodwin, Hunt, Key, and Samet (1987) demonstrated that being married predicts better medical outcome with cancer, whereas Ramirez et al. (1989) found that there is a higher probability of cancer recurrence associated with social stress such as divorce, loss of a job, and bereavement. The social network for cancer patients provided by support groups is extraordinarily meaningful, because it occurs at a time when patients may be experiencing an erosion in their natural support network and when more such support is needed.

Helper-Therapy Principle

The dual benefit of giving and receiving support that occurs in group therapy has been called the "helper-therapy principle" (Riessman, 1965, p. 27). Many cancer patients gain new self-esteem in using their experience with cancer to assist others undergoing similar distress. Thus, the random tragedy of a cancer diagnosis becomes an asset as one patient provides concrete help to another. Cancer patients experience other patients most beneficially when they model successful coping and surviving (Taylor & Dakof, 1988). This provides dual benefit: Those receiving information about coping acquire "tips" on living with the illness acquired by others who have firsthand experience, and those providing the information gain a sense of accomplishment from having learned something that allows them to help others in a similar situation.

For example, one woman who was a 10-year survivor of metastatic breast cancer, had been diagnosed with 29 positive lymph nodes, and had had 3 bone and skin metastases was viewed in her support group as a virtual model of survivorship and coping. The term the other group members used for her was *warrior*. Thus, she emerged from a difficult medical history with poor prognostic odds feeling proud of her ability to set a standard for others in her group. In addition, group therapy increases the probability of constructive compassion with and for other cancer patients (I. Yalom, 1995; I. D. Yalom & Greaves, 1977).

Cost-effectiveness

Group therapy is obviously more cost-effective than individual therapy in that it makes limited professional resources available to many more patients, including underserved populations. Group therapy may in fact be up to four times more affordable for patients and for institutions (V. Yalom & Yalom, 1990). An extensive literature demonstrates that psychoeducational (Devine, 1992) and psychotherapeutic (Mumford, Schlesinger, Glass, Patrick, & Cuerdon, 1984) interventions produce cost savings in medical treatment. Effects on medical practice resulting from such psychosocial interventions for medically ill patient populations include more rapid recovery from surgery (Devine, 1992), shorter hospital stays (Devine, 1992; Mumford et al., 1984; Strain et al., 1991), and reduced distress-related outpatient visits to doctors (Cummings & VandenBos, 1981; Hellman, Budd, Borysenko, McClelland, & Benson, 1990; Lorig, Lubeck, Kraines, Selesznick, & Holman, 1985). This is of vital importance to health care service delivery and cost, considering the current prevalence and incidence of cancer in the population.

The group format enables patients to give unique support to one other, provides an extended social network, allows patients to model coping with various aspects of the disease, and enhances patients' self-esteem as it creates an opportunity for them to provide concrete help to others dealing with similar circumstances.

Therapeutic Themes

Psychosocial intervention for cancer patients in our clinical research program, conducted in conjunction with appropriate psychopharmacologic, medical, and surgical treatment, consists of seven basic components.

Social Support

Psychotherapy, particularly in groups, can provide a heretofore unavailable social network with the common bond of confronting similar problems (Spiegel, 1993b). At a time when the illness makes a person feel removed from the flow of life and when others may retreat out of fear or awkwardness, psychotherapeutic support provides a new and important social connection. The level of caring and relatedness, therefore, is a given and develops rapidly from the beginning of most groups.

Emotional Expression

Emotion is important as a signal system that attracts attention to novel or threatening life situations. Thus, the diagnosis of cancer or recurrence naturally arouses strong feelings. At the same time, emotion can hamper coping ability, reducing comprehension of medical information, willingness to communicate, or ability to change behavior. The expression of emotion can be quite helpful in managing it, minimizing social isolation, and improving coping. However, expression of even quite appropriate disease-related emotion is often discouraged. Emotional suppression and avoidance are associated with poorer coping (Classen et al., 1996; Derogatis, Abeloff, & Melisartos, 1979; Greer, 1991; Greer, Morris, & Pettingale, 1979; Pettingale, 1984; Spiegel, 1993a; Temoshok, 1985). There is much that can be done in both group and individual psychotherapies to facilitate the expression of emotion appropriate to the illness. Doing so appears to decrease repressive coping, which reduces the expression of positive as well as negative emotion.

Detoxifying Dying

This component of treatment involves directly discussing and confronting anxiety about death rather than avoiding it. When worked through, even life-threatening problems can come to seem less overwhelming (Spiegel, 1993a). Following a diagnosis of cancer, a variety of coping strategies come into play, including positive reappraisal and cognitive avoidance (Jarrett, Ramirez, Richards, & Weinman, 1992). Facing life-threatening issues directly can help patients shift from emotion-focused to problem-focused coping (Moos & Schaefer, 1987; Spiegel, 1990). Direct discussion of death anxiety can help to divide the fear of death into a series of problems: loss of control over treatment decisions, fear of separation from loved ones, and anxiety about pain. The process of dying is often more threatening than death itself. Discussion of these concerns can lead to means of addressing, if not completely resolving, each of these issues. Even the specter of facing death can result in positive life changes.

One woman with metastatic breast cancer described her experience in this way:

> What I found is that talking about death is like looking down into the Grand Canyon (I don't like heights). You know that if you fell down, it would be a disaster, but you feel better about yourself because you're able to look. I can't say I feel serene, but I can look at it now. (Spiegel, 1993a, p. 148)

Even the process of grieving deaths among group members, although threatening, can be reassuring at the same time. The experience of grieving others who have died of the same condition constitutes a deeply personal experience of the depth of loss that will be experienced by others after one's own death.

Reordering Life Priorities

The acceptance of the possibility that illness may shorten one's life carries with it an opportunity for reevaluating life priorities. When cure is not possible, a realistic evaluation of the future can help those with life-threatening illness make the best use of their remaining time. One of the costs of unrealistic optimism is the loss of time for accomplishing life projects, communicating openly with family and friends, and setting affairs in order. Facing the threat of death can aid patients in making the most of their lives (Spiegel, 1993a; Spiegel et al., 1981; I. D. Yalom, 1980).

Facing death can help patients take control of those aspects of their lives they can influence, even as they grieve for and relinquish those they cannot. Defining a domain of realistic control can actually be reassuring.

Family Support

Psychotherapeutic interventions can also be quite helpful in improving communication; identifying needs; increasing role flexibility; and adjusting to new medical, social, vocational, and financial realities. There is evidence that an atmosphere of open and shared problem solving in families results in reduced anxiety and depression among cancer patients (Spiegel, Bloom, & Gottheil, 1983). Therefore, facilitating the development of such open addressing of common dilemmas is a useful therapeutic goal. The group format is especially helpful for such a task, in that the problems patients have in expressing their needs and wishes can be examined by group members, who may then model ways to clarify communication in the family.

In addition to enhancing communication, group participants are encouraged to develop role flexibility, a capacity to exchange roles or develop new ones as the pressures of the illness demand. One woman, for example, who became unable to carry out her usual household chores, wrote an "owner's manual" for the care of the house so that her husband could more effectively help her and carry on after her death. Others wrote letters to friends asking them to cook an extra bit of dinner on one evening a month to share with them and relieve them of the pressure of cooking.

Communication With Physicians

Facilitating communication with physicians can help to foster patients' sense of control and facilitate treatment adherence. Support groups can be extremely useful in facilitating better communication between patients and physicians as well as other health care professionals. Groups provide mutual encouragement to get questions answered, to participate more actively in treatment decisions, and to consider alternatives carefully. Research has shown that breast cancer patients are more satisfied with the results of intervention, such as lumpectomy as opposed to modified radical mastectomy, to the extent that they have been involved in making the decision about which type of treatment to have (Fallowfield, Baum, & Maguire, 1987; Fallowfield, Hall, & Maguire, 1990; Levy et al., 1992). Such groups must be mindful of not interfering with medical treatment or decisions; the emphasis should be on encouraging problem clarification and the development of a truly cooperative partnership between doctor and patient.

Symptom Control

Many group and individual psychotherapies teach specific coping skills designed to help patients decrease cancer-related symptoms such as anxiety, anticipatory nausea, vomiting, and pain. Techniques used include specific self-regulation skills such as self-hypnosis, meditation, biofeedback, and progressive muscle relaxation (Burish & Lyles, 1981; Hilgard & Hilgard, 1975; Morrow & Morrell, 1982; Spiegel, 1990; Spiegel & Bloom, 1983; Zeltzer & LeBaron, 1982).

Outcomes of Psychotherapeutic Intervention

Various types of group interventions have been tested. Some have lasted only 6 weeks and have been demonstrated to improve coping skills (Fawzy, Cousins, et al., 1990), whereas others have helped to reduce such symptoms as pain, nausea, and vomiting (Cain, Kohorn, Quinlan, Latimer, & Schwartz, 1986; Forester, Kornfeld, & Fleiss, 1985; Morrow & Morrell, 1982). Some interventions result in immediate improvement in psychosocial functioning (Telch & Telch 1986); with other interventions, the more obvious effects appeared at the 6-month follow-up (Fawzy, Cousins, et al., 1990; Fawzy, Kemeny, et al., 1990). Group interventions for cancer patients have been shown to significantly reduce psychological symptoms (Andersen, 1992; Fawzy, Fawzy, Arndt, & Pasnau, 1995), such as anxiety and depression (Ferlic, Goldman, & Kennedy, 1979; Gustafson & Whitman, 1978; Mulder et al., 1995; Spiegel et al., 1981; Wood, Milligan, Christ, & Liff, 1978); improve coping skills (Fawzy, Cousins, et al., 1990; Turns, 1988); and reduce symptoms such as pain, nausea, and vomiting (Cain et al., 1986; Forester et al., 1985; Morrow & Morrell, 1982; Spiegel & Bloom, 1983).

Many of the psychotherapies that have shown promise in improving emotional adjustment and influencing survival time involve encouraging open expression of emotion and assertiveness in assuming control over the course of treatment, life decisions, and relationships (Fawzy, Cousins, et al., 1990; Spiegel et al., 1981; Spiegel, Bloom, Kraemer, & Gottheil, 1989; Spiegel & Yalom, 1978). Adequate assessment of quality of life requires attention to multiple variables (Ganz, 1994). Recent research has shown that patients who believe that they have control over the cause of disease have poor outcomes, whereas those who believe that they control the course of the disease have better outcomes (Watson, Greer, Pruyn, & Van den Borne, 1990). Supportive–expressive group therapy for metastatic breast cancer patients has been shown to result in better mood, fewer maladaptive coping responses, fewer phobic symptoms (Spiegel et al., 1981), and reduced pain (Spiegel & Bloom, 1983). Supportive–expressive group psychotherapy has been compared in a randomized prospective trial with cognitive–behavioral treatment in a sample of HIV-positive patients (Kelly et al., 1993). This more emotionally expressive approach was found to be more effective in reducing mood disturbance.

Predictors of Response to Treatment

Those most in need of help are most likely to benefit from it when it is provided and tend to persist in doing poorly without it. Initial levels of mood disturbance are strong predictors of subsequent distress (Ell, Nishimoto, Morvay, Mantell, & Hamovitch, 1989). Other predictors are a history of depression (Maunsell, Brisson, & Deschenes, 1992), low self-esteem (Felton, Revenson, & Hinrichsen, 1984; Timko & Janoff-Bulman 1985), external locus of control (Northouse & Swain, 1987), and neuroticism (Morris, Greer, & White, 1977, as reviewed in Irvine et al., 1991). Those whose initial distress is greatest are likely to benefit the most from psychotherapeutic intervention.

The absence of social support should predict greater need for intervention, because social support has been shown to improve adjustment, promote emotional well-being, and reduce fear of recurrence in women with breast cancer (Irvine et al., 1991; Jamison, Wellisch, & Pasnau, 1978; Northouse, 1981; Reynolds & Kaplan, 1990; Woods & Earp, 1978). Bloom (1982) demonstrated that amount of social contact and perceived family cohesiveness directly affected coping and indirectly affected adjustment. Affect, affirmation, and reciprocity within families were associated with decreased depression and better family functioning (Primomo, Yates, & Woods, 1990).

Medical Treatment Adherence

One outcome of psychotherapeutic intervention for cancer patients may be adherence to difficult medical treatment. Adherence issues are particularly important for cancer patients because of treatment complexity and intensity, and these issues are particularly challenging because of the highly unpleasant side effects associated particularly with chemotherapy and radiation treatment. Adherence problems may include (Hoagland, Morrow, Bennett, & Carnike, 1983) failure to return following initial evaluation for recommended outpatient treatment, failure to keep subsequent appointments, patient refusal of the recommended inpatient and outpatient treatments, and nonadherence with prescribed home medication regimens (Itano et al., 1983). Nonadherence to treatment regimens is high among cancer patients. In one study, 23% of patients did not keep their appointments for the administration of chemotherapy (Itano et al., 1983). Withdrawal from the recommended treatment protocol is estimated to range from 16% to 33% (Glass et al., 1981; Laszlo & Lucas, 1981; Lee, 1983; Wilcox, Fetting, Nettesheim, & Abeloff, 1982). In a study of women with abnormal Pap smears requiring follow-up care, 29% did not return for screening follow-up (Marcus et al., 1992).

Variables that have been shown to affect adherence include demographics, patient perceptions of the illness and his or her role in its treatment, social support, the costs and benefits of adherence from the patient's perspective, and an intention to comply (Given & Given, 1989). All of the psychosocial factors in this model except demographics may be influenced by participating in a cancer support group. Participating in a group increases patients' knowledge, changes their attitudes about treatment, and may help them to overcome practical obstacles to adherence. Other factors, such as educating patients about the efficacy of treatments, produces better adherence with medication regimens (Beck et al., 1988; Ferguson & Bole, 1979). To the extent that groups help patients take an active and collaborative role in their medical treatment, there will be greater satisfaction and adherence (Eisenthal, Emery, Lazare, & Udin, 1979; Wyszynski, 1990). This literature provides evidence that participation in therapy groups improves treatment adherence by helping patients (a) better manage the anxiety that is intertwined with treatment, (b) better understand the reasoning behind treatment decisions, (c) feel more in control of the course of treatment through clearer communication with their physicians, and (d) more effectively mobilize support from friends and family for participating in treatment.

Quantity of Life

Recent research has emerged indicating that group psychotherapy may affect health status and the quantity as well as the quality of life. Providing social support interventions particularly for isolated individuals under stress has been related to improved health outcome (Fawzy, 1991; Raphael, 1977; Richardson, Shelton, Krailo, & Levine, 1990; Rodin, 1980, 1986; Spiegel et al., 1989; Turner, 1981). Social support has been shown to be an important factor in mediating individuals' ability to cope with stress. Rodin (1980, 1986) observed decreases in urinary free cortisol levels in geriatric patients exposed to education on stress management. Moreover, she found that patients who received this experimental coping intervention were not only rated as happier and more sociable, but also had longer survival times than others who were not treated. Forester et al. (1985) found that in a sample of 48 cancer patients, both mood disturbance and physical symptoms of anorexia, fatigue, and nausea and vomiting were significantly improved by individual psychotherapy compared with those of a matched control group.

Prior work in our laboratory (Spiegel et al., 1989) has shown that participation in psychosocial group treatment for metastatic cancer patients prolongs survival time twofold from the point of randomization, an average of 18 months. Fifty women with metastatic breast cancer were randomly assigned to a year of weekly support groups with training in self-hypnosis for pain control, and they survived an average of 18 months longer than 36 control patients who had been randomly assigned to routine care. This difference is clinically as well as statistically significant. These data were recently reviewed and supplemented by other researchers (Kogon, Biswas, Pearl, Carlson, & Spiegel, 1997). Differences in disease course between control metastatic breast cancer patients and those who received psychotherapeutic intervention in the earlier study were found to be independent of any differences in medical treatment they received.

Some studies show no effect of psychosocial treatment on medical outcome. The apparent beneficial effect of psychosocial support on survival time of 34 breast cancer patients in another study (Morgenstern, Gellert, Walter, Ostfeld, & Siegel,

1984) disappeared when time from cancer diagnosis to program entry was controlled. This lack of difference was recently confirmed in a long-term follow-up of the same sample (Gellert, Maxwell, & Siegel, 1993). Two trials, both randomized, also found no survival benefit to psychotherapy for cancer patients. Linn, Linn, and Harris (1982) offered individual psychotherapy to a group of patients with a variety of cancers, including those of lung and pancreas, in a randomized protocol. There was no difference in survival time. It may be that because virtually all of the patients died during the follow-up year, their disease was too far advanced to be significantly influenced by psychotherapeutic support. Similarly, Ilnyckyj, Farber, Cheang, & Weinerman (1994) found no survival advantage for breast cancer patients randomly assigned to one of several group psychotherapies (some of which were led by other patients), nor was there any demonstrable psychological benefit. In this particular case, the relative inefficacy of the intervention may account for the lack of medical effect.

However, two other randomized trials have demonstrated a psychosocial effect on survival time among cancer patients. Richardson et al. (1990) used a four-cell design among patients with lymphomas and leukemias. Patients were assigned to either a routine care condition or to one of three educational and home-visiting supportive interventions. The control group had significantly shorter survival time than patients allocated to the intervention. There were also differences in patients' adherence to medical treatment as measured by allopurinol intake. The survival differences held even when differences in medication adherence were controlled.

Fawzy and colleagues (Fawzy, Cousins, et al., 1990; Fawzy et al., 1993; Fawzy, Kemeny, et al., 1990) published psychosocial, immunological, recurrence, and survival results of a randomized trial involving 80 patients with malignant melanoma. This work is considered in more detail in the next chapter; we note by way of summary that initial reports (Fawzy, Cousins, et al., 1990) indicated significant reductions in mood disturbance and significant differences in immune function at the 3-month follow-up, and they predicted increases in natural killer cytotoxicity and in LEU56 cells in the intervention sample (Fawzy, Kemeny, et al., 1990). A 6-year follow-up (Fawzy, Kemeny, et al., 1990) showed lower rates of recurrence and mortality among intervention patients.

Conclusion

Distress, depression, and anxiety are problems for a substantial minority of cancer patients. Some experience a persistence of these problems for years after the initial diagnosis. Coping styles are related to adjustment and, in some studies, survival time. The nature of the patient–physician relationship has a considerable impact on adjustment to the disease, satisfaction with treatment outcome, and adherence to medical treatment protocols, which are positively correlated with relapse and survival.

A variety of studies suggest that serious life stress can adversely affect medical outcome. Social support by way of integration, availability of confidantes, and structured psychotherapy has been shown to positively affect adjustment and may even affect survival time. In combination, these studies show that the social, psychological, and medical environment of cancer patients is vital to their adjustment. Clear and open communication, expression of all emotion appropriate to their situation, and collaborative planning and problem-solving enhance adjustment and improve outcome. At the same time, circumstances that isolate cancer patients from others or undermine support can have deleterious medical and psychosocial consequences.

The literature makes it clear that cancer patients suffer considerable emotional and social distress and that a significant minority suffers persistent symptoms that produce considerable distress and interfere with medical treatment. Group interventions have been shown to be clinically efficacious and cost-effective, reducing mood disturbance and pain and improving adherence to treatment. Special populations of cancer patients with high initial levels of mood disturbance, recency and severity of medical condition, and poor social support are associated with poor subsequent adjustment. Therefore, these populations could be reasonably expected to benefit most from participation in an effective therapy program. The diagnosis and treatment of cancer constitutes a major life stressor for which few people are adequately prepared. The studies reviewed above did not screen patients for a threshold criterion of demonstrable psychopathology (e.g., an anxiety or depressive disorder) or problematic coping. Although some may benefit more than others, it is not clear that there is a subpopulation immune to potential benefit.

There is a clear and growing body of evidence that suggests that psychotherapeutic intervention for cancer patients, including those without a prior psychiatric diagnosis, is a powerful and important component of treatment, with marked psychological effects (distress reduction; improved coping; enhanced interaction with family, friends, and health care professionals) . Furthermore, provocative recent studies strongly suggest the possibility that such interventions may have physical effects that influence the course of cancer as well. Such techniques have shown themselves to be humane, effective, and cost-effective.

References

Andersen, B. L. (1992). Psychological interventions for cancer patients to enhance quality of life. *Journal of Consulting and Clinical Psychology, 60*(4), 552–568.

Beck, N. C., Parker, J. C., Frank, R. G., Geden, E. A., Kay, D. R., Gamache, M., Shivers, N., Smith, E., & Anderson, S. (1988). Patients with rheumatoid arthritis at high risk for noncompliance with salicylate treatment regimens. *Journal of Rheumatology, 15,* 1081–1084.

Berkman, L. F., & Syme, S. L. (1979). Social networks, host resistance, and mortality: A nine-year follow-up study of Alameda County residents. *American Journal of Epidemiology, 109*(2), 186–204.

Bloom, J. R. (1982). Social support, accommodation to stress and adjustment to breast cancer. *Social Science and Medicine, 16,* 1329–1338.

Browne, G. B., Arpin, K., Corey, P., Fitch, M., & Gafni, A. (1990). Individual correlates of health service utilization and the cost of poor adjustment to chronic illness. *Medical Care, 28*(1), 43–58.

Burish, T. G., & Lyles, J. N. (1981). Effectiveness of relaxation training in reducing adverse reactions to cancer chemotherapy. *Journal of Behavioral Medicine, 4*(1), 65–78.

Cain, E. N., Kohorn, E. I., Quinlan, D. M., Latimer, K., & Schwartz, P. E. (1986). Psychosocial benefits of a cancer support group. *Cancer, 57*(1), 183–189.

Chochinov, H. M., Wilson, K. G., Enns, M., Mowchun, N., Lander, S., Levitt, M., & Clinch, J. J. (1995). Desire for death in the terminally ill. *American Journal of Psychiatry, 152,* 1185–1191.

Classen, C., Koopman, C., Angell, K., & Spiegel, D. (1996). Coping styles associated with psychological adjustment to advanced breast cancer. *Health Psychology, 15,* 434–437.

Cummings, N. A., & VandenBos, G. R. (1981). The twenty years Kaiser-Permanente experience with psychotherapy and medical utilization: Implications for national health policy and national health insurance. *Health Policy Quarterly, 1*(2), 159–175.

Derogatis, L. R., Abeloff, M. D., & Melisartos, N. (1979). Psychological coping mechanisms and survival time in metastatic breast cancer. *Journal of the American Medical Association, 242,* 1504–1508.

Derogatis, L. R., Morrow, G. R., Fetting, J., Penman, D., Piasetsky, S., Schmale, A. M., Henrichs, M., & Carnicke, C. L., Jr. (1983). The prevalence of psychiatric disorders among cancer patients. *Journal of the American Medical Association, 249,* 751–757.

Devine, E. C. (1992). Effects of psychoeducational care for adult surgical patients: A meta-analysis of 191 studies. *Patient Education and Counseling, 19*(2), 129–142.

Ell, K., Nishimoto, R., Morvay, T., Mantell, J., & Hamovitch, M. (1989). A longitudinal analysis of psychological adaptation among survivors of cancer. *Cancer, 63*(2), 406–413.

Eisenthal, S., Emery, R., Lazare, A., & Udin, H. (1979). "Adherence" and the negotiated approach to patienthood. *Archives of General Psychiatry, 36,* 393–398.

Fallowfield, L., Baum, M., & Maguire, G. P. (1987). Effects of breast conservation on psychological morbidity associated with diagnosis and treatment of early breast cancer. *British Medical Journal, 239,* 1331–1334.

Fallowfield, L., Hall, A., Maguire, G. P., & Baum, M. (1990). Psychological outcomes in women with early breast cancer [Letter, Comment]. *British Medical Journal, 301*(6765), 1394.

Fawzy, F. (1991, October). *Effects of group support on malignant melanoma patients.* Paper presented at the Memorial Sloan-Kettering Conference on Psychosocial Oncology, New York.

Fawzy, F. I., Cousins, N., Fawzy, N. W., Kemeny, M. E., Elashoff, R., & Morton, D. (1990). A structured psychiatric intervention for cancer patients. I. Changes over time in methods of coping and affective disturbance. *Archives of General Psychiatry, 47,* 720–725.

Fawzy, F. I., Fawzy, N. W., Arndt, L. A., & Pasnau, R. O. (1995). Critical review of psychosocial interventions in cancer care. *Archives of General Psychiatry, 52,* 100–113.

Fawzy, F. I., Fawzy, N. W., Hyun, C. S., Elashoff, R., Guthrie, D., Fahey, J. L., & Morton, D. L. (1993). Malignant melanoma. Effects of an early structured psychiatric intervention, coping, and affective state on recurrence and survival 6 years later. *Archives of General Psychiatry, 50,* 681–689.

Fawzy, F. I., Kemeny, M. E., Fawzy, N. W., Elashoff, R., Morton, D., Cousins, N., & Fahey, J. L. (1990). A structured psychiatric intervention for cancer patients. II. Changes over time in immunological measures. *Archives of General Psychiatry, 47,* 729–735.

Felton, B. J., Revenson, T. A., & Hinrichsen, G. A. (1984). Stress and coping in the explanation of psychological adjustment among chronically ill adults. *Social Science and Medicine, 18,* 889–898.

Ferguson, K., & Bole, G. G. (1979). Family support, health beliefs, and therapeutic compliance in patients with rheumatoid arthritis. *Patient Counselling and Health Education, 1*(3), 101–105.

Ferlic, M., Goldman, A., & Kennedy, B. J. (1979). Group counseling in adult patients with advanced cancer. *Cancer, 43,* 760–766.

Forester, B., Kornfeld, D. S., & Fleiss, J. L. (1985). Psychotherapy during radiotherapy: Effects on emotional and physical distress. *American Journal of Psychiatry, 142*(1), 22–27.

Ganz, P. A. (1994). Quality of life and the patient with cancer. Individual and policy implications. *Cancer, 74*(Suppl. 4), 1445–1452.

Gellert, G. A., Maxwell, R. M., & Siegel, B. S. (1993). Survival of breast cancer patients receiving adjunctive psychosocial support therapy: A 10-year follow-up study. *Journal of Clinical Oncology, 11*(1), 66–69.

Given, B. A., & Given, C. W. (1989). Compliance among patients with cancer. *Oncology Nursing Forum, 16*(1), 97–103.

Glass, A., Wieand, H. S., Fisher, B., Redmond, C., Lerner, H., Wolter, J., Shibata, H., Plotkin, D., Foster, D., Margolese, R., & Wolmark, N. (1981). Acute toxicity during adjuvant chemotherapy for breast cancer: The National Surgical Adjuvant Breast and Bowel Project (NSABP) experience from 1717 patients receiving single and multiple agents. *Cancer Treatment Reports, 65*(5–6), 363–376.

Goodwin, J. S., Hunt, W. C., Key, C. R., & Samet, J. M. (1987). The effect of marital status on stage, treatment, and survival of cancer patients. *Journal of the American Medical Association, 258,* 3125–3130.

Greer, S. (1991). Psychological response to cancer and survival. *Psychological Medicine, 21*(1), 43–49.

Greer, S., Morris, T., & Pettingale, K. W. (1979). Psychological response to breast cancer: Effect on outcome. *Lancet, 2*(8146), 785–787.

Gustafson, J., & Whitman, H. (1978). Towards a balanced social environment on the oncology service. *Social Psychiatry, 13,* 147–152.

Hellman, C. J., Budd, M., Borysenko, J., McClelland, D. C., & Benson, H. (1990). A study of the effectiveness of two group behavioral medicine interventions for patients with psychosomatic complaints. *Behavioral Medicine, 16,* 165–173.

Hilgard, E. R., & Hilgard, J. R. (1975). *Hypnosis in the relief of pain.* Los Altos, CA: William Kauffman.

Hoagland, A. C., Morrow, G. R., Bennett, J. M., & Carnrike, C. L., Jr. (1983). Oncologists' views of cancer patient noncompliance. *American Journal of Clinical Oncology, 6,* 239–244.

Holland, J., & Rowland, J. (Eds.). (1990). *Handbook of psychooncology: Psychologic care of the patient with cancer.* Newark, NJ: Oxford University Press.

House, J. S., Landis, K. R., & Umberson, D. (1988). Social relationships and health. *Science, 241*(4865), 540–545.

Ilnyckyj, A., Farber, J., Cheang, M., & Weinerman, B. (1994). A randomized controlled trial of psychotherapeutic intervention in cancer patients. *Annals of the Royal College of Physicians and Surgeons of Canada, 27*(2), 93–96.

Irvine, D., Brown, B., Crooks, D., Roberts, J., & Browne, G. (1991). Psychosocial adjustment in women with breast cancer. *Cancer, 67,* 1097–1117.

Itano, J., Tanabe, P., Lum, J. L., Lamkin, L., Rizzo, E., Weiland, M., & Sata, P. (1983). Compliance of cancer patients to therapy. *Western Journal of Nursing Research, 5*(1), 5–20.

Jamison, K. R., Wellisch, D. K., & Pasnau, R. O. (1978). Psychosocial aspects of mastectomy: I. The women's perspective. *American Journal of Psychiatry, 135,* 432–436.

Jarrett, S. R., Ramirez, A. J., Richards, M. A., & Weinman, J. (1992). Measuring coping in breast cancer. *Journal of Psychosomatic Research, 36,* 593–602.

Kelly, J. A., Murphy, D. A., Bahr, G. R., Kalichman, S. C., Morgan, M. G., Stevenson, L. Y., & Koob, J. J. (1993). Outcome of cognitive–behavioral and support group brief therapies for depressed, HIV-infected persons. *American Journal of Psychiatry, 150,* 1679–1686.

Kogon, M. M., Biswas, A., Pearl, D., Carlson, R. W., & Spiegel, D. (1997). Effects of medical and psychotherapeutic treatment on the survival of women with metastatic breast carcinoma. *Cancer, 80,* 225–230.

Koopman, C., Hermanson, K., Diamond, S., Angell, K., & Spiegel, D. (1998). Social support, life stress, pain and emotional adjustment to advanced breast cancer. *Psycho-oncology, 7*(2), 101–111.

Laszlo, J., & Lucas, V., Jr. (1981). Emesis as a critical problem in chemotherapy [editorial]. *New England Journal of Medicine, 305,* 948–949.

Lee, Y. T. (1983). Adjuvant chemotherapy (CMF) for breast carcinoma. Patient's compliance and total dose achieved. *American Journal of Clinical Oncology, 6*(1), 25–30.

Levy, S. M., Haynes, L. T., Herberman, R. B., Lee, J., McFeeley, S., & Kirkwood, J. (1992). Mastectomy versus breast conservation surgery: Mental health effects at long-term follow-up. *Health Psychology, 11,* 349–354.

Linn, M. W., Linn, B. S., & Harris, R. (1982). Effects of counseling for late stage cancer. *Cancer, 49,* 1048–1055.

Lorig, K., Lubeck, D., Kraines, R. G., Sele52nick, M., & Holman, H. R. (1985). Outcomes of self-help education for patients with arthritis. *Arthritis and Rheumatism, 28,* 680–685.

Marcus, A. C., Crane, L. A., Kaplan, C. P., Reading, A. E., Savage, E., Gunning, J., Bernstein, G., & Berek, J. S. (1992). Improving adherence to screening follow-up among women with abnormal Pap smears: Results from a large clinic-based trial of three intervention strategies. *Medical Care, 30,* 216–230.

Maunsell, E., Brisson, J., & Deschenes, L. (1992). Psychological distress after initial treatment of breast cancer. Assessment of potential risk factors. *Cancer, 70,* 120–125.

Mermelstein, H. T., & Lesko, L. (1992). Depression in patients with cancer. *Psychooncology, 1,* 199–125.

Moos, R. H., & Schaefer, J. A. (1987). The crisis of physical illness: An overview and conceptual approach. In R. H. Moos (Ed.), *Coping with physical illness: Vol. 2. New perspectives* (pp. 3–25). New York: Plenum.

Morgenstern, H., Gellert, G. A., Walter, S. D., Ostfeld, A. M., & Siegel, B. S. (1984). The impact of a psychosocial support program on survival with breast cancer: The importance of selection bias in program evaluation. *Journal of Chronic Diseases, 37*(4), 273–282.

Morris, T., Greer, H. S., & White, P. (1977). Psychological and social adjustment to mastectomy: A two-year follow-up study. *Cancer, 40,* 2381–2387.

Morrow, G. R., & Morrell, C. (1982). Behavioral treatment for the anticipatory nausea and vomiting induced by cancer chemotherapy. *New England Journal of Medicine, 307,* 1476–1480.

Mulder, C. L., Antoni, M. H., Emmelkamp, P. M., Veugeiers, P. J., Sandfort, T. G., van de Vijver, F. A., & de Vries, M. J. (1995). Psychosocial group intervention and the rate of decline of immunological parameters in asymptomatic HIV-infected homosexual men. *Psychotherapy Psychosomatics, 63*(3–4), 185–192.

Mumford, E., Schlesinger, H. J., Glass, G. V., Patrick, C., & Cuerdon, T. (1984). A new look at evidence about reduced cost of medical utilization following mental health treatment. *American Journal of Psychiatry, 141,* 1145–1158.

Northouse, L. L. (1981). Mastectomy patients and the fear of cancer recurrence. *Cancer Nursing, 4,* 213–220.

Northouse, L. L., & Swain, M. A. (1987). Adjustment of patients and husbands to the initial impact of breast cancer. *Nursing Research, 36*(4), 221–225.

Omne-Ponten, M., Holmberg, L., & Sjoden, P. O. (1994). Psychosocial adjustment among women with breast cancer stages I and II: Six-year follow-up of consecutive patients. *Journal of Clinical Oncology, 12,* 1778–1782.

Pettingale, K. W. (1984). Coping and cancer prognosis. *Journal of Psychosomatic Research, 28,* 363–364.

Primomo, J., Yates, B. C., & Woods, N. F. (1990). Social support for women during chronic illness: The relationship among sources and types to adjustment. *Research in Nursing and Health, 13*(3), 153–161.

Ramirez, A. J., Craig, T. K., Watson, J. P., Fentiman, I. S., North, W. R., & Rubens, R. D. (1989). Stress and relapse of breast cancer. *British Medical Journal, 298*(6669), 291–293.

Raphael, B. (1977). Preventive intervention with the recently bereaved. *Archives of General Psychiatry, 34,* 1450–1454.

Reynolds, P., & Kaplan, G. A. (1990). Social connections and risk for cancer: Prospective evidence from the Alameda County Study. *Behavioral Medicine, 16,* 101–110.

Richardson, J. L., Shelton, D. R., Krailo, M., & Levine, A. M. (1990). The effect of compliance with treatment on survival among patients with hematologic malignancies. *Journal of Clinical Oncology, 8,* 356–364.

Riessman, F. (1965). The "helper" therapy principle. *Social Work, 10,* 27–32.

Rodin, J. (1980). *Managing the stress of aging: The role of control and coping.* New York: Plenum.

Rodin, J. (1986). *Health, control and aging.* Hillsdale, NJ: Erlbaum.

Spiegel, D. (1979). Psychological support for women with metastatic carcinoma. *Psychosomatics, 20,* 780–787.

Spiegel, D. (1990). Facilitating emotional coping during treatment. *Cancer, 66*(Suppl. 6), 1422–1426.

Spiegel, D. (1993a). *Living beyond limits: New help and hope for facing life-threatening illness.* New York: Times Books/Random House.

Spiegel, D. (1993b). Psychosocial intervention in cancer. *Journal of the National Cancer Institute, 85,* 1198–1205.

Spiegel, D. (1994). Health caring: Psychosocial support for patients with cancer. *Cancer, 74*(Suppl. 4), 1453–1457.

Spiegel, D. (1995). Essentials of psychotherapeutic intervention for cancer patients. *Support Care Cancer, 3,* 252–256.

Spiegel, D., & Bloom, J. R. (1983). Group therapy and hypnosis reduce metastatic breast carcinoma pain. *Psychosomatic Medicine, 45,* 333–339.

Spiegel, D., Bloom, J. R., & Gottheil, E. (1983). Family environment as a predictor of adjustment to metastatic breast carcinoma. *Journal of Psychosocial Oncology, 1*(1), 33–44.

Spiegel, D., Bloom, J. R., Kraemer, H. C., & Gottheil, E. (1989). Effect of psychosocial treatment on survival of patients with metastatic breast cancer. *Lancet, 2*(8668), 888–891.

Spiegel, D., Bloom, J. R., & Yalom, I. (1981). Group support for patients with metastatic cancer. A randomized outcome study. *Archives of General Psychiatry, 38,* 527–533.

Spiegel, D., & Yalom, I. (1978). A support group for dying patients. *International Journal of Group Psychotherapy, 28,* 233–245.

Strain, J. J., Lyons, J. S., Hammer, J. S., Fahs, M., Lebovits, A., Paddison, P. L., Snyder, S., Strauss, E., Burton, R., & Nuber, G. (1991). Cost offset from a psychiatric consultation-liaison intervention with elderly hip fracture patients. *American Journal of Psychiatry, 148,* 1044–1049.

Taylor, S., & Dakof, G. (1988). *Social support and the cancer patient.* Newbury Park, CA: Sage.

Telch, C. F., & Telch, M. J. (1986). Group coping skills instruction and supportive group therapy for cancer patients: A comparison of strategies. *Journal of Consulting and Clinical Psychology, 54,* 802–808.

Temoshok, L. (1985). Biopsychosocial studies on cutaneous malignant melanoma: Psychosocial factors associated with prognostic indicators, progression, psychophysiology and tumor–host response. *Social Science and Medicine, 20,* 833–840.

Timko, C., & Janoff-Bulman, R. (1985). Attributions, vulnerability, and psychological adjustment: The case of breast cancer. *Health Psychology, 4,* 521–544.

Turner, R. J. (1981). Social support as a contingency to psychological well-being. *Journal of Health Social Behavior, 22,* 357–367.

Turns, D. M. (1988). Psychosocial factors. In W. L. Donegan & J. S. Spratt (Eds.), *Cancer of the breast* (pp. 728–738). Philadelphia: W. B. Saunders.

Vinokur, A. D., Threatt, B. A., Caplan, R. D., & Zimmerman, B. L. (1989). Physical and psychosocial functioning and adjustment to breast cancer. Long-term follow-up of a screening population. *Cancer, 63,* 394–405.

Von Korff, M., Ormel, J., Katon, W., & Lin, E. H. (1992). Disability and depression among high utilizers of health care. A longitudinal analysis. *Archives of General Psychiatry, 49*(2), 91–100.

Watson, M., Greer, S., Pruyn, J., & Van den Borne, B. (1990). Locus of control and adjustment to cancer. *Psychological Reports, 66*(1), 39–48.

Wilcox, P. M., Fetting, J. H., Nettesheim, K. M., & Abeloff, M. D. (1982). Anticipatory vomiting in women receiving cyclophosphamide, methotrexate, and 5-FU (CMF) adjuvant chemotherapy for breast carcinoma. *Cancer Treatment Reports, 66,* 1601–1604.

Wood, P. E., Milligan, M., Christ, G., & Liff, D. (1978). Group counseling for cancer patients in a community hospital. *Psychosomatics, 19,* 555–561.

Woods, N. F., & Earp, J. A. (1978). Women with cured breast cancer: A study of mastectomy patients in North Carolina. *Nursing Research, 27*(5), 279–285.

Wyszynski, A. A. (1990). Managing noncompliance in the "difficult" medical patient: The contributions of insight. A case report. *Psychotherapy and Psychosomatics, 54*(4), 181–186.

Yalom, I. D. (1995). *Theory and practice of group psychotherapy.* New York: Basic Books.

Yalom, I. D. (1980). Existential psychotherapy. New York: Basic Books.

Yalom, I. D., & Greaves, C. (1977). Group therapy with the terminally ill. *American Journal of Psychiatry, 134,* 396–400.

Yalom, V., & Yalom, I. (1990). Brief interactive group psychotherapy. *Psychiatric Annals, 20,* 362–367.

Zeltzer, L., & LeBaron, S. (1982). Hypnosis and nonhypnotic techniques for reduction of pain and anxiety during painful procedures in children and adolescents with cancer. *Journal of Pediatrics, 101,* 1032–1035.

CHAPTER 13

Psychoeducational Intervention Programs for Patients With Cancer

Fawzy I. Fawzy

Nancy W. Fawzy

Andrea L. Canada

The American Cancer Society (2000) reported that there are over 8.4 million cancer survivors in the United States and that more than 59% have survived for 5 years or longer. Today there is an encouraging trend away from focusing only on terminal care and bereavement and toward helping people live as fully as possible with their cancer. A significant amount of research has been done that helps us to understand the psychological distress that patients with cancer and their families experience (Cohen, Cullen, & Martin, 1982; Weisman, 1979a). Numerous articles have also been published regarding differing interventions aimed at helping individuals deal with the diagnosis and treatment of cancer (F. I. Fawzy, Fawzy, Arndt, & Pasnau, 1995). Evidence is accumulating that some of these interventions may contribute to both psychological (reduction of distress and enhancement of coping and adjustment) and physical health outcomes (reduced side effects, lower rates of recurrence and improved survival; F. I. Fawzy et al., 1993; Greer, 1991; Ornish et al., 1992; Spiegel, Bloom, Kraemer, & Gottheil, 1989). We present an overview of this literature and offer a short-term structured, psychoeducational intervention program consisting of health education, stress management, coping skills training, and psychological support as an effective model of care for newly diagnosed patients with cancer. We also attempt to elucidate possible mechanisms underlying the positive outcomes of such interventions and discuss the continuing gaps in our knowledge base requiring future research.

Psychosocial Issues

The most frequently studied group in regard to psychosocial issues has been women with breast cancer. Breast cancer patients have been found to manifest greater anxiety and depression than general surgery patients (P. Maguire, 1976) or women with benign breast tumors (P. Maguire et al., 1978; Morris, Greer, & White, 1977). Worden and Weisman (1977) reported that among 40 newly diagnosed breast cancer patients, 20% were notably depressed according to psychological tests and clinical interviews. In addition to increased anxiety and depression, other life changes have been described in this patient population. For instance, P. Maguire et al. (1978) found that mastectomy patients experienced more sexual problems than did a control group of benign breast tumor patients at 4 and 12 months postsurgery. After comprehensively reviewing the literature on psychological correlates of breast cancer, Meyerowitz (1980) summarized the typical responses of this patient group as follows: (a) "Some degree of depression, anxiety and/or anger; (b) disruption in everyday life patterns, including marital and/or sexual relationships, and (c) considerable fear regarding the danger and mutilation of cancer and mastectomy" (p. 114).

Other cancer patient groups have been studied from a psychosocial viewpoint, although not nearly as extensively. Gordon et al. (1980) followed 308 breast, lung, and melanoma patients through the first 6 months of their disease. The most often noted problems at the time of initial hospitalization were in the area of worry about the disease itself. Negative affect became the predominant concern in the period following discharge. A broader array of problems such as physical discomfort, concern about medical treatment, dissatisfaction with health care service, lack of mobility, financial concerns, family and social problems, worry about the disease, negative affect, and body image difficulties was noted at 3 and 6 months postdischarge. Worden and Weisman (1977) found that site of cancer was a significant factor in adjustment. Peak distress periods occurred at different times during the first 3 months of illness for different site groups (lung, breast, colon, melanoma, Hodgkin's disease).

Liang, Dunn, Gorman, and Stuart-Harris (1990) asked 188 cancer patients (129 female, 59 male) with various solid tumors to rank areas of need. The patients ranked the areas of "worry" in the following order: dealing with family issues, coping with emotional stress, getting information, solving money problems, dealing with work issues, having a social life, sustaining a sex life, and dealing with hospital staff. Patients with head and neck or breast cancer reported the most distress, and female patients reported more distress than did male patients.

In another study, Dunkel-Schetter, Feinstein, Taylor, and Falke (1992) found that among 603 cancer patients, fear or uncertainty about the future was the number one concern (41%), followed by limited physical ability (24%) and pain (12%). This study also assessed how patients coped with cancer, and it identified five coping patterns: seeking and using social support, focusing on the positive, distancing, cognitive escape–avoidance, and behavioral escape–avoidance. One interesting finding was that specific concerns about cancer (i.e., fear, limited physical ability, and pain) were not associated with how patients coped. However, perceptions about the stressfulness of the situation were significantly associated with more coping through use of social support and cognitive and behavioral escape–avoidance.

Types of Interventions

Differing kinds of interventions have been used to help cancer patients and those with other catastrophic diseases deal with their psychosocial needs (Bloom, Ross, & Burnell, 1978). Many of these interventions are designed to help the person feel less helpless and hopeless, to take more responsibility for getting well or for complying with medical regimens. Holland (1982) described the goals of these interventions as follows: to decrease feelings of alienation by talking to others in a similar situation; reduce anxiety about the treatments; assist in clarifying misperception and misinformation; and lessen feelings of isolation, helplessness, and being neglected by others. The most common forms of psychosocial intervention for patients with cancer are education; behavioral training; and problem-solving and supportive therapy in both individual and group settings.

Education

Educational interventions vary in the amount of psychosocial information or coping instruction and behavioral training they provide, but their emphasis is generally on educating patients about their disease and its treatment. Brandberg et al. (1994) investigated the effects of an information program with 231 malignant melanoma patients. All patients were asked to indicate whether they were interested in participating in the information program or not. Interested patients were randomized to receive the program before the first visit (experimental group) or to receive no additional information before the first visit (control group). Those patients in the experimental group attended a single 1 ½-hour group meeting in which information was provided concerning melanoma, risk factors, prevention, and procedures at the medical examination. They also received a brochure on melanoma and skin cancer. Results indicate that patients in the information group were significantly more satisfied with information and had a higher level of knowledge regarding their disease compared with the control group at 3 months postbaseline.

Richardson, Shelton, Krailo, and Levine (1990) randomly assigned newly diagnosed hematology patients to either a control group or one of three educational intervention groups. Using regression analysis, they concluded that low severity of disease, assignment to any one of three educational programs, plus high allopurinol compliance were predictive of increased survival in patients with newly diagnosed hematological malignancy. Compliance was strongly associated with participation in any one of the education groups. However, Pruitt et al. (1992) did not report survival effects of intervention in a randomized trial with radiation therapy patients with mixed diagnoses. Some participated in a three-session intervention, and others were in a standard control group. The education consisted of information about radiation therapy and cancer, coping strategies, and communication skills. Knowledge levels were unchanged in both groups, and depression was the only measure of affective state found to improve. Ali and Khalil (1989) also found mood effects when they assessed the impact of a psychoeducational intervention program on reducing anxiety among a group of patients with bladder cancer. Compared with the control group, the experimental group showed significantly less anxiety 3 days after surgery and just before hospital discharge.

Gordon et al. (1980) examined the effects of a program of education combined with counseling on 157 patients with different types of cancer. Evaluations were conducted 3 and 6 months after hospital discharge. When compared with 151 patients in two control groups, patients who took part in the program were less depressed and anxious and were quicker to return to activities of daily living and activities outside the home; education alone did not show the same benefits. Education is an important component in any program designed to assist cancer patients, and representative studies have shown improvement in knowledge levels and treatment compliance. However, small and short-term improvements were seen in affective states. As early as 1970, Zimbardo and Ebbeson concluded that, in general, educational interventions are often insufficient for changing attitudes and improving coping.

Behavioral Training

Behavioral training includes hypnosis, guided imagery or visualization, relaxation training, and biofeedback that is often combined with problem-solving and coping instruction in what have been called *psychoeducational approaches* (see also Helgeson, Cohen, Schulz, and Yasko, this volume, chapter 14).

The behavioral training program for patients with cancer used by Baider, Uziely, and De-Nour (1994) was designed to increase self-control and improve quality of life. The treatment was conducted with 86 patients in groups of 8 to 10. Patients met weekly for 6 weeks, 90 minutes per session, and the treatment consisted of progressive muscle relaxation and guided imagery. Psychological distress and ability to cope with cancer were measured with three self-reports: the Multidimensional Health Locus of Control (Wallston, Strudler-Wallston, & DeVellis, 1978), the Impact of Event Scale (Horowitz, Wilner, & Alvarez, 1979), and the Brief Symptom Inventory (Derogatis, 1975). Assessments were made prior to therapy; before the final therapy session; and at 2, 4, and 6 months after therapy. Patients reported a substantial and statistically significant improvement following treatment. Their psychological distress lessened, as did their avoidance of the disease and its intrusiveness. The feeling that their health depended on outside factors also decreased.

Gruber et al. (1993) randomly assigned breast cancer patients to either an immediate treatment group that received relaxation, guided imagery, and biofeedback training or to a delayed treatment control group. Pre- and posttreatment measures included blood samples, psychological testing, and a computerized psychophysiological stress evaluation. Results showed that the only psychological difference was in anxiety levels, which were reduced shortly after each group began the intervention. Immune system parameters were significantly improved and directly correlated with the behavioral interventions.

Decker, Cline-Elsen, and Gallagher (1992) studied the impact of stress reduction by relaxation training and imagery in 63 outpatients who were undergoing radiotherapy. Patients were randomly assigned to a relaxation training condition ($n = 34$) as an adjunct to radiation or to a control condition ($n = 29$), which involved education and counseling along with radiation therapy. The experimental group was trained in progressive muscle relaxation, deep breathing, pairing the relaxed state with a self-induced cue word ("calm"), and coping with tension by self-administration of the cue-controlled relaxation response. Comparing scores on the Profile of Mood States (POMS; McNair, Lorr, & Droppleman, 1971), which was administered before and after the intervention, the researchers noted statistically significant reductions in the treatment group in tension, depression, anger, and fatigue. The results suggest that relaxation training substantially improves several psychological parameters associated with quality of life in patients who are undergoing radiation therapy for cancer.

Bridge, Benson, Pietroni, and Priest (1988) conducted a randomized study to determine whether relaxation and imagery training could decrease the level of distress in early stage (Stages I and II) breast cancer patients. The intervention program lasted 6 weeks, and patients were divided into three groups: (a) a control group in which patients were encouraged to talk about themselves, (b) a relaxation group in which patients were taught muscle relaxation techniques, and (c) a relaxation and imagery group in which patients were taught both muscle relaxation and guided imagery. In addition, both the second and third groups were given cassette tapes repeating the intervention instructions and told to practice once a day. At the end of the 6 weeks, there was significantly lower total mood disturbance in the intervention groups (with the relaxation and imagery group reporting less disturbance than the relaxation-only group) than in the control group.

Relaxation training and hypnosis have also been described as effective in reducing nausea, emotional distress, and physiological arousal following chemotherapy (Burish & Lyles, 1981; Burish, Snyder, & Jenkins, 1991). In addition, Arathuzik (1994) conducted a pilot study to examine the effects of a combination of behavioral and cognitive interventions on pain perception, mood, and pain control in metastatic breast cancer patients. A pretest–posttest experimental research design was used. Twenty-four patients were randomly assigned to a control group; a treatment group receiving relaxation and visual training; or a treatment group receiving relaxation, visualization, and cognitive coping skills training. Measures of the patients' pain intensity, pain distress, pain control, ability to decrease pain, and mood were taken before and after treatment. Scores for the ability to decrease pain scales were significantly greater for each of the treatment groups following both interventions. Of interest is that patients reported that they preferred the relaxation intervention to either the visualization or coping skills treatments.

As with education, behavioral training has shown some positive benefits in improving affective state and symptom control.

Problem-Solving and Supportive Therapy

There is definite evidence supporting the value of one-on-one supportive counseling for patients with cancer as well as for their spouses. In an investigation by Blanchard, Toseland, and McCallion (1996), 66 spouses of patients with cancer were randomly assigned either to a coping with cancer (CWC) intervention program ($n = 30$) or to usual services ($n = 36$). Spouses in the CWC group attended six 1-hour individual counseling sessions during which a short-term problem-solving model was used. The model was designed to increase spousal coping in the caregiving role. Spouses and patients were assessed for perceived health status, psychological well-being, social support, and coping behavior at baseline, 2 weeks postintervention, and 6 months postbaseline. Results indicate that patients whose spouses participated in the CWC program became significantly less depressed over the 6-month follow-up period than patients whose spouses did not. No other group differences were significant.

N. W. Fawzy (1996) investigated the efficacy of a psychoeducational nursing intervention to enhance coping and affective state in newly diagnosed malignant melanoma patients. The intervention consisted of 3 hours of individualized teaching and emotional support by an oncology nurse and included health education, stress management, and coping skills training. At the 3-month follow-up, patients in the intervention group demonstrated less psychological distress and decreases in Brief Symptom Inventory somatization, and they were using fewer ineffective passive resignation coping strategies than the control group.

In 1994, Moorey and colleagues completed a 1-year follow-up of patients with cancer who had received individual adjuvant psychological therapy (i.e., a brief cognitive–behavioral treatment). One year after completing treatment, the experimental patients exhibited less anxiety and depression than controls.

Linn, Linn, and Harris (1982) randomly assigned 120 men with end-stage cancer (various primary sites) to an intervention condition (ongoing, client-centered supportive therapy) or to a control condition (evaluation only). Patients were assessed before assignment to treatment and at 1, 3, 6, and 12 months. Measures included quality-of-life variables (depression, alienation, life satisfaction, and self-esteem), functional status, and survival time. Functional status and survival did not differ between groups, but patients receiving counseling showed significantly better quality-of-life scores at 3 months. Among those who survived, these differences held up through the 1-year follow-up. These findings are important because quality-of-life issues are key concerns for terminal patients.

The popularity of support groups has grown immensely in the past decade, and there is evidence to suggest that such groups are associated with better psychosocial adjustment to illness (Bloom, 1982; Cunningham & Tocco, 1989; F. I. Fawzy, Cousins, et al., 1990; F. I. Fawzy et al., 1993; F. I. Fawzy, Wellisch, & Yager, 1977; Gordon et al., 1980; Spiegel & Bloom, 1983; Spiegel, Bloom, & Yalom, 1981).

Researchers (Bottomley, Hunton, Roberts, Jones, & Bradley, 1996) evaluated the efficacy of group cognitive–behavioral therapy for psychologically distressed cancer patients versus a social support group and a standard-care nonintervention group. Thirty-one of 107 patients newly diagnosed with cancer were screened and identified as distressed; 9 of these were consecutively allocated to a cognitive–behavioral group, 8 to a social support group, and 14 to a standard-care nonintervention group. The two intervention groups lasted 8 weeks. The principal focus of the cancer-specific cognitive–behavioral group was on identifying negative, automatic thoughts and challenging those processes to induce a greater ability to cope with and reduce levels of psychological distress. The social support group had no specific psychotherapeutic intervention strategy except to allow honest and open expression of ideas. The therapist's role was to keep discussions focused or to assist and guide group members when needed. Patients were assessed at baseline, at the end of the intervention, and at 3-month follow-up using the Hospital Anxiety and Depression Scale (Zigmond & Snaith, 1979), the Mental Adjustment to Cancer scale (Watson et al., 1988), and the Bottomley Cancer Social Support Scale (Bottomley, 1995). Immediately following the intervention, those in the cognitive–behavioral group demonstrated significant differences in anxiety and fighting spirit, suggesting that these patients increased their use of coping skills to reduce their anxiety. No significant changes were found in the social support and nonintervention groups on any of the measures, although there was a trend for poorer psychological functioning on several scales for the nonintervention group.

In a preliminary study by Hosaka (1996), 20 Japanese breast cancer patients participated in a five-session intervention designed to decrease emotional distress and increase coping ability. The intervention included psychoeducation, problem-solving, psychological support, relaxation training, and guided imagery. Ten of the patients received the intervention individually, and the other 10 were treated in a group therapy setting. In order to investigate the short-term efficacy of the intervention, the patients were assessed at baseline and immediately following the intervention using the POMS and the Dealing with Illness Inventory (Namir, Wolcott, Fawzy, & Alumbaugh, 1987). A comparison of pre- and postintervention scores revealed a decrease in all categories of negative emotions in both the individual and group intervention cohorts. In particular, depression, fatigue, and total mood disturbance were significantly lowered. The intervention was less effective in changing the coping styles of these Japanese women; however, there was a positive tendency for active behavioral coping styles to increase and avoidance coping to decrease.

Cunningham, Edmonds, Jenkins, and Lockwood (1995) compared two different formats of a brief, group psychoeducational program for cancer patients. Patients were randomly assigned to either a standard (6 weekly 2-hour sessions) intervention or a "weekend intensive" intervention group. At 19 weeks following the intervention, effects on mood and quality of life were comparable in patients in both conditions. Quality-of-life improvement appeared to be somewhat greater for the standard 6-week intervention group.

Berglund, Bolund, Gustafsson, and Sjoden (1994) established a prospective randomized study with cancer patients who took part in a 7-week rehabilitation program. The intervention focused on "Starting Again" and consisted of physical training, coping skills, and information. Compared with patients in the control group, patients in the experimental condition improved significantly in physical training, physical strength, fighting spirit, body image, sufficient information, and decreased sleeping problems. All three goals of the intervention were met, and results indicated that the Starting Again program has many beneficial effects for cancer patients.

Cocker, Bell, and Kidman (1994) instigated a pilot project in preparation for a formal study on the effects of cognitive–behavioral therapy on emotional well-being and survival time with advanced breast cancer patients. Six patients were enrolled into a 12-week group cognitive–behavioral therapy program, which consisted of cognitive restructuring, relaxation and visualization, assertion training and communication including role-playing, self-instructional coping methods, and patient education; the study included a control group. Patients were assessed at baseline, at the end of the intervention, and at a 3-month follow-up using the Beck Depression Inventory (Beck, Rush, Shaw, & Emery, 1979), Beck Anxiety Inventory (Beck, Epstein, Brown, & Steer, 1988), Novaco Anger Inventory (Novaco, 1975), Spielberger State–Trait Anger Expression Inventory (Spielberger, 1991), and the Coopersmith Self-Esteem Inventory (Coopersmith, 1981). The results of this pilot study indicated that depression and anger management scores were improved by the program. Data regarding the effect of cognitive–behavior therapy on length of survival are included in the formal study.

Cella and associates (Cella, Sarafian, Snider, Yellen, & Winicour, 1993) detailed an 8-week support group for cancer patients in a local community. There was no random selection or a control group in this study. As expected, self-reported quality of life improved significantly by the final session, compared with reports completed at the start of the intervention. Community and peer support was noted by participants as the most helpful aspect of the program, and the group evaluations showed high satisfaction levels in all areas.

A prospective randomized study by Greer et al. (1992) found that adjuvant psychological therapy improved psychological distress among 174 cancer patients. The authors looked at anxiety, depression, and adjustment in patients with primary diagnosis or first recurrence of cancer. Compared with the control patients, the experimental patients scored significantly higher in fighting spirit and significantly lower in anxiety, anxious preoccupation, helplessness, and fatalism. Some of the effects were still observable at 4-months follow-up.

Another randomized study examined the effects of an early intervention program (immediately following diagnosis) versus later intervention (4-month delay) in newly diagnosed cancer patients and followed these patients for a 12-month period (Edgar, Rosberger, & Nowlis, 1992). The intervention consisted of five 1-hour sessions with a nurse in which problem-solving techniques, goal setting, cognitive reappraisal, relaxation training, and effective use of resources were taught. The intervention program, which was developed from a review of the literature and the authors' own clinical experiences, sought to decrease distress in cancer patients by increasing knowledge, enhancing personal control, strengthening coping skills, and reducing emotional arousal. No significant differences were found between the early intervention or the later intervention until the 8-month follow-up. The later intervention group ($n = 102$) scored significantly lower in depression, anxiety, and worry and felt more in control than the early intervention group ($n = 103$). At the 12-month follow-up, the later intervention group continued to worry less than the early intervention group.

Bos-Branolte, Zielstra, Rijshouwer, and Duivenvoorden (1988) evaluated the effects of psychotherapy in patients who were presumed to be cured of gynecological cancers. Eighty-three patients were offered psychotherapy; 26 accepted, 5 choosing individual and 21 group psychotherapy. The remaining nonacceptors were used for comparison. All patients were evaluated at baseline and at 6 and 9 months after initial assessment using the Basic Oncology Scale (BOS; Bos-Branolte et al., 1998), which measures anxiety, depression, body image, self-esteem, partner and proximity relation, and general feeling of well-being. Individual psychotherapy involved 45-minute weekly sessions, and themes surrounded the six areas assessed by the BOS. The number of individual sessions with each patient was not fixed and ranged from 4 to 22. Group psychotherapy consisted of eight 90-minute sessions spaced over the course of 10 weeks and was designed to generate favorable changes in patient quality of life. Also focusing on the six themes of the BOS, the group intervention included progressive muscle relaxation, role-playing, and learning by imitation. Results indicate that improvement of severe and moderate problems after 9 months across all six BOS variables was significantly higher in patients who participated in psychotherapy. In addition, patients in individual psychotherapy improved more than those in group therapy; however, the number of patients in individual treatment was too small to permit definitive conclusions in comparing the two groups.

Spiegel et al. (1981) reported improved mood, increased coping, and less fear in breast cancer patients who participated in group therapy once a week for a year, when compared with randomly selected control patients. The weekly discussion sessions focused on practical coping problems associated with terminal illness; feelings and attitudes toward death; and interpersonal relationships with family, friends, and physicians. In a 10-year follow-up, the authors found that patients in the experimental group had increased survival time (36.6 months) as compared with that of the patients in the control group (18.9 months).

Structured Psychoeducational Intervention Model

In reviewing the literature, it became clear that many of the above-mentioned therapeutic modalities had some positive benefits. However, the variance accounted for by each of these alone was not large. Therefore, portions of those interventions that were found to be effective and appropriate were selected and combined. This comprehensive intervention was first used in a group of 50 gay men with AIDS within 3 months of diagnosis (F. I. Fawzy, Namir, & Wolcott, 1989).

Experimental Design and Model Components

The intervention model was used for a group of newly diagnosed malignant melanoma patients (F. I. Fawzy, Cousins, et al., 1990; F. I. Fawzy, Kemeny, et al., 1990). Patients were randomly assigned to either a control group receiving routine medical care or to an experimental group receiving the same kind of routine medical care plus a 6-week structured psychoeducational group intervention. Groups of 7 to 10 patients met for 1½ hours weekly for 6 weeks. Outcome measures included both short- and long-term psychological and immunological parameters.

This comprehensive intervention consisted of four components: health education, stress management techniques, enhancement of coping skills (problem-solving techniques), and supportive group psychotherapy.

Health Education

The health education component of the intervention contained easily understood health care information specific to the diagnosis of skin cancer. Melanoma patients were taught about their disease, including information on risk factors that appear to be influencing the dramatic increase in skin cancer (e.g., ultraviolet radiation, skin pigmentation, genetic factors, hormonal factors, and immunological factors). They were informed about preventive measures to avoid future sun exposure by reducing ultraviolet radiation exposure (e.g., wearing protective clothing, using sunscreens). Finally, patients were presented with melanoma warning signs and the terms and definitions of malignant melanoma, and they were given booklets from the American Cancer Society and the National Cancer Institute on nutrition and the immune system.

Stress Management

The stress management component was divided into two sections: stress awareness and management techniques. Awareness had two subcategories: (a) identifying sources of stress; and (b) identifying personal reactions to stress, including physiological, psychological, and behavioral reactions. Worksheets covering signs and symptoms of stress as well as sources of stress were included in the intervention manual. The second component of stress awareness was the actual management of stress. This had four subcomponents: eliminating or modifying sources of stress through problem-solving, changing the attitude or perception toward the stressors by trying to look at the situations in a "new light," and changing the physical reaction to the stressors through relaxation response. Patients were taught simple relaxation exercises (e.g., progressive muscle relaxation followed by guided imagery of a pleasant scene) that took approximately 15–20 minutes to perform. Patients were encouraged to use these techniques on a daily basis (to help them relax, to learn what a state of relaxation feels like, and to learn how to achieve it) and to use them to help them fall asleep at night or to return to sleep if they should wake up during the night. In addition, patients were taught how to use an abbreviated form of this exercise when they found themselves in acutely stressful situations.

Coping Skills (Problem-Solving Techniques)

An important aim of the coping skills component is to increase the patient's awareness of what Weisman (1979a) termed the *key ingredients of good coping*: (a) optimism (the expectation of positive change); (b) practicality (learning that options and alternatives are seldom completely exhausted); (c) flexibility (changing strategies to reflect the changing nature of perceived problems); and (d) resourcefulness (developing the ability to call upon additional information and support to strengthen coping).

In the coping skills component of the intervention, patients were first taught the five steps of problem-solving: relaxing, identifying the problem, brainstorming for possible solutions, selecting and implementing a possible solution, and evaluating.

Patients were then introduced to the concept of coping methods that are commonly used by patients to deal with their cancer (Lazarus & Folkman, 1984). Three general theoretical methods of coping have been identified and are listed below; the first two are helpful, but the third is usually detrimental:

1. *Active behavioral methods.* One tries to improve some aspect of the illness by active means such as exercise, use of relaxation techniques, and frequent collaborative consultations with the physician.

2. *Active cognitive methods.* One tries to understand the illness and accepts its effect on life by focusing on positive rather than negative changes that have occurred since the onset of illness. In general, patients who use active behavioral and active cognitive coping methods report more positive affective states, higher levels of self-esteem, and fewer physical symptoms than patients who do not use these methods.

3. *Avoidance methods.* One avoids being with others, hides feelings about the illness, and refuses to think about the illness. Patients who use more

avoidance coping usually have higher levels of psychological distress such as anxiety, indirectly expressed anger, depression, and lower quality of life than patients who do not use these methods.

The final part of the coping skills component involves integrating the stress management and problem-solving techniques with the information on coping methods and strategies and applying these to specific situations. The method used was modeled after Project Omega (Sobel & Worden, 1982; Weisman, Worden, & Sobel, 1980), which teaches positive coping strategies as a way of diminishing stress and enhancing coping. It included learning an approach to problem-solving, practicing the approach theoretically, and applying the approach to personal problems through a series of pictures. The researchers at Project Omega developed and evaluated problem-solving interventions for cancer patients. They found that highly distressed patients used fewer and less effective coping strategies, had more problems and concerns, and achieved poor resolutions when attempting to solve critical illness-related concerns (Sobel & Worden, 1982; Weisman et al., 1980). The authors compared two interventions, one involving clarification, emotional expression, and individual problem identification and the other consisting of a cognitive skills training intervention. The results showed that compared with the control group condition, both interventions were effective in reducing emotional distress during a 6-month follow-up period.

A new series of pictures illustrating 10 common problems or situations encountered by patients with malignant melanoma were developed (F. I. Fawzy, Cousins, et al., 1990). The first of these situations deals with worries and concerns in the prediagnosis period. Next comes accepting the diagnosis and informing family and friends. Doctor–patient relationships are then explored, followed by issues involving treatment such as fear, feelings of isolation, overwhelming technological environments, body image changes, and depression. Communication issues with significant others and with extended groups such as friends and co-workers are covered. Finally, returning to "normal" by reentering everyday life and planning for the future by resuming a forward "life trajectory" are reviewed. Each situation is represented by two different pictures. The first picture generally shows the patient coping ineffectively, and the second picture depicts more effective coping behavior. The first picture was introduced and the patients were asked to identify the negative coping methods. Further discussion was encouraged to clarify why such coping is ineffective and to generate more positive options. The second picture of the patient coping more effectively was then introduced. Effective coping techniques identified by the group discussion were validated and reinforced. Any effective techniques not thought of by the group members were presented and explained by the group leader. The patients were then encouraged to apply these theoretical pictured situations to their own real-life situations. Patients were given a manual containing the coping scenarios and written descriptions of the situations and the coping techniques involved. They were given these manuals to keep so that they could review the scenarios as needed and to share them with significant others who may not have attended the meetings.

Supportive Group Psychotherapy

Psychological support from the staff was inherent throughout the intervention and was initiated with a series of talks on engendering hope and determination and mobilizing coping resources. There was also a great deal of within-group support provided by the patients themselves.

The advantages of this program are that the patients are taught to collaborate with the health team and to cope actively with increased responsibility for their own health care program. If the intervention is successful, another advantage would be that the patients take with them valuable skills that will enable them to deal more effectively with future problems.

Results

The first objective was to assess the impact of such an intervention on affective state. Affective state was measured using the POMS. This instrument measures affective state and distress and is divided into six factors: tension–anxiety, depression–dejection, anger–hostility, vigor–activity, fatigue–inertia, and confusion–bewilderment. A total mood disturbance score (TMD) is then obtained by summing the scores of the six factors.

All the patients in the melanoma study reported moderate to high levels of psychological distress at baseline comparable to other cancer patients. However, at the end of the 6-week structured group intervention, the patients in the experimental condition started showing some reduction in psychological distress as compared with the control patients. Six months following the intervention, the group differences were even more pronounced. The experimental group reported significantly lower levels of confusion, depression, fatigue, and total mood disturbance, and higher levels of vigor (Table 13.1). Participation in the group intervention appeared to reduce the psychological turmoil associated with cancer diagnosis. This reduction in distress was maintained throughout the follow-up period. Five years following the intervention, experimental patients still showed significantly lower levels of anxiety, depression, and total mood disturbance (Table 13.2).

Our second objective was to assess the impact of such an intervention on coping and adjustment. People use a variety of coping methods to deal with serious medical conditions, including cancer. Three general theoretical methods of coping have been identified: active behavioral coping, active cognitive coping, and avoidance. We used the Dealing with Illness Inventory (Namir et al., 1987), which is a modified version of an instrument developed by Lazarus and Folkman (1984) to measure coping.

Immediately following the 6-week structured intervention, the intervention group used active behavioral coping methods significantly more often than did the

TABLE 13.1

Mean POMS scores comparing control (n = 28) and experimental (n = 38) groups at baseline, Week 6, and Month 6

POMS	BASELINE			WEEK 6			MONTH 6		
	CONTROL GROUP	EXPERIMENTAL GROUP	p	CONTROL GROUP	EXPERIMENTAL GROUP	p	CONTROL GROUP	EXPERIMENTAL GROUP	p
Anxiety	7.25	11.11	.029*	7.98	6.15	.168	8.30	6.04	.074
Depression	4.79	10.13	.024**	5.99	4.64	.372	7.44	3.76	.017*
Anger	5.21	9.66	.015*	5.22	6.24	.555	6.67	4.92	.274
Lack of vigor	15.18	15.21	.986	14.29	11.05	.026*	14.33	10.39	.001**
Fatigue	7.07	9.38	.166	6.61	4.31	.060	7.77	4.88	.022*
Confusion	4.96	7.00	.069	5.24	4.34	.298	5.69	3.76	.013**
Total	44.46	62.48	.053*	45.77	36.40	.128	50.30	33.67	.006**

Note. Data are analyses of covariance for adjusted treatment means. POMS = Profile of Mood States.
*p < .05. **p < .01.

TABLE 13.2

Mean POMS scores comparing control (n = 28) and experimental (n = 38) groups at Year 1, Year 3, and Year 5

	YEAR 1			YEAR 3			YEAR 5		
POMS	CONTROL GROUP	EXPERIMENTAL GROUP	p	CONTROL GROUP	EXPERIMENTAL GROUP	p	CONTROL GROUP	EXPERIMENTAL GROUP	p
Anxiety	7.13	5.41	.154	8.68	3.50	.001**	8.81	4.81	.023*
Depression	5.08	3.70	.344	6.13	2.81	.091	8.57	3.09	.015*
Total	3.02	32.56	.071	48.78	23.49	.001**	51.73	29.53	.01**

Note. POMS = Profile of Mood States.
*p < .05. **p < .01.

249

control group. Six months after the intervention was completed, the intervention group continued to use significantly more active behavioral coping and was also using more active cognitive coping methods than was the control group (Table 13.3). At the 5-year follow-up, the intervention group continued to show a significantly higher level of active behavioral and active cognitive coping (Table 13.4).

Our third objective was to assess the impact of this intervention on certain aspects of the immune system. Several of the specific lymphocyte subsets assessed are shown in Table 13.5. In addition, we also examined a functional assay, interferon-alpha augmented natural killer (NK) cell cytotoxicity.

At the end of the 6-week intervention, there was a significant increase in the percentage of large granular lymphocytes (LGLs; defined as CD57 with Leu7; Table 13.6). Six months following the intervention, there continued to be an increase in the percentage of LGLs as well as increases in NK cells (defined as CD16 with Leu11 and CD56 with Leu19) and interferon alpha augmented NK cell cytotoxicity (Table 13.6). After 1 year no statistically significant immune differences were found between the two groups.

Our fourth objective was to assess the effects of this intervention on recurrence and survival 6 years later. The survival and recurrence distributions for each group were estimated using the Kaplan–Meier method and tested for equality by the log-rank test (Lawless, 1981; SAS Institute Inc., 1991). The Cox proportion hazards regression model (Lawless, 1981) was used to quantify the relationship between treatment and the outcomes adjusted by multiple covariates (age, sex, Breslow Depth, tumor site, baseline POMS TMD, baseline active behavioral coping, baseline natural killer cell activity [NKCA], and group intervention). The stepwise procedure was used for covariate selection. In the third part of the analysis, the Cox model was used to identify the role of baseline values as well as the changes over time and the result of the psychiatric intervention in survival and recurrence.

In the control group, 10 of the original 34 patients with Stage I disease died, and 3 others had local recurrences. In the experimental group, only 3 of the original 34 died; 4 had local recurrences. A log-rank test showed the number of deaths was significantly less in the experimental group ($p = .03$). A trend was also apparent for the number of recurrences ($p = .09$; Table 13.7).

The relationship between treatment and outcomes using a single covariate was examined. Four factors identified as significant for recurrence and survival are age, sex, initial Breslow depth, and site of the original tumor (Lee, 1989). Specifically, being older, being male, having a Breslow depth of greater than 1.5 mm, and having the initial melanoma lesion on the trunk of the body all indicate poorer prognosis. These four factors were used as single covariates in the Cox regression model. Age was not a significant factor in outcome; neither was the site of the original tumor. However, sex (i.e., being male) was significant for both greater recurrence ($p = .01$) and poorer survival ($p = .01$). The initial Breslow depth was also significant

TABLE 13.3

Mean coping scores comparing control (n = 28) and experimental (n = 38) groups at baseline, Week 6, and Month 6

METHOD	BASELINE			WEEK 6			MONTH 6		
	CONTROL GROUP	EXPERIMENTAL GROUP	p	CONTROL GROUP	EXPERIMENTAL GROUP	p	CONTROL GROUP	EXPERIMENTAL GROUP	p
Active behavioral	52.00	56.42	.08	52.13	60.50	.0001**	49.59	59.88	.0001**
Active cognitive	49.96	52.84	.116	49.11	52.02	.063	49.18	52.19	.03*

Note. Data are analyses of covariance for adjusted treatment means.
$*p < .05$. $**p < .01$.

TABLE 13.4

Mean coping scores comparing control (n = 28) and experimental (n = 38) groups at Year 1, Year 3, and Year 5

METHOD	YEAR 1			YEAR 3			YEAR 5		
	CONTROL GROUP	EXPERIMENTAL GROUP	p	CONTROL GROUP	EXPERIMENTAL GROUP	p	CONTROL GROUP	EXPERIMENTAL GROUP	p
Active behavioral	51.97	59.02	.003**	53.32	65.23	.0001**	50.85	66.04	.0001**
Active cognitive	48.75	51.94	.072	50.01	53.71	.03*	49.86	59.93	.05*

$*p < .05$. $**p < .01$.

TABLE 13.5

Lymphocyte subsets assessed

CD DESIGNATION (MONOCLONAL ANTIBODY)	LYMPHOCYTE SUBSET	MAJOR FUNCTION
CD16 (Leu11)	Fc-receptor-bearing cell including most NK cells	Nonspecific killing of viral-infected cells
CD56 (Leu19)	Population including NK cells	Nonspecific killing of viral-infected cells
CD57 (Leu7)	Large granular lymphocytes	Includes cells capable of both specific and nonspecific killing

Note. NK = natural killer.

for recurrence ($p = .001$) and survival ($p = .001$). The greater the Breslow depth, the poorer the prognosis (Table 13.8).

The relationship between treatment and outcomes using multiple covariates was also studied. Using all of the covariates identified as potentially pertinent in the Cox model and using stepwise regression with inclusion of treatment (group intervention), we found that only Breslow depth and treatment were significant for recurrence and survival (Table 13.9). Adjusting for Breslow depth, we found that treatment was still significant.

A parametric model was devised and applied to the data. Once again the results indicate that Breslow depth and treatment were significant for both recurrence and survival (Table 13.10).

Finally, the relationship of baseline scores and change over 6 months for Breslow depth, POMS, Coping, and NKCA to recurrence and survival were studied (Table 13.11). The result shows the effect of baseline values for Breslow depth, affective state (POMS TMD), coping (active behavioral), and NKCA on recurrence and survival. It also shows the effects of changes in POMS TMD, active behavioral coping, and NKCA over time on outcome. It is clear that greater Breslow depth continues to be a significant factor for higher rates of both recurrence and death. Higher baseline distress (POMS TMD) scores and higher baseline coping scores (active behavioral) are related to a lower rate of recurrence and death. Higher NKCA at baseline is also related to lower recurrence rates but not to survival. Neither changes in POMS TMD nor NKCA over the 6 months showed any relationship to the outcomes, but an increase in active behavioral coping scores was significantly related to better survival ($p = .03$), and a trend was apparent for recurrence ($p = .06$).

TABLE 13.6

Mean immune variables comparing control and intervention groups at Week 6, Month 6, and Year 1

IMMUNE VARIABLE	WEEK 6					MONTH 6					YEAR 1				
	CONTROL GROUP		INTERVENTION GROUP			CONTROL GROUP		INTERVENTION GROUP			CONTROL GROUP		INTERVENTION GROUP		
	M	N	M	N	P	M	N	M	N	P	M	N	M	N	P
CD16 (Leu11)	10.7	26	10.7	35	.955	10.0	26	13.0	35	.022*	10.5	26	12.0	34	.231
CD56 (Leu19)	12.8	21	13.1	24	.787	9.9	21	14.7	24	.005**	11.2	21	12.4	24	.456
CD57 (Leu7)	10.7	26	12.7	35	.025*	11.5	26	13.8	35	.038*	N/A	N/A	N/A	N/A	N/A
Augmented NK	42.4	17	45.7	19	.556	43.4	17	53.1	17	.034*	54.2	18	57.8	18	.541

Note. Data are analyses of covariance for adjusted treatment scores. NK = natural killer; NA = data not available.
°The reduced sample size for the functional tests results from elimination of certain assays.
*p < .05. **p < .01.

TABLE 13.7

Recurrence and survival

OUTCOME	CONTROL GROUP	EXPERIMENTAL GROUP	LOG-RANK TEST (P)
Recurrence			.09
Yes	13	7	
No	21	27	
Survival			.03*
Dead	10	3	
Alive	24	31	

*$p < .05$.

Discussion

Presumed Mechanisms

The survival analysis indicates that patients who participated in the structured, 6-week, psychiatric intervention had a statistically significantly ($p = .03$) better survival rate than the control group patients at 5 to 6 years follow-up. Only 3 out of 34 experimental group patients died, whereas 10 of the 34 control group patients died. There was also a definite trend in the same direction for recurrence ($p = .09$). Seven of the 34 experimental group patients and 13 of the 34 control group patients experienced recurrence. Our control sample was compared with a historical sample matched for stage, Breslow depth, gender, and medical treatment. There was no difference in survival between the historical matched sample and the control sample, suggesting that our control group was representative of the norm. Because our control and experimental groups were well-matched groups that had been randomly assigned, these results suggest that the intervention could well have played some role in the differential recurrence and survival outcomes (Fox, 1992).

A number of explanations are possible. These encompass educational benefits including increased compliance, enhanced coping and adjustment, decreased distress, improved social support, and a possible positive impact on the immune system.

The intervention may have fostered improved health habits (through increased knowledge and encouragement), specifically sun protection (i.e., sun avoidance, protective clothing, broad spectrum sun blocks), better nutrition, and exercise regimens. Richardson et al. (1990) found that "the use of special educational and supportive programs designed to improve patient compliance were associated with significant prolongation of patient survival due to, as well as independent of, their effects on compliance" (p. 356).

Patients may have learned to manage their stress better by eliminating or altering their personal stressors through problem-solving, changing their attitudes toward

TABLE 13.8

Cox regression model, single covariate

VARIABLE	n	RECURRENCE			SURVIVAL		
		ESTIMATED β	ESTIMATED SE	P	ESTIMATED β	ESTIMATED SE	P
Age	68	.02	.02	.28	.01	.02	.61
Sex	68	-1.34	.52	.01*	-1.91	.77	.01**
Breslow depth	64	.71	.19	.0001**	.98	.24	.0001**
Site	68			.71			.30
Trunk		.55	.56	.32	1.22	.80	.13
Arm		-.004	.84	.99	.20	1.23	.87
Head and neck		.49	.67	.46	1.20	.91	.19

Note. Estimated β = regression coefficient. Each site listed is compared with the leg site. SE = standard error.
*p < .05. **p < .01.

255

TABLE 13.9

Cox regression model, multiple covariates

VARIABLE	RECURRENCE			SURVIVAL		
	ESTIMATED β	ESTIMATED SE	p	ESTIMATED β	ESTIMATED SE	p
Breslow depth (n = 64)	.80	.20	.0001**	1.24	.28	.0001**
Treatment (group intervention)	−.98	.48	.0438*	−1.93	.71	.0066**

Note. Estimated β = regression coefficient; SE = standard error.
*p < .05. **p < .01.

TABLE 13.10

Weibull regression model

VARIABLE	RECURRENCE			SURVIVAL		
	ESTIMATED β	ESTIMATED SE	p	ESTIMATED β	ESTIMATED SE	p
Treatment (group intervention)	.69	.34	.04*	.79	.29	.0064**
Breslow depth	−.57	.16	.0003**	−.49	.13	.0002**
Intercept	5.42	.37	.0001**	5.30	.33	.0001**
Scale	.68	.14		.38	.09	

Note. Data are multiple covariates (parametric). Estimated β = regression coefficient; SE = standard error.
*p < .05. **p < .01.

TABLE 13.11

Cox/stepwise regression model

VARIABLE	RECURRENCE			SURVIVAL		
	ESTIMATED β	ESTIMATED SE	p	ESTIMATED β	ESTIMATED SE	p
Breslow depth	1.12	.30	.0002**	3.13	1.04	.0025**
POMS TMD (baseline)	-.03	.02	.0519*	-.08	.04	.0521*
Coping (baseline)	-.06	.03	.0398**	-.19	.08	.0193*
NKCA (baseline)	-.18	.09	.0434**	.06	.12	.5882
POMS TMD (change)	-.02	.02	.2512	-.03	.04	.4488
Coping (change)	-.09	.05	.0606	-.28	.13	.0306**
NKCA (change)	.10	.09	.2848	.21	.18	.2401

Note. Data are multiple covariates (n = 54). POM TMD = Profile of Mood States, total mood disturbance; NKCA = natural killer cell activity; estimated β = regression coefficient; SE = standard error.
*p < .05. **p < .01.

minor daily stressors (e.g., perceiving them as less important and therefore less stressful) and altering their physiological response to stress through relaxation techniques. Effective coping may have been enhanced, resulting in such things as improved doctor–patient partnerships, positive mental attitudes, and greater compliance with treatment and follow-up regimens.

Adjustment and coping are factors that directly affect mood. When people feel they can cope with a new event or problem, then affective state is positively affected. Conversely, people feel bad when they believe they are helpless, out of control, or powerless to improve a situation. The group intervention patients had the opportunity to practice their coping skills in the group. Coping is greatly enhanced by sharing concerns with other group members. Patients receive firsthand information on how to deal with the specific problems that each of them is facing. Furthermore, although it may be helpful to receive coping information from an objective health care professional, it is probably much more powerful coming subjectively from a fellow patient and likely to have a more enduring effect. In summary, these patients learned to cope better in the group setting through interaction and practice. This enhancement in coping may then have led to an improvement in affective state. A number of researchers have explored the role of coping and emphasized its importance in relation to health outcomes (Lazarus & Folkman, 1984; Rogentine et al., 1979; Temoshok & Fox, 1984).

Another possible factor may be the emotional support that patients received during the group sessions. They were able to express their feelings freely to an understanding and sympathetic audience. They had the benefit of hearing how others were dealing with stresses of the same disease. By about the third session, total strangers were able to form a cohesive group. Everyone knew everyone else's name, illness stories had been shared, and people were getting to know about each other's families, problems, and concerns. With each group meeting, the feeling of camaraderie increased. Missing members were quickly identified and asked about. Individuals were able to put aside their own issues for a time and reach out to others in the group. Hand holding, hugging, and verbal encouragement were common. This emotional support continued outside the groups. Telephone numbers were exchanged so members could continue to talk with each other. A number of members formed ongoing relationships, meeting for meals and social events. This social support was clearly an important component in decreasing emotional distress. Social support has also been reported by others to be related to health outcomes (Rabkin & Streuning, 1976; Sklar & Anisman, 1981; Soloman & Amkrant, 1981).

Our research also highlighted the importance of looking at individual baseline scores for both mood and coping as well as change over time. This analysis is based on the entire sample. To our surprise we found that baseline distress appeared to be a critical measure of awareness and behavioral motivation, rather than being a negative factor. Survivors averaged a higher score on baseline distress (POMS TMD) than those who died later. Furthermore, premorbid coping behavior of individuals and the effectiveness of coping in dealing with life-threatening situations were also critical factors.

In our study the mean baseline active behavioral coping score for survivors was higher than the mean for patients who died. Those with active behavioral coping ability, whether or not they participated in the intervention, seemed to have the best health outcomes. It was also apparent that positive coping behavior can be learned or enhanced (F. I. Fawzy, Cousins, et al., 1990), and if implemented, can improve health outcomes.

Therefore, knowledge about levels of both affective state and coping at baseline is essential for identifying members of each subgroup and the tailoring of interventions to meet specific needs. For instance, those patients with high levels of distress and low levels of baseline coping were in need of interventions aimed at enhancing their resources and improving their coping behavior. Those with high levels of distress and high levels of coping need interventions aimed at reinforcing the importance of this mobilization. These two groups are likely to be receptive to such interventions as a means of reducing their distress.

On the other hand, those who minimize the importance and threat of cancer to their well-being appear to be at the greatest risk. These individuals present with low levels of baseline distress and coping. They apparently lack the required stimulus for mobilization of their coping resources. This lack of mobilization leaves them woefully unprepared to deal with the myriad of psychological and physical issues associated with the diagnosis and treatment of their cancer.

Interventions for this group need to focus on helping these individuals understand and accept the realistic nature of the threat to their well-being and mobilize their resources. The theme for interventions in this subgroup should be, "Don't minimize, mobilize!" Although this group is at the highest risk, they are not likely to be receptive to any intervention because they do not perceive its necessity.

Changes in the immune system through neuro-endocrine processes may be a primary link between psychological state and the course of cancer. More in-depth reviews of these mechanisms appear elsewhere in this text. However, a few findings are worthy of mention here. For instance, the stress-induced release of the hormone corticotropin-releasing factor (CRF) mediates a reduction of splenic NKCA through activation of the sympathetic nervous system. This reduction in splenic NKCA is independent of CRF-induced activation of the pituitary adrenal axis (Irwin, Hauger, Jones, Provencio, & Britton, 1990; Irwin, Vale, & Rivier, 1990). Clinical studies have also found that chronic activation of sympathetic outflow may suppress immune function during life stress and depression. Specifically, the increased sympathetic nervous system activity and the release of neuropeptide Y appears to be associated with modulation of NKCA (Irwin et al., 1991). Ben-Eliyahu, Yirmiya, Liebeskind, Taylor, and Gale (1991) reported that rats exposed to acute stress showed a substantial decrease in NKCA against a syngeneic mammary tumor in vitro. These same mice showed a twofold increase in surface lung metastases when injected with this tumor. Conversely, a number of other researchers have reported enhancement of immune functions in humans as a result of psychosocial interventions (Gruber, Hall, Hersh, & Dubois, 1988; Kiecolt-Glaser et al., 1985; Kiecolt-Glaser et al., 1986).

Conceptual Model

Over the past two decades, a wealth of information about the needs of cancer patients and ways of meeting those needs has begun to emerge. However, there are still a number of significant gaps in our knowledge base. We propose the following conceptual model (Figure 13.1) as a framework to fill in those gaps and to help in postulating the future priorities for the field of psychooncology.

We believe that the following should be the focus of psychoeducational intervention research with cancer patients:

- Develop a better understanding of the impact of the independent variables (i.e., cancer diagnosis and treatment) on individual patients,
- Identify the specific mediating variables that could contribute to both positive and negative outcomes for cancer patients,
- Clearly define and standardize interventions to allow for study replication and clinical implementation,
- Agree on the important outcome variables for the interventions, and
- Identify or develop valid and reliable measurements for those outcome variables.

Conclusion

The psychological and medical problems encountered by cancer patients are numerous and unique. On the basis of a review of the literature and our clinical and research experience, we believe that cancer patients may benefit from a variety of psychological intervention programs. A structured, psychiatric intervention consisting of health education, stress management–behavioral training, coping including problem-solving techniques, and psychosocial group support offers the greatest potential benefit for patients newly diagnosed or in the early stages of their treatment. Patients are usually distressed, anxious, and unable to effectively use their normal coping styles. A structured intervention offered early on during the course of cancer diagnosis and treatment may be less stigmatizing and more readily accepted by both patients and staff and easily integrated into the comprehensive medical care of cancer patients. The advantages of such a program include easy implementation and replication, promotion of important illness-related problem-solving skills, and increased participation in decision making and active coping.

A short-term, structured, psychoeducational group intervention is the model that the authors propose to be used for newly diagnosed patients and patients with

FIGURE 13.1

Model for psychiatric intervention research in oncology

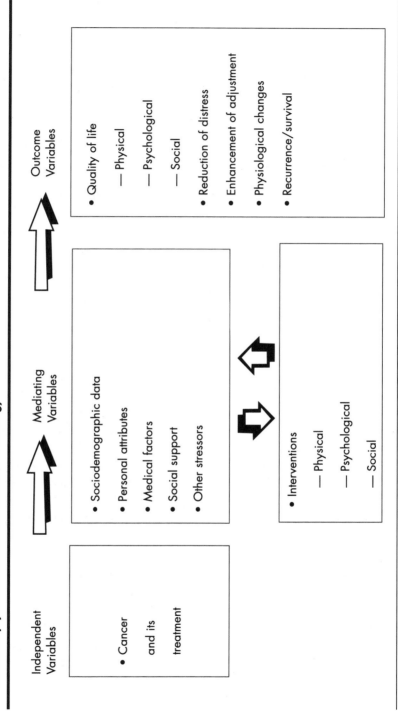

Independent Variables
- Cancer and its treatment

Mediating Variables
- Sociodemographic data
- Personal attributes
- Medical factors
- Social support
- Other stressors

- Interventions
  — Physical
  — Psychological
  — Social

Outcome Variables
- Quality of life
  — Physical
  — Psychological
  — Social
- Reduction of distress
- Enhancement of adjustment
- Physiological changes
- Recurrence/survival

a good prognosis. The focus is on learning how to live with cancer. We also encourage the development of ongoing weekly group support programs for patients with advanced metastatic disease, drawn from Speigel et al. (1981; Spiegel et al., 1989), that focus on daily coping, managing pain, and dealing with the existential issues related to death and dying. Psychiatric interventions should be used as an integral part of competent, comprehensive medical care and not as an independent treatment modality for cancer.

References

Ali, N., & Khalil, H. (1989). Effects of psychoeducational intervention on anxiety among Egyptian bladder cancer patients. *Cancer Nursing, 12*(4), 236–242.

American Cancer Society. (2000). *Cancer facts and figures—1992.* Atlanta, GA: Author.

Arathuzik, D. (1994). Effects of cognitive behavioral strategies on pain in cancer patients. *Cancer Nursing, 17*(3), 207–214.

Baider, L., Uziely, B., & De-Nour, A. K. (1994). Progressive muscle relaxation and guided imagery in cancer patients. *General Hospital Psychiatry, 16,* 340–347.

Beck, A. T., Epstein, N., Brown, G., & Steer, R. A. (1988). An inventory for measuring clinical anxiety: Psychometric properties. *Journal of Consulting and Clinical Psychology, 56,* 893–897.

Beck, A. T., Rush, A. J., Shaw, B. F., & Emery, G. (1979). *Cognitive therapy of depression.* New York: Guilford.

Ben-Eliyahu, S., Yirmiya, R., Liebeskind, J., Taylor, A., & Gale, R. (1991). Stress increases metastatic spread of a mammary tumor in rats: Evidence for mediation by the immune system. *Brain Behavior Immunology, 5,* 193–205.

Berglund, G., Bolund, C., Gustafsson, U., & Sjoden, P. O. (1994). A randomized study of a rehabilitation program for cancer patients: The "Starting Again" group. *Psycho-Oncology, 3,* 109–120.

Blanchard, C., Toseland, R., & McCallion, P. (1996). The effect of a problem-solving intervention with spouses of cancer patients. *Journal of Psychosocial Oncology, 14*(2), 1–21.

Bloom, J. R. (1982). Social support systems and cancer: A conceptual view. In J. Cohen, J. Cullen, & R. L. Martin (Eds.), *Psychosocial aspects of cancer* (pp. 129–149). New York: Raven Press.

Bloom, J. R., Ross, R. D., & Burnell, G. M. (1978). Effect of social support on patient adjustment following breast surgery. *Patient Counsel on Health Education, 1,* 50–59.

Bos-Branolte, G., Rijshouwer, Y. M., Zielstra, E. M., & Duivenvoorden, H. J. (1998). Psychologic morbidity in survivors of gynaecologic cancer. *European Journal of Guynaecological Oncology, 9*(2), 168–177.

Bos-Branolte, G., Zielstra, E., Rijshouwer, Y., & Duivenvoorden, H. (1988). Psychotherapy inpatients cured of gynecological cancers. *Recent Results in Cancer Research, 108,* 277–288.

Bottomley, A. (1995). The development of the Bottomley Cancer Support Scale. *European Journal of Cancer Care, 4,* 127–131.

Bottomley, A., Hunton, S., Roberts, G., Jones, L., & Bradley, C. (1996). A pilot study of cognitive behavioral therapy and social support group interventions for newly diagnosed cancer patients. *Journal of Psychosocial Oncology, 14*(4), 65–83.

Brandberg, Y., Bergenmar, M., Bolund, C., Michelson, H., Mansson-Brahme, E., Ringborg, U., & Sjoden, P. O. (1994). Information to patients with malignant melanoma: A randomized group study. *Patient Education and Counseling, 23,* 97–105.

Bridge, L. R., Benson, P., Pietroni, P. C., & Priest, R. G. (1988). Relaxation and imagery in the treatment of breast cancer. *British Medical Journal, 297,* 1169–1172.

Burish, T. G., & Lyles, J. N. (1981). Effectiveness of relaxation training in reducing adverse reactions to cancer chemotherapy. *Journal of Behavioral Medicine, 4,* 65–78.

Burish, T. G., Snyder, S. L., & Jenkins, R. A. (1991). Preparing patients for cancer chemotherapy: Effect of coping preparation and relaxation interventions. *Journal of Consulting and Clinical Psychology, 59,* 518–525.

Cella, D. F., Sarafian, B., Snider, P. R., Yellen, S. B., & Winicour, P. (1993). Evaluation of a community-based cancer support group. *Psycho-Oncology, 2,* 123–132.

Cocker, K., Bell, D., & Kidman, A. (1994). Cognitive behaviour therapy with advanced breast cancer patients: A brief report of a pilot study. *Psycho-Oncology, 3,* 233–237

Cohen, J., Cullen, J., & Martin, L. (1982). *Psychosocial aspects of cancer.* New York: Raven Press.

Coopersmith, S. (1981). *Coopersmith Self-Esteem Inventories manual.* Palo Alto, CA: Consulting Psychologists Press.

Cunningham, A. J., Edmonds, C. V. I., Jenkins, G., & Lockwood, G. A. (1995). A randomized comparison of two forms of a brief, group, psychoeducational program for cancer patients: Weekly sessions versus a "weekend intensive." *International Journal of Psychiatry in Medicine, 25,* 173–189.

Cunningham, A. J., & Tocco, E. K. (1989). A randomized trial of group psychoeducational therapy for cancer patients. *Patient Education and Counseling, 14,* 101–114.

Decker, T., Cline-Elsen, J., & Gallagher, M. (1992). Relaxation therapy as an adjunct in radiation oncology. *Journal of Clinical Psychology, 48,* 388–393.

Derogatis, L. R. (1975). *Brief Symptom Inventory (BSI).* Baltimore: Clinical Psychometric Research.

Dunkel-Schetter, C., Feinstein, L. G., Taylor, S. E., & Falke, R. L. (1992). Patterns of coping with cancer. *Health Psychology, 11*(2), 79–87.

Edgar, L., Rosberger, Z., & Nowlis, D. (1992). Coping with cancer during the first year after diagnosis: Assessment and intervention. *Cancer, 69,* 817–828.

Fawzy, F. I., Cousins, N., Fawzy, N. W., Kemeny, M. E., Elashoff, R., & Morton, D. (1990). A structured psychiatric intervention for cancer patients: I. Changes over time in methods of coping and affective disturbance. *Archives of General Psychiatry, 47,* 720–725.

Fawzy, F. I., Fawzy, N. W., Arndt, L. A., & Pasnau, R. O. (1995). Critical review of psychosocial interventions in cancer care. *Archives of General Psychiatry, 52,* 100–113.

Fawzy, F. I., Fawzy, N. W., Hyun, C. S., Guthrie, D., Fahey, J. L., & Morton, D. L. (1993). Malignant melanoma: Effects of an early structured psychiatric intervention, coping, and affective state on recurrence and survival 6 years later. *Archives of General Psychiatry, 50,* 681–689.

Fawzy, F. I., Kemeny, M. E., Fawzy, N. W., Elashoff, R., Morton, D., Cousins, N., & Fahey, J. L. (1990). A structured psychiatric intervention for cancer patients: II. Changes over time in immunologic measures. *Archives of General Psychiatry, 47,* 729–735.

Fawzy, F. I., Namir, S., & Wolcott, D. L. (1989). Structured group intervention model for AIDS patients. *Psychiatric Medicine, 7*(2), 35–46.

Fawzy, F. I., Wellisch, D., & Yager, J. (1977). Psychiatric liaison to the bone-marrow transplant project. In C. E. Hollingsworth & R. O. Pasnau (Eds.), *The family in mourning* (pp. 181–189). New York: Grune & Stratton.

Fawzy, N. W. (1996). A psychoeducational nursing intervention to enhance coping and affective state in newly diagnosed malignant melanoma patients. *Cancer Nursing, 18,* 427–438.

Fox, B. (1992). LeShan's hypothesis is provocative, but is it plausible? *Advances Journal of Mind–Body Health, 8,* 82–84.

Gordon, W. A., Freidenbergs, I., Diller, L., Hibbard, M., Wolf, C., Levine, L., Lipkins, R., Ezrachi, O., & Lucido, D. (1980). Efficacy of psychosocial intervention with cancer patients. *Journal of Consulting and Clinical Psychology, 48,* 743–759.

Greer, S. (1991). Psychological response to cancer and survival. *Psychological Medicine, 21*(1), 43–49.

Greer, S., Moorey, S., Baruch, J. D. R., Watson, M., Robertson, B. M., Mason, A., Rowden, L., Law, M. G., & Bliss, J. M. (1992). Adjuvant psychological therapy for patients with cancer: A prospective randomized trial. *British Medical Journal, 304,* 675–680.

Gruber, B., Hall, N., Hersh, S., & Dubois, P. (1988). Immune system and psychological changes in metastatic cancer patients using relaxation and guided imagery: A pilot study. *Scandinavian Journal of Behavior Therapy, 17,* 25–35.

Gruber, B. L., Hersh, S. P., Hall, N. R. S., Waletzky, L. R., Kunz, J. F., Carpenter, J. K., Kverno, K. S., & Weiss, S. M. (1993). Immunological responses of breast cancer patients to behavioral interventions. *Biofeedback and Self-Regulation, 18*(1), 1–21.

Holland, J. C. (1982). Psychologic aspects of cancer. In J. F. Holland & E. Frei III (Eds.), *Cancer Medicine* (2nd ed., pp. 1175–1203, 2325–2331). Philadelphia: Lee & Febiger.

Horowitz, M., Wilner, N., & Alvarez, E. (1979). Impact of Events Scale: A measure of subjective stress. *Psychosomatic Medicine, 41,* 209–218.

Hosaka, T. (1996). A pilot study of a structured psychiatric intervention for Japanese women with breast cancer. *Psycho-Oncology, 5,* 59–65.

Irwin, M., Brown, M., Patterson, T., Hauger, R., Mascovic, A., & Grant, I. (1991). Neuropeptide Y and natural killer cell activity: Findings in depression and Alzheimer caregiver stress. *FASEB Journal, 5,* 3100–3107.

Irwin, M., Hauger, R., Jones, L., Provencio, M., & Britton, K. (1990). Sympathetic nervous system mediates central corticotropin releasing factor induced suppression of natural killer toxicity. *Journal of Pharmacological Experimental Therapy, 255,* 101–107.

Irwin, M., Vale, W., & Rivier, C. (1990). Central corticotropin-releasing factor mediates the immunosuppressive effect of stress on natural killer toxicity. *Endocrinology, 126,* 2837–2844.

Kiecolt-Glaser, J. K., Glaser, R., Strain, E., Stout, J., Tarr, K., Holliday, J., & Speicher, C. E. (1986). Modulation of cellular immunity in medical students. *Journal of Behavioral Medicine, 9,* 5–21.

Kiecolt-Glaser, J. K., Glaser, R., Williger, D., Stout, J., Messick, G., Sheppard, S., Ricker, D., Romisher, S., Briner, W., Bonnell, G., & Donnerberg, R. (1985). Psychosocial enhancement of immunocompetence in a geriatric population. *Health Psychology, 4,* 25–41.

Lawless, J. (1981). *Statistical models and methods for lifetime data.* New York: Wiley.

Lazarus, R., & Folkman, S. (1984). *Stress, appraisal, and coping.* New York: Springer.

Lee, J. (1989). The relationship between malignant melanoma of the skin and exposure to sunlight. *Photochemistry and Photobiology, 50,* 493–496.

Liang, L. P., Dunn, S. M., Gorman, A., & Stuart-Harris, R. (1990). Identifying priorities of psychosocial need in cancer patients. *British Journal of Cancer, 62,* 1000–1003.

Linn, M. W., Linn, B. S., & Harris, R. (1982). Effects of counseling for late stage cancer patients. *Cancer, 49,* 1048–1055.

Maguire, P. (1976). The psychological and social sequelae of mastectomy. In J. G. Howells (Ed.), *Modern perspectives in the psychiatric aspects of surgery* (pp. 390–421). New York: Brunner/Mazel.

Maguire, P., Lee, E. G., Bevington, D. J., Kuchemann, C., Crabtree, R. J., & Cornell, C. E. (1978). Psychiatric problems in the first year after mastectomy. *British Medical Journal, 1,* 963–965.

McNair, D., Lorr, M., & Droppleman, L. (1971). Profile of Mood States instrument. In D. McNair, M. Lorr, & L. Droppleman (Eds.), *Manual for the Profile of Mood States.* San Diego, CA: Educational and Industrial Testing Service.

Meyerowitz, B. E. (1980). Psychosocial correlates of breast cancer and its treatment. *Psychological Bulletin, 87,* 108–131.

Moorey, S., Greer, S., Watson, M., Baruch, J. D. R., Robertson, B. M., Mason, A., Rowden, L., Tunmore, R., Law, M., & Bliss, J. M. (1994). Adjuvant psychological therapy for patients with cancer: Outcome at one year. *Psycho-Oncology, 3,* 39–46.

Morris, T., Greer, H. S., & White, P. (1977). Psychological and social adjustment to mastectomy: A two-year follow-up study. *Cancer, 43,* 1613–1618.

Namir, S., Wolcott, D. L., Fawzy, F. I., & Alumbaugh, M. J. (1987). Coping with AIDS: Psychological and health implications. *Journal of Applied and Social Psychology, 17,* 308–328.

Novaco, R. W. (1975). *Anger control—the development and evaluation of an experimental treatment.* Lexington, MA: Heath.

Ornish, D., Brown, S. E., Scherwitz, L. W., Billings, J. H., Armstrong, W. T., Ports, T. A., McLanahan, S. M., Kirkeeide, R. L., Brand, R. J., & Gould, K. L. (1992). Can lifestyle changes reverse coronary heart disease? *Lancet, 336*(8708), 129–133.

Pruitt, B. T., Waligora-Serafin, B., McMahon, T., Byrd, G., Besselman, L., Kelly, G. M., Drake, D. A., & Cueller, D. (1992). An educational intervention for newly-diagnosed cancer patients undergoing radiotherapy. *Psycho-Oncology, 2*, 55–62.

Rabkin, J., & Streuning, E. (1976). Life events, stress, and illness. *Science, 194*, 1013–1020.

Richardson, J. L., Shelton, D. R., Krailo, M., & Levine, A. M. (1990). The effect of compliance with treatment on survival among patients with hematologic malignancies. *Journal of Clinical Oncology, 8*, 356–364.

Rogentine, G., Van Kammen, D., Fox, B., Docherty, J., Rosenblatt, J., Boyd, S., & Bunney, W. (1979). Psychological factors in the prognosis of malignant melanoma: A prospective study. *Psychosomatic Medicine, 41*, 647–655.

SAS Institute, Inc. (1991). *SAS/STAT software: The PHREG procedure. Version 6* (SAS Technical Report P-217). Cary, NC: Author.

Sklar, L., & Anisman, H. (1981). Stress and cancer. *Psychological Bulletin, 89*, 369–406.

Sobel, H. J., & Worden, J. W. (1982). *Helping cancer patients cope: Practitioner's manual.* New York: Guilford.

Soloman, G., & Amkrant, A. (1981). Psychoneuroendocrinological effects on the immune response. *Annual Review of Microbiology, 35*, 155–184.

Spiegel, D., & Bloom, J. R. (1983). Pain in metastatic breast cancer. *Cancer, 52*, 341–345.

Spiegel, D., Bloom, J. R., Kraemer, H. C., & Gottheil, E. (1989). Effect of psychosocial treatment on survival of patients with metastatic breast cancer. *Lancet, 2*(8668), 888–891.

Spiegel, D., Bloom, J. R., & Yalom, I. D. (1981). Group support for metastatic cancer patients: A randomized prospective outcome study. *Archives of General Psychiatry, 38*, 527–533.

Spielberger, C. D. (1991). *State–Trait Anger Expression Inventory manual.* Lutz, FL: Psychological Assessment Resources.

Temoshok, L., & Fox, B. (1984). Coping styles and other psychosocial factors related to medical status and to prognosis in patients with cutaneous malignant melanoma. In B. Fox & B. Newberry (Eds.), *Impact of psychoendocrine systems in cancer and immunity* (pp. 258–287). Lewiston, NY: C. J. Hogrefe.

Wallston, K. A., Strudler-Wallston, B., & DeVellis, R. (1978). Development of the Multidimensional Health Locus of Control (MHLC) scales. *Health Education Monographs, 6*, 160–171.

Watson, M., Greer, S., Young, J., Inayat, Q., Burgess, C., & Robertson, B. (1988). Development of a questionnaire of adjustment to cancer: The MAC scale. *Psychological Medicine, 18*, 203–209.

Weisman, A. D. (1979a). *Coping with cancer.* New York: McGraw-Hill.

Weisman, A. D. (1979b). A model for psychosocial phasing in cancer. *General Hospital Psychiatry, 1*(3), 187–195.

Weisman, A. D., Worden, J. W., & Sobel, H. J. (1980). *Psychosocial screening and intervention with cancer patients* (Project Omega, Grant No. CA-19797). Boston: Harvard Medical School, Massachusetts General Hospital.

Worden, J. W., & Weisman, A. D. (1977). The fallacy in postmastectomy depression. *American Journal of Medical Science, 273*(2), 169–175.

Zigmond, A., & Snaith, R. P. (1979). The Hospital Anxiety and Depression Scale. *Acta Psychiatrica Scandinavica, 67,* 367–370.

Zimbardo, P., & Ebbeson, E. B. (1970). *Influencing attitudes and changing behavior.* Reading, MA: Addison Wesley.

CHAPTER 14

Group Support Interventions for People With Cancer

Benefits and Hazards

Vicki S. Helgeson
Sheldon Cohen
Richard Schulz
Joyce Yasko

In this chapter we discuss group support interventions for people with cancer. We examine the value of a group-level approach for intervention and discuss the strengths and weaknesses of the existing literature. We present our own group-level intervention, briefly summarize the findings of our study (Helgeson, Cohen, Schulz, & Yasko, 1999), and use the results to discuss important issues that should be considered in this kind of research. We discuss in depth the development of our intervention and the implications of our findings for the field of research. Finally, we conclude by raising issues for future research to consider.

Why Study Group Interventions?

There are a number of reasons to evaluate group interventions for people with cancer. Cancer is the second leading cause of death in the United States and affects one out of three Americans (American Cancer Society, 1997). The disease and treatment affect a wide array of domains of functioning (psychological, social, vocational, physical). If a group-level intervention is effective in improving quality or quantity of life, it has the potential to be more cost-effective than individually tailored

This research was funded by National Institutes of Health (NIH) Grant R01 CA61303, NIH Senior Scientist Development Award MH00721, and an American Cancer Society Junior Investigator Award from the Pittsburgh Cancer Institute.

interventions. That is, group-level treatments reach a larger number of people at a reduced cost compared with individual-level treatments.

Second, group support interventions are widely used in the community. These interventions, typically referred to as *support groups,* are often assumed to be beneficial by the people conducting the groups and by the people referring patients to such groups. There are a number of group-level programs that exist at the national level. Programs such as I Can Cope and Reach to Recovery, sponsored by the American Cancer Society, and Us Too, sponsored by the American Foundation for Urologic Disease, are commonly found in larger communities. Although participants rate these programs favorably, the effectiveness of such programs has rarely, if at all, been evaluated.

A final reason to evaluate the efficacy of group support interventions is that benefits from a few scientific studies of peer support groups have been popularized by the media to encourage people to join support groups. Many people with cancer and many health care professionals are familiar with the findings from David Spiegel's study (Spiegel, Bloom, Kraemer, & Gottheil, 1989) of women with breast cancer or Fawzy's study (Fawzy et al., 1990) of people with melanoma, both of which documented survival benefits of attending a group support intervention. People may be less familiar with the particulars of these interventions. The Spiegel psychotherapeutic group lasted 1 year, was limited to women with metastatic breast cancer, and was conducted by trained therapists. Fawzy's intervention lasted only 6 weeks but was multifaceted and included coping skills, education, cognitive–behavioral therapy, and group discussion. Although the results from these two very different studies are certainly encouraging, they do not provide a sufficient basis on which to base an unequivocal recommendation that cancer patients should join community support groups, particularly under the guise that doing so increases longevity.

Research on Group Interventions

Despite popular belief about the benefits of support groups for people with cancer, few evaluations of support group interventions have been undertaken. Many of the few studies that do exist suffer from methodological flaws or conceptual weaknesses. Some studies do not include a control group, partly from the belief that withholding treatment (i.e., the support group) would be harmful to patients. Such studies typically use a pre–post design, often demonstrating that patients' quality of life improves or psychological distress diminishes after attending a group. These findings, however, cannot be interpreted because the passage of time is a strong predictor of improved quality of life. A comparison group is critical to the evaluation of a support intervention. Other studies do not randomly assign patients to conditions, which means that patients can "select" into the intervention group. The problem with this design is that the benefit of the intervention may be unique to the patients who selected into the group. Alternatively, these "self-selectors" may have been the kind of people to improve without the intervention. Because group interventions are difficult to conduct, studies often have very small sample sizes. The typical group intervention study compares one intervention group with one control group. Thus, the modal number of groups being compared is one. Because the dynamics of a particular group of patients can influence individuals' response to treatment, it is necessary to include multiple groups within each level of treatment to evaluate the effectiveness of a group intervention.

Interventions that have been evaluated often lack a theoretical basis for their design. Historically, health care professionals such as nurses and social workers were the ones conducting and evaluating support groups. The design of those groups is likely to have been based on the nurse's clinical experience of what would be helpful to people with cancer. The difficulty with this kind of procedure is that one cannot determine why a particular intervention was effective. It is difficult to replicate the effects of an intervention without understanding its theoretical underpinnings. Previous research has rarely examined explanatory mechanisms for an intervention's effect. For example, Spiegel et al. (1989) hypothesized that their intervention increased feelings of mastery; provided emotional support; and decreased isolation, helplessness, and feelings of worthlessness. Yet, most of these mechanisms were not evaluated. Among those that were examined (self-esteem, locus of control), intervention effects were not observed. Fawzy et al. (1993) found effects of their intervention on immune function, but the immune changes did not account for the mortality benefit. Sophisticated studies by David Spiegel and Barbara Anderson, however, are evaluating a wide array of psychological and physiological mechanisms.

Previous group interventions, especially those that have been successful, also have provided patients with multiple resources—information, coping skills, relaxation training, hypnosis, and social support (Fawzy et al., 1990). The difficulty with this approach is that the particular component of the intervention responsible for its benefits is not clear. It may be that only a single component is necessary, that all components are necessary, or that there is a synergy among components. In a recent meta-analytic review of the literature on psychosocial interventions (mostly individual level) for people with cancer, Meyer and Mark (1995) concluded that psychosocial interventions can improve adjustment to cancer and that there is no evidence that one approach is more effective than another. Interventions, however, are rarely compared with one another. Meyer and Mark suggested that future research should attempt to tease apart the effective components of psychosocial interventions and determine who benefits most from which kind of intervention.

Helgeson and Cohen (1996) reviewed the literature on group interventions for people with cancer. They found more evidence for the effectiveness of interventions that contained an educational component than interventions based on peer discussion only. To be fair, however, the authors also concluded that few sound evaluations have been conducted of the peer discussion intervention and that studies have not compared the effectiveness of these two components of group interventions. In this era of rising health care costs, it is important to know the components of a group intervention that are critical to its success.

We attempted to address many of the previously raised issues by designing a group-level intervention for women with Stages I and II breast cancer that included a no-treatment control group, randomized patients to condition, and included multiple groups within each treatment. We had a conceptual framework for the development of the intervention and identified mechanisms by which we expected the intervention to improve adjustment to breast cancer. We also designed these interventions to be cost-effective and easily transportable to the community. The interventions lasted 8 weeks and were conducted by oncology nurses and social workers, the people who are usually in charge of hospital support groups.

Our Study

Method

Interventions

We used the literature on psychosocial issues women confront when faced with breast cancer as the basis for the two interventions we designed. The literature suggests that the diagnosis and treatment of cancer is associated with a loss of control and an assault on self-esteem (Fobair, Hoppe, Bloom, Cox, & Varghese, 1986; Lesko, Ostroff, & Smith, 1991). People tend to perceive control over the events that happen to them (Taylor & Brown, 1988). A traumatic event threatens this perception of control. A diagnosis of breast cancer threatens our perceptions of control over our lives in general and our bodies in particular. Rarely are there warning signs of breast cancer. Most women with breast cancer do not have a family history of the disease. The first sign of the cancer is a lump in the breast or a suspicious routine mammogram. Because it is difficult to identify a single cause of the disease, it is difficult for women to gain a sense of control over the illness or perceive that they can prevent a recurrence of disease. Instead, women struggle with the question of "why me?"

The treatment for breast cancer also challenges perceptions of control. The treatment and accompanying side effects are disruptive and often unpredictable. For example, chemotherapy treatments are frequently postponed because women's white blood cell counts do not reach acceptable limits to tolerate the next dose of treatment. Thus, even on a day-to-day basis, it can be difficult for women to feel any control over their bodies or daily activities.

The diagnosis of and treatment for breast cancer also affects self-image. Cancer is still associated with a stigma in our society. People with cancer are often labeled as victims. Interactions with network members can be awkward because people are afraid of cancer, may fear it is contagious, or find it unpleasant to be reminded of the existence of a life-threatening disease (Peters-Golden, 1982). The treatment for breast cancer also influences self-esteem. Women diagnosed with early stage disease felt healthy prior to their diagnosis and then feel sick as the treatment (e.g., surgery, radiation therapy, chemotherapy) debilitates them. The loss of a breast through surgery, the loss of hair through chemotherapy, and the fatigue associated with radiation are assaults to self-image.

Thus, we designed group-level interventions to improve quality of life by ameliorating these two psychological threats—loss of perceived control and loss of self-esteem. We designed two support interventions, both patterned after the kinds of interventions that exist in the community. One was based on the provision of informational support through education, and one was based on the provision of emotional support through peer discussion. The ways in which we thought the interventions would influence quality of life are shown in Figure 14.1.

The first intervention was education based. We thought that by providing women with information about their disease and treatment and some ways of coping with their illness, perceptions of control over the illness experience would be enhanced. We also thought that such information would reduce women's feelings of confusion surrounding their illness. To the extent that the information addressed women's unanswered questions and enabled them to make sense of the experience, unwanted disturbing intrusive thoughts about the illness should diminish.

The second intervention was peer discussion. We expected that this intervention would influence self-esteem in three ways. First, we expected that sharing experiences with others facing the same common stressor would help to normalize the cancer experience and reduce feelings of deviance (Coates & Winston, 1983; Lieberman, 1993; Spiegel, Bloom, & Yalom, 1981). Women should receive validation from one another. Second, we thought the discussion group would influence self-esteem and subsequently promote adjustment by providing opportunities for women to help one another. The "helper-therapy" principle has long been thought to be a way that group interventions benefit participants (Rosenberg, 1984). By helping one another, women gain a sense of competence. The third process—social comparison—was an implicit rather than an explicit process. When people are faced with threat, such as the diagnosis of a serious illness, one way that they cope is by comparing themselves with other people. The social comparison literature suggests that the most prevalent kind of comparison among people faced with threat (cancer, in particular) is a downward comparison, a comparison with others who are worse off (Buunk, Collins, Taylor, Van Yperen, & Dakof, 1990; Wood, Taylor, & Lichtman, 1985). Such downward comparisons are usually thought to be positive, meaning one feels lucky in comparison with less-fortunate others. Positive downward comparisons have been shown to increase self-esteem (Reis, Gerrard, & Gibbons, 1993; Wills, 1981). We thought that the mere presence of the group would lead women to make such comparisons with one another. In addition, women in the group could compare the entire group favorably with other people (e.g., "At least we

FIGURE 14.1

Processes by which education and peer support interventions were expected to influence adjustment to breast cancer. The arrows indicate the pathways that we expected the interventions to take to influence adjustment.

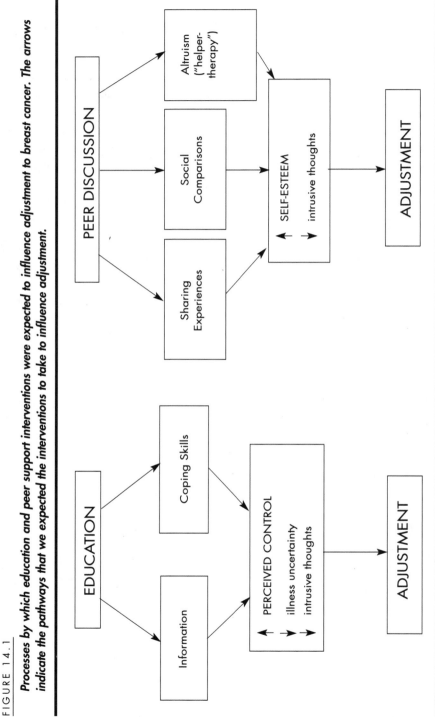

caught our breast cancer in time!"). We also expected that sharing experiences and expressing emotions in a warm and accepting atmosphere would reduce disturbing intrusive thoughts about the illness.

The content of the education and peer discussion interventions have been previously described (Helgeson et al., 1999) but are summarized here. Each of the interventions consisted of eight weekly meetings. The education intervention addressed the following topics: what breast cancer is, symptom management, nutrition, exercise, body image, communication, future health care issues, and relationships–sexuality. Each of these topics was addressed by either a facilitator or an expert in the area. The theme of the group was fostering perceptions of control—control over the illness experience rather than control over the illness. The intervention was conducted in a classroom-like atmosphere to minimize interaction among patients. Although patients could not be prevented from talking with one another, facilitators attempted to minimize such interactions by starting and ending the groups on time.

The peer discussion intervention focused on the expression of feelings and sharing of experiences. Women were provided with workbooks each week, wherein they recorded personal experiences and problems related to the illness. Workbooks were used as a way to begin each group and guide discussion. Facilitators were told not to offer information in this group. Although they could answer patients' questions and were ethically bound to correct misinformation, they were told to encourage patients to focus on their own experiences and feelings. Facilitators encouraged patients to help one another.

Study Design

Women who were diagnosed with Stage I or Stage II breast cancer and were treated with surgery and adjuvant chemotherapy were eligible to participate in the intervention. Nurses from over 40 medical oncologists' offices identified eligible patients. Groups were run in three locations around the Pittsburgh area to maximize accrual rates. Once 10–12 women at a given site agreed to participate in the study, the group was randomized to one of four conditions: education, peer discussion, combined (education followed by peer discussion), and control. The three intervention groups met for 8 consecutive weeks. Education sessions lasted 45 minutes, peer discussion sessions lasted 1 hour, and combined sessions lasted 1 hour, 45 minutes. We convened seven separate groups in each of the four conditions. An oncology nurse and an oncology social worker facilitated the interventions. Each pair of facilitators conducted each of the three interventions so that facilitator was not confounded with intervention.

We measured quality of life with the Medical Outcome Survey Short Form 36 (MOS SF–36; Ware & Sherbourne, 1992). We also used the positive and negative affect scales from the PANAS (Watson, Clark, & Tellegen, 1988). Instruments were administered before random assignment to condition, immediately after the intervention, and 6 months after the intervention. We are continuing to follow women on an annual basis.

Results

The results of the study showed clear benefits of the education intervention and no benefits of the peer discussion intervention. On some outcomes (negative affect and a couple of the SF-36 scales), the peer discussion intervention led to worse outcomes. The combined intervention seemed to reflect the positive benefits of education and the null effects (and sometimes adverse effects) of peer discussion. All of these findings appeared immediately after the intervention and held up for 6 months. We also analyzed the data by using the particular group of women as the unit of analysis. For these analyses, the sample size was 28. Using the conservative group-level analysis, the findings were the same. We sought to explain the positive effects of the education intervention and the null—and sometimes negative—effects of the peer discussion intervention.

Discussion

The primary mechanism by which the education intervention benefited patients— in the short-term (1–2 weeks after intervention) and long-term (6 months after intervention)—centered on self-image. The education intervention enhanced self-esteem and body image. This was unexpected. In fact, self-image was hypothesized to be the mechanism by which the peer discussion intervention would promote adjustment. The information women received may have made them feel better about themselves by normalizing their experiences. The information also may have provided women with the tools to make themselves feel better. For example, women were provided with information about how to enhance appearance, what to eat during chemotherapy, how to regain arm motion, and what precautions to take against lymphedema. To the extent that they used this information in their daily life, feelings of competence may have been promoted.

In the short term, the education intervention also reduced feelings of confusion over the illness and increased discussion about the illness with network members. The information gained from the educational sessions may have been used as a safe and positive way to promote discussions about the illness with network members. In the long term, the education intervention increased feelings of control over the illness experience and reduced intrusive thoughts about the disease. Control was hypothesized as the primary mechanism by which the intervention would enhance adjustment. It is interesting that the effects of the intervention on feelings of control were not realized until 6 months after the intervention ended.

One reason why the peer discussion intervention was not effective and led to an increase in negative affect was that these women increased their rate of negative downward comparisons. We expected the peer discussion intervention to promote downward comparisons—comparison with worse-off others—but we expected those comparisons to be positive in nature (e.g., feeling lucky). Instead, women in the peer discussion intervention reported feeling anxious and concerned about their own condition when they faced worse-off others.

This finding was disturbing to us because negative downward comparisons were sometimes cited by women as a reason for not wanting to participate in the study. During recruitment, some women expressed concern about seeing other women who were dying or not coping well in the peer discussion condition. We naively assured women that the group was homogeneous with respect to diagnosis (i.e., all had a relatively good prognosis) and that facilitators would make sure a single distressed group member did not detract from the entire group. Given that no woman had metastatic disease and no one had died or faced a recurrence while a group convened, we were surprised that negative downward comparisons emerged.

In retrospect, however, we realize that there were other dimensions upon which women could have made negative downward comparisons. One dimension upon which women varied was the number of positive lymph nodes they had. We observed that women often introduced themselves by reporting their number of positive lymph nodes. In the first peer discussion group that we convened, facilitators told us that women reported their lymph node status at the first meeting and arranged themselves in the circle by lymph node status at subsequent meetings. That is, women with no positive lymph nodes sat on one side of the circle, and women with positive lymph nodes sat on the other side of the circle. Another dimension upon which women could compare was side effects of chemotherapy. Hair loss in particular was an important topic of group discussions, and women varied on this dimension.

That negative downward comparisons were problematic in this study suggests there could be even more difficulties with community support groups for people with different kinds of cancer and different stages of the disease. It may be, however, that women for whom negative downward comparisons were a problem would be unlikely to attend a "support group" or would drop out from a group early on. Nevertheless, our findings suggest that health care providers should think twice before encouraging a woman to join a support group if she expresses a reluctance to do so.

A second reason why peer discussion groups led to an increase in negative affect was that women reported an increase in negative interactions with network members during the period in which the group convened. Previous research has found an association between attending a support group and lack of support from family and friends (Taylor, Falke, Shoptaw, & Lichtman, 1986). This cross-sectional finding has often been interpreted to mean that people who lack social support are most likely to join support groups. Our results suggest that the reverse causal interpretation is viable. Attending a support group may adversely affect the social network.

How could a support group adversely affect one's relationships with social network members? First, attending the support group may have only altered group members' perceptions of their social relations. By listening and sharing experiences with one another, women may come to believe that network members were not as supportive as they once thought they were. Alternatively, attending the group may actually alter interactions with network members. Network members may feel excluded from the group. In our study we did not permit family and friends to participate in the group. Women may feel that it is no longer necessary to share feelings with family and friends because they have a group of people with whom they can do so. We cannot distinguish between these two explanations with our data. We do note, however, that the peer discussion group did not alter discussions about the illness with network members, whereas the education group increased discussion with network members. Thus, the peer support condition did not facilitate discussions with network members in the same way that the education condition did. The information in the educational intervention may have been used as a source of discussion with network members.

Six months after groups ended, the peer discussion group led to an increase in intrusive and avoidant thoughts about the illness. The education group, by contrast, led to a decrease in intrusive thoughts about the illness. The peer discussion group may have raised issues that could not be resolved in 8 weeks. The length of two previous beneficial peer discussion interventions was 1 year (Kriss & Kraemer, 1986; Spiegel et al., 1989). Issues also may not have been resolved in our peer discussion intervention because the group was not designed in a way to resolve them. Although group members were encouraged to help one another solve problems, it is not clear that one can depend on group members to have the skills to provide effective help. A group receiving structured psychotherapy may have addressed emotional issues more effectively. This study suggests that venting feelings alone, presumably in a warm and accepting atmosphere, is not sufficient to reduce intrusive thoughts about one's illness and that the form of ventilation we provided actually increased intrusive thoughts.

Who Benefits From What?

The final question that we sought to address in this study was who would benefit most from which kind of intervention (Helgeson, Cohen, Schulz, & Yasko, 2000). We hypothesized that women who lacked emotional support might benefit most from the intervention designed to provide emotional support—peer discussion. To our surprise, reports of emotional support at the onset of the study interacted with each of the three interventions to predict adjustment. It appeared that women who lacked emotional support were buffered by all of the interventions from the deterioration in physical functioning observed in the control group. However, women who scored high on support at the beginning of the study reacted differently to the three interventions. In the education group, their functioning did not change over time. In the peer discussion group, their functioning deteriorated over time. The results in the combination group, not surprisingly, fell somewhere between the two—a slight deterioration over time. Thus, the adverse effects of the peer discussion intervention may be limited to the women with high levels of support. These may be the women who reported more negative interactions with network members after attending the peer discussion group. Thus, women with emotional support from network members not only do not benefit from the peer discussion intervention but may actually be harmed by it.

We also examined whether personal resources, such as high self-esteem and feelings of control at the start of the study, would influence responsiveness to the interventions. We created a personal resource index that comprised feelings of control over the illness situation, high self-esteem, high body image, and reduced uncertainty about the illness. This index interacted with the education intervention only, such that women who had low personal resources were buffered by the education intervention from the deterioration in physical functioning observed in the control group.

Implications of Findings

To our knowledge, this is the largest randomized group intervention for people with cancer conducted to date. The results clearly showed support for benefits of education that were maintained for 6 months after the intervention. No benefits of peer discussion were observed. There were some adverse effects of peer discussion on negative affect and some of the specific SF-36 domains of functioning. These findings remained even when we used the conservative group unit of analysis, strengthening our confidence in the results. The results are consistent with Helgeson and Cohen's (1996) review of group interventions for people with cancer. In that review, they found more evidence for the effectiveness of education compared with peer discussion interventions. They also discussed a number of difficulties that may occur in peer discussion interventions, some of which were borne out in this research.

One of the major strengths of this study is that we were able to tease apart two of the common components of support interventions that exist in the community. Peer discussion is typically the focus of support groups in the community. Community support groups may or may not include an informational component. Peer discussion alone did not seem to benefit women, nor did it confer any special benefit when combined with education. In this era of limited health care resources, our data suggest that communities ought to emphasize education over peer discussion. The education intervention was easy to implement after it was developed because the materials were standardized. It is difficult to "standardize" a peer discussion, which may explain why it is harder to conduct.

The extent to which the benefits of the education intervention are due to the specific information provided rather than the group context is not clear. Future research could provide women with the same information through mail or video to discern the impact of the "group" on the effectiveness of the intervention. The group context may have influenced the delivery of the information. Hearing someone else's question may trigger a question of one's own. People who are afraid to raise issues or have difficulty articulating their concerns may find that others raise their questions. Participating in a group also could have increased people's motivation to pay attention and to think about the information provided. In these ways, the presence of the group could have contributed to a greater knowledge gain.

The group context also could have inadvertently conveyed emotional support. The mere presence of other people facing the same situation may have provided some reassurance and validation. Although women in the education intervention were not encouraged to talk to one another and structural barriers to group discussion were created, some women did find ways to talk to one another—if not in the group, then in the parking lot after the group! If those kinds of exchanges were supportive and contributed to the positive effects of the education intervention, one would have to question the usefulness of structured support interactions compared with the usefulness of more naturally occurring support interactions.

Why Wasn't the Peer Discussion Intervention Effective?

At first glance, the ineffectiveness of the peer discussion intervention appears to be inconsistent with the existing correlational research on social support among people with cancer. Correlational studies suggest that emotional support is the most frequently sought support by people with cancer and that emotional support has the strongest effects on quality-of-life outcomes (see Helgeson & Cohen, 1996, for a review). However, the sources of support in these studies are family and friends—not a group of strangers who share the same problem. The literature also suggests that there are barriers to family and friends being effective emotional support providers when one is diagnosed with cancer, which leads to the suggestion that peers—people who are experiencing the same stressor—might be able to remedy any emotional support deficits.

This group may not have had the intended benefits for a number of reasons. First, perhaps these women did not perceive the group as supportive. We have some data to indicate that this was not the case. Women in all intervention conditions rated the groups favorably. Women in the peer discussion condition reported feeling closer to one another and were more likely to get together with one another after the group ended than women in the education condition. However, this does not negate the possibility that there were some unsupportive exchanges in these group sessions. We are currently conducting a content analysis of the peer discussion sessions to obtain more information about the nature of the group discussions.

Second, the question arises as to whether peers can compensate for emotional support deficits from network members. Because women who reported a lack of emotional support from network members benefited from the peer discussion intervention, peer group members may be able to compensate in the case of problematic network relations. However, in cases where women were satisfied with the support they received from network members (which was the majority of women), peer discussion was not useful. One could conclude from this study that only women with support deficits should be referred to community support groups. Although these might be the only women who would benefit from the experience, the character of a support group composed only of women with support deficits is worrisome. People who lack social support might also lack some of the social skills needed to acquire support from other people or may have other major problems besides their cancer. It may be difficult for group leaders to facilitate naturalistic supportive exchanges among these people.

Third, the prognosis of the disease may influence the effectiveness of peer discussion. The vast majority of women were diagnosed with Stages I and II breast cancer, and none of the women had metastatic disease. An emotional support intervention may be more beneficial under more severe illness circumstances, as in the Spiegel et al. (1981) study. The kind of support that is most effective must match the needs of the situation (Cohen & Wills, 1985; Cutrona, 1990). Information may be most needed by people who are initially diagnosed with cancer and undergoing treatment. The information can be used to understand and cope with the disease and the treatment. Emotional support may be more beneficial when treatment is completed and one has the opportunity to reflect on the meaning of the illness for one's future. It is also possible that information is more helpful to people with a favorable prognosis because there is greater potential for control of the disease, and emotional support is more beneficial for those with advanced disease who have limited capacities to control the disease course. This latter hypothesis stems from Folkman's (1984) argument that problem-focused coping is more helpful when the circumstances are controllable, and emotion-focused coping is more helpful when the circumstances are uncontrollable. One could view Stages I and II breast cancer as a relatively more controllable situation (i.e., potential for cure) than Stage IV disease. The education intervention more directly maps onto problem-focused coping (i.e., providing women with information that they can use to influence how they are feeling), and the peer discussion intervention more directly maps onto emotion-focused coping (i.e., discussing feelings with the goal of changing how they feel about the situation).

The duration of the intervention—8 weeks—may not have been long enough for the peer discussion intervention to be beneficial. It may have taken women several weeks to warm up to the group discussion and to begin disclosing illness-related concerns. By the time these women were ready to discuss their hopes and fears, the group may have ended. Women who started the group by denying their illness may fall into this category. For these women, the group may have eventually challenged their denial and allowed them to express feelings of distress. Shedler, Mayman, and Manis (1993) discussed the possibility that one reason why therapeutic interventions do not appear effective is that discussions decrease distress for those who are initially willing to admit distress and increase distress for those who are initially unwilling to admit distress. In the end, it appears as if the intervention has no effect on the group as a whole.

Finally, it also is possible that the group discussion was not helpful and possibly harmful because discussing the illness with other women increased women's awareness of their own levels of distress. The intervention was not designed to teach women how to cope with the distress. The underlying premise of the intervention was that the ventilation of feelings and the sharing of experiences, in and of themselves, would be beneficial. Similar issues were recently raised by Frasure-Smith et al. (1997) to explain why their home-based nursing intervention for cardiac patients was associated with an increase in mortality among women. The authors suggested that frequent visits and telephone calls may have reminded women of their psychological distress and that the nurses, although equipped to provide emotional support, did not have the psychotherapeutic skills to resolve major difficulties.

It is possible that group discussion in and of itself is not sufficient to produce changes in the ways one thinks about and copes with an illness. The aim of the discussion was to provide emotional support, to reduce feelings of uniqueness, and to create bonds of similarity. However, more psychotherapeutic changes may need to occur for a support group to be effective. If that is the case, it is essential that such changes are documented and shown to explain the benefit of psychotherapeutic groups. Spiegel's psychotherapy group not only improved quality of life but extended longevity by 18 months among a group of women with metastatic breast cancer. We incorporated many of Spiegel's principles into our group discussion intervention (i.e., encouraging the expression of affect, both negative and positive; encouraging women to help one another; encouraging the sharing of feelings), but Spiegel referred to his intervention as *supportive-expressive therapy* rather than *peer discussion*. One difference between the two studies is that in the Spiegel et al. (1981) study, therapists taught specific coping skills, such as how to manage pain. According to Carkhuff (1973), support groups are not effective unless skills are provided to participants to cope with the problem. He argued that groups that meet to discuss problems and share experiences, with the occasional insight from the group leader, could leave participants worse off at the end of the group. Participants return to their unchanged problems, with hopes having been raised that they will be able to cope more effectively with those problems.

Regardless of which of the above reasons account for the null effects of the peer discussion intervention, the implications for community intervention are the same. Health care professionals should be cautious about advising women to join their local community support group.

Future Directions

The lack of effects for the peer discussion intervention along with women's high needs for emotional support suggest to us that researchers might benefit from creating different vehicles to deliver emotional support. Interventions could be aimed at families, in particular the patient–spouse relationship. The spouse is viewed as the most important source of support (Coyne & DeLongis, 1986; Jamison, Wellisch, & Pasnau, 1978). One could identify sources of miscommunication that arise among family members during the illness and deliver an intervention to reduce those miscommunications. Alternatively, a peer-dyad intervention might be more effective than a peer-group intervention in delivering emotional support. It is certainly the case that some women in support groups form close ties with one another and that the illness provides a common basis for discussion. Peers could be matched on characteristics of the disease (e.g., type of surgery, type of treatment) and demographic variables that provide a common basis for discussion, such as marital status and the presence of children. A newly diagnosed patient might benefit the most from a peer who has completed treatment. A study of patients awaiting coronary artery bypass surgery showed that patients preferred to be assigned a roommate who had already had bypass surgery rather a roommate who was awaiting the surgery (Kulik & Mahler, 1989). The nature of the interactions could be more closely controlled and monitored in a peer-dyad rather than a peer-group intervention. To the extent that peer role models are carefully selected and trained to deliver the intervention, unanticipated unsupportive interactions should be minimized.

We may still be at the point where successful intervention studies raise more questions than they answer. One broad question that continues to be raised is this: What kind of intervention is beneficial for whom? We have attempted to examine one dimension of "what"—education versus peer discussion. We have addressed a couple of dimensions of "whom"—the helpfulness of the interaction depends on people's naturally existing support and personal resources. Researchers should more explicitly examine the dimension of disease severity or prognosis. Several researchers (e.g., Andersen, 1992) have suggested that disease severity may be a potentially important moderating variable of the effectiveness of a support intervention. Another potentially important moderator is gender. The majority of support intervention studies focus on breast cancer, and thus women. To what extent do these findings generalize to men with cancer? To date, there has been one evaluation of a support intervention that focused exclusively on men with prostate cancer (Lepore & Helgeson, 1998). It showed that combined education and peer discussion confers benefits. In the area of bereavement, Schut, Stroebe, van den Bout, and de Keijser (1997) examined whether men or women would benefit from a problem-focused coping or emotion-focused coping intervention. They argued that women had greater needs for how to cope with concrete problems, such as finances, after bereavement and that men had greater emotional support needs because they had lost their sole source of emotional support. The findings showed that women benefited more from the problem-focused coping intervention and that men benefited more from the emotion-focused coping intervention.

One issue that all intervention researchers should keep in mind is cost-effectiveness and community implementation. The two issues are related. Communities are more likely to implement short-term, low-cost interventions. Thus, to the extent that we can identify the most effective components of support interventions that can be delivered in a low-cost format, the more likely it will be that our intervention will be implemented in the community. The educational intervention tested in this study meets these criteria. It is short-term, structured, and delivered in group format. All of these features make the intervention low-cost and easily transferred to the community. An effective peer discussion intervention is likely to be of higher cost if it requires more qualified leaders (e.g., clinical psychologists or psychiatrists rather than oncology nurses and social workers) and more time (e.g., 1 year). This does not mean that the latter intervention would not be cost-effective, however. The outcome must be taken into consideration. Obviously, if a more complicated intervention or a longer lasting intervention can influence disease progression, the intervention could be cost-effective.

References

American Cancer Society. (1997). *Cancer facts and figures.* Atlanta, GA: Author.

Andersen, B. L. (1992). Psychological interventions for cancer patients to enhance quality of life. *Journal of Consulting and Clinical Psychology, 60,* 552–568.

Buunk, B. P., Collins, R. L., Taylor, S. E., Van Yperen, N. W., & Dakof, G. A. (1990). The affective consequence of social comparison: Either direction has its ups and downs. *Journal of Personality and Social Psychology, 59,* 1238–1249.

Carkhuff, R. R. (1973, January). A human technology for group helping processes. *Educational Technology,* 31–38.

Coates, D., & Winston, T. (1983). Counteracting the deviance of depression: Peer support groups for victims. *Journal of Social Issues, 39,* 169–194.

Cohen, S., & Wills, T. A. (1985). Stress, social support, and the buffering hypothesis. *Psychological Bulletin, 98,* 310–357.

Coyne, J. C., & DeLongis, A. (1986). Going beyond social support: The role of social relationships in adaptation. *Journal of Consulting and Clinical Psychology, 54,* 454–460.

Cutrona, C. E. (1990). Stress and social support—In search of optimal matching. *Journal of Social and Clinical Psychology, 9*(1), 3–14.

Fawzy, F. I., Cousins, N., Fawzy, N. W., Kemeny, M. E., Elashoff, R., & Morton, D. (1990). A structured psychiatric intervention for cancer patients: I. Changes over time in methods of coping and affective disturbance. *Cancer Intervention, 47,* 720–725.

Fawzy, F. I., Fawzy, N. W., Hyun, C. S., Elashoff, R., Guthrie, D., Fahey, J. L., & Morton, D. L. (1993). Malignant melanoma: Effects of an early structured psychiatric intervention, coping, and affective state on recurrence and survival 6 years later. *Archives of General Psychiatry, 50,* 681–689.

Fobair, P., Hoppe, R. T., Bloom, J., Cox, R., & Varghese, A. (1986). Psychosocial problems among survivors of Hodgkin's disease. *Journal of Clinical Oncology, 4,* 805–814.

Folkman, S. (1984). Personal control and stress and coping processes: A theoretical analysis. *Journal of Personality and Social Psychology, 40,* 839–852.

Frasure-Smith, N., Lesperance, F., Prince, R. H., Verrier, P., Garber, R. A., Juneau, M., Wolfson, C., & Bourassa, M. G. (1997). Randomized trial of home-based psychosocial nursing intervention for patients recovering from myocardial infarction. *Lancet, 350,* 473–479.

Helgeson, V. S., & Cohen, S. (1996). Social support and adjustment to cancer: Reconciling descriptive, correlational, and intervention research. *Health Psychology, 15,* 135–148.

Helgeson, V. S., Cohen, S., Schulz, R., & Yasko, J. (1999). Education and peer discussion group interventions and adjustment to breast cancer. *Archives of General Psychiatry, 56,* 340–347.

Helgeson, V. S., Cohen, S., Schulz, R., & Yasko, J. (2000). Group support interventions for people with cancer: Who benefits from what? *Health Psychology, 19,* 107–114.

Jamison, K. R., Wellisch, D. K., & Pasnau, R. O. (1978). Psychosocial aspects of mastectomy: I. The woman's perspective. *American Journal of Psychiatry, 135,* 432–436.

Kriss, R. T., & Kraemer, H. C. (1986). Efficacy of group therapy for problems with postmastectomy self-perception, body image, and sexuality. *Journal of Sex Research, 22,* 438–451.

Kulik, J. A., & Mahler, H. I. M. (1989). Stress and affiliation in a hospital setting: Preoperative roommate preferences. *Personality and Social Psychology Bulletin, 15,* 183–193.

Lepore, S. J., & Helgeson, V. S. (1998). Social constraints, intrusive thoughts, and mental health after prostate cancer. *Journal of Social and Clinical Psychology, 17*(1), 89–106.

Lesko, L. M., Ostroff, J., & Smith, K. (1991). Life after cancer treatment: Survival and beyond. In J. C. Holland, L. M. Lesko, & M. H. Massie (Eds.), *Current concepts in psycho-oncology* (Vol. 4, pp. 47–53). New York: Memorial Sloan-Kettering Cancer Center.

Lieberman, M. A. (1993). Self-help groups. In H. I. Kaplan & B. J. Sadock (Eds.), *Comprehensive group psychotherapy* (pp. 292–304). Baltimore: Williams & Wilkins.

Meyer, T. J., & Mark, M. M. (1995). Effects of psychosocial interventions with adult cancer patients: A meta-analysis of randomized experiments. *Health Psychology, 14,* 101–108.

Peters-Golden, H. (1982). Breast cancer: Varied perceptions of social support in the illness experience. *Social Science and Medicine, 16,* 483–491.

Reis, T. J., Gerrard, M., & Gibbons, F. X. (1993). Social comparison and the pill: Reactions to upward and downward comparison of contraceptive behavior. *Personality and Social Psychology Bulletin, 19,* 13–20.

Rosenberg, P. P. (1984). Support groups: A special therapeutic entity. *Small Group Behavior, 15*(2), 173–186.

Schut, H. A. W., Stroebe, M. S., van den Bout, J., & de Keijser, J. (1997). Intervention for the bereaved: Gender differences in the efficacy of two counselling programmes. *British Journal of Clinical Psychology, 36,* 63–72.

Shedler, J., Mayman, M., & Manis, M. (1993). The illusion of mental health. *American Psychologist, 48,* 1117–1131.

Spiegel, D., Bloom, J. R., Kraemer, H. C., & Gottheil, E. (1989). Effect of psychosocial treatment on survival of patients with metastatic breast cancer. *The Lancet, 2,* 888–891.

Spiegel, D., Bloom, J., & Yalom, I. (1981). Group support for patients with metastatic cancer: A randomized prospective outcome study. *Archives of General Psychiatry, 38,* 527–533.

Taylor, S. E., & Brown, J. D. (1988). Illusion and well-being: A social psychological perspective on mental health. *Psychological Bulletin, 103,* 193–210.

Taylor, S. E., Falke, R. L., Shoptaw, S. J., & Lichtman, R. R. (1986). Social support, support groups, and the cancer patients. *Journal of Consulting and Clinical Psychology, 54,* 608–615.

Ware, J. E., & Sherbourne, C. D. (1992). The MOS 36-item short-form health survey (SF-36): I. Conceptual framework and item selection. *Medical Care, 30,* 473–483.

Watson, D., Clark, L. A., & Tellegen, A. (1988). Development and validation of brief measures of positive and negative affect: The PANAS Scales. *Journal of Personality and Social Psychology, 54,* 1063–1070.

Wills, T. A. (1981). Downward comparison principles in social psychology. *Psychological Bulletin, 90,* 245–271.

Wood, J. V., Taylor, S. E., & Lichtman, R. R. (1985). Social comparison in adjustment to breast cancer. *Journal of Personality and Social Psychology, 49,* 1169–183.

CHAPTER 15

Psychosocial Interventions for Women at Increased Risk for Breast Cancer

Marc D. Schwartz

Caryn Lerman

Barbara Rimer

reast cancer is the most common cancer among American women; more than 180,000 new cases and 46,000 deaths are expected this year (American Cancer Society, 1997). Researchers have identified a number of risk factors for breast cancer. Reproductive risk factors such as early age at menarche, nulliparity, or having a first child after the age of 25 have been found to increase a woman's risk for breast cancer (Gail et al., 1989). Environmental factors such as exposure to exogenous estrogens also increase breast cancer risk (Hoskins et al., 1995), and lifestyle factors such as excessive alcohol use and postmenopausal weight gain have also been implicated in breast cancer etiology (Kelsey & Bernstein, 1996).

A positive family history of breast cancer is perhaps the most important risk factor for breast cancer (Gail et al., 1989; Slattery & Kerber, 1993). Women with a single affected first-degree relative have a twofold to threefold increased breast cancer risk (Anderson, Duffy, Hallett, & Marcus, 1992; Slattery & Kerber, 1993). Those from families with multiple cases of breast or ovarian cancer may be at even higher risk, particularly if the breast cancers were premenopausal or bilateral. About 5–10% of breast cancer cases are attributable to inheritance of a mutation in a breast cancer susceptibility gene (e.g., BRCA1 or BRCA2). Women who have inherited BRCA1 or BRCA2 mutations have a lifetime breast cancer risk of 55–85% (Ford et al., 1994; Struewing et al., 1997), and they are also at increased risk for developing ovarian cancer (Struewing et al., 1997).

Researchers have categorized women with a family history of breast cancer into at least two risk groups. Women with a limited family history of breast cancer have low to moderate risk for developing breast cancer, particularly if the cancers were diagnosed later in life and there are no cases of ovarian cancer in the family (Hoskins et al., 1995). Women who have family histories consistent with hereditary breast cancer have been characterized as high risk (Hoskins et al., 1995; Offit & Brown,

1994). Psychoeducational interventions have targeted women from both of these risk categories (e.g., Kash, Holland, Osborne, & Miller, 1995).

The first three chapters in this section address interventions for cancer patients, which is clearly notable in the extent to which they experience stress and other psychosocial pressures. This chapter addresses different groups of people who also experience considerable distress and worry. In this chapter, we review the literature on psychosocial interventions targeted to women with varying risk of breast cancer. After presenting available data on the psychological and health behavior patterns of low- and moderate-risk women, we present evidence on three types of interventions: (a) breast cancer risk counseling (BCRC), (b) psychosocial interventions, and (c) genetic counseling interventions. We review the existing literature and describe our experiences in evaluating the impact of these interventions, and we discuss future directions for research in these areas.

Perceived Risk, Distress, and Adherence Among Women at Increased Risk

Considerable evidence suggests that women with a family history of breast cancer have inaccurate perceptions of their breast cancer risk. In a study of women who were patients in a high-risk breast cancer surveillance clinic, Kash and colleagues (1992) reported that more than 80% of their sample overestimated their risk of developing breast cancer. Similarly, among 969 women with one or more affected first-degree relatives, 86% overestimated their lifetime breast cancer risk (Daly et al., 1996). Furthermore, perceived risk was unrelated to the presence of objective risk factors. Although the majority of women at high risk for breast cancer overestimate their risk, a substantial minority appear to underestimate their risk. For example, in a study of women with at least one affected relative, Audrain and colleagues (1995) found that 25% of their sample perceived their breast cancer risk to be the same or less than that of women with no family history of breast cancer. Similarly, among women attending a clinic for women with a family history of breast cancer, 88% of the sample exhibited inaccurate risk perceptions (Evans, Burnell, Hopwood, & Howell, 1993). Although 47% of the sample overestimated their risk for breast cancer, 41% underestimated their risk. Despite some inconsistencies regarding the direction of the inaccuracies, evidence clearly demonstrates that first-degree relatives of breast cancer patients do not have an adequate understanding of their own breast cancer risk.

In addition to poor risk comprehension, first-degree relatives of breast cancer patients may also be at risk for psychological distress (Lerman & Schwartz, 1993). For example, in the Kash et al. (1992) study of women attending a high-risk breast cancer surveillance program, 27% of the participants exhibited clinically elevated distress as measured by the Brief Symptom Inventory (Derogatis, 1992). Valdimarsdottir et al. (1995) compared a similar group of high-risk women with a normal risk control group. They found that the high-risk women exhibited elevated distress in anticipation of a screening mammogram. Furthermore, distress remained elevated even after notification of negative screening results. It is possible that only the most distressed individuals are referred to or self-refer to high-risk surveillance programs. Thus, the women in these studies may not be representative of the average woman with a family history of breast cancer (Valdimarsdottir et al., 1995). However, studies in which a more representative sample is recruited by obtaining permission from breast cancer patients to contact their unaffected first-degree relatives have also demonstrated increased distress. Among women with one or more affected relatives, Lerman et al. (1993) found that 53% reported severe intrusive ideation. In separate studies we have found levels of distress that are comparable to those reported by breast cancer patients (Lerman & Schwartz, 1993; Schwartz et al., 1998). Our data suggest that first-degree relatives who overestimate their risk are particularly vulnerable to psychological distress (Audrain et al., 1997; Schwartz, Lerman, Miller, Daly, & Masny, 1995). Thus, intervening to reduce exaggerated risk perceptions could affect psychological distress.

Although inaccurate risk perceptions and elevated psychological distress are important intervention targets in their own right, they may be particularly important because of their association with breast cancer screening utilization. Several studies have documented an inverse association between psychological distress and adherence to breast cancer screening guidelines (Lerman & Schwartz, 1993). For example, in their study of high-risk women, Kash and colleagues (1992) reported that those with elevated distress were less likely to adhere to breast self-examination and clinical breast examination. Lerman et al. (1993) found that high levels of cancer-specific intrusive ideation led to decreased mammography adherence among first-degree relatives of breast cancer patients. In a more recent study of women at moderately increased breast cancer risk, Schwartz, Taylor, et al. (1999) found that high levels of cancer-specific distress were most strongly associated with decreased mammography adherence among women with low levels of conscientiousness.

The results of these studies suggest that women with a family history of breast cancer could benefit from psychosocial interventions designed to improve their risk comprehension, reduce elevated levels of psychological distress, and enhance adherence to breast cancer screening guidelines. With the advent of genetic testing for individuals from high-risk families, even greater attention must be paid to these factors so that individuals can make informed decisions regarding genetic testing. Inaccurate risk comprehension or excessive breast cancer related anxiety could lead individuals to make ill-informed testing decisions.

Breast Cancer Risk Counseling

Breast cancer risk counseling (BCRC) programs were developed prior to the availability of genetic testing for BRCA1 and BRCA2 mutations. Based on the classic genetic counseling model, BCRC was originally intended for women from moderate- and high-risk families. More recently researchers have suggested that BCRC may be most appropriate for women at low to moderate risk (Hoskins et al., 1995). Components of BCRC include a discussion of individual risk factors and recommendations for breast cancer screening. However, the central feature of BCRC is the communication of an individualized breast cancer risk estimate. This risk estimate is typically based on one of two validated quantitative models (Bondy, Lustbader, Halabi, Ross, & Vogel, 1994; Claus, Risch, & Thompson, 1994; Gail et al., 1989). The model developed by Gail et al. considers family history along with other epidemiological risk factors such as age of the respondent, age at menarche, age at first live birth, and previous breast biopsies. The model developed by Claus et al. relies solely on family history information. Both models provide risk estimates for given time intervals (e.g., lifetime risk or risk over the next 10 years). Because of its emphasis on risk factors other than family history, the Gail et al. model is considered more appropriate for moderate-risk women, whereas the emphasis of the Claus et al. model on family history may make it more appropriate for high-risk families (Hoskins et al., 1995). Each model has some limitations. For example, the Gail et al. model was validated on predominantly White women who were getting regular mammograms. Thus, its risk estimates are most applicable to this group. Similarly, the Claus et al. model focuses on familial risk factors and may therefore be less applicable to women without a significant family history of breast cancer (Hoskins et al., 1995).

A Review of the Literature

To date, there has been limited research directly evaluating the impact of BCRC. Two early studies evaluated the impact of providing nonquantitative risk information to first-degree relatives of breast cancer patients. Houts, Wojtkowiak, Simmonds, Weinberg, and Heitjan (1991) conducted telephone counseling sessions in which they informed first-degree relatives of their increased breast cancer risk, provided them with information about breast cancer, and made specific recommendations for breast cancer screening. These individuals ($N = 611$) were compared with a control group of participants who had not yet received a counseling telephone call ($N = 395$). Counseled participants exhibited increased breast cancer knowledge relative to the control group. In terms of breast cancer screening behavior, counseled participants were significantly more likely to perform breast self-exam (49% vs. 39%; odds ratio [OR] = 1.53, 95% confidence interval [CI] = 1.08, 2.17) and more likely to have obtained a mammogram since their counseling session (39% vs. 30%; OR = 1.57, 95% CI = 1.03, 2.40). The authors did not investigate the impact of the intervention on risk comprehension or psychological distress.

Similarly, Curry, Taplin, Anderman, Barlow, and McBride (1993) tested the impact on mammography rates of providing individualized breast cancer risk information. Although participants ($N = 2,076$) included women with and without a family history of breast cancer, the investigators examined the impact of the intervention among women with a positive breast cancer family history. They found that first-degree relatives who received mammography invitations that included personalized risk information had a higher rate of subsequent mammography (67%) compared with women who received general risk information (43%). The investigators did not examine the impact of this information on perceived risk or psychological distress.

More recent studies have provided participants with quantitative risk estimates. Evans and colleagues (Evan, Blair, Greenhalgh, Hopwood, & Howell, 1994) evaluated the impact of BCRC on risk perception among a group of women attending a breast cancer family history clinic. Some of the women were referred by a physician, but the majority were self-referred. All participants had at least one first-degree relative with breast cancer. However, many had multiple affected relatives. Participants were interviewed by a geneticist or oncologist, and a family pedigree was constructed. Lifetime risk estimates were generated using the Claus et al. (1994) model and communicated to participants in the form of a probability (e.g., your lifetime risk of breast cancer is 1 in 8). Perceived risk was assessed by asking participants to select their lifetime risk from one of 13 possible risk levels (ranging from inevitable to less than 1 in 100). Although the total study sample consisted of 517 women, only 78 had completed both the baseline and follow-up surveys at the time of publication. At baseline, less than 8% of this sample chose the correct level of risk, and only 46% of this sample chose a risk level within 50% of their true risk. However, following counseling, 39% of the sample chose the correct risk level and 67% were within 50% of their true risk level. The investigators also reported high rates of clinic reattendance for mammography screening. The impact of this intervention on psychological distress was not evaluated.

Report of Our Research

We have conducted the only published randomized clinical trial of BCRC. We compared BCRC with a general health counseling (GHC) control intervention (Lerman, Rimer, et al., 1994). Participants were women with at least one affected first-degree relative. The majority of study participants had a single affected relative, although 11% had two or more affected relatives. Patients were asked for permission to contact their unaffected first-degree relatives. First-degree relatives of those patients who provided permission were contacted for a baseline telephone interview during which we assessed the following variables: breast cancer risk factors, sociodemographic characteristics, risk perceptions, psychological distress, and breast cancer screening utilization. Following the interview participants were invited to attend a free individual counseling session. All participants who accepted were randomized to either the BCRC intervention or the GHC control intervention. Follow-up interviews were conducted 3 and 12 months after intervention.

The single-session BCRC intervention was conducted by a nurse educator and included the following elements: (a) discussion of individual risk factors, (b) presentation of individualized Gail et al. model risk estimates, and (c) recommendation for annual mammography, clinical breast exam, and monthly breast self-examination. Risk figures were presented to participants as absolute risks (e.g., you have an X% risk of developing breast cancer by the age of 70) and as relative risks (e.g., your risk of developing breast cancer by the age of 70 is 1 in X).

The GHC control intervention was chosen to control for the effects of having an individual session with a nurse educator and consisted of the following elements: (a) interview assessment of current health practices, (b) age-specific recommendations for a variety of cancer screening tests, (c) encouragement to quit smoking (if she smokes), (d) suggestions for reducing dietary fat to no more than 30% of daily calories, and (e) recommendations for regular aerobic exercise.

Although the final sample included 430 women who completed a counseling visit and a 12-month follow-up interview, interim analyses conducted at the 3-month follow-up assessment included fewer participants. The final sample was predominantly White and well-educated. Compared with individuals who had declined participation or who did not attend their scheduled counseling session, those who completed the study were more likely to be married, more highly educated, more likely to be between ages 40–49, and more concerned about their risk for breast cancer (Lerman, Rimer, et al., 1994).

The first outcome that we evaluated was risk comprehension (Lerman et al., 1995). During the baseline and follow-up interviews, we assessed risk perception by asking participants to rate their chances of getting breast cancer during their lifetimes on a scale from 0 (*definitely will not get it*) to 100 (*definitely will get it*). We created a categorical risk comprehension variable by (a) subtracting each participant's perceived risk rating from her estimated objective risk and (b) classifying individuals into the following categories: extreme overestimators (perceived risk higher than the highest possible Gail score for someone of the same age); overestimators (perceived risk more than 10% higher than objective score, but not higher than the highest possible Gail score); accurate (perceived risk within 10% in either direction of estimated objective risk); and underestimator (perceived risk more than 10% below objective risk).

At baseline, the BCRC group ($N = 90$) and the GHC group ($N = 110$) did not differ on risk comprehension; nearly 90% of the sample fell into the overestimator or extreme overestimator categories. To evaluate the impact of the BCRC intervention, we examined improvements in risk comprehension (i.e., movement into a more accurate risk comprehension category) from baseline to the 3-month follow-up. After controlling for confounding demographic and risk factor variables, group assignment was associated with improvement in risk comprehension. BCRC participants were significantly more likely to have improved risk comprehension compared with GHC participants (OR = 3.49, 95% CI = 1.28, 9.48). Despite this significant effect, the majority of individuals in both groups (GHC = 89%; BCRC = 82%) continued to overestimate their risk. Furthermore, there was evidence that BCRC was less effective among women who had high levels of baseline cancer-related distress.

Next, we evaluated the impact of the BCRC intervention on psychological distress at the 3-month follow-up (Lerman et al., 1996). We measured general distress with the Profile of Mood States (POMS; McNair, Lorr, & Droppleman, 1971) and cancer-specific distress with the intrusion subscale of the Impact of Event Scale (IES; Horowitz, Wilner, & Alvarez, 1979). We conducted two hierarchical multiple regression analyses to evaluate the impact of BCRC versus GHC on each of these outcomes. After controlling for baseline IES score, perceived risk, and the index patients' age at diagnosis, treatment group was marginally associated with cancer-specific distress. Individuals in the BCRC group exhibited less distress than those in the GHC group (R^2 change = .01, p = .06). However, this effect was modified by an interaction with education level (R^2 change = .02, p < .05). Simple effects analysis revealed that BCRC was particularly effective among less educated participants (see Figure 15.1). Using an identical analytic strategy, we did not find a significant effect of BCRC on general psychological distress.

FIGURE 15.1

Impact of breast cancer risk counseling and education (ed) level on cancer-specific distress, measured at baseline and 3 months (mos). IES = Impact of Event Scale. From "Psychological Impact of Breast Cancer Risk Counseling: Interacting Effects of Coping Style and Education," by C. Lerman, M. Schwartz, S. Miller, M. Daly, Sands, C., and B. Rimer, 1996, Health Psychology, 15, p. 80. Copyright 1996 by the American Psychological Association. Reprinted with permission.

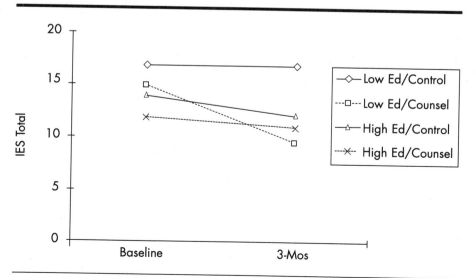

Finally, we evaluated the impact of BCRC on mammography utilization among the sample of 430 participants who completed the baseline and 12-month follow-up assessments (Schwartz, Rimer, Daly, Sands, & Lerman, 1999). The two intervention groups did not differ in their baseline mammography use [BCRC = 75%; GHC = 71%; $\chi(1, N = 430) = 1.2, p > .10$] or follow-up use [BCRC = 69%; GHC = 75%; $\chi(1, N = 430) = 2.3, p > .10$]. We conducted a logistic regression analysis to determine whether BCRC affected mammography after adjusting for potential confounding variables (baseline mammography utilization, ethnicity, age, time since diagnosis, education). We found a significant main effect for group (OR = 0.4, 95% CI = 0.2, 0.8) that was modified by education level (OR = 2.6, 95% CI = 1.1, 6.3). As shown in Figure 15.2, BCRC was less effective than GHC among less educated participants (OR = 0.4, 95% CI = 0.2, 0.8). In an unpublished analysis from this same dataset, we compared mammography utilization in the two intervention groups with that of individuals who had declined participation in the study (including those who had agreed to participate but did not attend their scheduled counseling session). These groups did not differ in mammography adherence at

FIGURE 15.2

Impact of breast cancer risk counseling (BCRC) and education level on mammography utilization. GHC = general health counseling. From "A Randomized Trial of Breast Cancer Risk Counseling: The Impact Upon Mammography Utilization," by M. D. Schwartz, B. K. Rimer, M. Daly, C. Sands, and C. Lerman, 1999, American Journal of Public Health, 89, p. 925. Copyright 1999 by the American Public Health Association. Reprinted with permission.

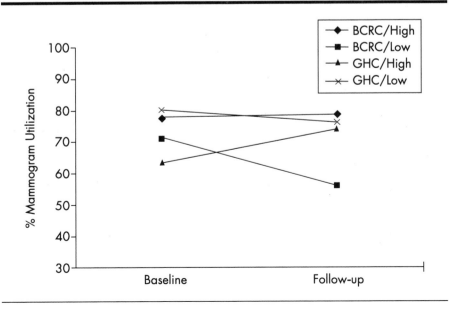

baseline. However, at the 12-month follow-up, participants in both the BCRC (OR = 2.2, 95% CI = 1.2, 3.9) and GHC (OR = 2.4, 95% CI = 1.4, 4.7) groups exhibited significantly higher adherence compared with decliners.

The results of these studies suggest moderate effects for BCRC. Following BCRC, participants in both the Lerman et al. (1993) and Evans et al. (1994) studies demonstrated improved risk comprehension. However, the majority of participants in both of these studies continued to report inaccurate breast cancer risk perceptions. Although this is consistent with research suggesting that individuals have great difficulty interpreting quantitative risk figures (Fischhoff, Bostrom, & Quadrel, 1993), it clearly demonstrates the need for research that focuses on new methods for enhancing risk comprehension in this population. Similarly, BCRC also had a modest impact upon distress, but the effect was considerably stronger among less educated participants. It is not clear why BCRC had stronger effects on less educated participants. However, the importance of education as a moderator of BCRC is further underscored by the finding that BCRC was particularly ineffective at enhancing mammography utilization among less educated participants. It is possible that this group experienced false reassurance, which led to both decreased distress and decreased screening utilization. However, we could not find evidence for such mediation in our follow-up analyses.

Psychosocial Interventions

We were able to identify only two published studies of psychoeducational interventions for women at high risk for breast cancer (Kash et al., 1995; Schwartz et al., 1998). Compared with published examples of BCRC, these interventions focused primarily on distress reduction rather than risk communication. Both studies used coping skills training to promote active coping and reduce avoidant coping. One of these studies also focused on provision of social support. The central premise of these interventions is that by fostering adaptive coping, distress can be reduced and screening adherence improved. Although risk information was provided to participants in both studies, the emphasis was on the psychosocial rather than risk-communication aspects of the intervention.

Kash and colleagues (Kash, Holland, Osborne, & Miller, 1995) conducted a preliminary investigation of a group psychoeducational intervention for women at high risk for breast cancer. Participants (N = 40) were randomly assigned to receive the experimental intervention or to a nonintervention control condition. The experimental intervention was a structured 6-week group intervention consisting of the following components: (a) breast cancer education and risk communication using individualized risk estimates from the Claus model, (b) coping skills training, and (c) group social support.

Preliminary results of this trial were promising. Participants who received the experimental intervention exhibited significant improvements in knowledge and risk comprehension and a significant decrease in perceived barriers to mammography relative to the control participants. In terms of screening, participants in the experimental intervention group exhibited increased mammography, clinical breast examination, and breast self-examination in the year following the intervention.

We have recently completed a randomized clinical trial comparing a brief coping skills intervention with a GHC control intervention among women with a recently diagnosed first-degree relative. Participants were randomly assigned to receive brief problem-solving training (PST) or GHC. Counseling sessions were conducted individually during a 2-hour session with a health educator. Both groups received identical information about breast cancer risk factors and breast cancer screening guidelines. However, individualized risk estimates were not provided to either group. In addition to the standard discussion of risk factors, PST participants received PST as outlined by D'Zurilla (1988). PST consists of four components: (a) training in problem definition, (b) brainstorming for potential coping strategies, (c) evaluation of potential coping strategies, and (d) implementation of chosen coping strategy and evaluation of its effectiveness.

First, we evaluated the impact of PST on cancer-specific and general psychological distress (Schwartz et al., 1998). We measured cancer-specific distress with the intrusion and avoidance scales of the IES. We measured general distress with the POMS Total Mood Disturbance score. The baseline and follow-up means and standard deviations of these variables are displayed in Table 15.1. We conducted three separate 2 (group) $\times$ 2 (time of assessment) mixed-factor analyses of variance to evaluate the impact of PST on each of our outcome variables. There was a significant effect for time of assessment on each of the three outcomes, suggesting overall declines in distress from baseline to the 3-month follow-up. However, the absence of the predicted group by time interaction effects suggested that PST did not have a beneficial impact relative to GHC (Schwartz et al., 1998). However, when PST

TABLE 15.1

Psychological distress at baseline and follow-up

	IES		POMS	
GROUP	**M**	**SD**	**M**	**SD**
GHC (N = 197)				
Baseline	19.6	14.2	29.5	30.9
3 months	15.6	12.2	22.6	29.1
PST (N = 144)				
Baseline	20.0	14.4	24.5	32.1
3 months	14.0	12.9	22.6	29.1

Note. IES = Impact of Event Scale; POMS = Profile of Mood States; GHC = general health counseling; PST = problem-solving training.

participants were divided into those who reported using the PST techniques ($N =$ 72) and those who reported that they did not use the techniques ($N = 72$), significant effects emerged. Using 3 (PST users vs. PST nonusers vs. GHC) $\times$ 2 (time of assessment) mixed-factor analyses of variance, we found significant Group $\times$ Time interactions for both intrusive ideation, $F(1, 71) = 9.2$, $p = .003$, and avoidant ideation, $F(1, 71) = 4.9$, $p = .008$. These interactions are displayed in Figures 15.3 and 15.4. Post hoc comparisons revealed that PST users exhibited significantly greater decreases in both intrusive and avoidant ideation than did PST nonusers and GHC participants ($p < .05$). There was no effect of PST practice on general psychological distress. Furthermore, analyses examining the impact of PST on cancer screening behaviors revealed no significant effects of the treatment of breast self-examination (Audrain et al., 1998) or mammography.

These studies suggest that a single-session coping skills intervention may be effective at reducing distress for only the most motivated participants. Future inter-

FIGURE 15.3

Impact of problem-solving training (PST) on cancer-specific distress, measured at baseline and 3 months (mos). GHC = general health counseling; IES = Impact of Event Scale. From "The Impact of a Brief Problem-Solving Training Intervention for Relatives of Recently Diagnosed Breast Cancer Patients," by M. D. Schartz, C. Lerman, J. Audrain, D. Cella, J. Garber, B. Rimer, T. Lin, M. Stefanek, and V. Vogel, 1998, Annals of Behavioral Medicine, 20, *p. 10. Copyright 1998 by the Society of Behavioral Medicine. Reprinted with permission.*

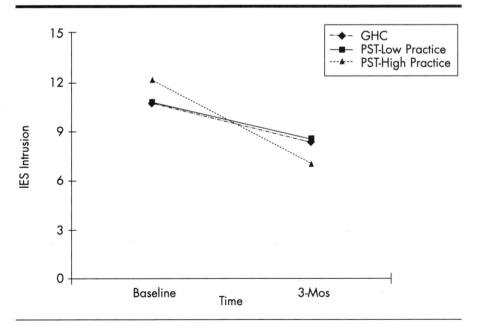

FIGURE 15.4

Impact of problem-solving training (PST) on general distress, measured at baseline and 3 months (mos). GHC = general health counseling; IES = Impact of Event Scale. From "The Impact of a Brief Problem-Solving Training Intervention for Relatives of Recently Diagnosed Breast Cancer Patients," by M. D. Schartz, C. Lerman, J. Audrain, D. Cella, J. Garber, B. Rimer, T. Lin, M. Stefanek, and V. Vogel, 1998, Annals of Behavioral Medicine, 20, *p. 10. Copyright 1998 by the Society of Behavioral Medicine. Reprinted with permission.*

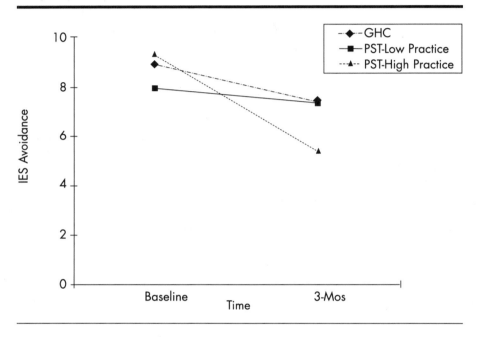

ventions could focus on those individuals who are at the most risk for psychological distress. The relative success of the intervention by Kash et al. (1995) could be partially due to the motivation of the participants as well as the higher intensity of the intervention. Participants in this study were individuals who had self-selected into a breast cancer high-risk program. These individuals may have been more motivated to participate in six-session psychosocial intervention.

Genetic Counseling Interventions

In response to the isolation of the BRCA1 and BRCA2 genes, biotechnology companies are already marketing genetic tests to health care providers and to the public. Initial studies indicate strong interest in BRCA1 testing in the general public and in populations at high risk (Chaliki et al., 1995; Lerman, Daly, et al., 1994; Tambor, Rimer, & Strigo, 1997). However, the optimal strategies for educating and counseling individuals have yet to be determined.

We conducted a study to evaluate the impact of alternate strategies for pretest education and counseling on decision making regarding BRCA1 and BRCA2 testing among women at low to moderate risk of breast cancer (Lerman, Biesecker, et al., 1997). A randomized trial design was used to evaluate the effects of education only (educational approach) and education plus counseling (counseling approach), as compared with a waiting-list (control) condition ($N = 400$ for all groups combined). The educational approach reviewed information about personal risk factors; inheritance of cancer susceptibility; the benefits, limitations, and risks of BRCA1 and BRCA2 testing; and cancer screening and prevention options. The counseling approach included this information, as well as a personalized discussion of experiences with cancer in the family and the potential psychological and social impact of testing. Data on knowledge of inherited cancer and BRCA1 and BRCA2 test characteristics, perceived risk, perceived benefits, limitations and risks of BRCA1 and BRCA2 testing, and testing intentions were collected by use of structured telephone interviews at baseline and at 1-month follow-up. Provision of a blood sample for future testing served as a proxy measure of intention to be tested (in the education and counseling arms of the study).

The effects of intervention group on study outcomes were evaluated by use of hierarchical linear regression modeling and logistic regression modeling (for the blood sample outcome). The educational and counseling approaches both led to significant increases in knowledge, relative to the control condition ($R^2 = .18$, $p < .001$, for both). The counseling approach, but not the educational approach, was superior to the control condition in producing significant increases in perceived limitations and risks of BRCA1 and BRCA2 testing ($R^2 = .18$, $p < .01$) and decreases in perceived benefits ($R^2 = .01$, $p < .05$). However, neither approach produced changes in intentions to have BRCA1 and BRCA2 testing. Prior to and following both education only and education plus counseling, approximately one-half of participants stated that they intended to be tested; after the session, 52% provided a blood sample.

Thus, the results of this initial study suggest that standard educational approaches may be as effective as expanded counseling approaches in enhancing knowledge. Because knowledge is a key aspect of medical decision making, standard education may be adequate in situations where genetic testing must be streamlined. On the other hand, it has been argued that optimal decision making requires not only knowledge but also a reasoned evaluation of the positive and negative consequences of alternate decisions. Although the counseling approach is more likely to achieve this goal, it may not diminish interest in testing, even among women at low to moderate risk.

In a follow-up analysis, we investigated ethnic differences in responses to the alternate BRCA1 and BRCA2 pretest education strategies (Lerman et al., 1999): African American women were found to differ from White women in the effects of the interventions on testing intentions, provision of a blood sample, and psychological distress. Specifically, use of the expanded counseling model with African American women led to greater increases than education only in intentions to be tested and provision of a blood sample. Marginally greater increases in cancer-specific distress were also found for African American women who received the expanded counseling. These effects were independent of socioeconomic status and referral mechanisms. In White women, there were no differential effects of the interventions on these outcomes. Thus, in low- to moderate-risk African American women, pretest education may motivate, rather than deter, BRCA1 and BRCA2 testing.

Evidence suggesting individual differences in responses to genetic counseling has prompted investigation of the use of tailored messages in this context. Rimer and colleagues are conducting a randomized trial in which probands (women who have had breast or ovarian cancer) and their relatives are randomized to receive either standard pretest education printed materials or tailored materials. The tailored print materials are individually created booklets that not only give women personalized and individualized estimates of the risk of having a mutation but also respond to a variety of personal concerns and situations. The data collected to date suggest a significant difference in knowledge between women in the tailored and standard materials conditions. Women who received the tailored materials were significantly more knowledgeable about genetic testing at the 2-week follow up.

Future Directions

The results of the studies conducted to date on BCRC with high-risk relatives and women who had breast or ovarian cancer are promising. There is some evidence that BCRC can have a positive impact on several important outcomes, including knowledge (e.g., Kash et al, 1995), understanding of personal risk (Evans et al., 1994; Lerman et al., 1995), and certain aspects of psychological distress (Lerman et al., 1996). Certainly, the results of these and other studies, although modest, suggest that in-person counseling approaches deserve further exploration.

Yet, in-person counseling strategies can be delivered to only a small proportion of the people who need and want information. Thus, other strategies should be developed to augment the small number of genetic counselors available in the United States today. Two methods that may be applicable are tailored print communications and tailored telephone counseling. Both tailored print communications and tailored telephone counseling are based on the assumption that counseling and education can be individualized to people on the basis of information that is known about them (e.g., their risk of having a BRCA1 and BRCA2 mutation, their reasons to be tested or not tested, and their personal health history).

Tailored print communications are print materials designed especially for an individual on the basis of information known or obtained about that person (Rimer & Glassman, 1999). More than 12 of these studies now have been reported, and most have shown either main effects or significant interactions. Moreover, there is evidence that tailored print communications may be especially appealing to African Americans (Skinner, Strecher, & Hospers, 1994). In the area of BCRC, these can provide information about a woman's chances of having a genetic mutation, the benefits and limitations of testing for her, and other sources of information. Such a strategy could be used to help women develop more realistic assessments of personal risk, perhaps decreasing the burden on scarce medical resources, including genetic counselors. Moreover, the use of tailored print communications may have additional advantages because they can be used by a woman on her own, at her own pace, and shared with significant others.

Tailored telephone counseling is another strategy that can be used to extend scarce resources and to provide counseling in a manner that is personalized, convenient, and cost-effective. Telephone counseling strategies can be used to deliver services without requiring women to take time from work or family or drive long distances. Telephone counseling has been proven effective in a number of areas, including mammography (Houts et al., 1991; King, Rimer, Seay, Balshem, & Engstrom, 1994), cervical cancer screening, and colposcopy use (Lerman et al., 1992; Miller et al., 1997). In at least one study, the combination of tailored print communications and tailored telephone counseling increased the proportion of women who were on schedule for cancer screening (Rimer et al., 1999).

Among the many future challenges are the development of cost-effective strategies to reach diverse populations of women with personalized information about breast cancer risk and options for genetic testing. Although in-person counseling may be the gold standard, a menu of options should be available to meet the needs of women at higher risk for breast cancer.

References

American Cancer Society. (1997). *Cancer facts and figures—1997.* Atlanta, GA: Author.

Anderson, D. M., Duffy, K., Hallett, C. D., & Marcus, A. C. (1992). Cancer prevention counseling on telephone helplines. *Public Health Reports, 107,* 278–283.

Audrain, J., Lerman, C., Rimer, B., Cella, D., Steffens, R., & Gomez-Caminero, A. (1995). Awareness of heightened breast cancer risk among first degree relatives of newly diagnosed breast cancer patients. *Cancer Epidemiology, Biomarkers and Prevention, 4,* 561–565.

Audrain, J., Rimer, B., Cella, D., Stefanek, M., Garber, J., Pennanen, M., Helzlsouer, K., Vogel, V., Lin, T. H., & Lerman, C. (1998). The impact of a coping skills intervention on breast-self examination in relatives of newly diagnosed breast cancer patients. *Psycho-Oncology, 8,* 220–229.

Audrain, J., Schwartz, M. D., Lerman, C., Hughes, C., Peshkin, B. N., & Biesecker, B. (1997). Psychological distress in women seeking genetic counseling for breast-ovarian cancer risk: The contributions of personality and appraisal. *Annals of Behavioral Medicine, 19,* 370–377.

Bondy, M. L., Lustbader, E. D., Halabi, S., Ross, E., & Vogel, V. G. (1994). Validation of a breast cancer risk assessment model in women with a positive family history. *Journal of the National Cancer Institute, 86,* 620–625.

Chaliki, H., Lauder, S., Levenkron, J., Logan-Young, W., Hall, W. J., & Rowley, P. T. (1995). Women's receptivity to testing for a genetic susceptibility to breast cancer. *American Journal of Public Health, 85,* 1133–1135.

Claus, E. R., Risch, N., & Thompson, W. D. (1994). Autosomal dominant inheritance of early onset breast cancer. *Cancer, 73,* 643–651.

Curry, S. J., Taplin, S. H., Anderman, C., Barlow, W. E., & McBride, C. (1993). A randomized trial of the impact of risk assessment and feedback on participation in mammography screening. *Preventive Medicine, 22,* 350–360.

Daly, M. B., Lerman, C., Ross, E., Schwartz, M. D., Sands, C., & Rimer, B. K. (1996). Gail model breast cancer risk components are poor predictors of risk perception and screening behavior. *Breast Cancer Research and Treatment, 41,* 59–70.

Derogatis, L. R. (1992). *Brief Symptom Inventory: Administration, scoring, and procedures manual–II.* Baltimore: Clinical Psychometric Research.

D'Zurilla,T. J. (1988). *Problem-solving therapy: A social competence approach to clinical intervention.* New York: Springer.

Evans, D. G., Blair, V., Greenhalgh, R., Hopwood, P., & Howell, A. (1994). The impact of genetic counseling on risk perception in women with a family history of breast cancer. *British Journal of Cancer, 70,* 934–938.

Evans, D. G. R., Burnell, L. D., Hopwood, P., & Howell, A. (1993). Perception of risk in women with a family history of breast cancer. *British Journal of Cancer, 67,* 612–614.

Fischhoff, B., Bostrom, A., & Quadrel, M. J. (1993). Risk perception and communication. *Annual Review of Public Health, 14,* 183–203.

Ford, D., Easton, D. F., Bishop, D. T., Narod, S. A., Goldgar, D. E., & the Breast Cancer Linkage Consortium. (1994). Risks of cancer in BRCA1-mutation carriers. *Lancet, 343,* 692–695.

Gail, M. H., Brinton, L. A., Byar, D. P., Corle, D. K., Green, S. B., Schairer, C., & Mulvihill, J. J. (1989). Projecting individualized probabilities of developing breast cancer for white females who are being screened annually. *Journal of the National Cancer Institute, 81,* 1879–1886.

Horowitz, M., Wilner, N., & Alvarez, W. (1979). Impact of Event Scale: A measure of subjective stress. *Psychosomatic Medicine, 41,* 209–218.

Hoskins, K. F., Stopfer, J. E., Calzone, K. A., Merajver, S. D., Rebbeck, T. R., Garber, J. E., & Weber, B. L. (1995). Assessment and counseling for women with a family history of breast cancer. *Journal of the American Medical Association, 273,* 577–585.

Houts, P. S., Wojtkowiak, S. L., Simmonds, M. A., Weinberg, G. B., & Heitjan, D. F. (1991). Using a state cancer registry to increase screening behaviors of sisters and daughters of breast cancer patients. *American Journal of Public Health, 81,* 386–388.

Kash, K. M., Holland, J. C., Halper, M. S., & Miller, D. G. (1992). Psychological distress and surveillance behaviors in women with a family history of breast cancer. *Journal of the National Cancer Institute, 84,* 24–30.

Kash, K. M., Holland, J. C., Osborne, M. P., & Miller, D. G. (1995). Psychological counseling strategies for women at risk for breast cancer. *Journal of the National Cancer Institute Monographs, 17,* 73–80.

Kelsey, J. L., & Bernstein, L. (1996). Epidemiology and prevention of breast cancer. *Annual Review of Public Health, 17,* 47–67.

King, E., Rimer, B. K., Seay, J., Balshem, A., & Engstrom, P. F. (1994). Promoting mammography use through progressive interventions: Is it effective? *American Journal of Public Health, 84,* 104–106.

Lerman, C., Biesecker, B., Benkendorf, J. L., Kerner, J., Gomez-Caminero, A., Hughes, C., & Reed, M. R. (1997). Controlled trial of pretest education approaches to enhance informed decision-making for BRCA1 gene testing. *Journal of the National Cancer Institute, 89,* 148–157.

Lerman, C., Daly, M., Masny, M., & Balshem, A. (1994). Attitudes about genetic testing for breast–ovarian cancer susceptibility. *Journal of Clinical Oncology, 12,* 843–850.

Lerman, C., Daly, M., Sands, C., Balshem, A., Lustbader, E., Heggan, T., Goldstein, L., James, J., & Engstrom, P. (1993). Mammography adherence and psychological distress among women at risk for breast cancer. *Journal of the National Cancer Institute, 85,* 1074–1080.

Lerman, C., Hanjani, P., Caputo, C., Miller, S., Delmoor, E., Nolte, S., & Engstrom, P. (1992). Telephone counseling improves adherence to colposcopy among lower income minority women. *Journal of Clinical Oncology, 27,* 283–286.

Lerman, C., Hughes, C., Benkendorf, J. L., Biesecker, B., Kerner, J., Willison, J., Eads, N., Hadley, D., & Lynch, J. (1999). Racial differences in testing motivation and psychological distress following pre-test education for BRCA1 gene testing. *Cancer Epidemiology Biomarkers and Prevention, 8,* 361–367.

Lerman, C., Lustbader, E., Rimer, B., Daly, M., Miller, S., Sands, C., & Balshem, A. (1995). Effects of individualized breast cancer risk counseling: A randomized trial. *Journal of the National Cancer Institute, 87,* 286–292.

Lerman, C. L., Rimer, B. K., Daly, M., Lustbader, E., Sands, C., Balshem, A., Masny, A., & Engstrom, P. (1994). Recruiting high risk women into a breast cancer health promotion trial. *Cancer Epidemiology, Biomarkers, and Prevention, 3,* 271–276.

Lerman, C., & Schwartz, M. (1993). Adherence and psychological adjustment in women at high risk for breast cancer. *Breast Cancer Research and Treatment, 28,* 145–155.

Lerman, C., Schwartz, M., Miller, S., Daly, M., Sands, C., & Rimer, B. (1996). Psychological impact of breast cancer risk counseling: Interacting effects of coping style and education. *Health Psychology, 15,* 75–83.

McNair, D., Lorr, M., & Droppleman, L. (1971). *Profile of Mood States.* San Diego, CA: Educational and Industrial Testing Service.

Miller, S. M., Siejak, K. K., Schroeder, C. M., Lerman, C., Hernandez, E., & Helm, C. W. (1997). Enhancing adherence following abnormal Pap smears among low-income minority women: A preventive telephone counseling strategy. *Journal of the National Cancer Institute, 89,* 703–708.

Offit, K., & Brown, K. (1994). Quantitating familial cancer risk: A resource for clinical oncologists. *Journal of Clinical Oncology, 12,* 1724–1736.

Rimer, B. K., Conaway, M., Lyna, P., Glassman, B., Yarnall, K., Lipkus, I., & Barber, T. (1999). The impact of tailored interventions on a community health center population. *Patient Education & Counseling, 37,* 171–178.

Rimer, B. K., & Glassman, B. (1999). Is there a use for tailored print communications in cancer risk communication? *Journal of the National Cancer Institute Monographs, 25,* 140–148.

Schwartz, M. D., Lerman, C., Audrain, J., Cella, D., Garber, J., Rimer, B., Lin, T., Stefanek, M., & Vogel, V. (1998). The impact of a brief problem-solving training intervention for relatives of recently diagnosed breast cancer patients. *Annals of Behavioral Medicine, 20,* 7–12.

Schwartz, M. D., Lerman, C., Miller, S., Daly, M., & Masny, A. (1995). Coping disposition, perceptions of risk, and psychological distress among women at high risk for ovarian cancer. *Health Psychology, 14,* 232–235.

Schwartz, M. D., Rimer, B. K., Daly, M., Sands, C., & Lerman, C. (1999). A randomized trial of breast cancer risk counseling: The impact upon mammography utilization. *American Journal of Public Health, 89,* 924–926.

Schwartz, M. D., Taylor, K. L., Lamdan, R., Seigal, J., Willard, K., & Moran, K. (1999). Distress, personality and mammography utilization among women at risk for breast cancer. *Health Psychology, 18,* 327–332.

Skinner, C. S., Strecher, V. J., & Hospers, H. (1994). Physician recommendations for mammography: Do tailored messages make a difference? *American Journal of Public Health, 84,* 43–49.

Slattery, M. L., & Kerber, R. A. (1993). A comprehensive evaluation of family history and breast cancer risk: The Utah population database. *Journal of the American Medical Association, 270,* 1563–1568.

Struewing, J. P., Hartge, P., Wacholder, S., Baker, S. M., Berlin, M., McAdams, M., Timmerman, M. M., Brody, L. C., & Tucker, M. A. (1997). The risk of cancer associated with specific mutations of BRCA1 and BRCA2 among Ashkenazi Jews. *New England Journal of Medicine, 15,* 1401–1408.

Tambor, E. S., Rimer, B. K., & Strigo, T. S. (1997). Genetic testing for breast cancer susceptibility: Awareness and interest among women in the general population. *American Journal of Medical Genetics, 68,* 43–49.

Valdimarsdottir, H. B., Bovbjerg, D. H., Kash, K. M., Holland, J. C., Osborne, M. P., & Miller, D. G. (1995). Psychological distress in women with a familial risk of breast cancer. *Psycho-Oncology, 4,* 133–141.

CHAPTER 16

Interventions for Healthy Individuals at Familial Risk for Cancer

Biobehavioral Mechanisms for Health Benefits

Dana H. Bovbjerg
Heiddis B. Valdimarsdottir

There is now overwhelming evidence that heredity plays a significant role in an individual's risk of cancer. One compelling example is breast cancer. Healthy women with a history of breast cancer in one or more first-degree relatives are now widely known to be at increased risk of developing the disease themselves. Indeed, family history is the strongest predictor that a woman will develop the disease at some point during her life. For breast cancer (as for a growing number of other cancers recognized to have a hereditary component), specific genetic abnormalities are increasingly known but not yet translated into clinically useful tools for widespread screening. The vast majority of women who have family histories of breast cancer must thus live with the threat that their health and even life may be claimed at any time. The psychological reactions of women to that stressor may result in additional risks to their health through at least three basic pathways (as shown in Figure 16.1): (a) high levels of fear and distress may have negative consequences on immune defenses against cancer; (b) high levels of fear and distress may have negative effects on health behaviors thought to affect cancer incidence (e.g., increased alcohol consumption); and (c) high levels of fear and distress may inhibit appropriate breast cancer screening behaviors, resulting in late detection and reduced likelihood of curative treatment. Cognitive–behavioral interventions designed to reduce fear and distress about cancer could thus have beneficial effects on health by influencing one or more of these pathways.

In this chapter, we briefly highlight the largely independent research literatures that provide the current evidence supporting this biobehavioral stress model. We begin by providing an overview of the now voluminous literature linking family histories of breast cancer with increased cancer incidence. We then review the

FIGURE 16.1

Schematic of pathways by which stress associated with having a family history of cancer may influence health.

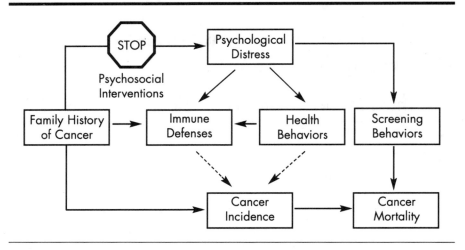

accumulating evidence that familial risk of breast cancer is associated with increased levels of distress, which can have a negative influence on health and screening behaviors known to affect cancer risk. The large literature indicating that distress can affect immune function is then highlighted. We then examine the evidence indicating that healthy individuals with family histories of cancer may have deficits in immune function, which according to theories of immune surveillance may lead to increased risk of developing cancer. We discuss the possibility that these deficits in immune function, previously attributed to inherited deficits in the immune system, may be due to higher levels of distress in women at familial risk. We conclude by noting the importance of additional research to concurrently examine these pathways to explore causal relations and possible health benefits, and we note the importance of developing effective cognitive–behavioral interventions.

Family History as a Risk Factor for Breast Cancer

The strongest predictor of a woman's lifetime risk of developing breast cancer is a family history of the disease (consistent with risk estimates for most common cancers; (see Figure 16.1; Harris, Lippman, Veronesi, & Willett, 1992). The risk that a healthy woman will develop breast cancer increases with the number of affected individuals in her family. For example, the relative risk of breast cancer for a woman with a single first-degree relative with breast cancer has been estimated as 1.5 to 2; with two first-degree relatives, estimates range from 4 to 6 relative risk. The relative risk is increased still further if the breast cancer in the affected relative was bilateral or occurred at an early age (Anderson, 1992; Harris et al., 1992). The individuals at highest risk are those with particular patterns of cancer in their family consistent with Mendelian segregation of autosomal dominant gene (Ford, Easton, & Peto, 1995). Recent molecular studies have identified two genes, BRCA1 on chromosome 17 and BRCA2 on chromosome 13, and it is now believed that mutations in these genes account for the majority of breast cancer cases in families with multiple affected relatives (Ford et al., 1995).

However, even in families with multiple instances of cancer associated with a known mutation in BRCA1 or BRCA2, the presence of the mutation may be necessary but not sufficient to account for the development of breast cancer; the presence of other genes and environmental factors may also be important (Schatzkin, Goldstein, & Freedman, 1995). Consistent with this possibility, there have been reports of BRCA2 mutation carriers who are still cancer-free over the age of 70 as well as data suggesting that entire families may show a consistent pattern of late-onset breast cancer in mutation carriers (Friend, 1996; Thorlacius et al., 1996). The factors that determine why some mutation carriers develop breast cancer late in life, or not at all, are not yet known (Friend, 1996). Because the immune system plays a role in eliminating cells expressing neoplastic mutations, it is possible that strong immune defenses may protect against the development of breast cancer in these women.

The role of mutations in BRCA1 and BRCA2 in women from families with less than four affected relatives is not yet clear (Ford & Easton, 1995). Nearly all data on the effects of mutations in these primary susceptibility genes have come from families with large numbers of affected relatives, which may introduce ascertainment bias, making it difficult to extrapolate to the population at large (Ford & Easton, 1995; Schatzkin et al., 1995). Indeed, recent data suggest that these genes may account for only 40–50% of hereditary cases, much lower than previously thought (Couch et al., 1997). Although epidemiological data indicate that a woman with even one first-degree relative with breast cancer (under the age of 50) has a significantly increased risk, the genetic mechanisms are not known (Ford & Easton, 1995; Ford et al., 1995). In some cases, mutations in BRCA1 or BRCA2 may be involved, but other genes and shared environmental influences are likely to play a more central role in these women's familial risk of breast cancer (Ford & Easton, 1995; Ford et al., 1995). Genetic investigators have speculated that the increased risk of breast cancer in these families may be due to more common susceptibility genes with low penetrance (Ford & Easton, 1995; Ford et al., 1995), such as inherited alterations in systemic factors, including immune defenses (Bodmer, 1994).

Psychological Distress in Women With Family Histories of Breast Cancer

Considering the increasing recognition of the role of family history in women's risk of developing breast cancer, one might expect that women at familial risk would experience chronic psychological distress. With rare exception, the literature supports this hypothesis. For example, Kash and colleagues found that women with a family history of breast cancer showed high levels of general emotional distress on the Brief Symptom Inventory (BSI; Derogatis & Spencer, 1982) compared with population norms for that scale (Kash, Holland, Halper, & Miller, 1992). High levels of intrusive thoughts about breast cancer have also been reported in women at familial risk. Lerman and colleagues (1993) found that 56% of women with breast cancer in first-degree relatives reported having intrusive thoughts about breast cancer; 30% of these women reported that these thoughts interfered with their daily functioning. Confirming these findings, a recent larger study found levels of intrusive thoughts in these women similar to those seen in posttraumatic stress disorder (Lerman, Kash, & Stefanek, 1994). In a recent study from our group (Valdimarsdottir et al., 1995), one of the few to include a normal risk comparison group, we found higher levels of intrusive thoughts about breast cancer as well as higher levels of general distress (as reflected in BSI scores) in women at familial risk. In a subsequent study, with a different sample of women, we found that intrusive thoughts about breast cancer were highest among women whose parents had died of cancer, raising the possibility that psychosocial interventions might profitably focus on bereavement issues (Zakowski et al., 1997). As one might expect, high levels of cancer-specific distress (e.g., intrusive thoughts about breast cancer) have also been reported in women with family histories of breast cancer who know that they carry a mutation in a breast cancer susceptibility gene (Lerman et al., 1996).

Stress as a Barrier to Breast Cancer Screening

One important negative consequence of stress in women with family histories of cancer is indicated by studies revealing that, in addition to other barriers, high levels of psychological distress may reduce the likelihood that women follow appropriate breast cancer screening practices, including mammography, clinical breast examination, and breast self-examination, as well as interest in genetic testing (see Figure 16.1). Appropriate breast cancer screening remains the single most important step women can take to reduce their risk of dying of the disease, because tumors detected at a later stage are less likely to be successfully treated. It is less well-established that health behaviors (e.g., drinking, smoking, exercise) affect women's risk of developing breast cancer (Mezzetti et al., 1998); therefore, the well-established link between distress and those behaviors (Taylor, Repetti, & Seeman, 1997) is not reviewed here.

A number of studies suggest that cancer fears and anxieties may be a barrier to appropriate breast cancer screening behavior. For example, Kash and colleagues (1992) found that among women with family histories of breast cancer, those with higher levels of distress were less likely to perform breast self-exams. Lerman and colleagues (1993) have reported that worries and intrusive thoughts about breast cancer are associated with reduced adherence to mammography screening guidelines in women with family histories of breast cancer, a negative relation that was particularly strong among individuals with lower educational levels. Miller and Hailey (1994) have reported preliminary data consistent with their hypothesis that the negative effects of anxiety on adherence to mammography guidelines may be particularly important in American women of African descent, for whom the threat of cancer may be especially pronounced because of the higher mortality rates in this population. On the other hand, McCaul, Branstetter, Schroeder, and Glasgow (1996) conducted a meta-analysis and found that higher levels of distress were predictive of increased mammography screening among normal-risk women. Among high-risk women, Lerman, Schwartz, Narod, and Lynch (1997) found that higher levels of distress were associated with increased likelihood that the women would request the results of their genetic testing for breast cancer susceptibility.

One possible explanation for these apparently inconsistent findings is that there may an inverse "U" relationship between distress and breast cancer screening. Studies have found that "moderate" levels of anxiety were associated with increased adherence to mammography screening guidelines (Stefanek & Wilcox, 1991). In addition, we have recently found that women with moderate levels of intrusive thoughts about breast cancer are more likely to undergo genetic testing for breast cancer susceptibility, as compared with women with either lower or higher levels of cancer-specific distress (Valdimarsdottir et al., 1999). These findings are consistent with fear arousing communications theory, which posits that some degree of cancer-specific distress may be necessary to motivate screening behaviors, whereas very high levels of anxiety about breast cancer may result in avoidance (Lerman & Schwartz, 1993). To date, little research has explored the factors involved in determining the transition points at which cancer-specific distress begins to motivate and then to inhibit screening, which may differ across individuals and populations. Another possible explanation for discrepant findings in studies linking stress and screening behaviors is that women who overperform screening behaviors are included in the "adherent" group in most studies. Recent evidence, both from our and others' studies, suggests that overperformance and underperformance of screening behaviors may be predicted by high levels of cancer-specific distress (Epstein et al., 1997; Erblich, Bovbjerg, & Valdimarsdottir, 2000).

The mechanisms linking distress and screening behaviors have yet to be elucidated. One possible mechanism is suggested by the work of Millar and Millar (1995), who have hypothesized that thinking about screening behaviors may elicit considerable distress because screening involves the threat that cancer will be detected. Supporting their hypothesis, these investigators demonstrated in an experimental study that imagining the performance of a cancer screening procedure resulted in increased negative affect in a college student sample (Millar & Millar, 1995). On the basis of emotional processing theory (Lang, 1993), it could be hypothesized that the experience of these aversive effects may serve to punish (in operant learning terms) behaviors required for the performance of breast cancer screening. The possibility that cognitions and images involving breast cancer may also elicit aversive psychobiological effects in women at familial risk has not yet been examined.

The Influence of Psychological Variables on Immune Function

Another potentially important negative consequence of stress associated with having a family history of breast cancer is raised by a growing literature indicating that stress affects the activity of the immune system (see Figure 16.1). Research approaches in this literature have included correlational investigations of the immune effects of exposure to chronic and acute environmental stressors, correlations between self-reported emotional distress and immune measures, psychosocial intervention studies, and experimental studies of the immunological consequences of controlled exposure to laboratory stressors.

A wide variety of stressful life events have been reported to affect the activity of the immune system, even after controlling for behavioral variables (e.g., drinking, smoking) known to affect immune function (Herbert & Cohen, 1993). Life events in these studies have included living close to Three-Mile Island following the nuclear accident (McKinnon, Weisse, Reynolds, Bowles, & Baum, 1989); surviving the death of a spouse (Irwin, Daniels, Bloom, Smith, & Weiner, 1987); enduring marital problems and divorce (Kiecolt-Glaser, Kennedy, Malkoff, Fisher, Speicher, & Glaser, 1988); taking care of sick relatives (Kiecolt-Glaser, Dura, Speicher, Trask, & Glaser, 1991); being unemployed (Arnetz et al., 1987); working at the site of an airplane crash (Delahanty, Dougall, Craig, Jenkins, & Baum, 1997); experiencing earthquakes (Solomon, Segerstrom, Grohr, Kemeny, & Fahey, 1997) and hurricanes (Ironson et al., 1997); and taking academic examinations (Glaser et al., 1992). The most consistently reported immunological changes in these studies are reductions in in vitro measures of cell-mediated immune function (e.g., proliferative responses to T-cell mitogens and natural killer [NK] cell activity). There is currently considerable interest in the clinical significance of these distress-induced immune changes, because they could contribute to increased risks for a variety of illnesses, including infectious disease and cancer (Andersen, Kiecolt-Glaser, & Glaser, 1994; Bovbjerg & Stone, 1996).

The temporal association of life stressor, emotional distress, and alterations in immune measures in these naturalistic studies has supported the view that it is the emotional distress induced by the stressor that influences the activity of the immune system (Herbert & Cohen, 1993). Additional support for this view has come from several studies in which the relations between psychological factors and measures of immune function in vitro have been statistically examined and significant relations found

(Bovbjerg & Valdimarsdottir, 1993; Glaser et al., 1992). Recent examples of this approach include our study indicating that NK cell activity is inversely correlated to negative mood, an effect that is buffered by the experience of positive mood at some time during the day of assessment (Valdimarsdottir & Bovbjerg, 1997).

Another recent report indicated that individuals' levels of intrusive thoughts about a stressful event (a hurricane) were associated with lower levels of NK cell activity (Ironson et al., 1997). Relationships between distress levels and individuals' immune responses to in vivo immune challenges (vaccination) have also been reported (Glaser et al., 1992).

The evidence from naturalistic studies indicates associations between stress (e.g., exposure to stressors and emotional distress) and immune function, which are consistent with a causal pathway. Further evidence that stress causes the immune changes comes from studies indicating that cognitive–behavioral interventions to reduce distress have effects on the immune system. Several intervention techniques have been found to alter immune measures (Ironson, Antoni, & Lutgendorf, 1995); examples include relaxation (Van Rood, Bogaards, Goulmy, & van Houwelingen, 1993), hypnosis (Zachariae, Bjerring, & Arendt-Nielsen, 1989), biofeedback (McGrady, Conran, & Dickey, 1992), and self-disclosure (Christensen et al., 1996).

Most of the studies in this literature have been based on the responses of healthy individuals. For example, Kiecolt-Glaser and colleagues (1985) observed increases in NK cell activity and lymphocyte proliferation as well as lower levels of antibody to herpes simplex virus in geriatric residents who received training in relaxation three times a week for a month. No change was observed in the group of individuals who had been assigned to a social contact group or to a no-treatment condition. Suggesting an interaction between personality variables and response to the intervention, Christensen and colleagues (1996) found that individuals characterized as high in cynical hostility had higher levels of NK cell activity after speaking about traumatic experience than individuals classified as low in cynical hostility.

The few studies of individuals with cancer have also found that cognitive–behavioral interventions can affect various parameters of the immune system (as described in more detail in Spiegel & Diamond, this volume, chapter 12). Fawzy, Fawzy, and Hyun (1994), for example, evaluated the immediate and long-term effects of a structured psychiatric intervention on psychosocial adjustment, coping, and immune function in cancer patients with Stage I or II malignant melanoma. After the 6-week intervention, participants in the group sessions had less distress; increases in active behavioral coping strategies; and increases in the percentage of large granular lymphocytes (the NK cell phenotype), NK cell numbers, and alpha interferon-augmented NK activity. Although not without exceptions, these studies suggest that such interventions can have beneficial effects on the immune system.

The mechanisms through which these interventions affect the immune system are not yet clear. It is possible that the interventions affect subjective distress and correlated physiological reactions (e.g., sympathetic arousal) that affect the immune system, or alternatively they may affect health behaviors (e.g., smoking) known to affect the immune system (see Figure 16.1). Some of the investigators included measures of subjective distress and found that changes in distress correlated with changes in immune measures, whereas others found no correlations (Ironson et al., 1995). Such effects may be complex. Following their intervention with cancer patients, Schedlowski and colleagues observed increases in absolute numbers of white blood cells, which were paralleled by decreases in plasma levels of cortisol; however, there were no correlations between these endocrine and immune measures (Schedlowski, Tewes, & Schmoll, 1994). Few of these studies have included assessments of health behaviors to determine their possible contribution to any effects of the intervention on immune function (Andersen et al., 1994; Kiecolt-Glaser & Glaser, 1988).

The naturalistic studies and randomized intervention trials reviewed above provide strong support for the hypothesis that there are relations between stressful life events, emotional distress, and alterations in immune function; however, naturalistic studies have several limitations, including a lack of control over immunomodulatory factors such as nutrition, drug use, or sleep disturbances, as well as difficulties in studying the underlying biological mechanisms (Kiecolt-Glaser & Glaser, 1988). One solution to these concerns is the use of randomized experimental designs in which participants are subjected to standard acute stressors in a controlled laboratory setting. This approach has been used in cardiovascular research for decades and, more recently, has been extended to include immune assessments (Cacioppo, 1994; Kiecolt-Glaser, Cacioppo, Malarkey, & Glaser, 1992). In addition to eliminating confounds associated with correlational studies, this experimental approach also facilitates the study of individual differences in reactivity.

The laboratory stressors in these studies have primarily included brief active coping tasks (e.g., mental arithmetic, the Stroop color word task) and passive coping tasks (e.g., watching a film of combat surgery), developed by cardiovascular researchers. Acute changes in a number of immune measures (e.g., NK cell counts and activity, white cell counts) have been consistently reported in several studies (Benschop et al., 1998; Cacioppo et al., 1998), although the generalizability of the experimental model to the effects of naturally occurring stressors has yet to be established. Consistent with the naturalistic studies, experimental studies have repeatedly found decreases in peripheral blood mitogen responses; however, unlike naturalistic studies, brief laboratory stressors have been reported in most studies, although not all, to result in acute increases in NK cell activity and the numbers of NK cells (Cacioppo et al., 1998; Kiecolt-Glaser et al., 1992). The most likely explanation for this apparent discrepancy is that some of the immunologic changes after stress may show a biphasic response such that early increases are followed by later decreases in response. Consistent with this possibility, Schedlowski, Jacobs, et al. (1993) found that increases in NK cell counts and NK cell activity seen immediately after a parachute jump were followed by significant decreases in both measures 1 hour later.

The mechanisms underlying distress-induced immune changes are not yet well understood. Considerable biological research indicates that there are many direct and indirect pathways that could mediate the relations between psychological variables and alterations in immune function. Among the many efferent connections between the brain and immune system are autonomic pathways (sympathetic and parasympathetic), as well as classic neuroendocrine pathways (e.g., the hypothalamic-pituitary-adrenal [HPA] axis; Madden & Felten, 1995). For example, sympathetic nerve fibers in lymphoid organs have catecholamine-containing terminals in close proximity to leukocytes, which have been shown to bear adrenergic receptors (Madden & Felten, 1995). Selective modulation of various aspects of immune function may occur as a result of differences in adrenergic receptor numbers and affinity on different subpopulations of leukocytes (Landmann, 1992). Indeed, recent studies have raised the possibility that glucocorticoid and adrenergic responses may have selective effects on T helper (T_H1 and T_H2) subsets, which play a critical role in determining the balance between cell-mediated and humoral effector mechanisms (Sredni et al., 1996).

Stressors are classically viewed as activating both the sympathetic adrenal medullary and hypothalamic pituitary adrenal responses (Henry, 1992), and both these pathways have been proposed as possible mediators of the immune changes induced by stressors (Madden & Felten, 1995). Several studies have shown that infusions of epinephrine and norepinephrine result in acute reductions in lymphocyte proliferative responses to T-cell mitogens, whereas acute increases are observed in measures of NK cell activity (Schedlowski, Falk, et al., 1993). On the other hand, infusions of glucocorticoids result in reduced levels of both proliferative responses to T mitogens and NK cell activity (Bateman, Singh, Kral, & Solomon, 1989). Further support for the hypothesis that sympathetic activation may contribute to the acute effects of stressors on immune measures in experimental studies has come from several reports that individuals with heightened catecholamine and cardiovascular reactions ("sympathetic reactors") to laboratory stressors also show larger immunologic effects (e.g., reduced T-cell mitogen responses and increased NK cell numbers or activity; Sgoutas-Emch et al., 1994). These reports of individual differences suggest the potential heuristic benefits of the experimental approach to understanding adrenergic influences. However, given the short duration of most of the experimental stressor studies, the possible influences of increases in cortisol levels on immune measures are not yet clear. Unlike catecholamines, which rise within 5 minutes following the stressor, cortisol responses take significantly longer to reach their peak (Henry, 1992). This temporal pattern of neuroendocrine response could provide a mechanism for a biphasic pattern of alterations in some immune measures (e.g., initial increases in NK cell activity followed by subsequent decreases).

Immune Alterations Reported in Individuals With Family Histories of Cancer

Investigations of immune function in individuals at familial risk for cancer have been rare, but several studies have found reductions in NK cell activity in individuals with family histories of a variety of different types of cancer (see Figure 16.1; Hersey, Edwards, Honeyman, & McCarthy, 1979; Strayer, Carter, & Brodsky, 1986; Strayer, Carter, Mayberry, Pequignot, & Brodsky, 1984). For example, Hersey and colleagues (1979) reported lower NK cell activity in individuals with a family history of melanoma. Strayer and colleagues (1984) reported lower NK cell activity in healthy individuals with a family history of a variety of different types of cancer, including colorectal, lung, prostate, and uterine cancer, and melanoma. In a subsequent study, Strayer and colleagues (1986) found that healthy women with family histories of breast cancer had lower NK cell activity than women without cancer in their families even after controlling for behavioral variables (e.g., smoking). It is not yet clear whether the reduction in NK cell activity represents a selective deficit in this one cell type or is a manifestation of a more pervasive deficit in multiple effector mechanisms, which could be driven by changes in the balance between T_H1 and T_H2 subsets (Sredni et al., 1996). Consistent with immune surveillance theories against cancer (Bovbjerg & Valdimarsdottir, 1998; see also Finn, this volume, chapter 10), several researchers have speculated that the increased cancer risk in individuals with family histories of cancer may, in part, be due to inherited deficits in NK cell activity, which has been cited as a principal effector mechanism of immune surveillance by a number of investigators (Trinchieri, 1990). It is important to note, however, that researchers have yet to conduct the large-scale study necessary to determine the potential contribution of deficits in immune defenses to the actual development of cancer in individuals with a family history. The impact of immune defenses on cancer risk for individuals with family histories, or for those who carry mutations in susceptibility genes, is therefore not yet known.

The possibility that stress effects on the immune system could contribute to the reduced levels of NK cell activity in individuals with family histories of cancer has received little research attention. Studies in the immunological literature have not included measures of stress or even described the circumstances under which participants were recruited (e.g., at the time the relative was diagnosed) or under which blood was drawn (e.g., when they were visiting the hospital to see the affected relative). Even without such stressors, these individuals are likely to have chronic fear and anxiety about their own cancer risk. In a recent study, we examined the possibly that the lower levels of NK cell activity in individuals with family histories of cancer could be due to their higher levels of stress (Bovbjerg & Valdimarsdottir, 1993). Measures of distress were completed immediately prior to a blood draw, which was collected for blind assessment of NK cell activity. Results confirmed previous reports of lower NK cell activity in individuals with family histories of cancer and showed a trend for higher levels of distress, which were inversely related to levels of NK cell activity. Statistically controlling for the contribution of distress to variability in NK cell activity reduced but did not eliminate the relation between family history of cancer and lower NK cell activity (Bovbjerg & Valdimarsdottir, 1993). Similar results were obtained in a subsequent study of healthy women with and without family histories of breast cancer (Bovbjerg et al., 2000). Consistent with the literature indicating that chronically stressed individuals are more psychobiologically reactive to acute stress (Lepore, Miles, & Levy, 1997), we have found that experimental stressors elicited stronger psychological, cardiovascular, and immune changes in women with family histories of breast cancer than in women without familial risk (Valdimarsdottir et al., 2000).

Our repeated finding from the naturalistic studies that the reduced levels of NK cell activity in individuals at familial risk for cancer cannot be entirely attributed to psychological influences may indicate that stress was not adequately assessed in these studies. Alternatively, the reduced NK cell activity in individuals at familial risk may be due to psychological influences superimposed on underlying inherited deficits in immune function. It is tempting to speculate that stress-induced changes in immune function may synergize with inherited deficits, resulting in a "double-whammy" such that stress-induced reductions in immune defenses against cancer, which might go undetected in individuals at normal risk for cancer, may be particularly pronounced in this population. Any large-scale investigation of the relations between immune defenses and the development of cancer among individuals at familial risk could profitably include appropriate psychological assessments to explore this possibility.

Conclusion

In this brief overview, we have highlighted three potential negative consequences of the stress associated with having a family history of cancer, which may further increase the risk of developing the disease for this population. First, to the extent that stress reduces adherence to cancer screening guidelines, cancer is more likely to be detected at a later stage when treatment is less effective. Second, to the extent that stress alters health or risk behaviors known to affect the development of cancer (e.g., smoking, drinking), cancer is more likely to develop. Third, to the extent that the immune system is important in defending against cancer, stress-induced immune suppression may increase the risk of developing cancer. As we have tried to indicate in the chapter, evidence supports each of these consequences of stress, but the results are not yet definitive. Additional research clearly is needed. It would be inappropriate, however, to ignore the potential benefits of reducing fear and anxiety about cancer. Effective cognitive–behavioral interventions for individuals at familial risk for cancer may not only improve their quality of life, but may also reduce their risk of developing and dying of the disease.

References

Andersen, B. L., Kiecolt-Glaser, J. K., & Glaser, R. (1994). A biobehavioral model of cancer stress and disease course. *American Psychologist, 49,* 389–404.

Anderson, D. E. (1992). Familial versus sporadic breast cancer. *Cancer, 70,* 1740–1746.

Arnetz, B. B., Wasserman, J., Petrini, B., Brenner, S. O., Levi, L., & Eneroth, P. (1987). Immune function in unemployed women. *Psychosomatic Medicine, 49(1),* 3–12.

Bateman, A., Singh, A., Kral, T., & Solomon, S. (1989). The immune–hypothalamic–pituitary–adrenal axis. *Endocrine Reviews, 10(1),* 92–112.

Benschop, R. J., Geenen, R., Mills, P. J., Naliboff, B. D., Kiecolt-Glaser, J. K., Herbert, T. B., van der Pompe, G., Miller, G. E., Matthews, K. A., Godaert, G. L. R., Gilmore, S. L., Glaser, R., Heijnen, C. J., Dopp, J. M., Bijlsma, W. J., Solomon, G. F., & Cacioppo, J. T. (1998). Cardiovascular and immune responses to acute psychological stress in young and old women: A meta-analysis. *Psychosomatic Medicine, 60,* 290–296.

Bodmer, W. F. (1994). Cancer genetics. *British Medical Bulletin, 50,* 517–526.

Bovbjerg, D., & Stone, A. (1996). Psychological stress and upper respiratory illness. In H. Friedman, T. Klein, & A. Friedman (Eds.), *Psychoneuroimmunology, stress, and infection* (pp. 195–213). Boca Raton, FL: CRC Press.

Bovbjerg, D. H., & Valdimarsdottir, H. (1993). Familial cancer, emotional distress, and low natural cytotoxic activity in healthy women. *Annals of Oncology, 4,* 745–752.

Bovbjerg, D. H., & Valdimarsdottir, H. B. (1998). Psychoneuroimmunology: Implications for psycho-oncology. In J. C. Holland (Ed.), *Psycho-Oncology* (pp. 125–134). New York: Oxford University Press.

Bovbjerg, D. H., Valdimarsdottir, H. B., Lubin, M. B., Borgen, P., Holland, J., Kash, K., Miller, D., & Osborne, M. (2000). *Familial risk of breast cancer, psychological distress, and lower natural killer cell activity in healthy women.* Manuscript submitted for publication.

Cacioppo, J. T. (1994). Social neuroscience: Autonomic, neuroendocrine, and immune responses to stress. *Psychophysiology, 31,* 113–128.

Cacioppo, J. T., Kiecolt-Glaser, J. K., Malarkey, W. B., Burleson, M. H., Berntson, G. G., & Glaser, R. (1998). Cellular immune responses to acute stress in female caregivers of dementia patients and matched controls. *Health Psychology, 17,* 182–189.

Christensen, A. J., Edwards, D. L., Wiebe, J. S., Benotsch, E. G., McKelvey, L., Andrews, M., & Lubaroff, D. M. (1996). Effect of verbal self-disclosure on natural killer cell activity: Moderating influence of cynical hostility. *Psychosomatic Medicine, 58,* 150–155.

Couch, F. J., DeShano, M. L., Blackwood, M. A., Calzone, K., Stopfer, J., Campeau, L., Ganguly, A., Rebbeck, T., & Weber, B. L. (1997). BRCA1 mutations in women attending clinics that evaluate the risk of breast cancer. *New England Journal of Medicine, 336,* 1409–1415.

Delahanty, D. L., Dougall, A. L., Craig, K. J., Jenkins, F. J., & Baum, A. (1997). Chronic stress and natural killer cell activity after exposure to traumatic death. *Psychosomatic Medicine, 59,* 467–476.

Derogatis, L. R. & Spencer, P. (1982). *The Brief Symptom Inventory (BSI): Administration, scoring, and procedures manual-1.* Unpublished copyrighted manuscript.

Epstein, S. A., Lin, T. H., Audrain, J., Stefanek, M., Rimer, B. K., Lerman, C., & The High-Risk Breast Cancer Consortium. (1997). Excessive breast self-examination among first-degree relatives of newly diagnosed breast cancer patients. *Psychosomatics, 38,* 253–261.

Erblich, J., Bovbjerg, D. H., & Valdimarsdottier, H. B. (2000). Psychological distress, health beliefs, and frequency of breast self-examination. *Journal of Behavioral Medicine, 23,* 277–292.

Fawzy, F. I., Fawzy, N. W., & Hyun, C. S. (1994). Short-term psychiatric intervention for patients with malignant melanoma: Effects on psychological state, coping, and the immune system. In C. E. Lewis, C. O'Sullivan, & J. Barraclough (Eds.), *The psychoimmunology of cancer* (pp. 292–319). New York: Oxford University Press.

Ford, D., & Easton, D. F. (1995). The genetics of breast and ovarian cancer. *British Journal of Cancer, 72,* 805–812.

Ford, D., Easton, D. F., & Peto, J. (1995). Estimates of the gene frequency of BRCA1 and its contribution to breast and ovarian cancer incidence. *American Journal of Human Genetics, 57,* 1457–1462.

Friend, S. H. (1996). Breast cancer susceptibility testing: Realities in the post-genomic era. *Nature Genetics, 13,* 16–17.

Glaser, R., Kiecolt-Glaser, J. K., Bonneau, R. H., Malarkey, W., Kennedy, S., & Hughes, J. (1992). Stress induced modulation of the immune response to recombinant Hepatitis B vaccine. *Psychosomatic Medicine, 54,* 22–29.

Harris, J. R., Lippman, M. E., Veronesi, U., & Willett, W. (1992). Breast cancer. *New England Journal of Medicine, 327*(5), 319–328.

Henry, J. P. (1992). Biological basis of the stress response. *Integrative Physiological and Behavioral Science, 27,* 66–83.

Herbert, T. B., & Cohen, S. (1993). Stress and immunity in humans: A meta-analytic review. *Psychosomatic Medicine, 55,* 364–379.

Hersey, P., Edwards, A., Honeyman, M., & McCarthy, W. H. (1979). Low natural killer cell activity in familial melanoma patients and their relatives. *British Journal of Cancer, 40,* 113–122.

Ironson, G., Antoni, M., & Lutgendorf, S. (1995). Can psychological interventions affect immunity and survival? Present findings and suggested targets with a focus on cancer and human immunodeficiency virus. *Mind/Body Medicine, 1,* 85–113.

Ironson, G., Wynings, C., Schneiderman, N., Baum, A., Rodriguez, M., Greenwood, D., Benight, C., Antoni, M., LaPerriere, A., Huang, H., Klimas, N., & Fletcher, M. A. (1997). Posttraumatic stress symptoms, intrusive thoughts, loss, and immune function after Hurricane Andrew. *Psychosomatic Medicine, 59,* 128–141.

Irwin, M., Daniels, M., Bloom, E. T., Smith, T. L., & Weiner, H. (1987). Life events, depressive symptoms, and immune function. *American Journal of Psychiatry, 144,* 437–441.

Kash, K. M., Holland, J. C., Halper, M. S., & Miller, D. G. (1992). Psychological distress and surveillance behaviors of women with a family history of breast cancer. *Journal of National Cancer Institute, 84,* 24–30.

Kiecolt-Glaser, J. K., Cacioppo, J. T., Malarkey, W. B., & Glaser, R. (1992). Editorial comment: Acute psychological stressors and short term immune changes: What, why, for whom, and to what extent? *Psychosomatic Medicine, 54,* 680–685.

Kiecolt-Glaser, J. K., Dura, J. R., Speicher, C. E., Trask, O. J., & Glaser, R. (1991). Spousal caregivers of dementia victims: Longitudinal changes in immunity and health. *Psychosomatic Medicine, 53,* 345–362.

Kiecolt-Glaser, J. K., & Glaser, R. (1988). Methodological issues in behavioral immunology research with humans. *Brain Behavior and Immunity, 2,* 67–78.

Kiecolt-Glaser, J. K., Glaser, R., Williger, D., Stout, J., Messick, G., Sheppard, S., Ricker, D., Romisher, S. C., Briner, W., Bonnell, G., & Donnerberg, R. (1985). Psychosocial enhancement of immunocompetence in a geriatric population. *Health Psychology, 4,* 25–41.

Kiecolt-Glaser, J. K., Kennedy, S., Malkoff, S., Fisher, L., Speicher, C. E., & Glaser, R. (1988). Marital discord and immunity in males. *Psychosomatic Medicine, 50,* 213–229.

Landmann, R. (1992). Beta-adrenergic receptors in human leukocyte subpopulations. *European Journal of Clinical Investigation, 22*(Suppl. 1), 30–36.

Lang, P. J. (1993). From emotional imagery to the organization of emotion in memory. In N. Birbaumer & A. Ohman (Eds.), *The structure of emotion: Psychophysiological, cognitive and clinical aspects* (pp. 69–92). Seattle, WA: Hogrefe & Huber.

Lepore, S. J., Miles, H. J., & Levy, J. S. (1997). Relation of chronic and episodic stressors to psychological distress, reactivity and health problems. *International Journal of Behavioral Medicine, 4,* 39–59.

Lerman, C., Daly, M., Sands, C., Balshem, A. M., Lustbader, E., Heggan, T., Goldstein, L., James, J., & Engstrom, P. (1993). Mammography adherence and psychological distress among women at risk for breast cancer. *Journal of National Cancer Institute, 85,* 1074–1080.

Lerman, C., Kash, K., & Stefanek, M. (1994). Younger women at increased risk for breast cancer: Perceived risk, psychological well-being, and surveillance behavior. *Monograph of the National Cancer Institute, 16,* 171–176.

Lerman, C., Narod, S., Schulman, K., Hughes, C., Gomez-Caminero, A., Bonney, G., Gold, K., Trock, B., Main, D., Lynch, J., Fulmore, C., Snyder, C., Lemon, S. J., Conway, T., Tonin, P., Lenoir, G., & Lynch, H. (1996). BRCA1 testing in families with breast–ovarian cancer: A prospective study of patient decision-making and outcomes. *Journal of the American Medical Association, 275,* 1885–1892.

Lerman, C. L., & Schwartz, M. (1993). Adherence and psychological adjustment among women at high risk for breast cancer. *Breast Cancer Research and Treatment, 28,* 145–155.

Lerman, C., Schwartz, M. D., Narod, S., & Lynch, H. T. (1997). The influence of psychological distress on use of genetic testing for cancer risk. *Journal of Consulting and Clinical Psychology, 65,* 414–420.

Madden, K. S., & Felten, D. L. (1995). Experimental basis for neural-immune interactions. *Physiological Reviews, 75,* 77–106.

McCaul, K. D., Branstetter, A. D., Schroeder, D. M., & Glasgow, R. E. (1996). What is the relationship between breast cancer risk and mammography screening? A meta-analytic review. *Health Psychology, 6,* 423–429.

McGrady, A., Conran, P., & Dickey, D. (1992). The effects of biofeedback-assisted relaxation on cell mediated immunity, cortisol, and white blood cell count in healthy adult subjects. *Behavioral Medicine, 15,* 343–354.

McKinnon, W., Weisse, C. S., Reynolds, C. P., Bowles, C. A., & Baum, A. (1989). Chronic stress, leukocyte subpopulations, and humoral response to latent viruses. *Health Psychology, 8,* 389–402.

Mezzetti, M., La Vecchia, C., Decarli, A., Boyle, P., Talamini, R., & Franceschi, S. (1998). Population attributable risk for breast cancer: Diet, nutrition, and physical exercise. *Journal of the National Cancer Institute, 90,* 389–394.

Millar, M. G., & Millar, K. (1995). Negative affective consequences of thinking about disease detection behaviors. *Health Psychology, 14,* 141–146.

Miller, L. Y., & Hailey, B. J. (1994). Cancer anxiety and breast cancer screening in African-American women: A preliminary study. *Womens Health Issues, 4,* 170–174.

Schatzkin, A., Goldstein, A., & Freedman, L. S. (1995). What does it mean to be a cancer gene carrier? Problems in establishing causality from the molecular genetics of cancer. *Journal of the National Cancer Institute, 87,* 1126–1130.

Schedlowski, M., Falk, A., Rohne, A., Wagner, T. O. F., Jacobs, R., Tewes, U., & Schmidt, R. E. (1993). Catecholamines induce alterations of distribution and activity of human natural killer (NK) cells. *Journal of Clinical Immunology, 13,* 344–351.

Schedlowski, M., Jacobs, R., Stratmann, G., Richter, S., Hadicke, A., Tewes, U., Wagner, T. O. F., & Schmidt, R. E. (1993). Changes of natural killer cells during acute psychological stress. *Journal of Clinical Immunology, 13,* 119–126.

Schedlowski, M., Tewes, U., & Schmoll, H. J. (1994). The effects of psychological intervention on cortisol levels and leukocyte numbers in the peripheral blood of breast cancer patients. In C. E. Lewis, C. O'Sullivan, & J. Barraclough (Eds.), *The psychoimmunology of cancer* (pp. 336–348). New York: Oxford University Press.

Sgoutas-Emch, S. A., Cacioppo, J. T., Uchino, B. N., Malarkey, W., Pearl, D., Kiecolt-Glaser, J. K., & Glaser, R. (1994). The effects of an acute psychological stressor on cardiovascular, endocrine, and cellular immune response: A prospective study of individuals high and low in heart rate reactivity. *Experimental Immunology, 31,* 264–271.

Solomon, G. F., Segerstrom, S. C., Grohr, P., Kemeny, M., & Fahey, J. (1997). Shaking up immunity: Psychological and immunologic changes after a natural disaster. *Psychosomatic Medicine, 59,* 114–127.

Sredni, B., Tichler, T., Shani, A., Catane, R., Kaufman, B., Strassmann, G., Albeck, M., & Kalechman, Y. (1996). Predominance of TH1 response in tumor bearing mice and cancer patients treated with AS101. *Journal of the National Cancer Institute, 88,* 1276–1284.

Stefanek, M. E., & Wilcox, P. (1991). First degree relatives of breast cancer patients: Screening practices and provision of risk information. *Cancer Detection and Prevention, 15,* 379–384.

Strayer, D. R, Carter, W. A., & Brodsky, I. (1986). Familiar occurrence of breast cancer is associated with reduced natural killer cytotoxicity. *Breast Cancer Research Treatment, 7,* 187–192.

Strayer, D. R., Carter, W. A., Mayberry, S. D., Pequignot, E., & Brodsky, I. (1984). Low natural cytotoxicity of peripheral blood mononuclear cells in individuals with high familial incidences of cancer. *Cancer Research, 44,* 370–374.

Taylor, S. E., Repetti, R. L., & Seeman, T. (1997). Health psychology: What is an unhealthy environment and how does it get under the skin? *Annual Review of Psychology, 48,* 411–447.

Thorlacius, S., Olafsdottir, G., Tryggvadottir, L., Neuhausen, S., Jonasson, J. G., Ogmundsdottir, H. M., & Eyfjord, J. E. (1996). A single BRCA2 mutation in male and female breast cancer families from Iceland with varied cancer phenotypes. *Nature Genetics, 13,* 117–119.

Trinchieri, G. (1990). Biology of natural killer cells. *Advances in Immunology, 47,* 187–376.

Valdimarsdottir, H., & Bovbjerg, D. H. (1997). Positive and negative mood: Association with natural killer cell activity. *Psychology and Health, 12,* 319–327.

Valdimarsdottir, H. B., Bovbjerg, D. H., Brown, K., Jacobsen, P., Schwartz, M. D., Bleiker, E., & Offit, K. (1999). Cancer-specific distress is related to women's decisions to undergo BRCA1 testing. *Cancer Research, Therapy, and Control, 8,* 61–68.

Valdimarsdottir, H. B., Bovbjerg, D. H., Kash, K. M., Holland, J. C., Osborne, M. P., & Miller, D. G. (1995). Psychological distress in women with a familial risk of breast cancer. *Psycho-Oncology, 4,* 133–141.

Valdimarsdottir, H. B., Bovbjerg, D. H., Zakowski, S. G., Gerin, W., Mamakos, J., & Pickering, T. G. (2000). *Heightened psychobiological reactivity to laboratory stressors in healthy women at familial risk for breast cancer.* Manuscript submitted for publication.

Van Rood, V. R, Bogaards, M., Goulmy, E., & van Houwelingen, H. C. (1993). The effects of stress and relaxation on the in vitro immune response in man: A meta-analytic study. *Journal of Behavioral Medicine, 16,* 163–181.

Zachariae, R., Bjerring, P., & Arendt-Nielsen, L. (1989). Modulation of type I immediate and type IV delayed immunoreactivity using direct suggestion and guided imagery during hypnosis. *Allergy, 44,* 537–542.

Zakowski, S. G., Valdimarsdottir, H. B., Bovbjerg, D. H., Borgen, P., Holland, J., Kash, K., Miller, D., Mitnick, J., Osborne, M., & Van Zee, K. (1997). Predictors of intrusive thoughts and avoidance in women with family histories of breast cancer. *Annals of Behavioral Medicine, 19,* 362–369.

17

Targets for Interventions to Reduce Cancer Morbidity

Lorenzo Cohen
Andrew Baum

A s has been amply noted and discussed in earlier chapters of this book, cancer remains a major threat to health and well-being despite the advances of the past two decades in understanding the causes, detection, and treatment of neoplastic disease. The second leading cause of death worldwide, cancer claims more lives each year, and its treatment accounts for a substantial portion of spiraling health care costs in the United States. In the United States, cancer-related mortality increased 7.1% between 1967 and 1992, and cancer care accounted for $35 billion in direct medical costs, $12 billion in lost productivity, and $57 billion in mortality costs in 1990 (Bal, Nixon, Foerster, & Brownson, 1995; Garfinkel, 1995; Parker, Tong, Bolden, & Wingo, 1997). Reducing mortality and health care expenditures is critical, and new emphasis on cancer prevention and control offers ways to go about reducing these costs. We consider behaviors that are associated with cancer risk, detection, or progression of disease and the implications of preventing or modifying them. We briefly describe some recent trends in tobacco control, modification of diet, and exercise as strategies for cancer risk management. Although we do not intend this to be an exhaustive review, we consider some of the most promising efforts to modify risk for cancer or progression of disease and those investigations that have begun to produce positive results.

Doll and Preto (1981) estimated that 75–80% of all cancers are preventable through behavioral and environmental modifications that include smoking cessation; changes in diet (moderating fat and alcohol intake); and decreasing exposure to environmental carcinogens such as the sun, radiation, pesticides, and other carcinogens. More conservative estimates of preventable cancers are still substantial, suggest-

Partial funding was received from the National Cancer Institute of Canada with funds from the Terry Fox Run.

ing that smoking and smokeless tobacco accounts for at least 35% of total cancers, whereas diet and alcohol account for 35% or more of some cancers, and sun exposure determines 80% or more of all skin cancers (Reizenstein, Modan, & Kuller, 1994).

The Scope of Cancer Prevention

Suggesting that some or even many cancers can be prevented does not mean that all cancers are avoidable or that risk for cancer can be eliminated. Many major risk factors associated with cancer etiology are not modifiable. Age is perhaps the most influential risk for cancer, presumably because of age-related increases in mutogenic activity and declines in immune, nervous system, and DNA repair systems in the body. Up to 85% of all new cancers diagnosed in 1990 were in people ages 50 or older (Dodd, 1991). Heritable factors are also major risk factors for cancer that may not be susceptible to change. However, many causes of cancer are modifiable behaviors (Greenwald & Sondik, 1986). Moreover, current technology allows us to detect some types of cancer growth early in the disease process, with 5-year survival rate as high as 90% in some forms (Garfinkel, 1995). Prevention of modifiable sources of risk is a powerful weapon against cancer, but prevention and early detection programs have had mixed success and have been marred by delays in the application of new knowledge and technology (Breslow, Agran, Breslow, Morganstern, & Ellwin, 1977).

Renewed emphasis on behavior change in health psychology and behavioral medicine and lessons learned from applications of behavioral theory research on prevention of HIV transmission have greatly enhanced the science and practice of preventive behavior modification (Lichtenstein & Glasgow, 1992; Schneiderman et al., 1992). At the same time, more powerful techniques, better appreciation of the complexity of relapse, and new approaches to education and motivation have resulted in larger, more lasting changes in targeted health-impairing behaviors (Fisher & Fisher, 1992; Schwartz, 1992). The development of prevention programs has focused on cancer-associated behaviors, particularly smoking, diet, use of screening, and sun protection.

Early detection of cancer is also important. For cancers that can be detected at early stages with screening, the weighted average 5-year survival rates are 90% for localized disease, 61% for regional disease, and 18% for distant or metastasized disease (Garfinkel, 1995). Although there is a clear relationship between stage of disease and life expectancy and good evidence that early detection conveys an advantage, a significant portion of detectable cancers are discovered at an advanced stage. This is particularly true for skin cancer, where early detection only necessitates vigilant observation.

Recent evidence suggests that stress may be related to the development and progression of some cancers (Chen et al., 1995; Funch & Marshall, 1984; Ramirez et al., 1989; Scherg & Blomke, 1988). Although the influence of stress as an etiological factor for cancer is disputed (Burke & Goodkin, 1997; Cassileth, 1996; Roberts, Newcomb, Trentham-Dietz, & Storer, 1996), there is more substantial evidence that stress contributes to the progression of disease (Burke & Goodkin, 1997; Cassileth, 1996; Funch & Marshall, 1984; Ramirez et al., 1989; Roberts et al., 1996). Chronic stress produces physiological changes that may affect disease course and influence vulnerability to and progression of disease (Van der Pompe et al., 1994). Moreover, stress can interfere with compliance (Curry & Emmons, 1994; Lerman et al., 1993; Sellick, Charles, Woodbeck, & Kyle, 1995) and increase health-damaging behaviors such as smoking or drug use (Baum & Singer, 1987; Grunberg & Baum, 1985), both of which might influence progression of disease. Recent intervention research suggests that psychosocial stress management programs may influence quality of life, physiological parameters, and cancer mortality (Fawzy et al., 1993; Spiegel, Bloom, Kraemer, & Gottheil, 1989).

Prevention Is Not That Easy

Perhaps because the contribution of some behavioral risk factors to cancer are so great, preventing cancer is difficult. As we have suggested, many risk factors are not behaviorally mediated or modifiable. However, some causes or promoters of cancer are modifiable and can be altered to reduce or eliminate risk (Greenwald & Sondik, 1986). The contributions of some individual behavioral risk factors are likely to be small, and many of these behaviors are difficult to change. However, treatments for cancer are often not effective and are typically toxic and expensive; as a result, any reduction of morbidity through prevention is valuable. This suggests that we should continue to try to modify unhealthy behaviors and other sources of cancer risk or develop better ways of detecting cancer early. First, sources of risk must be identified, a slow and costly process that often requires critical analysis of contradictory and small effects. Modifiable risks may account for fewer than half of all cases, they may be correlated with other irrelevant factors that must be eliminated, or several different sources of modifiable risk may exist independently of each other. These make appropriate evaluation of risks or causes of disease difficult to disentangle.

A second problem, more specific to primary prevention of cancer, is how the effectiveness of an intervention is evaluated. Cancer develops over variable, often long periods of time. The behaviors or exposures at one point in time may not be manifest as detectable disease for 10 to 15 years. Prospective evaluation of risk is very costly, and it is readily apparent that in a healthy population where the average risk for cancer is less than 30% over a lifetime (Parker et al., 1997), evaluation of risk factors or prevention efforts requires very large samples and long follow-ups. The expense, time, and funding needed to conduct these studies have been formidable barriers to systematic evaluation of behavior change as a way to prevent cancer.

Modification of Behavioral Sources of Cancer Risk

Tobacco Use

Tobacco use is the most potent single modifiable risk factor for many cancers, and the smoking prevention and cessation literature is extensive. More than 30% of all cancer deaths in the United States are attributable to smoking (Centers for Disease Control and Prevention, 1989). Even though the prevalence of smoking has declined in recent years, approximately 48 million adults are current smokers, and the major decline in smoking rates appears to have stabilized (Skaar et al., 1997). The Agency for Health Care Policy and Research recently published the *Smoking Cessation Clinical Practice Guideline*, which reviewed more than 300 randomized trials of smoking cessation interventions (Fiore et al., 1996). Although the estimated cessation rates ranged from 9.3% to 25.5%, there was a clear dose–response relationship between the amount of clinical contact and the effectiveness of the intervention. Brief cessation treatments are effective, but optimal effects are seen with relatively intensive interventions that include approximately 4 to 7 sessions over as many weeks and multiple cessation modalities (e.g., nicotine replacement therapy, social support, and skills-training–problem-solving (Skaar et al., 1997). We do not consider this literature here because it warrants more attention than space permits. Interested readers are referred to excellent reviews by Gritz (1994), Lichtenstein and Glasgow (1992), and Schwartz (1992).

Exercise

Epidemiological evidence suggests that exercise decreases the relative risk of developing cancer (Francis, 1996; Kampert, Blair, Barlow, & Kohl, 1996; Shephard, 1993; Thune, Brenn, Lund, & Gaard, 1997). The strength of the association varies across studies; a sedentary lifestyle is associated with an approximate 1.5 risk ratio for all cancers (Shephard, 1993). Researchers have examined the protective effects of both occupational and leisure activities, and both have consistently been associated with a decreased relative risk of developing colon cancer (Shephard, 1993). This relationship is stronger for men than for women and remains significant after controlling for other known risk factors such as age, body mass index, smoking, diet, and family history. This is particularly relevant because colon cancer is the third leading cause of cancer deaths (Parker et al., 1997).

More consistent evidence is starting to emerge on the relationship between exercise and the development of breast and reproductive cancers in women, although there are some studies that find no association (Bernstein, Henderson, Hanisch, Sullivan-Halley, & Ross, 1994; Friedenreich & Rohan, 1995; Kramer & Wells, 1996; Mink, Folsom, Sellers, & Kushi, 1996; Paffenbarger, Hyde, & Wing, 1987; Thune et al., 1997; Vena, Graham, Zielezny, Brasure, & Swanson, 1987). There is less evidence linking exercise and prostate cancer, although a recent study did find a moderate association (Thune & Lund, 1994). A definitive causal relationship between exercise and a reduced risk of cancer, however, has yet to be determined; therefore, we do not review research in this area.

Diet

One focus of efforts to reduce cancer risk has been on what people eat. Diet is important "locally"; cancers related to diet, alcohol consumption, and general nutrition are often localized in the digestive tract, including the esophagus, stomach, liver, colon, and rectum. Dietary factors may also affect cancers of the breast, prostate, endometrium, and ovary (Weisberg & Williams, 1995). Diets rich in vegetables and fruits and low in fat have been recommended, and increasing consumption of the former while reducing fat to 30% or less of one's calories should decrease incidence of some cancers (Greenwald & Sondik, 1986).

One problem in understanding the association between diet and cancer is the complexity of these effects. For example, research suggests that estrogen levels are associated with estrogen receptor-positive breast cancers, and use of oral contraceptives, age of first birth, age at menarche and menopause, and other factors linked to lifetime estrogen exposure are components of risk for breast cancer (Henderson, 1995). Estrogen levels are also positively associated with fat intake (Longcope et al., 1987). Furthermore, dietary fat intake in women diagnosed with estrogen receptor-positive tumors predicted recurrence of breast cancer in a dose–response pattern, and carbohydrate and vitamin C consumption were positively related to disease-free status (Holm et al., 1993). The association between diet and cancer was also evident in the severity of tissue changes observed in mammographic data. Women with mammogram patterns indicating greatest risk reported the highest fat intake and lowest fiber, carbohydrate, and calcium intake, whereas women with patterns indicating lower risk consumed less fat and more fiber, carbohydrates, and calcium (Nordevang, Azavedo, Svane, Nilsson, & Holm, 1993). Although these findings are provocative, recent studies have challenged the notion that dietary fat is associated with breast cancer (Negri et al., 1996), and additional study is warranted.

Maintaining a healthy diet can be difficult, particularly in older individuals where habits are more entrenched. Many people find that the foods they like best are not healthy ones, and both social and psychologically derived aspects of eating behavior have made effective dietary intervention difficult. Several large-scale clinical trials are currently under way to examine the effects of diet modification on cancer incidence, and a number of successful modifications of diet have been reported. The majority of these studies seek to decrease the percentage of total calories derived from fat, and some try to increase dietary fiber.

Dietary interventions have successfully modified behaviors thought to be risk factors for cancer. This is particularly true for randomized intervention trials seeking to decrease the percentage of total energy from dietary fat in people's diet. Most studies find that participants are able to modify dietary fat intake so that it is close to or at recommended levels, and these changes are reflected in overall weight loss (Heber et al., 1992; Meyskens, Alberts, & Earnest, 1985; Prentice et al., 1988; Schapira, Kumar, Lyman, & Baile, 1991; White et al., 1992). In addition, some interventions have also been successful at increasing fiber intake (Atwood et al., 1992; Schapira et al., 1991).

Community intervention trials have also been successful, although long-term adherence has been more difficult to assess (Potter et al., 1990; van Assema, Steenbak- kers, Kok, Eriksen, & de Vries, 1994). Some community trials have also targeted young children and adolescents with the belief that increasing healthy dietary habits in children may result in long-term adherence, with a corresponding decrease in cancer incidence. The Know Your Body program, a comprehensive school health promotion program for kindergarten through Grade 6, had some success at modifying health-related behaviors (Williams, Arnold, & Wynder, 1977). Initial findings showed a reduction in consumption of saturated fats and a reduction in cholesterol levels among children in the intervention group (Wynder, 1991). Three years into the program, the intervention was associated with lower systolic blood pressure and serum cholesterol and increased self-reported intake of healthy foods (Resnicow et al., 1992). After 5 years, some schools reported changes in cholesterol, diastolic blood pressure, and percentage of kilocalories from fat, whereas others did not (Resnicow, Cross, & Wynder, 1993). The Gimme 5 program, implemented with 4th- and 5th-grade students, also has some encouraging findings (Domel et al., 1993). This school-based curriculum intervention, including newsletters and videotapes for parents and point-of-purchase education at local grocery stores, was associated with an increase in both fruit and vegetable consumption (Domel et al., 1993). Although the changes were small, increasing consumption of healthy foods may have a long- term impact on future health.

Most dietary intervention programs have been successful in reducing the per- centage of calories from dietary fat and in increasing dietary fiber levels when this was part of the intervention. Although community trials have not had as much success at producing dietary behavior changes as clinical trials, this may in part be due to methodological factors as well as a lower level of intensity of the interventions. Education, skills, opportunities for modeling, and support have been common elements of these dietary events and appear to be necessary but insufficient by themselves in producing behavior change. Further study is needed to determine long-term adherence to dietary changes and their effects on cancer incidence.

Sun Exposure

Rapidly increasing rates of skin cancer have led to concern about sun exposure and protection and interest in preventing skin cancer. Cumulative exposure to sun and ultraviolet light over long periods of time increases the risks of nonmelanoma skin cancers (basal cell and squamous cell carcinomas), and an intense exposure sufficient to cause sunburn increases one's risk for malignant melanoma (Urist, Miller, & Maddox, 1995). Lifetime risk of melanoma is at least doubled by having had one or more severe sunburns during adolescence, and excessive exposure to the sun early in life (i.e., prior to age 20) is the best predictor of later development of nonmelanoma and melanoma skin cancers (Urist et al., 1995; Weinstock et al., 1989). Because of these findings, children and adolescents have been identified as a key group for primary prevention (Consensus Development Panel, 1991).

Exposure to sunlight should be an easily modifiable risk factor for the development of skin cancer. Although certain individuals may have an increased risk of developing skin cancer, the majority of skin cancers appear to be preventable through use of shaded areas when outside, wearing protective clothing, and appropriate use of sunscreen. The impact of sun exposure and the ready availability of methods for protecting oneself belie the difficulty in changing these behaviors. Overwhelming publicity about the link between sun exposure and skin cancer has not produced large-scale behavior change. Even though the dangers of excessive sun exposure are well-known to the public, social norms of the 20th century still associate a suntan with a healthy appearance. Advertising reinforces the view that having a tan looks good, and there are many reports in the popular press on safe methods of achieving a tan (Arthey & Clarke, 1995).

Although it is relatively easy to identify sun exposure risk factors, it has been more difficult to increase sun protection behaviors. Age is the best predictor of sun protective behaviors, but because early life exposures are important, resistance to behavior change by younger adults and adolescents is a major concern (Campbell & Birsell, 1994; Hill et al., 1992; Rosenman, Gardiner, Swanson, Mullan, & Zhu, 1995). A recent survey of 3,843 people indicated that only 45% of those surveyed believed that sun exposure affected the chances of getting cancer, and fewer than 50% used any sun protective measures (Campbell & Birsell, 1994). Skin cancer knowledge and number of people one knew with cancer predicted sunscreen use in one study (Keesling & Friedman, 1987); in another study (Marlenga, 1995), farmers (a group at particularly high risk for skin cancer) reported appropriate levels of skin cancer knowledge, believed that their susceptibility to skin cancer was higher than average, believed that skin cancer is a serious disease, and believed in the efficacy of daily protection from the sun, but few of them protected themselves from the sun.

Skin cancer knowledge and knowledge of protection techniques appear to be necessary but insufficient for behavior change (Keesling & Friedman, 1987). They are related to protective behaviors and to perceived risk, but they have not been consistently predictive of avoiding exposure or protecting oneself from sun exposure (Marlenga, 1995; Mermelstein & Riesenberg, 1992). Individuals may not have the education or knowledge to screen for or decrease cancer risk, or they may not have the means to pay for such information and services, but knowledge appears to be a necessary condition for effective behavior change. Strong counter influences related to appearance and outdoor activity also mitigate against meaningful behavior change.

Randomized trials and community-based trials have increased skin cancer knowledge and awareness of protection, but increasing preventive behaviors has not been as successful in at-risk groups (Borland, Hill, & Noy, 1990; Girgis, Sanson-Fisher, & Watson, 1994; Lombard, Neubauer, Canfield, & Winett, 1991; Rassaby, Larcombe, Hill, & Wake, 1983). Some programs were effective in increasing protective behaviors in children and should decrease cancer incidence (Buller, Loescher, & Buller, 1994; Girgis, Sanson-Fisher, Tripodi, & Golding, 1993), but long-term adherence and changes in incidence of skin cancers have not been assessed. Part of the problem is that the models guiding interventions to decrease sun exposure do not adequately capture the power of immediate sensual and social influences on behavior.

Intervention with children and adolescents is of particular significance. Sun exposure at an early age appears to be important in the development of skin cancer. Interventions that consider social norms and peer pressures may have the greatest impact on sun exposure if they can counter these influences. What is needed is a fundamental shift in the way society views tanned skin, not as an indication of health and good looks, but as a risk factor for skin cancer. The excesses of suntanning and indiscriminant exposure to the sun must be revealed and the immediacy of rewards for "looking good," strong enough to overwhelm concerns about the possibility of disease at some remote time in the future, need to be countered (Baum & Cohen, 1998). Effective increases in sun protective behaviors are difficult to achieve until we can modify the beliefs that having a suntan looks healthy and that people with tans look better than people without them. Further studies are needed to assess long-term behavior changes and the effects on cancer incidence (Baum & Cohen, 1998).

Screening and Surveillance

Another important activity that has been difficult to foster in the general population is surveillance for early signs of disease. Early-stage detection and diagnosis of cancer increases the probability of successful treatment (Parker et al., 1997) and also is a major component of secondary prevention. In some cases early detection permits effective excision of the cancer, whereas in others, it improves the odds that adjuvant and primary treatment will eliminate the cancer.

Patients and nonpatients are advised to become active in monitoring bodily changes and signs of cancer, and they are taught to perform regular self-exams of the skin, breast, testes, and oral cavity, where knowledgeable self-exams can be the best means for early detection. However, self-exams are not feasible for many cancers and are ordinarily not practiced regularly when they are possible. Consequently, screening by health care providers is also important and may include the fecal occult blood test and sigmoidoscopy for detection of colon cancer, digital rectal exam and monitoring of prostate-specific antigen levels for prostate cancer, mammography for breast cancer, and the Papanicolaou Stain Test (Pap smear) for cervical cancer. The recommended frequency of these procedures varies with age, previous cancer history, family history, and other risk factors. For some cancers, risk determined through genetic testing also influences the frequency of screening.

Early detection of tumor growth not only increases one's chances of survival but may also decrease medical cost by lowering the need for extraordinary or intensive treatments (Bal et al., 1995). Attempts to characterize people who are more or less likely to conduct self-examinations or participate in recommended screening have been useful in designing interventions for individuals at risk for noncompliance. However, even people who have previously been diagnosed with cancer do not subscribe to screening programs and general cancer surveillance, nor do they participate in early detection activities (Robinson, 1990).

Some of the variables that predict screening behaviors are not readily modifiable (e.g., age, previous health care, income, education), but some factors, including cancer knowledge, perceived risk, and support from physicians, can be changed and are consistently associated with screening (Lerman, Rimer, Trock, Balshem, & Engstrom, 1990; Rimer, Keintz, Kessler, Engstrom, & Rosan, 1989; Sellick et al., 1995). Fear and anxiety of developing cancer interfere with screening behaviors, and efforts to decrease this distress may increase cancer surveillance (Sellick et al., 1995). Providing accurate expectations and realistic perceptions of risk through increased cancer knowledge may decrease fear and anxiety, as can support from a health care provider.

Interventions to increase screening and surveillance behaviors with patients can be effective. Interventions that increase cancer risk information as well as cancer screening knowledge increase screening behaviors or the intent to be screened (Lerman et al., 1992; Meyers et al., 1994; Rothman, Salovey, Turvey, & Fishkin, 1993; Yancey, Tanjasiri, Klein, & Tunder, 1995). Low-cost interventions such as letters, telephone calls, or videotapes have met with limited success in increasing screening behaviors (King, Rimer, Seay, Balshem, & Engstrom, 1994; Lerman, Kash, & Stefanek, 1994; Meyers et al., 1994; Yancey et al., 1995). Moreover, message framing appears to be important; messages emphasizing negative consequences of not screening or providing internal attributions of responsibility were most effective in increasing surveillance behaviors (Meyerowitz & Chaiken, 1987; Rothman et al., 1993).

Increased screening publicity and availability of health fairs and free clinics has led to an earlier average stage of melanoma at diagnosis, an increased percentage of thin tumors detected, and a progressive increase in survival rates (Herd et al., 1995; Koh, Geller, Miller, Grossbart, & Lew, 1996). Patients who indicated that they were influenced by the publicity had a higher percentage of thin tumors detected (85%) compared with patients who said they were not influenced by the publicity

(57%; Herd et al., 1995). Encouraging results have been obtained from the free melanoma and skin cancer education and skin cancer screening programs sponsored by the American Academy of Dermatology (AAD) (Koh et al., 1996). Results indicated decreases in advanced melanoma detected, and patients diagnosed with melanoma in the AAD program indicated that they would not have had a physician examine their skin without the free program. Both studies suggest that screening is effective at diagnosing melanoma at an earlier stage and might result in increases in survival rates.

Two studies provided important evidence that enhanced screening can translate into better medical outcomes, indicating not only that interventions increase screening, but also that they are associated with a decrease in the severity of cancers detected, a decrease in overall medical costs, and an increase in lives saved (Cristofolini et al., 1993; Theobald, Marks, Hill, & Dorvitch, 1991). Although more research is needed to determine whether cancer incidence and mortality are affected, even slight increases in the percentage of cancers detected at an early stage should have an impact on cancer outcomes and a decreased burden on the health care system.

Stress and Stress Management

As described in several of the preceding chapters, cancer is a very stressful disease, and relevant sources of threat include fear of death or of progression or recurrence of disease, uncertainty, and concerns about changes in quality of life and social relationships (Aaronson et al., 1991; Andersen, Kiecolt-Glaser, & Glaser, 1994; Dunkel-Schetter, Feinstein, Taylor, & Falke, 1992). Stress is best thought of as a psychophysiological process, usually experienced as a negative emotional state, that is both a product of appraisal of situational and psychological factors and an impetus for coping (Baum, Cohen, & Hall, 1993). Stressors, events posing threat, harm, or challenge, are judged in light of personal disposition factors and environmental factors, and if appraised as menacing or challenging, specific responses directed at reducing the stress occur (Lazarus & Folkman, 1984).

Psychological and behavioral consequences of stress may include increased negative affect, posttraumatic stress disorder, narrowing of attention, increases in health-impairing behaviors (poor diet, lack of exercise, substance abuse), poor sleep, and decreased quality of life (Baum & Singer, 1987; Glass, Singer, & Friedman, 1969; Grunberg & Baum, 1985; Ironson et al., 1997; Irwin, Smith, & Gillin, 1992). Research has shown that stress can also interfere with compliance (Curry & Emmons, 1994; Lerman et al., 1993; Sellick et al., 1995). Sustained stress may also cause persistent increases in sympathetic nervous system activity, including increased blood pressure, heart rate, catecholamine secretion, and platelet aggregation and decreased immune function (Baum et al., 1993; Irwin et al., 1990; Patterson et al., 1994; Yehuda, Resnick, Kahana, & Giller, 1993). Both acute and chronic stressors produce changes in the number and function of a variety of immune cells (Cohen, Delahanty, Schmitz, Jenkins, & Baum, 1993; Kiecolt-Glaser et al., 1984; Kiecolt-

Glaser et al., 1987; Manuck, Cohen, Rabin, Muldoon, & Bachen, 1991; Sieber et al., 1992). This is presumed to be one of the mechanisms responsible for negative health consequences of stress. In addition, stress-induced immune suppression may be detrimental to survival for patients with cancer (Adler, Stein, & Ben-Efraim, 1980a, 1980b; Fawzy et al., 1993; Head, Elliott, & McCoy, 1993; Levy, Herberman, Lippman, & d'Angelo, 1987). Although controversial, this new area of research demonstrates that psychological factors can result in behavioral and regulatory system changes and may affect future health or course of disease.

Several studies indicate that stress may contribute to the etiology and progression of cancer (Gehde & Balthrusch, 1990; Greer, Morris, & Pettingale, 1979; Morris, Greer, Pettingale, & Watson, 1981; Ramirez et al., 1989). Although this research is controversial, stress-induced decreases in natural killer (NK) cell activity (Cohen et al., 1993; Kiecolt-Glaser et al., 1984; Sieber et al., 1992), a primary defense against metastatic tumor growth (Herberman & Ortaldo, 1981), have been linked to tumor growth in animals (Ben-Eliyahu, Yirmiya, Liebeskind, Taylor, & Gale, 1991). Other studies suggest that immune function, including NK cell function and T-lymphocyte proliferation, is predictive of prognostic indicators, recurrence, and survival time for patients with breast cancer and malignant melanoma (Adler et al., 1980a, 1980b; Fawzy et al., 1993; Head et al., 1993; Levy et al., 1987; Levy, Herberman, Maluish, Schlien, & Lippman, 1985; Reynier, Bazin, Bizzini, Chany, & Leandri, 1988). These findings suggest that stress-induced changes in immune function may be associated with the onset of neoplastic growth and may contribute to the progression of disease.

There is mounting evidence that psychosocial and psychoeducational interventions are valuable in reducing stress among cancer patients (Andersen, 1992; Baum, Herberman, & Cohen, 1995; see also chapters 12 and 13, this volume). Quality of life, survival, and in some cases immune status are enhanced by these programs that provide support and skills useful in managing stress (Fawzy, Fawzy, Arndt, & Pasnau, 1995; Spiegel, 1992). The extent to which stress-focused interventions can reduce the incidence of cancer remains to be evaluated.

Conclusion

In the past two decades, efforts to prevent cancer have dramatically increased. Behavioral interventions have generally been successful in increasing healthy dietary habits, and more modest results have been obtained from efforts to increase sun protective behaviors or increase adherence to cancer screening and surveillance. It is not yet clear whether these behavioral changes can be maintained for long periods of time or whether they have salutary effects on cancer outcomes. Two studies did find that early detection of skin cancer was cost-effective and saved lives (Cristofolini et al., 1993; Theobald et al., 1991). Future studies will more definitively determine the costs and benefits of these behavioral interventions.

The implications of these efforts are broad. First, they may reduce overall cancer morbidity and mortality. Reduction or elimination of risk caused by poor diet, smoking, alcohol use, and exposure to carcinogens would substantially affect cancer rates. This should also have a substantial effect on medical costs and on the acceptability or importance of prevention in capitated health systems. Finally, this research and intervention has important implications for models of health care and for the development of behavioral medicine.

Intervention programs that modify diet, sun exposure, cancer screening behaviors, and stress levels of people living with cancer have been somewhat successful. To date, there is no definitive indication of whether these behavioral modifications result in reduced disease or disease progression. However, data suggest that these programs should result in decreased cancer incidence, a less advanced stage of disease at diagnosis, increased quality of life, and attenuation of disease progression. Lowering the overall cancer burden and the stage of disease at diagnosis has clear cost implications, because there will be less need for extensive medical treatments. As this research continues to evolve, the inclusion of behavioral medicine in models of health care becomes more imperative. Behavioral intervention programs can be useful adjuncts at all stages of the disease process as well as help decrease overall disease incidence.

People adhere to or maintain healthy lifestyles for complex reasons, and it is difficult to determine variables that consistently predict health-enhancing behaviors that may prevent cancer. Individuals may not have the education or knowledge to screen for or decrease cancer risk, or they may not have the means to pay for such information and services (and knowledge appears to be a necessary condition for effective behavior change). Moreover, individual risk perception may vary greatly, and individual difference variables such as anxiety and self-efficacy may also play a role. Message framing may also be an important determinant of the efficacy of interventions. Screening and surveillance were increased by negatively framed messages (Meyerowitz & Chaiken, 1987) or messages targeting internal attributions of responsibility (Rothman et al., 1993). This complexity may in part explain why the success of some interventions has been limited.

Studies that examine the effects of behavioral interventions to prevent cancer take decades to complete. Available data cannot answer the question of whether behavioral interventions prevent cancer or prolong the life of individuals with cancer. Behavioral research has found that people can alter behaviors that increase their risk for cancer, that they can, for example, modify their diets and adhere to a program that should decrease cancer incidence. Behavioral interventions also are helpful in increasing cancer prevention knowledge as well as screening behaviors. The extent to which these interventions produce long-term behavioral modification is not known. Even though behavioral changes must be maintained over long periods of time to prevent disease, short-term changes may have a dramatic effect on the health care system by decreasing the extent of disease when first diagnosed. Interventions should provide cost-effective means for reinforcing individuals to maintain health-enhancing behaviors and should target younger populations. Adoption of good dietary habits and sun protective behaviors at an early age are easier to maintain later in life and may be the best strategy to decrease cancer incidence.

References

Aaronson, N. K., Meyerowitz, B. E., Bard, M., Bloom, J. R., Fawzy, F. I., Feldstein, M., Fink, D., Holland, J. C., Johnson, J. E., & Lowman, J. T. (1991). Quality of life research in oncology. Past achievements and future priorities. *Cancer, 67*(Suppl. 3), 839–843.

Adler, A., Stein, J. A., & Ben-Efraim, S. (1980a). Immunocompetence, immunosuppression, and human breast cancer: II. Further evidence of initial immune impairment by integrated assessment effect of nodal involvement (N) and primary tumor size (T). *Cancer, 45,* 2061–2073.

Adler, A., Stein, J. A., & Ben-Efraim, S. (1980b). Immunocompetence, immunosuppression, and human breast cancer: III. Prognostic significance of initial level of immunocompetence in early and advanced disease. *Cancer, 45,* 2074–2083.

Andersen, B. L. (1992). Psychological interventions for cancer patients to enhance the quality of life. *Journal of Consulting and Clinical Psychology, 60,* 552–568.

Andersen, B. L., Kiecolt-Glaser, J. K., & Glaser, R. (1994). A biobehavioral model of cancer, stress, and disease course. *American Psychologist, 49,* 389–404.

Arthey, S., & Clarke, V. A. (1995). Suntanning and sun protection: A review of the psychological literature. *Social Science and Medicine, 40*(2), 265–274.

Atwood, J. R., Aickin, M., Giordano, L., Benedict, J., Bell, M., Ritenbaugh, C., Rees-McGee, S., Sheehan, E., Ho, E., Meyskens, E., & Alberts, D. (1992). The effectiveness of adherence intervention in a colon cancer prevention field trial. *Preventive Medicine, 21,* 637–653.

Bal, D. G., Nixon, D. W., Foerster, S. B., & Brownson, R. C. (1995). Cancer prevention. In G. P. Murphy, J. W. Lawrence, & R. E. Lenhard (Eds.), *Clinical oncology* (pp. 40–63). Washington, DC: American Cancer Society.

Baum, A., & Cohen, L. (1998). Successful behavioral interventions to prevent cancer: The example of skin cancer. *Annual Review of Public Health, 19,* 319–333.

Baum, A., Cohen, L., & Hall, M. H. (1993). Control and intrusive memories as possible determinants of chronic stress. *Psychosomatic Medicine, 55,* 274–286.

Baum, A., Herberman, H., & Cohen, L. (1995). Managing stress and managing illness: Survival and quality of life in chronic disease. *Journal of Clinical Psychology in Medical Settings, 2,* 309–333.

Baum, A., & Singer, J. E. (Eds.). (1987). *Handbook of psychology and health* (Vol. 5). Hillsdale, NJ: Erlbaum.

Ben-Eliyahu, S., Yirmiya, R., Liebeskind, J. C., Taylor, A. N., & Gale, R. P. (1991). Stress increases metastatic spread of a mammary tumor in rats: Evidence for mediation by the immune system. *Brain, Behavior, and Immunity, 5,* 193–205.

Bernstein, L., Henderson, B. E., Hanisch, R., Sullivan-Halley, J., & Ross, R. K. (1994). Physical exercise and reduced risk of breast cancer in young women. *Journal of the National Cancer Institute, 86*, 1403–1408.

Borland, R., Hill, D., & Noy, S. (1990). Being sun smart: Changes in community awareness and reported behavior following a primary prevention program for skin cancer control. *Behavioral Change, 7*, 126–135.

Breslow, L., Agran, L., Breslow, D. M., Morganstern, M., & Ellwin, L. (1977). Cancer control: Implications from history. *Journal of the National Cancer Institute, 59*(Suppl. 2), 671–686.

Buller, M. K., Loescher, L. J., & Buller, D. B. (1994). "Sunshine and Skin Health": A curriculum for skin cancer prevention education. *Journal of Cancer Education, 9*, 155–162.

Burke, M. A., & Goodkin, K. (1997). Stress and the development of breast cancer: A persistent and popular link despite contrary evidence. *Cancer, 79*, 1055–1058.

Campbell, H. S., & Birsell, J. M. (1994). Knowledge, beliefs, and sun protection behaviors of Alberta adults. *Preventive Medicine, 23*, 160–166.

Cassileth, B. R. (1996). Stress and the development of breast cancer: A persistent and popular link despite contrary evidence. *Cancer, 77*, 1015–1016.

Centers for Disease Control and Prevention. (1989). *Reducing the health consequences of smoking: 25 years of progress: A report of the Surgeon General* (CDC 89-8411). Rockville, MD: U.S. Public Health Service.

Chen, C. C., David, A. S., Nunnerley, H., Michell, M., Dawson, J. L., Berry, H., Dobbs, J., & Fahy, T. (1995). Adverse life events and breast cancer: Case-control study. *British Medical Journal, 311*, 1527–1530.

Cohen, L., Delahanty, D., Schmitz, J. B., Jenkins, F. J., & Baum, A. (1993). Mild stress and natural killer cell activity in healthy men. *Journal of Applied Biobehavioral Research, 1*(2), 120–132.

Consensus Development Panel. (1991). National Institutes of Health summary of the consensus development conference on sunlight, ultraviolet radiation, and the skin. *Journal of the American Academy of Dermatology, 24*, 608–612.

Cristofolini, M., Bianchi, R., Boi, S., Decarli, A., Hanau, C., Micciolio, R., & Zumiani, G. (1993). Analysis of the cost-effectiveness ratio of the health campaign for the early diagnosis of cutaneous melanoma in Trentino, Italy. *Cancer, 71,* 370–374.

Curry, S. J., & Emmons, K. M. (1994). Theoretical models for predicting and improving compliance with breast cancer screening. Mini-Series: Advances in behavioral medicine research on breast cancer. *Annals of Behavioral Medicine, 16*, 302–316.

Dodd, G. D. (1991). Cancer control and the older person. *Cancer, 68*, 2493–2495.

Doll, R., & Preto, R. (1981). The causes of cancer: Quantitative estimates of avoidable risk of cancer in the United States today. *Journal of the National Cancer Institute, 66*, 1191–1308.

Domel, S. B., Baranowski, T., Davis, H., Thompson, W. O., Leonard, S. B., Riley, P., Baranowski, J., Dudovitz, B., & Smyth, M. (1993). Development and evaluation of a school intervention to increase fruit and vegetable consumption among 4th and 5th grade students. *Journal of Nutrition Education, 25b*, 345–349.

Dunkel-Schetter, C., Feinstein, L., Taylor, S., & Falke, R. L. (1992). Patterns of coping with cancer. *Health Psychology, 11,* 79–87.

Fawzy, F. I., Fawzy, N. W., Arndt, L. A., & Pasnau, R. O. (1995). Critical review of psychosocial interventions in cancer care. *Archives of General Psychiatry, 52,* 100–113.

Fawzy, F. I., Fawzy, N. W., Hyun, C. S., Elashoff, R., Guthrie, D., Fahey, J. L., & Morton, D. L. (1993). Malignant melanoma: Effects of an early structured psychiatric intervention, coping, and affective state on recurrence and survival 6 years later. *Archives of General Psychiatry, 50,* 681–689.

Fiore, M. C., Bailey, W. C., Cohen, S. J., Dorfman, S. F., Goldstein, M. G., Gritz, E. R., Heyman, R. B., Holbrook, J., Jaén, C. R, Kottke, T., Lando, H. A., Mecklenberg, R., Mullen, P. D., Nett, L. M., Robinson, L., Stitzer, M. L., Tommasello, A. L., Villego, L., Wewers, M. E. (1996). *Smoking cessation* (Clinical Practice Guideline No. 18, Agency for Health Care Policy and Research No. 96-0692). Rockville, MD: U.S. Department of Health and Human Services, U.S. Public Health Service.

Fisher, J. D., & Fisher, W. A. (1992). Changing AIDS-risk behavior. *Psychological Bulletin, 111,* 455–474.

Francis, K. (1996). Physical activity: Breast and reproductive cancer. *Comprehensive Therapy, 22*(2), 94–99.

Friedenreich, C. M., & Rohan, T. E. (1995). A review of physical activity and breast cancer. *Epidemiology, 6,* 311–317.

Funch, D. P., & Marshall, J. R. (1984). Measuring life stress: Factors affecting fall-off in the reporting of life events. *Journal of Health and Social Behavior, 25,* 453–464.

Garfinkel, L. (1995). Cancer statistics and trends. In G. P. Murphy, J. W. Lawrence, & R. E. Lenhard (Eds.), *Clinical oncology* (pp. 1–11). Washington, DC: American Cancer Society.

Gehde, E., & Balthrusch, H. J. F. (1990). Early experience and development of cancer in later life: Implications for psychoimmunologic research. *International Journal of Neuroscience, 51,* 257–260.

Girgis, A., Sanson-Fisher, R. W., Tripodi, D. A., & Golding, T. (1993). Evaluation of intentions to improve solar protection in primary schools. *Health Education Quarterly, 20,* 275–287.

Girgis, A., Sanson-Fisher, S., & Watson, A. (1994). A workplace intervention for increasing outdoor workers' use of solar protection. *American Journal of Public Health, 84,* 77–81.

Glass, D. C., Singer, J. E., & Friedman, L. N. (1969). Psychic cost of adaptation to an environmental stressor. *Journal of Personality and Social Psychology, 12,* 200–210.

Greenwald, P., & Sondik, E. J. (Eds.). (1986). *Cancer control objectives for the nation: 1985–2000.* Bethesda, MD: National Cancer Institute.

Greer, S., Morris, T., & Pettingale, K. W. (1979). Psychological response to breast cancer: Effect on outcome. *Lancet, 2,* 1239–1248.

Gritz, E. R. (1994). Reaching toward and beyond the year 2000 goals for cigarette smoking. Research and public health priorities. *Cancer, 74*(Suppl. 4), 1423–1432.

Grunberg, N. E., & Baum, A. (1985). Biological commonalities of stress and substance abuse. In S. Shiffman & T. Wills (Eds.), *Coping and substance abuse* (pp. 25–65). Orlando, FL: Academic Press.

Head, J. F., Elliott, R. L., & McCoy, J. L. (1993). Evaluation of lymphocyte immunity in breast cancer patients. *Breast Cancer Research and Treatment, 26,* 77–88.

Heber, D., Ashley, J. D., McCarthy, W. J., Solares, M. E., Leaf, D. A., Chang, L. J. C., & Elashoff, R. M. (1992). Assessment of adherence to a low-fat diet for breast cancer prevention. *Preventive Medicine, 21,* 218–227.

Henderson, I. C. (1995). Breast cancer. In G. P. Murphy, J. W. Lawrence, & R. E. Lenhard (Eds.), *Clinical oncology* (pp. 198–219). Washington, DC: American Cancer Society.

Herberman, R., & Ortaldo, J. (1981). Natural killer cells: Their role in defenses against disease. *Science, 214,* 24–29.

Herd, R. M., Cooper, E. J., Hunter, J. A., McLaren, A., Chetty, U., Watson, A. C. H., & Gollock, J. (1995). Cutaneous malignant melanoma. Publicity, screening clinics and survival—The Edinburgh experience 1982–90. *British Journal of Dermatology, 132,* 563–570.

Hill, D., White, V., Marks, R., Theobald, T., Borland, R., & Roy, C. (1992). Melanoma prevention: Behavioral and nonbehavioral factors in sunburn among an Australian urban population. *Preventive Medicine, 21,* 654–669.

Holm, L. E., Nordevang, E., Hjalmar, M. L., Lidbrick, E., Callmer, E., & Nilsson, B. (1993). Treatment failure and dietary habits with breast cancer. *Journal of the National Cancer Institute, 85,* 32–36.

Ironson, G., Wynings, C., Schneiderman, N., Baum, A., Rodriquez, M., Greenwood, D., Benight, C., Antoni, M., LaPerriere, A., Huang, H., Klimas, N., & Fletcher, M. (1997). Post-traumatic stress symptoms, intrusive thoughts, loss and immune function after Hurricane Andrew. *Psychosomatic Medicine, 59*(2), 128–141.

Irwin, M., Patterson, T., Smith, T. L., Caldwell, C., Brown, S. A., Gillin, J. C., & Grant, I. (1990). Reduction of immune function in life stress and depression. *Biological Psychiatry, 27,* 22–30.

Irwin, M., Smith, T. L., & Gillin, J. C. (1992). Electroencephalographic sleep and natural killer activity in depressed patients and control subjects. *Psychosomatic Medicine, 54,* 10–21.

Kampert, J. B., Blair, S. N., Barlow, C. E., & Kohl, H. W., III. (1996). Physical activity, physical fitness, and all-cause and cancer mortality: A prospective study of men and women. *Annals of Epidemiology, 6,* 452–457.

Keesling, B., & Friedman, H. S. (1987). Psychosocial factors in sunbathing and sunscreen use. *Health Psychology, 6,* 463–477.

Kiecolt-Glaser, J. K., Garner, W., Speicher, C., Penn, G., Holliday, J., & Glaser, R. (1984). Psychosocial modifiers of immunocompetence in medical students. *Psychosomatic Medicine, 46,* 7–14.

Kiecolt-Glaser, J. K., Glaser, R., Shuttleworth, E. C., Dyer, C. S., Ogrocki, P., & Speicher, C. E. (1987). Chronic stress and immunity in family caregivers of Alzheimer's disease victims. *Psychosomatic Medicine, 49,* 523–535.

King, E. S., Rimer, B. K., Seay, J., Balshem, A., & Engstrom, P. F. (1994). Promoting mammography use through progressive interventions: Is it effective? *American Journal of Public Health, 84*(1), 104–106.

Koh, H. K., Geller, A. C., Miller, D. R., Grossbart, T. A., & Lew, R. A. (1996). Prevention and early detection strategies for melanoma and skin cancer. *Archives of Dermatology, 132*(4), 436–443.

Kramer, M. M., & Wells, C. L. (1996). Does physical activity reduce risk of estrogen-dependent cancer in women? *Medicine & Science in Sports & Exercise, 28,* 322–334.

Lazarus, R. S., & Folkman, S. (1984). *Stress, appraisal, and coping.* New York: Springer.

Lerman, C., Daly, M., Sands, C., Balshem, A., Lustbader, E., Heggan, T., Goldstein, L., James, J., & Engstrom, P. F. (1993). Mammography adherence and psychological distress among women at risk for breast cancer. *Journal of the National Cancer Institute, 85,* 1074–1080.

Lerman, C., Hanjani, P., Caputo, C., Miller, S., Delmoor, E., Nolte, S., & Engstrom, P. (1992). Telephone counseling improves adherence to colposcopy among lower-income minority women. *Journal of Clinical Oncology, 10,* 330–333.

Lerman, C., Kash, K., & Stefanek, M. (1994). Younger women at increased risk for breast cancer: Perceived risk, psychological well-being, and surveillance behavior. *Monographs of the National Cancer Institute, 16,* 171–176.

Lerman, C., Rimer, B. K., Trock, B., Balshem, A., & Engstrom, P. F. (1990). Factors associated with repeat adherence to breast cancer screening. *Preventive Medicine, 19,* 279–290.

Levy, S., Herberman, R., Lippman, M., & d'Angelo, T. (1987). Correlations of stress factors with sustained depression of natural killer cell activity and predicted prognosis in patients with breast cancer. *Journal of Clinical Oncology, 5,* 348–353.

Levy, S., Herberman, R., Maluish, A., Schlien, B., & Lippman, M. (1985). Prognostic risk assessment in primary breast cancer by behavioral and immunological parameters. *Health Psychology, 4,* 99–113.

Lichtenstein, E., & Glasgow, R. E. (1992). Smoking cessation: What have we learned over the past decade? *Journal of Consulting and Clinical Psychology, 60,* 518–527.

Lombard, D., Neubauer, T. E., Canfield, D., & Winett, R. A. (1991). Behavioral community intervention to reduce the risk of skin cancer. *Journal of Applied Behavioral Analysis, 24,* 677–686.

Longcope, C., Gorbach, S., Goldin, B., Woods, M., Dwyer, J., Morrill, A., & Warram, J. (1987). The effects of a low-fat diet on estrogen metabolism. *Journal of Clinical Endocrinology and Metabolism, 64,* 1246–1250.

Manuck, S. B., Cohen, S., Rabin, B. S., Muldoon, M. F., & Bachen, E. A. (1991). Individual differences in cellular immune response to stress. *Psychological Science, 2,* 111–115.

Marlenga, B. (1995). The health beliefs and skin cancer prevention practices of Wisconsin dairy farmers. *Oncology Nursing Forum, 22,* 681–686.

Mermelstein, R. J., & Riesenberg, L. A. (1992). Changing knowledge and attitudes about skin cancer risk factors in adolescents. *Health Psychology, 11,* 371–376.

Meyerowitz, B. E., & Chaiken, S. (1987). The effects of message framing on breast self-examination attitudes, intentions, and behavior. *Journal of Personality and Social Psychology, 52,* 500–510.

Meyskens, F. L., Alberts, D., & Earnest, D. (1985). *The Colon Cancer Prevention Project: National Institutes of Health* (PO1 CA41108). Bethesda, MD: National Cancer Institute.

Mink, P. J., Folsom, A. R., Sellers, T. A., & Kushi, L. H. (1996). Physical activity, waist-to-hip ratio, and other risk factors for ovarian cancer: A follow-up study of older women. *Epidemiology, 7*(1), 38–45.

Morris, T., Greer, S., Pettingale, K. W., & Watson, M. (1981). Patterns of expression of anger and their psychological correlates in women with breast cancer. *Journal of Psychosomatic Research, 25,* 111–117.

Myers, R. E., Ross, E., Jepson, C., Wolf, T., Balshem, A., Millner, L., & Leventhal, H. (1994). Modeling adherence to colorectal cancer screening. *Preventive Medicine, 23,* 142–151.

Negri, E., LaVecchia, C., Franceschi, S., D'Avanzo, B., Talamini, R., Parpinel, M., Filiberti, R., Montella, M., Falcini, F., Conti, E., & Decarli, A. (1996). Intake of selected micronutrients and risk of breast cancer. *International Journal of Cancer, 65*(2), 140–144.

Nordevang, E., Azavedo, E., Svane, G., Nilsson, B., & Holm, L. E. (1993). Dietary habits and mammographic patterns in patients with breast cancer. *Breast Cancer Research and Treatment, 26,* 207–215.

Paffenbarger, R. S., Hyde, R. T., & Wing, A. L. (1987). Physical activity and incidence of cancer in diverse populations: A preliminary report. *American Journal of Clinical Nutrition, 45,* 312–317.

Parker, S. L., Tong, T., Bolden, S., & Wingo, P. A. (1997). Cancer statistics, 1997. *CA: A Cancer Journal for Clinicians, 46,* 5–27.

Patterson, S. M., Zakowski, S. G., Hall, M. H., Cohen, L., Wollman, K., & Baum, A. (1994). Psychological stress and platelet activation: Differences in platelet reactivity in healthy men during active and passive stressors. *Health Psychology, 13,* 34–38.

Potter, J. D., Graves, K., Finnegan, J. R., Mullis, R. M., Baxter, J. S., Crockett, S., Elmer, P. J., Gloeb, B. D., Hall, N. J., Hertog, J., Pirie, P., Richardson, S. L., Rooney, B., Slavin, J., Snyder, M. P., Splett, P., & Viswanath, K. (1990). The Cancer and Diet Intervention Project: A community based intervention to reduce nutrition-related risk and cancer. *Health Education Research, 5,* 489–503.

Prentice, R. L., Kakar, F., Hursting, S., Sheppard, L., Klein, R., & Kushi, L. H. (1988). Aspects of the rationale for the Women's Health Trial. *Journal of the National Cancer Institute, 80,* 788–790.

Ramirez, A. J., Craig, T. K. J., Watson, J. P., Fentiman, I. S., North, W. R. S., & Rubens, R. D. (1989). Stress and relapse of breast cancer. *British Medical Journal, 298,* 291–293.

Rassaby, J., Larcombe, I., Hill, D., & Wake, F. R. (1983). Slip! slop! slap! Health education about skin cancer. *Cancer Forum, 7,* 63–69.

Reizenstein, P., Modan, B., & Kuller, L. H. (1994). The quandary of cancer prevention. *Journal of Clinical Epidemiology, 47,* 575–581.

Resnicow, K., Cohn, L., Reinhardt, J., Cross, D., Futterman, R., Kirscher, E., Wynder, E. L., & Allegrante, J. P. (1992). A three-year evaluation of the Know Your Body Program in inner-city school children. *Health Education Quarterly, 19,* 463–480.

Resnicow, K., Cross, D., & Wynder, E. Y. (1993). The Know Your Body Program: A review of evaluation studies. *Bulletin of the New York Academy of Medicine, 70,* 188–207.

Reynier, J., Bazin, J. C., Bizzini, V. R., Chany, C., & Leandri, S. (1988). An experimental and clinical study of immunocompetence and immunostimulation in breast cancer. *Internal Surgery, 73*, 10–15.

Rimer, B. K., Keintz, M. K., Kessler, H. B., Engstrom, P. F., & Rosan, J. R. (1989). Why women resist screening mammography: Patient-related barriers. *Radiology, 172,* 243–246.

Roberts, F. D., Newcomb, P. A., Trentham-Dietz, A., & Storer, B. E. (1996). Self-reported stress and risk of breast cancer. *Cancer, 77*, 1089–1093.

Robinson, J. K. (1990). Behavior modification obtained by sun protection education coupled with removal of a skin cancer. *Archives of Dermatology, 29*(2), 135–139.

Rosenman, K. D., Gardiner, J., Swanson, G. M., Mullan, P., & Zhu, Z. (1995). Use of skin-cancer prevention strategies among farmers and their spouses. *American Journal of Preventive Medicine, 11*, 342–347.

Rothman, A. J., Salovey, P., Turvey, C., & Fishkin, S. A. (1993). Attributions of responsibility and persuasion: Increasing mammography utilization among women over 40 with an internally oriented message. *Health Psychology, 12*, 39–47.

Schapira, D. V., Kumar, N. B., Lyman, G. H., & Baile, W. F. (1991). The effect of duration of intervention and locus of control on dietary change. *American Journal of Preventive Medicine, 7*, 341–347.

Scherg, H., & Blomke, M. (1988). Associations between selected life events and cancer. *Behavioral Medicine, 14*, 119–124.

Schneiderman, N., Antoni, M. H., Ironson, G., LaPerriere, A., & Fletcher, M. A. (1992). Applied psychological science and HIV-1 spectrum disease. *Applied and Preventive Psychology, 1*(2), 67–82.

Schwartz, J. L. (1992). Methods of smoking cessation. *Medical Clinics of North America, 76*, 451–476.

Sellick, S. M., Charles, K., Woodbeck, H., & Kyle, M. J. (1995). Factors influencing nonadherence to mobile breast screening. *Psycho-Oncology, 4*, 223–230.

Shephard, R. J. (1993). Exercise in the prevention and treatment of cancer: An update. *Sports Medicine, 15*, 258–280.

Sieber, W. J., Rodin, J., Larson, L., Ortega, S., Cummings, N., Levy, S., Whiteside, T., & Herberman, R. (1992). Modulation of natural killer cell activity by exposure to uncontrollable stress. *Brain, Behavior, and Immunity, 6*, 141–156.

Skaar, K. L., Tsoh, J. Y., McClure, J. B., Cinciripini, P. M., Friedman, K., Wetter, D. W., & Gritz, E. R. (1997). Smoking cessation: 1. An overview of research. *Behavioral Medicine, 23*, 5–13.

Spiegel, D. (1992). Effects of psychosocial support on patients with metastatic breast cancer. *Journal of Psychosocial Oncology, 10*(2), 113–120.

Spiegel, D., Bloom, J. R., Kraemer, H. C., & Gottheil, E. (1989). Effect of psychosocial treatment on survival of patients with metastatic breast cancer. *Lancet, 11*, 888–891.

Theobald, T., Marks, R., Hill, D., & Dorvitch, A. (1991). "Goodbye Sunshine": The effects of a television program about melanoma on beliefs, behavior, and melanoma thickness. *Journal of the American Academy of Dermatology, 25*, 717–723.

Thune, I., Brenn, T., Lund, E., & Gaard, M. (1997). Physical activity and the risk of breast cancer. *New England Journal of Medicine, 336,* 1269–1275.

Thune, I., & Lund, E. (1994). Physical activity and the risk of prostate and testicular cancer: A cohort study of 53,000 Norwegian men. *Cancer Causes and Control, 5,* 549–556.

Urist, M. M., Miller, D. M., & Maddox, W. A. (1995). Malignant melanoma. In G. P. Murphy, J. W. Lawrence, & R. E. Lenhard (Eds.), *Clinical oncology* (pp. 304–312). Washington, DC: American Cancer Society.

van Assema, P., Steenbakkers, M., Kok, G., Eriksen, M., & de Vries, H. (1994). Results of the Dutch community Project "Healthy Bergeyk." *Preventive Medicine, 23,* 394–401.

Van der Pompe, G., Antoni, M. H., Mulder, C. L., Heijnen, C., Goodkin, K., De Graeff, A., Garssen, B., & De Urics, M. J. (1994). Psychoneuroimmunology and the course of breast cancer: An overview. The impact of psychosocial factors on progression of breast cancer through immune and endocrine measures. *Psycho-Oncology, 3,* 271–288.

Vena, J. E., Graham, S., Zielezny, M., Brasure, J., & Swanson, M. (1987). Occupational exercise and risk of cancer. *American Journal of Clinical Nutrition, 45,* 318–327.

Weinstock, M. A., Colditz, G. A., Willett, W. C., Stampfer, M. J., Bronstein, B. R., Mihm Jr., M. C., & Speizer, F. E. (1989). Non-familial cutaneous melanoma incidence in women associated with sun exposure before 20 years of age. *Pediatrics, 84*(2), 199–204.

Weisberg, J. H., & Williams, G. M. (1995). Causes of cancer. In G. P. Murphy, J. W. Lawrence, & R. E. Lenhard (Eds.), *Clinical oncology* (pp. 10–39). Washington, DC: American Cancer Society.

White, E., Shattuck, A. L., Kristal, A. R., Urban, N., Prentice, R. L., Henderson, M. M., Insull, W., Jr., Moskowitz, M., Goldman, S., & Woods, M. N. (1992). Maintenance of a low-fat diet: Follow-up of the Women's Health Trial. *Cancer Epidemiology, Biomarkers and Prevention, 1,* 315–323.

Williams, C. L., Arnold, C. B., & Wynder, E. L. (1977). Primary prevention of chronic disease beginning in childhood: The Know Your Body Program: Design of study. *Preventive Medicine, 6,* 344–357.

Wynder, E. L. (1991). Primary prevention of cancer: The case for comprehensive school health education. *Cancer, 67,* 1820–1823.

Yancey, A. K., Tanjasiri, S. P., Klein, M., & Tunder, J. (1995). Increased cancer screening behavior in women of color by culturally sensitive video exposure. *Preventive Medicine, 24,* 142–148.

Yehuda, R., Resnick, H., Kahana, B., & Giller, E. L. (1993). Long-lasting hormonal alterations to extreme stress in humans: Normative or maladaptive? *Psychosomatic Medicine, 55,* 287–297.

PART 4

Conclusions

CHAPTER 18

Tailoring Psychosocial Interventions to the Individual's Health Information-Processing Style

The Influence of Monitoring Versus Blunting in Cancer Risk and Disease

Suzanne M. Miller

Carolyn Y. Fang

Michael A. Diefenbach

Christina B. Bales

Technological advances in oncology are progressively increasing the patient's access to innovative cancer prevention and control regimens (Lerman, 1998; Shoda et al., 1998). It is becoming clear, however, that simply informing patients about the availability of cancer screening and management options does not automatically translate into improved health outcomes (Miller, Shoda, & Hurley, 1996; Miller, Mischel, O'Leary, & Mills, 1996). Consider two possible modes of response among women undergoing genetic counseling because of a family history of breast cancer. In one case, the individual may react by becoming highly distressed and pessimistic about her prospects. Convinced that her fate has already been determined, she may be less inclined to follow her physician's recommendations for annual mammography and monthly breast self-exams (Kash, Holland, Halper, & Miller, 1992). In contrast, in the other case, the individual may feel less distressed and more confident that adherence to screening recommendations will enable her to detect disease at the earliest possible stage (Stefanek & Wilcox, 1991).

Preparation of this chapter was supported in part by American Cancer Society Grant PBP-89318; Department of Defense Grants BC971638 and OC970004; National Institute of Health Grants CA58999, CA61280, CA06927, CA76644, and HG01766; and appropriations from the Commonwealth of Pennsylvania.

We are indebted to Rob Sipps, Lloyd Ohls, and Jennifer Driscoll for their technical assistance.

343

These divergent patterns of response point to the need to assess and address patient differences in the processing of cancer-relevant feedback. In particular, previous research has shown that individuals differ greatly not just in what they see and define as stressful, but also in how attentively and pervasively they look for threat, how readily they find it, how tenaciously they maintain and relive it, and how they ultimately deal with it (Miller, 1995). However, in order to tailor psychosocial interventions to the individual's needs for cancer risk and disease information in a cost- and time-effective manner, it is important to go beyond the ideographic case level to identify and target broader cognitive–affective subtypes of responses.

In this chapter, we begin by presenting an overarching cognitive–social model, based on cumulative research and findings in the behavioral medicine field (Miller, Shoda, & Hurley, 1996). This approach provides an integrative framework for delineating the cognitive and affective processes that determine how individuals react to cancer threats. We then describe two prototypic psychological profiles for coping with threat and specify how individuals characterized by these profiles typically respond to cancer-related feedback (Miller, 1995). Finally, we consider the implications of the cognitive–social model for the development of psychosocial interventions designed to facilitate adherence, adjustment, and decision making that are tailored to the individual's distinctive profile.

Cognitive–Affective Patterns of Response to Cancer Risk and Disease Feedback: Monitoring Versus Blunting

The recently developed cognitive–social health information-processing (C–SHIP) model provides a conceptual framework for the organization of the relevant individual difference parameters that play a role in the process of coping with cancer threat and disease (Miller, Shoda, & Hurley, 1996). The C–SHIP framework highlights five main cognitive–affective mediating units that become active in the processing of cancer-relevant information (see Exhibit 18.1). Collectively, these units represent the primary theoretical constructs that have emerged from studies in the cognitive, social, and health sciences. These units include the individual's encoding and self-construals of cancer-relevant feedback (Champion, 1985, 1987, 1988; Lazarus & Folkman, 1984; Leventhal, 1970, 1983, 1989); the individual's generation of cancer-related self-efficacy beliefs and outcome expectations (Bandura, 1986; Leventhal, 1970, 1983, 1989; Scheier & Carver, 1985); the individual's cancer-related values and goals (Lau, Hartman, & Ware, 1986); the individual's affective and emotional responses to cancer threats (Horowitz, 1991; Leventhal, 1970, 1983, 1989); and the individual's repertoire of self-regulatory and coping skills and strategies (Carver, Scheier, & Weintraub, 1989). The dynamic interplay among these units determines the individual's subsequent decision making, adjustment, and behavior with respect to cancer risk and disease.

EXHIBIT 18.1

Overview of psychological factors involved in processing and responding to cancer prevention and control messages

Cancer-Relevant Encodings and Self-Construals

Strategies and constructs for appraising one's own health and wellness, personal cancer risks and vulnerabilities, and illness and disease (e.g., the individual's perceived likelihood of developing cancer, based on his or her genetic pedigree and behavioral risk factors).

Cancer-Relevant Beliefs and Expectancies

Specific beliefs and expectations activated in health-information processing. Includes expectancies about cancer outcomes (e.g., the individual's optimistic or pessimistic beliefs about available prevention and control options) and self-efficacy expectancies (e.g., the individual's confidence about his or her ability to adhere to recommended cancer screening, diagnostic, and treatment regimens).

Cancer-Relevant Affects and Emotions

Affective and emotional states activated in cancer-related information processing and behavioral responses (e.g., anxiety, depression, anger, intrusive and avoidant thinking).

Cancer-Relevant Goals and Values

Desired and valued health outcomes and their subjective importance (e.g., whether or not the individual believes that it is critical to be healthy) and goals for achieving health-relevant life projects (e.g., the individual's intention to diet and exercise regularly).

Cancer-Relevant Self-Regulatory Competencies and Skills

Knowledge and strategies for dealing with barriers to cancer prevention and control behaviors and for the construction and maintenance of effective behavioral scripts over time. Includes coping skills for executing, maintaining, and adhering to long-term, health-protective behavioral and medical regimens (e.g., planning, self-reward, anxiety management).

Note. From "Applying Cognitive–Social Theory to Health-Protective Behavior: Breast Self-Examination in Cancer Screening," by S. M. Miller, Y. Shoda, and K. Hurley, 1996, *Psychological Bulletin*, 119, p. 73. Copyright 1996 by the American Psychological Association. Adapted with permission.

From the C–SHIP perspective, individuals differ in the ease with which they typically activate and process threat-relevant cognitions and affects when faced with cancer-relevant feedback (Miller, Shoda, & Hurley, 1996; Miller, Mischel, et al., 1996). We have focused on two dispositional attentional styles that influence adaptation, by orienting and selectively filtering information about the patient's disease prospects and options (Miller, 1987, 1989, 1990, 1995). The first profile, *monitoring*, is characterized by scanning for, and amplification of, threatening cancer cues. In contrast, the second profile, *blunting*, involves distraction from and minimizing of threatening information. The correlates and consequences of these signature response styles have been explored in a variety of cancer risk and disease contexts (Miller, 1995). In this work, attentional styles are measured by the Monitor–Blunter Style Scale (MBSS; Miller, 1987), an instrument for which extensive evidence has accumulated with regard to its reliability, validity, and utility in medical settings (e.g., Miller, 1987, 1995). We now systematically review the literature on each of the mediating units elucidated by the C–SHIP, focusing on the differences between monitors and blunters.

Cancer-Relevant Encodings and Self-Construals

The first mediating unit, cancer-relevant encoding and self-construals, encompasses how the individual appraises incoming threat and disease-relevant information (e.g., genetic risk feedback, disease prognosis, treatment recommendations). As information is encountered, the individual forms a mental representation by linking new details to existing schematic and conceptual memory structures. Schematic memories derive from the individual's own emotional, behavioral, or social experience with prior illnesses or illness threats (Miller & Diefenbach, 1998). For example, for a woman with a history of benign lumps, detection of a suspicious lump in her breast elicits a schematic memory of a good outcome (i.e., finding out that the tumor is noncancerous; Berrenberg, 1989). In contrast, for a woman with a previous history of breast cancer, the same experience elicits a schematic memory of a negative outcome (i.e., focusing on the severity of the disease and the aversiveness of treatment; Miller, Shoda, & Hurley, 1996).

Conceptual memories involve the individual's inferences, judgments, and abstractions about past health threats and illnesses (Miller & Diefenbach, 1998). If a patient has a history of breast lumps, she is likely to remember that she attributed her previous biopsy results to her healthy lifestyle and her rigorous performance of breast self-exams (Strauss, Solomon, Costanza, Worden, & Foster, 1987). In contrast, a breast cancer survivor is likely to remember that she attributed her disease to genetic factors (Sheley & Lessan, 1986). The retrieval of conceptual memories is associated with the process of labeling and evaluating novel events. It is therefore instrumental in determining the types of decisions that the individual makes. For example, the woman with a history of benign lumps may be more likely to exhibit proactive behaviors (e.g., scheduling a clinical exam or mammogram) in response to a new lump, because she is able to retrieve the conceptual memories of assuming personal responsibility for her prior healthy results (Berrenberg, 1989). The breast cancer survivor may be less likely to display these behaviors, because she retrieves conceptual memories of attributing her illness to a genetic predisposition that cannot be changed (Sheley & Lessan, 1986).

Previous research has found that individuals' subjective perceptions of their cancer risk are related to their objective cancer risk in one of three ways. First, the individual's perceived risk may have little or no association with his or her objective risk. For example, among women at risk for breast cancer, a number of studies have reported low correlations between indices of patients' objective cancer risk and their own subjective ratings of cancer vulnerability (Aiken, West, Woodward, & Reno, 1994; Calnan & Rutter, 1988). Second, individuals' risk perceptions may be exaggerated in comparison to their objective level of risk (Dolan, Lee, & McDermott, 1997; Lerman et al., 1995). For example, in one study, two-thirds of women with a family history of breast cancer extremely overestimated their lifetime risk for disease (Lerman et al., 1995). Finally, some individuals underestimate their cancer susceptibility (Blalock, DeVellis, Afifi, & Sandler, 1990; Kash et al., 1992). For example, 24% of women at familial risk for breast cancer reported that they were at minimal risk for developing the disease (Kash et al., 1992).

Individual differences in encoding appear to influence the relationship between the individual's objective cancer risk status and his or her perceived susceptibility to the disease. Because monitors tend to seek out and focus on threatening cues, they are more likely than blunters to develop threat-laden encodings when dealing with potentially stressful situations. In particular, monitors are more inclined to amplify the threatening aspects of incoming information and to focus on the aversive elements of past. In a study of first-degree relatives (FDRs) of ovarian cancer patients, monitors perceived themselves to be at greater risk for developing the disease than blunters, independent of their true levels of risk (Schwartz, Lerman, Miller, Daly, & Masny, 1995). Hence, their construals of their personal cancer risk are characterized by elevated perceptions of vulnerability (Schwartz et al., 1995). Increased perceptions of risk can ultimately undermine adaptive health-protective behaviors (Kash et al., 1992; Lerman, Daly, Sands, et al., 1993).

Cancer-Relevant Expectancies and Beliefs

Expectancies refer to the individual's self-efficacy beliefs (e.g., "I can perform routine breast self-exam [BSE]"), as well as to the anticipated consequences of particular courses of action (e.g., "I can reduce my breast cancer risk through vigilant BSE screening"; Bandura, 1986; Lau, Bernard, & Hartman, 1989; Leventhal & Diefenbach, 1991; Leventhal, Diefenbach, & Leventhal, 1992). These expectancies can have profound consequences for health behaviors (Stefanek & Wilcox, 1991). For example, optimists—who have general expectancies for good outcomes—are more likely to engage in health behaviors (e.g., exercising, eating healthy foods, not smoking) than are pessimists (Scheier & Carver, 1985).

Patients' expectancies also affect their emotional responses. In a study of breast cancer patients undergoing surgical treatment, optimism was related to lower levels of distress, both before and after surgery (Carver et al., 1993). Thus, individuals who have negative expectancies regarding the controllability of disease risks and the potential consequences of management and treatment options have a more adverse response in comparison with those who hold greater expectancies of control and more positive expectancies of their cancer management and treatment options.

Research has shown that monitors and blunters are characterized by different expectations and beliefs about the nature and consequences of health threats. Notably, monitors are more likely than blunters to have negative expectations about the severity (Miller, Leinbach, & Brody, 1989; Miller, Roussi, Altman, Helm, & Steinberg, 1994) and consequences (Gattuso, Litt, & Fitzgerald, 1992; Lerman, Kash, & Stefanek, 1994; Muris, van Zuuren, & Kindt, 1994) of medical stressors. For example, in a study of women undergoing follow-up for an abnormal Pap smear (i.e., colposcopy), monitors considered their condition to be more serious than their blunting counterparts (Miller et al., 1994). Monitors were also more likely to blame themselves for their health problem and to believe that they had responsibility for its course over time. However, they were less convinced that effective solutions to their condition could be found. Thirty-nine percent of monitors versus 28% of blunters believed that the physician could exert only minimal to moderate control over their prognosis.

Furthermore, monitors are characterized by lower self-efficacy expectations than are blunters. For example, in a study of patients undergoing an aversive medical procedure, monitors had lower expectations than blunters about their ability to cope with the procedure, in terms of limiting its physical impact on them (Gattuso et al., 1992). Consistent with these findings, monitors are more likely than blunters to believe that they will experience adverse psychological consequences in response to cancer threats (Lerman, Daly, Masny, & Balshem, 1994). For example, in a study of women at risk for breast-ovarian cancer, monitors were more inclined to expect that genetic testing feedback would lead to feelings of depression, anxiety, or guilt (Lerman, Daly, et al., 1994).

Taken together, the results indicate that monitors are inclined to attend to, and amplify, the threatening elements of cancer-relevant cues and experiences. This focus can promote pessimistic expectations about their condition and its consequences, as well as about their own self-efficacy to deal with the stressor. These negative expectancies, in turn, can further reinforce the focus on threat and thereby intensify the stressful nature of the experience.

Cancer-Relevant Affects and Emotions

Individuals have been shown to differ in their affective and emotional reactions to cancer-relevant threats (Horowitz, 1991; Leventhal, 1970, 1983, 1989). Affect encompasses a variety of emotions, including anxiety, frustration, anger, and guilt. It interacts with cognitions in a reciprocal cycle in which particular emotions are triggered by certain thoughts and vice versa (Miller & Diefenbach, 1998). For example, a woman who is aware of her genetic risk for breast cancer may experience elevated distress (Lerman, 1998). Her cancer worry may trigger thoughts that she should schedule a mammogram, which in turn may activate additional anxiety. This reciprocal sequence of activation can occur so rapidly that affects and cognitions appear to arise simultaneously. Indeed, *cancer* is such an emotionally charged word that the term itself may elicit a negative affective response that instantaneously triggers a cascade of negative beliefs and expectations about disease outcome (e.g., exposure to painful, futile treatments).

Affective responses to cancer risk feedback have been particularly well-documented in the breast cancer context. A number of studies have demonstrated that women with a history of breast cancer manifest a constellation of distress symptoms, including elevated levels of anxiety (Kash et al., 1992), cancer-specific worries (Lerman, Kash, & Stefanek, 1994), and intrusive ideation (Lerman, Daly, Sands, et al., 1993; Lerman, Miller, et al., 1991; Lerman, Trock, et al., 1991). These responses not only have the potential to undermine daily functioning (Lerman, Kash, & Stefanek, 1994), but they can also interfere with the execution of recommended adherence behaviors (Lerman, Daly, Sands, et al., 1993; Lerman, Kash & Stefanek, 1994; Lerman et al., 1990). For example, studies of high-risk women have shown that high levels of intrusive ideation are associated with lower levels of adherence to mammography regimens (Kash et al., 1992; Lerman, Daly, Sands, et al., 1993; Lerman, Kash & Stefanek, 1994).

Across a number of disease contexts, monitors have been shown to exhibit higher levels of distress and anxiety than blunters at the psychological, behavioral, and physical levels (Davis et al., 1994; Miller et al., 1994; Wardle, 1995; Wardle et al., 1993; Wardle, Pernet, Collins, & Bourne, 1994). For example, among women undergoing diagnostic follow-up for an abnormal Pap smear, monitors are more likely than blunters to manifest signs and symptoms of distress during the examination itself. They also experience higher levels of discomfort and pain during the 5 days following the visit. Monitors have also been found to be more likely than blunters to anticipate, and worry about, experiencing pain, discomfort, and embarrassment during the colposcopic procedure (Miller, Roussi, et al., 1994).

Similarly, among at-risk women participating in a screening program to detect early familial ovarian cancer by ultrasound scan, monitors were more adversely affected by positive (i.e., abnormal) results (Wardle, 1995; Wardle et al., 1993; Wardle et al., 1994). Specifically, prior to undergoing the scan, both monitors and blunters showed equivalent levels of overall psychological well-being, anxiety, and cancer-specific anxiety and concerns. Immediately after the scan, monitors who had received (false) positive results reported experiencing greater anxiety and cancer-specific concerns, as well as reduced psychological wellness, when compared with blunters who had received (false) positive results and when compared with patients who had received negative results (Wardle et al., 1993). These effects were found to persist at a 1-year follow-up (Wardle, 1995; Wardle et al., 1994). Elevated levels of distress among monitors are often characterized by high levels of intrusive ideation (Borkovec & Lyonfields, 1993; Meichenbaum, 1992), a stress response that entails repetitive reliving of the threatening experience (Miller et al., 1994; Miller et al., 1999; Miller, Rodoletz, Schroeder, Mangan, & Sedlacek, 1996; Muris, de Jongh, van Zuuren, & ter Horst, 1994; Muris & van Zuuren, 1992).

Monitoring–blunting differences in distress have been demonstrated in response to treatment regimens, as well as in response to diagnostic regimens (Christensen, Moran, Lawton, Stallman, & Voigts, 1997; Davis et al., 1994; Gard, Edwards, Harris, & McCormack, 1988; Lerman et al., 1990; Miller & Mangan, 1983; Steptoe & O'Sullivan, 1986). For example, among cancer patients undergoing chemotherapy, monitors were more likely than blunters to experience anxiety prior to treatment and to report higher levels of depression during the administration of chemotherapeutic agents (Lerman et al., 1990). In addition, monitors were more likely than blunters to experience nausea before and during treatment (Gard et al., 1988; Lerman et al., 1990). Strikingly, monitors also manifested more severe and prolonged episodes of nausea in comparison with blunters (Gard et al., 1988).

These findings suggest that monitors are particularly vulnerable to high levels of cancer-related distress and intrusive thinking when confronted with threatening cancer feedback and cancer diagnostic and treatment procedures. These responses can lead to heightened attempts to avoid the threat, thereby potentially undermining adherence and effective coping (Kash et al., 1992; Lerman, Daly, Sands, et al., 1993).

Cancer-Relevant Values and Goals

Values involve the degree of personal importance that individuals assign to their health and their goals with respect to cancer-relevant feedback and management recommendations. In particular, individuals differ considerably in their desire for information and in the role they desire to play in their cancer care. For example, although some research shows that patients want to be informed about their cancer risk (Croyle & Lerman, 1993; Gautaum & Nijhawan, 1987; Henriques, Stadil, & Baden, 1980; Lerman, Daly, Masny, & Balshem, 1994), other research indicates that patients sometimes prefer to remain uninformed (Jones, 1981; McIntosh, 1976). Similarly, whereas some patients want to be integrally involved with medical decision making (Cassileth, Zupkis, Sutton-Smith, & March, 1980), other patients prefer to adopt a more passive role (Degner & Sloan, 1992; Sutherland, Llewellyn-Thomas, Lockwood, Tritchler, & Till, 1989).

Results from a number of studies indicate that monitoring and blunting styles influence the individual's health-relevant values and goals. Whereas monitors tend to desire and seek out elaborate information about their health, blunters prefer to obtain more minimal details (Lerman, Daly, Walsh, et al., 1993; Miller, 1987; Miller, Brody, & Summerton, 1988; Miller & Mangan, 1983; Steptoe & O'Sullivan, 1986; Steptoe, Sutcliffe, Allen, & Coombes, 1991; Watkins, Weaver, & Odegaard, 1986). For example, monitors are more apt to desire extensive information about their general health status, the etiology of their medical condition, the side effects of any recommended medications, and any steps they can take to prevent future health problems (Miller et al., 1988). Given their high need for voluminous detail, monitors tend to be less satisfied with the standard amount of information provided in routine medical care (Miller & Mangan, 1983; Steptoe & O'Sullivan, 1986).

In addition to requiring voluminous information, monitors are generally more demanding than blunters (Miller, Brody, & Summerton, 1988). Specifically, monitors are more inclined to place a high level of importance on receiving kindness, respect, and reassurance from their physicians. They are also more likely to desire greater technological interventions (e.g., diagnostic tests, prescriptions). Despite their need for voluminous information and attention, monitors often want to play a less active role than blunters in decisions about their medical care (Miller, Brody, & Summerton, 1988). Hence, they are more (not less) inclined to yield control to the identified experts. This may reflect the fact that monitors are more factually aware of the medical complexities of different screening and management options (Steptoe & O'Sullivan, 1986).

The informational and emotional needs of monitors can be particularly challenging to meet in the oncologic context, where screening and management regimens often entail a high degree of uncertainty (Steptoe et al., 1991). A study of Stage I and II breast cancer patients revealed that monitors were more likely than blunters to report problems communicating with the physician treatment team (Lerman, Daly, Walsh, et al., 1993). Similar results were found among patients with metastatic cancer (Steptoe et al., 1991), where a higher proportion of monitors expressed dissatisfaction with physician communications regarding needed tests and treatments. Moreover, low ratings of satisfaction with the physician were highly correlated with increased levels of distress and anxiety.

Overall, monitors and blunters diverge in the amount and type of information they desire. This research suggests that it may be beneficial to tailor interventions to their distinctive profiles of health-related values and goals (Miller et al., 1988).

Cancer-Relevant Self-Regulatory and Coping Strategies

In order to effectively execute cancer prevention and control behaviors, individuals must be able to easily access and implement a broad range of self-regulatory strategies for overcoming diverse barriers (Carver et al., 1989; Miller & Diefenbach, 1998). The C–SHIP model highlights two strategies that are central to successful adjustment and adherence over time: (a) the ability to plan effectively (e.g., developing a strategy for obtaining recommended cancer screenings) and (b) the ability to manage anxiety in the service of executing desired behavioral scripts (Miller, Mischel, et al., 1996; Miller, Shoda, & Hurley, 1996). For example, among breast cancer patients, the utilization of emotionally positive coping strategies (e.g., use of humor, acceptance) was found to be associated with lower distress (Carver et al., 1993).

The ability to successfully perform self-regulatory strategies has been shown to vary as a function of attentional style. Because monitors are more likely than blunters to attend to health-related threats and to feel more vulnerable to disease, they tend to be more motivated to adhere to recommended regimens. In particular, under relatively low threat or routine medical conditions, monitors are more inclined than blunters to schedule and undertake routine cancer screening (e.g., mammography, Pap smears, colorectal exams; Christensen, Smith, Turner, & Cundick, 1994; Steptoe & O'Sullivan, 1986). For example, monitors have been shown to be more likely to adhere to annual cervical screening and to practice breast self-examination with greater frequency than blunters (Steptoe & O'Sullivan, 1986). In contrast, blunters are less attentive to threat and more likely to feel invulnerable. Consequently, they are less likely to participate in routine cancer screening behaviors (Christensen et al., 1994; Steptoe & O'Sullivan, 1986).

However, under conditions of high threat (e.g., a cancer diagnosis), adherence to recommended medical regimens can become difficult, even for monitors. For monitors, intense threats can lead to sustained distress and high levels of intrusive ideation (Lerman et al., 1996; Miller et al., 1994; Miller, Rodoletz, et al., 1996). Moreover, monitors believe that they cannot easily suppress their negative thoughts (Muris, de Jongh, et al., 1994). Therefore, in an effort to limit their distress, monitors attempt to actively avoid situations or cues that remind them of the threat. For example, among a sample of women who were infected with human papillomavirus, high levels of intrusive ideation among monitors triggered the increased use of avoidant ideation (Miller et al., 1994; Miller, Mischel, et al., 1996). Avoidant ideation, in turn, led to high levels of denial and disengagement (Miller, Rodoletz, et al., 1996). Furthermore, as the severity of the disease threat increases, the likelihood that intrusive ideation triggers avoidance and denial increases (Miller, Rodoletz, et al., 1996).

This type of defensive pattern can ultimately undermine appropriate health-protective behaviors and interfere with adjustment to the realities of the situation (Miller, Rodoletz, et al., 1996; Schwartz et al., 1995). Thus, there are two main routes to nonadherence. Blunters do not adhere from the outset, because they downplay the personal relevance of cancer threats. Monitors, on the other hand, may initially adhere to routine screening but, under conditions of high threat, heightened levels of intrusive ideation can activate avoidance and even denial-type strategies.

Psychosocial Interventions Tailored to the Patient's Attentional Style

Given the challenges of preventing and reducing cancer disease, disability, and death in the face of evolving technologies, it may be beneficial to incorporate our knowledge of individual differences into psychosocial interventions and communications. We now provide some examples of how to tailor interventions to the cognitive–affective profile of the patient, with a view to improving adjustment, adherence, and informed decision making (Miller, 1995).

Improving Adjustment and Adherence: Amount and Type of Cancer-Relevant Information

There is evidence that tailoring preparatory interventions to the different informational preferences of monitors and blunters can promote psychological adjustment and adherence in medical contexts. For example, monitors undergoing diagnostic follow-up (colposcopy) for an abnormal Pap smear have been found to benefit from receiving detailed preparatory information about the forthcoming experience (Miller, Combs, & Stoddard, 1989). Specifically, when monitors viewed a short video providing detailed procedural and sensory information (including what to expect to feel during and after the examination), they experienced less psychological distress and physiological arousal than monitors who viewed a distracting video. In contrast, blunters were found to fare better when they received a standard level of information and instead viewed a distracting video on nutrition. Similar findings have been found among patients facing other potentially severe and chronic medical conditions (e.g., Ludwick-Rosenfeld & Neufeld, 1993; Watkins et al., 1986).

In addition to interventions that vary the amount of information, interventions designed to enhance self-efficacy have been shown to have beneficial effects for monitors and blunters (Gattuso et al., 1992; Muris, de Jongh, et al., 1994). For example, prior to undergoing an aversive diagnostic procedure, when monitors (who have lower expectations about their coping skills) received positive feedback regarding their ability to relax (i.e., enhanced self-efficacy beliefs), they manifested better adjustment during the procedure (Gattuso et al., 1992; see also Jacob, Penn, Kulik, & Spieth, 1992; Litt, Nye, & Shafer, 1995).

For monitors, these types of preparatory interventions have an impact on their cognitive–affective processing dynamics by changing the "if–then" conditionals about what to expect in the face of the procedure. That is, receiving voluminous information and self-efficacy communications addresses and modifies construals of the self as fragile and vulnerable, alters beliefs about what can be expected (from more negative to less negative), reduces worry and uncertainty, and provides cues for planning, coping, and managing anxiety. For the blunter, the same types of information only force them to deal, cognitively and affectively, with facts that they prefer not to face (Miller, 1995).

Research has also shown that patients differentially benefit from how information is framed. In a recent study (Miller et al., 1999), women who were undergoing follow-up for cervical dysplasia were presented with screening recommendations that were either loss framed (i.e., emphasizing the cost associated with nonadherence), positively framed (i.e., emphasizing the benefit of adherence), or neutrally framed (i.e., no emphasis). The results showed that monitors fared worse at the affective level (in terms of increased levels of intrusive ideation) when the message was presented in a loss frame. Their levels of adherence and knowledge were not affected by the loss frame. Monitors are typically more negatively biased about their health.

Hence, exposure to loss framing only heightens their sense of risk, without promoting a more adaptive cognitive and behavioral response. Blunters, on the other hand, manifested greater adherence and knowledge when information was presented in a loss-framed manner, without experiencing an affective cost in terms of increased intrusive ideation. Blunters tend to distract from cancer-relevant cues. Therefore, they fare better with messages that increase the salience of threat and motivate health-protective actions.

In summary, these findings highlight the importance of matching the amount and type of preparatory information to the patient's processing style. When there is a mismatch between processing style and information provision, patients become emotionally upset, preoccupied with their distress, less cooperative, and less likely to follow the doctor's recommendations in the future (Ludwick-Rosenthal & Neufeld, 1993). This can be problematic, because at-risk individuals and cancer patients generally need to be tracked over time.

Cognitive-Affective Processing for Informed Decision Making

Although individuals are characterized by stable cognitive–affective processing patterns, they are often unaware of their own pattern of response, particularly when the health threat is unfamiliar and uncertain. Hence, targeted interventions are needed that assess and address how the individual processes cancer-relevant information, both cognitively and emotionally. Specifically, individuals need to be helped to realistically anticipate, and plan for, the consequences for them personally of various cancer screening, prevention, and management options, given their signature processing style (Shoda et al., 1998). Guided by the cognitive–social framework, we have developed a cognitive–affective preparation (CAP) procedure, designed to enable patients to anticipate the scenarios that might develop from different options, thereby providing a more informed basis for decision making and dealing with the consequences.

The goal of the CAP procedure is to facilitate deep processing of the experience by pre-living it, emotionally as well as cognitively, in a supportive environment, thereby potentially attenuating or decreasing adverse reactions (Foa & Kozak, 1986). Toward this end, individuals are encouraged to self-assess and pre-live their experience in a safe, nonthreatening context. Prior research has shown that the pre-living of a stressful experience under supportive conditions enhances the person's ability to integrate and come to terms with the experience and to prevent the development of cognitive–affective disorganization and chronic posttraumatic stress disorder (Foa & Kozak, 1986; Meichenbaum, 1992).

The CAP procedure allows patients to vividly anticipate, observe, and enact in specific detail, through structured protocols, the scenarios that might develop in the cancer prevention and control context, and their potential cognitive–affective reactions to them. This, in turn, provides a more fully and deeply processed basis for making cancer-relevant decisions, dealing with the consequences, and maximizing health-protective behaviors. The CAP procedure thus applies well-established cognitive–behavioral assessment and intervention methods widely used in clinical psychology to enable individuals to anticipate and manage their own probable reactions to the stressors in the cancer prevention and control context.

The CAP procedure entails three phases:

1. *Activation of relevant cognitive–affective reactions.* The CAP intervention begins with an assessment of the individual's distinctive pattern of thoughts and feelings by vividly acting out the situation as if it were occurring in vivo. As part of this procedure, participants are presented with a realistic representation or simulation of the potential stressor (e.g., obtaining feedback from BRCA1 and BRCA2 testing) in a safe, supportive role-play environment. This procedure thus allows individuals to anticipate and sample the particular thoughts and feelings that they are likely to experience in the relevant oncologic context.

   Within the context of pre-living the experience, the individual's cognitions and emotions regarding each aspect of the experience are sensitively probed. The individual is prompted to express the various reactions that are triggered, such as the belief that cancer will (or will not) inevitably develop and the impact of this belief for subsequent cancer behaviors (e.g., adherence to cancer screening regimens, decisions about prophylactic options). The CAP procedure is designed to identify and address any maladaptive response patterns (e.g., feelings of pessimism, hopelessness, and despair caused by one's cancer risk) that are likely to undermine planful problem solving and adherence to recommended regimens. The identification of these response patterns thereby allows for the targeted application of various therapeutic techniques to overcome specific barriers and help the individual to deal with medical options without becoming overwhelmed.

2. *Appraisal of cognitive–affective reactions: Self-selecting courses of action designed to take account of these reactions.* This phase consists of an appraisal of the thoughts and feelings that are likely to be significant when the patient actually encounters the situation, so as to enable the individual to choose a course of action that is psychologically (as well as medically) appropriate. For example, if the pre-living role-play exercise reveals that the individual is a high monitor who is likely to react to cancer-risk feedback (i.e., genetic testing) with a maladaptive cognitive–affective profile (i.e., characterized by self-construals of vulnerability to cancer, expectations of poor health and a loss of control, and high levels of distress), the individual can more realistically appraise whether undergoing genetic

testing is a viable option. If the individual decides that he or she is still a candidate for genetic testing, the use of cognitive–behavioral strategies to modulate distress and maintain adaptive cancer-protective behaviors can be explored.

3. *From assessment to adherence: Providing coping strategies to enhance conse-quential cancer-protection behaviors.* Following the identification of poten-tially problematic thoughts and emotions, the CAP protocol is designed to help each individual plan and rehearse strategies for coping with these reactions. Furthermore, the individual is assisted in making informed decisions and health-protective plans that take into account her cognitive and affective reactions. In this phase, a wide array of coping and self-management strategies are used, including cognitive restructuring and self-dialogue to re-encode the experiences that provoked anxiety or discomfort during the pre-living exercise; relaxation techniques to manage intrusive thoughts; enhancement of self-efficacy expectations; and problem-solving and planning to manage any practical barriers identified (e.g., Foa & Kozak, 1986; Meichenbaum, 1992).

Conclusion

The C–SHIP model provides a theoretical framework that delineates the cognitive and affective processes involved in cancer-relevant information processing. In this chapter, we focused on two prototypic cognitive–affective profiles for coping with cancer threats. In comparison with blunters, monitors were shown to manifest a cognitive–affective profile characterized by greater perceptions of threat, lower self-efficacy expectations, and greater cancer-related distress. Given their greater atten-tiveness to threat, monitors have been found to fare better when provided with detailed information and enhanced self-efficacy expectations. Furthermore, framing cancer-relevant information in a less negative, nonthreatening manner leads to reduced distress among monitors. In contrast, blunters fare better when provided with more minimal information, framed to emphasize the costs of not adhering to recommended screening regimens.

Finally, we described a cognitive–affective preparatory procedure, developed to facilitate adjustment, adherence, and decision making, by making the individual's probable reactions to different options more accessible. In this procedure, the individ-ual's reactions are activated, in a proactive fashion, by "pre-living" the scenarios that are likely to unfold, so that potential reactions can be assessed in a safe, supportive role-play environment. In this context, they can be used by the individual to experi-ence and plan for his or her own cognitive–affective response, potentially attenuating or preventing unanticipated adverse reactions.

In future studies, it will be important to continue to systematically delineate the nature and correlates of the cognitive–affective processing dynamics that become activated in response to different types of cancer threats and challenges. This should allow for progressively more fine-grained tailoring of informational and preparatory interventions, designed to improve adjustment and adherence. It will also be useful to carefully explore the benefits of the cognitive–affective preparation approach and to progressively refine it. In particular, research is needed to evaluate whether this type of pre-living exercise facilitates more accurate self-assessments and better planning for decisions made. The exercise should also lead patients to feel more confident about, and satisfied with, their decisions, as well as promote better adjustment to the consequences.

References

Aiken, L., West, S., Woodward, C., & Reno, R. (1994). Health beliefs and compliance with mammography-screening recommendations in asymptomatic women. *Health Psychology*, 13, 122–129.

Bandura A. (1986). *Social foundations of thought and action: A social cognitive theory*. Englewood Cliffs, NJ: Prentice-Hall.

Berrenberg, J. (1989). Attitudes towards cancer as a function of experience with the disease: A test of three models. *Psychology and Health*, 3, 233–243.

Blalock, S., DeVellis, B., Afifi, R., & Sandler, R. (1990). Risk perceptions and participation in colorectal cancer screening. *Health Psychology*, 9, 792–806.

Borkovec, T. D., & Lyonfields, J. D. (1993). Worry: Thought suppression of emotional processing. In H. W. Krohne (Ed.), *Attention and avoidance: Strategies in coping with aversiveness* (pp. 255–273). Gottingen, Germany: Hogrefe & Huber.

Calnan, M., & Rutter, D. (1988). Do health beliefs predict health behavior? A follow-up analysis of breast self-examination. *Social Science and Medicine*, 26, 463–465.

Carver, C. S., Pozo, C., Harris, S. D., Noriega, V., Scheier, M. F., Robinson, D. S., Ketcham, A. S., Moffat, F. L., Jr., & Clark, K. C. (1993). How coping mediates the effect of optimism on distress: A study of women with early stage breast cancer. *Journal of Personality and Social Psychology, 65,* 375–390.

Carver, C., Scheier, M., & Weintraub, J. K. (1989). Assessing coping strategies: A theoretically based approach. *Journal of Personality and Social Psychology*, 56, 267–283.

Cassileth, B. R., Zupkis, R. V., Sutton-Smith, K., & March, V. (1980). Information and participation preferences among cancer patients. *Annals of Internal Medicine*, 92, 832–836.

Champion, V. (1985). Use of the health belief model in determining frequency of breast self-exam. *Research in Nursing and Health*, 8, 373–379.

Champion, V. (1987). The relationship of breast self-examination to health belief model variables. *Research in Nursing and Health*, 10, 375–382.

Champion, V. (1988). Attitudinal variables related to intention, frequency, and proficiency of breast self-examination in women 35 and over. *Research in Nursing and Health, 11,* 283–291.

Christensen, A. J., Moran, P. J., Lawton, W., Stallman, D., & Voigts, A. (1997). Monitoring attentional style and medical regimen adherence in hemodialysis patients. *Health Psychology, 16,* 256–262.

Christensen, A. J., Smith, T. W., Turner, C. W., & Cundick, K. E. (1994). Patient adherence and adjustment in renal dialysis: A person by treatment interactive approach. *Journal of Behavioral Medicine, 17,* 549–566.

Croyle, R., & Lerman, C. (1993). Interest in genetic testing for colon cancer susceptibility: Cognitive and emotional correlates. *Preventive Medicine, 22,* 284–292.

Davis, T., Maguire, T., Haraphongse, M., & Schaumberger, M. (1994). Undergoing cardiac catheterization: The effects of informational preparation and coping style on patient anxiety during the procedure. *Heart and Lung, 23,* 140–150.

Degner, L. F., & Sloan, J. A. (1992). Decision making during serious illness: What role do patients really want to play? *Journal of Clinical Epidemiology, 45,* 941–950.

Dolan, N. C., Lee, A. M., & McDermott, M. M. (1997). Age-related differences in breast carcinoma knowledge, beliefs, and perceived risk among women visiting an academic general medicine practice. *Cancer, 80,* 413–420.

Foa, E. B., & Kozak, M. J. (1986). Emotional processing of fear: Exposure to corrective information. *Psychological Bulletin, 99,* 20–35.

Gard, D., Edwards, P. W., Harris, J., & McCormack, G. (1988). Sensitizing effects of pretreatment measures on cancer chemotherapy nausea and vomiting. *Journal of Consulting Clinical Psychology, 56,* 80–84.

Gattuso, S. M., Litt, M. D., & Fitzgerald, T. E. (1992). Coping with gastrointestinal endoscopy: Self-efficacy enhancement and coping style. *Journal of Consulting and Clinical Psychology, 60,* 133–139.

Gautaum, S., & Nijhawan, M. (1987). Communicating with cancer patients. *British Journal of Psychiatry, 150,* 760–764.

Henriques, B., Stadil, F., & Baden, H. (1980). Patient information about cancer: A prospective study of patients' opinion and reaction to information about cancer diagnosis. *Acta Chirurgica Scandanavia, 146,* 309–311.

Horowitz, M. (Ed.). (1991). *Person schemas and maladaptive interpersonal patterns.* Chicago: University of Chicago Press.

Jacob, T. C., Penn, N. E., Kulik, J. A., & Speith, L. E. (1992). Effects of cognitive style and maintenance strategies on breast self-examination (BSE) practiced by African-American women. *Journal of Behavioral Medicine, 15,* 589–609.

Jones, J. S. (1981). Telling the right patient. *British Medical Journal, 283,* 291–292.

Kash, K., Holland, J., Halper, M., & Miller, D. (1992). Psychological distress and surveillance behaviors of women with a family history of breast cancer. *Journal of the National Cancer Institute, 84,* 24–30.

Lau, R. R., Bernard, T. M., & Hartman, K. A. (1989). Further explorations of common-sense representations of common illnesses. *Health Psychology, 8,* 195–219.

Lau, R., Hartman, K., & Ware, J. (1986). Health as a value: Methodological and theoretical considerations. *Health Psychology, 5,* 25–43.

Lazarus, R., & Folkman, S. (1984). *Stress, appraisal, and coping.* New York: Springer.

Lerman, C. (1998). Psychological aspects of genetic testing for cancer susceptibility. In D. Krantz & A. Baum (Eds.), *Technology and methods in behavioral medicine* (pp. 15–28). Mahwah, NJ: Erlbaum.

Lerman, C., Daly, M., Masny, A., & Balshem, A. (1994). Attitudes about genetic testing for breast-ovarian cancer susceptibility. *Journal of Clinical Oncology, 12,* 843–850.

Lerman, C., Daly, M., Sands, C., Balshem, A., Lustbader, E., Heggan, T., Goldstein, L., James, J., & Engstrom, P. E. (1993). Mammography adherence and psychological distress among women at risk for breast cancer. *Journal of the National Cancer Institute, 85,* 1074–1080.

Lerman, C., Daly, M., Walsh, W. P., Resch, N., Seay, J., Barsevick, A., Birenbaum, L. Heggan, T., & Martin, G. (1993). Communication between patients with breast cancer and health care providers: Determinants and implications. *Cancer, 72,* 2612–2620.

Lerman, C., Kash, K., & Stefanek, M. (1994). Younger women at increased risk for breast cancer: Perceived risk, psychological well-being, and surveillance behavior. *Journal of the National Cancer Institute Monographs, 16,* 171–176.

Lerman, C., Lustbader, E., Rimer, B., Daly, M., Miller, S., Sands, S., & Balshem, A. (1995). Effects of individualized breast cancer risk counseling: A randomized trial. *Journal of the National Cancer Institute, 87,* 286–292.

Lerman, C., Miller, S. M., Scarborough, R., Hanjani, P., Nolte, S., & Smith, D. (1991). Adverse psychologic consequences of positive cytologic cervical screening. *American Journal of Obstetrics and Gynecology, 165,* 658–662.

Lerman, C., Rimer, B., Blumberg, B., Cristinzio, S., Engstrom, P. F., MacElwee, N., O-Conner, K., & Seay, J. (1990). Effects of coping style and relaxation on cancer chemotherapy side-effects and emotional responses. *Cancer Nursing, 13,* 308–315.

Lerman, C., Schwartz, M. D., Miller, S. M., Daly, M., Sands, C., & Rimer, B. K. (1996). A randomized trial of breast cancer risk counseling: Interacting effects of counseling, education level, and coping style. *Health Psychology, 15,* 75–83.

Lerman, C., Trock, B., Rimer, B., Boyce, A., Jepson, C., & Engstrom, P. E. (1991). Psychological and behavioral implications of abnormal mammograms. *Annals of Internal Medicine, 114,* 657–661.

Leventhal, H. (1970). Findings and theory in the study of fear communications. In L. Berkowitz (Ed.), *Advances in experimental social psychology* (Vol. 5, pp. 120–186). New York: Academic Press.

Leventhal, H. (1983). Behavioral medicine: Psychology in health care. In D. Mechanic (Ed.), *Handbook of health, healthcare, and the health professions* (pp. 709–743). New York: Free Press.

Leventhal, H. (1989). Emotional and behavioral processes in the study of stress during medical procedures. In M. Johnston & L. Wallace (Eds.), *Stress and medical procedures* (pp. 3–35). Oxford, England: Oxford Science and Medical Publications.

Leventhal, H., & Diefenbach, M. (1991). The active side of illness cognition. In J. A. Skelton & R. T. Croyle (Eds.), *Mental representation in health and illness* (pp. 247–272). New York: Springer-Verlag.

Leventhal, H., Diefenbach, M., & Leventhal, E. (1992). Illness cognition: Using common sense to understand treatment adherence and affect cognition interaction. *Cognitive Therapy and Research, 16,* 143–163.

Litt, M., Nye, C., & Shafer, D. (1995). Preparation for oral surgery: Evaluating elements of coping. *Journal of Behavioral Medicine, 18,* 435–459.

Ludwick-Rosenthal, R., & Neufeld, R. W. (1993). Preparation for undergoing an invasive medical procedure: Interacting effects of information and coping style. *Journal of Consulting & Clinical Psychology, 61,* 156–164.

McIntosh, J. (1976). Patients' awareness and desire for information about the diagnosed but undisclosed malignant disease. *Lancet, 2,* 300–303.

Meichenbaum, D. (1992). Stress inoculation training: A twenty year update. In R. L. Woolfolk & P. M. Lehrer (Eds.), *Principles and practice of stress management* (pp. 373–406). New York: Guilford Press.

Miller, S. M. (1987). Monitoring and blunting: Validation of a questionnaire to assess styles of information-seeking under threat. *Journal of Personality and Social Psychology, 52,* 345–353.

Miller, S. M. (1989). Cognitive informational styles in the process of coping with threat and frustration. *Advances in Behaviour Research and Therapy, 11,* 223–234.

Miller, S. M. (1990). To see or not to see: Cognitive informational styles in the coping process. In M. Rosenbaum (Ed.), *Learned resourcefulness: On coping skills, self-regulation and adaptive behavior* (pp. 95–126). New York: Springer Press.

Miller, S. M. (1995). Monitoring versus blunting styles of coping with cancer influence the information patients want and need about their disease. *Cancer, 76,* 167–177.

Miller, S. M., Brody, D. S., & Summerton, J. (1988). Styles of coping with threat: Implications for health. *Journal of Personality and Social Psychology, 54,* 142–148.

Miller, S. M., Buzaglo, J. S., Green, V., Simms, S. L., Bales, C., Mangan, C. E., & Sedlacek, T. V. (1999). Monitoring styles in women at risk for cervical cancer: Implications for the framing of health-relevant messages [Special issue]. *Annals of Behavioral Medicine, 21,* 91–99.

Miller, S. M., Combs, C., & Stoddard, E. (1989). Information, coping, and control in patients undergoing surgery and stressful medical procedures. In A. Steptoe & A. Appels (Eds.), *Stress, personal control and health* (pp. 107–130). New York: Wiley.

Miller, S. M., & Diefenbach, M. A. (1998). The cognitive–social health information processing (C-SHIP) model: A theoretical framework for research in behavioral oncology. In D. Krantz (Ed.), *Perspectives in behavioral medicine* (pp. 219–244). Hillsdale, NJ: Erlbaum.

Miller, S. M., Leinbach, A., & Brody, D. S. (1989). Coping style in hypertensive patients: Nature and consequences [invited article]. *Journal of Consulting and Clinical Psychology, 57,* 333–337.

Miller, S. M., & Mangan, C. E. (1983). The interacting effects of information and coping style in adapting to gynecologic stress: Should the doctor tell all? *Journal of Personality and Social Psychology, 45,* 223–236.

Miller, S. M., Mischel, W., O'Leary, A., & Mills, M. (1996). From human papillomavirus (HPV) to cervical cancer: Psychological processes in infection, detection, and control. *Annals of Behavioral Medicine, 18,* 219–228.

Miller, S. M., Rodoletz, M., Schroeder, C. M., Mangan, C. E., & Sedlacek, T. V. (1996). Applications of the monitoring process model to coping with severe long-term medical threats. *Health Psychology, 15,* 216–225.

Miller, S. M., Roussi, P., Altman, D., Helm, W., & Steinberg, A. (1994). The effects of coping style on psychological reactions to colposcopy among low-income minority women. *Journal of Reproductive Medicine, 39,* 711–718.

Miller, S. M., Shoda, Y., & Hurley, K. (1996). Applying cognitive social theory to breast self-examination in cancer screening: Breast self-examination in cancer screening. *Psychological Bulletin, 119,* 70–94.

Muris, P., de Jongh, A., van Zuuren, F., & ter Horst, G. (1994). Coping style and anxiety, cognitions, and cognitive control in dental phobia. *Personality and Individual Differences, 17,* 143–145.

Muris, P., & van Zuuren, F. (1992). Monitoring medical fears and physical symptoms. *British Journal of Clinical Psychology, 31,* 360–362.

Muris, P., van Zuuren, F., & Kindt, M. (1994). Monitoring coping style, fear of AIDS, and attitudes towards AIDS prevention. *Social Behavior and Personality, 22,* 137–144.

Scheier, M., & Carver, C. (1985). Optimism, coping, and health: Assessment and implications of generalized outcome expectancies. *Health Psychology, 4,* 219–247.

Schwartz, M., Lerman, C., Miller, S. M., Daly, M., & Masny, A. (1995). Coping disposition, perceived risk, and psychological distress among women at increased risk for ovarian cancer. *Health Psychology, 14,* 232–235.

Sheley, J., & Lessan, G. (1986). Limited impact of the breast self-examination movement: A Latin American illustration. *Social Science and Medicine, 23,* 905–910.

Shoda, Y., Mischel, W., Miller, S. M., Diefenbach, M. A., Daly, M. B., & Engstrom, P. F. (1998). Psychological interventions and genetic testing: Facilitating informed decisions about BRCA1/2 cancer susceptibility. *Journal of Clinical Psychology in Medical Settings, 5,* 3–17.

Stefanek, M. E., & Wilcox, P. (1991). First degree relatives of breast cancer patients: Screening practices and provision of risk information. *Cancer Detection and Prevention, 15,* 379–384.

Steptoe, A., & O'Sullivan, J. (1986). Monitoring and blunting coping styles in women prior to surgery. *British Journal of Clinical Psychology, 25,* 143–144.

Steptoe, A., Sutcliffe, I., Allen, B., & Coombes, C. (1991). Satisfaction with communication, medical knowledge, and coping style in patients with metastatic cancer. *Social Science and Medicine, 32,* 627–632.

Strauss, L., Solomon, L., Costanza, M., Worden, J., & Foster, R. (1987). Breast self-examination practices and attitudes of women with and without a history of breast cancer. *Journal of Behavioral Medicine, 10,* 337–350.

Sutherland, H. J., Llewellyn-Thomas, H. A., Lockwood, G. A., Tritchler, D. L., & Till, J. E. (1989). Cancer patients: Their desire for information and participation in treatment decisions. *Journal of the Royal Society of Medicine, 82,* 260–263.

Wardle, F. J. (1995). Women at risk for ovarian cancer. *Journal of the National Cancer Institute Monographs, 17,* 81–85.

Wardle, F. J., Collins, W., Pernet, A. L., Whitehead, M. I, Bourne, T. H., & Campbell, S. (1993). Psychological impact of screening for familial ovarian cancer. *Journal of the National Cancer Institute, 85,* 653–657.

Wardle, F. J., Pernet, A., Collins, W., & Bourne, T. (1994). False positive results in ovarian cancer screening: One year follow-up of psychological status. *Psychology and Health, 10,* 33–40.

Watkins, L. O., Weaver, L., & Odegaard, V. (1986). Preparation for cardiac catheterization: Tailoring content of instruction to coping style. *Heart Lung, 15,* 382–389.

Preventive Psychosocial Intervention in Cancer Treatment

Implications for Managed Care

Gerald P. Koocher

Irene S. Pollin

The landscapes of most human lives are permanently altered by a cancer diagnosis. Even when some positive changes or insights result, returning to "the way things were" is simply not possible. This does not mean that restoring a sense of normalcy is impossible. Rather, patients must come to a new understanding of what constitutes "normal" for them (Shapiro & Koocher, 1996). Said another way: The goal of the medical crisis counseling (MCC) is to help the patient optimize social and occupational functioning and manage medical aspects of the disease. In this chapter we demonstrate the effectiveness of MCC to help such patients and their families set realistic goals and address them using a time-effective preventive counseling approach. First, however, we review the MCC approach and summarize its use with cancer patients in an HMO-based randomized clinical trial.

Intervention During Medical Crises

Restoring some patients to a prior level of functioning may be feasible, but it is an inadequate if not unrealistic goal for most patients facing a prolonged course of cancer treatment. People with cancer may face arduous chemotherapy, radiation treatment, surgery, newer experimental therapies, or any combination of these. Even when medical intervention yields optimal outcomes, these patients live with years of uncertainty regarding potential recurrence or late effects of treatment under emotional pressures that have been termed a kind of Damocles syndrome (Koocher & O'Malley, 1981). A psychotherapist who approaches these patients with the goal of restoring them to a prior level of functioning denies the very real life-changing nature of the medical crises they face and risks alienating patients by minimizing these challenges or, worse, by communicating unrealistic expectations.

Basic Assumptions of the MCC Paradigm

We have four primary clinical assumptions when working with patients struggling with cancer and other medical crises. First, we assume, as did Caplan (1960), that psychological responses to medical crises rarely represent pathology. Rather, anyone facing the extreme stress of life-threatening chronic illness may react with a host of psychiatric symptoms, including those frequently associated with mental illness, such as dissociation, denial, and the vegetative symptoms indicative of anxiety disorders and major depression. These responses, however, do not warrant the same treatment approach as the patient experiencing the same symptoms independent of medical distress (Pollin, 1995).

Second, we assume that there is a continuum of social, occupational, and biomedical functioning along which coping progress can be demonstrated. Imagine two patients with identical social, occupational, and educational backgrounds diagnosed with the same type of malignancy undergoing identical treatment protocols. One patient may cope by writing letters to friends, taking walks, and engaging in some active mind-occupying process. Meanwhile, the other patient quietly and passively wastes away emotionally in bed staring at the cracks in the ceiling. Although they are similar people with similar backgrounds and have the same illness and prognosis, the patients' functional coping responses may be radically different.

Third, individuals' responses to serious medical illness cannot be understood in a social or interpersonal vacuum. The patients' relationships at home, work, and school and in the local neighborhood are often affected by illness. As in systems theory, we assume that changes in one part of the patient's ecology (e.g., the onset of illness) resonate throughout the entire system (McDaniel, Hepworth, & Doherty, 1992, 1997; Minuchin & Fishman, 1981). Therefore, it is necessary to assess and work toward optimal functioning in every social system in which the patient interacts. Although this observation may be obvious to those who routinely work with medical patients, it has only recently been called to the attention of psychotherapists more broadly. McDaniel and her colleagues (1992) recognized as much when they noted that "powerful benefits that can emerge when therapists acknowledge illness as a vital part of everyone's psychology" (p. XIX).

Fourth, we assume that the duration of a given crisis varies from disease to disease and from person to person. Many medical crises can be broken into a series of turbulent periods broken up by periods of relative calm. Others are acute and short-lived. In cancer treatment, the diagnosis, onset of treatment side effects, or relapse are examples of turbulent periods, contrasted with longer uneventful yet tense intervals of waiting with the hope that nothing worse will happen. The number of permutations is infinite. This unfolding natural history or course of the illness has significant implications for the frequency, duration, and intensity of treatment. Offering counseling outside of such context sensitivity is ineffective.

The ultimate goal of MCC treatment is to limit impediments to optimal functioning and promote active coping. The consistent question asked of each patient during the first session and throughout treatment is this: "Given the realistic confines of your illness how can you create or modify your life to optimize functioning and enjoyment?" (Pollin, 1994, p. 104). This is a complex question. It requires that the patient and counselor distinguish unchangeable limitations induced by the illness from impediments that can be addressed in treatment. In summary, the goal is to help the patient mourn losses incurred by the disease and to simultaneously take steps to optimize functioning in social, occupational, and biomedical realms.

Common Impediments to Optimal Functioning

MCC typically addresses and describes eight fears or issues commonly encountered in the struggle to cope with chronic illness. These include loss of control, loss of self-image, dependency, stigma, abandonment, anger, isolation, and death. A full discussion may be found in Pollin (1994, 1995). A few are discussed here for illustrative purposes in the context of other investigators' findings.

Isolation

The powerful stress-buffering effects of social support have been widely acknowledged (e.g., Dunkel-Schetter, Folkman, & Lazarus, 1987; Sarason, Levine, Basham, & Sarason, 1983; Spiegel, 1990, 1992). Social support has been found to improve quality of life and longevity (Neale, Tilley, & Vernon, 1986). Yet for many medical patients, emotional isolation is the norm. In medical populations there are a number of powerful impediments that contribute to isolation. Many ill patients avoid talking to friends and family about their illnesses. A common and understandable motive is fear of burdening loved ones (Ell, Nishimoto, Mantell, & Hamovitch, 1988). Avoidance also maintains the status quo. As strategic theorists have maintained, most systems strive to maintain homeostasis at all costs. In fact, avoidance is very common in medical samples (Suls & Fletcher, 1985). As a result of this silence, patients may often feel emotionally starved at a virtual banquet of social support. MCC addresses both sources of social support and the importance of communication as strategies to advance coping.

There are a number of other factors that contribute to the prevalence of avoidance among cancer patients. Cancer invariably assaults one's appearance: hair loss, dramatic weight changes, mood swings, cushinoid body features as the direct result of chemotherapy, fatigue, and changes in sexual functioning are typical experiences. As a result, patients are often unwilling to enthusiastically embrace previously enjoyed social activities. Dependence on medication routines, fear of embarrassing or frightening symptoms, and anxiety about being away from medical help for any length of time can also hamper social connections.

Differences in coping styles within relationships can also impede open communication. Although the stresses of chronic illness have been found to be roughly equivalent in patients and their families (e.g., Cassileth & Hamilton, 1979; Ell et al., 1988), there is a growing body of literature to suggest that patients often cope differently from family members (Carter, Carter, & Prosen, 1992; Gotay, 1984). For example, a husband might adopt a cheerful optimism, whereas his wife prefers to prepare for the worst-case scenario. These differences in coping styles can be problematic. Although estimates vary, in cancer populations a full one fourth of patients have been found to experience serious problems in previously stable relationships, and a much larger proportion report some rejection or social withdrawal from social supports (Lichtmann, Taylor, & Wood, 1987). These results probably can be generalized to other populations.

Losses and Dependency

Medical crises are rife with loss. In concrete terms, medical patients frequently lose their original appearance, their freedom of movement, freedom from pain, strength, sensory acuity, and ability to communicate or even think clearly. More abstractly, but easily as powerful, such patients may grieve loss of independence, financial security, occupational identity, family roles, expectations, dreams, hobbies, and even a personal sense of meaning.

Adverse changes in physical appearance are an obvious loss and concern for many patients. Social psychologists have long known that physical appearance has powerful interpersonal effects. Attractive people are often judged to hold higher social status, are less likely to be considered maladjusted, and are hired more often than equally qualified less attractive people (Baron & Bryne, 1981; Bersheid & Walster, 1978; Wrightsman & Deaux, 1981). The severity of the reactions to changes in appearance appear to be correlated with the severity of the perceived deformity. For example, difficult but short-lived reactions have been described by breast cancer patients recovering from mastectomies (Ganz, Schag, Polinsky, Heinrich & Flack, 1987), whereas more severe, longer term reactions have been observed in burn patients with pervasive injury (Andreasen, Noyes, Hartford, Brodland, & Proctor, 1972).

The loss of freedom of movement cannot be underestimated. Patients who were recently able to hop into a shower, gulp down a cup of coffee, and ride a bicycle across town to work may suddenly have to plan each step toward the bathroom. Speed and ease of life are usually the first sacrifices to illness and signals of dependency. As patients adjust they must alter their expectations for what they can reasonably do in a given period of time.

Although they may be less overtly visible, losses of life expectancy or goals are also powerful. The patient who had every expectation of having a family or reaching a particular life milestone may be forced to abandon these expectations, resulting in grief for these losses.

Loss of Control in the Medical System

Patients in medical systems face two common impediments to optimal functioning. First, they often have problems communicating with medical staff. They report feeling "left out," uncared for as individuals, unaware of their current medical status, and unable to access information (Adamson, Teschann, Gullion, & Oppenberg, 1989; Faden, Becker, Lewis, Freeman, & Faden, 1981; Waitzkin, 1985). Second, they are frequently surprised at the level of dehumanization, vulnerability, and powerlessness they experience (Liss-Levinson, 1982; Seligman, 1975).

Being a patient demands specialized skills. Unfortunately, success in the patient role demands exercising those skills precisely when patients feel their most vulnerable and least able to muster personal resources. Some of the most important instructions we get in our lifetime (such as how to comply with medical regimens that may save our lives) come to us at times when we are the most anxious, distracted, physically disabled, and feeling out of control (Shapiro, Boggs, Melamed, & Rodriguez, 1992).

Overview of the Intervention:
Assessment and Intervention Structure

As in any form of psychotherapy, building an effective alliance and creating a safe environment are critical. Unlike many patients encountered in mental health settings, most medical patients have usually had little contact with mental health professionals. The stigma of seeing a professional for help with emotional matters is often an acute obstacle. For this reason it is frequently useful to explain the four basic assumptions of medical crisis treatment directly to the patient. Emphasizing the normalizing assumption, that medical diseases are stressful for everyone, is often particularly useful (Pollin, 1995).

The consistent question asked of the patient during the first session and through-out treatment is this: "Given the realistic confines of your illness, how can you create or modify your life to optimize functioning and enjoyment?" Before establishing any goals, it is helpful to assess the patient's perspective regarding the illness and its ramifications. Asking patients to tell the story of their illness, starting from just prior to diagnosis and leading to the present, is usually illustrative. This narrative provides the clinician with insights into the patient's perceived losses and changes in social, occupational, and biomedical functioning. In turn, these initial perceptions are likely to help the clinician generate hypotheses regarding impediments to optimal functioning.

By the first session the clinician should have an understanding of the patient's medical history and current social, occupational, and biomedical functioning. Clearly, as in any clinical setting, the treater should also inquire about substance use and any history of suicidal or homicidal ideation, intent, plans, or actions.

The following questions are provided to help focus the treater on relevant topics. First, medical issues should be discussed from the patient's perspective, even if the medical record has already been carefully reviewed (e.g., "When were you diagnosed? How did you know you were ill? How many times have you been hospitalized? Had surgery? Other treatments? What medications do you take? What are their side effects? How do the symptoms of your illness influence your life?"). Second, current social functioning should be addressed (e.g., "How much time do you spend with your family, friends, engaged in social activities? How much do others important to you in your daily life know about what you are going through?"). Third, occupational functioning should be discussed (e.g., "How has work or school been impacted by your illness? Start from when you wake up and take me through your day. What are your hobbies and interests? How have they been affected?"). Functioning within the medical system should be assessed (e.g., "How satisfied are you with your treaters? How often do you see them? How involved are you in making decisions regarding your treatment? What side effects and symptoms do you regularly experience?"). Some clinicians also find it useful to explore any family history of crisis and previous experience with services from mental health professionals.

After the initial assessment, the therapist should provide patients with an idea of what to expect in treatment. Medical crisis clinicians must use flexibility and creativity in time management. The traditional 50-minute hour may be too much or little treatment for patients struggling with medical crises. Unfortunately, there are little scientific data to help guide clinicians grappling with the ideal frequency and intensity for a given patient. There are a few competing time models that can provide guidance. The patients referred to medical crisis clinicians tend to fall in one of three categories: those bearing life-threatening diagnoses as a result of illness or accidents; patients with chronic or relapse and remitting diseases who are in distress or not complying with medical advice; and patients who are either preparing for an intervention (i.e., surgery or organ transplantation) or have just undergone such an intervention.

Method

Participants

As part of a larger study involving four diagnostic categories (Koocher, Curtiss, Pollin, & Patton, in press), adult patients of the Fallon Community Health Care (FCHC) system who had recently begun treatment for a newly diagnosed malignancy were identified as potential participants. Cancer patients were selected for special attention because they represent a relatively common chronic illness with powerful life-changing aspects. The diagnosis triggers a medical crisis in the sense that patients must accommodate abruptly changed medical circumstances that require ongoing medical attention and self-care components.

Recruitment

FCHC physicians, nurses, and other direct care staff were educated about the project through briefings with the investigators at departmental or treatment team meetings and by mail. They were invited to nominate qualified patients as participants. In addition, management information system files were actively searched on a monthly basis to identify individuals who had recently been assigned an eligible diagnosis. In each case the primary care physician was contacted in writing regarding any contraindications to participating in the study (e.g., preexisting major psychopathology or rapidly deteriorating medical status). Those patients referred were screened by the research department at FCHC using record reviews and fact checking to confirm that diagnoses were accurate and that the patients met the study eligibility criteria.

Eligible patients were prerandomized to either the MCC condition or a standard care control (SCC) group. The purpose of prerandomization was twofold. First, we did not want to disappoint some patients who might agree to enroll in the study because they hoped to be assigned to a particular group, thus resulting in emotional distress or premature termination of participation if they were subsequently assigned to (in their view) a less desirable arm of the study. Second, we did not want to increase personal distress experienced by people newly diagnosed with cancer by telling them that they were not eligible for a special intervention program. We feared that such a message would be experienced as an incremental loss following their recent serious medical diagnosis. When contacted about the study, each patient was offered information only about the arm of the study for which he or she was eligible. This procedure was reviewed and approved by the Institutional Review Board of FCHC.

Of patients invited to enter the MCC (i.e., treatment arm) program, 36% agreed, whereas 63% of those invited to enter the SCC group accepted the offer. The relative resistance to accepting an offer of counseling in contrast with the higher enrollment rate for the SCC condition is of interest and seems to reflect a degree of social stigma associated with mental health services, even when MCC was described from a normalizing (as opposed to pathologizing) perspective. Many of the patients who turned down offers of the MCC program commented that they "did not need or want psychotherapy," despite explanations of the unique nonpathologizing approach.

A total of 45 individuals with cancer enrolled in the study, and 38 participants completed the full research protocol. The breakdown of participants by clinical trial group appears in Table 19.1. Two patients in the MCC group dropped out of the study before follow-up. Another 5 patients (4 in the SCC group and 1 in the MCC group) died prior to the 6-month follow-up.

Outcome Measures

Dependent measures focused on four domains: self-reported psychiatric symptoms, quality of life, consumer satisfaction, and cost-offset data. The Brief Symptom Inven-

TABLE 19.1

Group Composition

GROUP	N	MEAN AGE (YEARS)	MEAN EDUCATION (YEARS)	MEAN DAYS POSTDIAGNOSIS AT ENTRY
MCC	20	57.5	13.6	96.7
Control	18	54.6	13.11	113.3

Note. MCC = medical crisis counseling. The MCC group had 12 women and 8 men; the control group had 12 women and 6 men.

tory (BSI; Derogatis, 1992; Derogatis & Melisaratos, 1983) was used as a measure of psychiatric symptoms. The BSI is a shorter (i.e., 53-item) version of the SCL-90 (Symptom Checklist-90; Derogatis & Melisaratos, 1983) and has been widely used in psychotherapy outcome studies where repeated measurements with good reliability are desired. The instrument yields nine subscales (i.e., Somatization, Obsessive–Compulsive thinking, Interpersonal sensitivity, Depression, Anxiety, Hostility, Phobic anxiety, Paranoid ideation, and Psychoticism) and Global measures of distress.

The measure used to approximate quality-of-life issues was the Customer Reported Outcomes and Satisfaction Scales (CROSS; Mason, 1995). The CROSS is a 76-item self-administered questionnaire designed to measure the health status of patients in a multidimensional fashion using 14 specific scales. Most patients are able to complete the scale in about 10 minutes. Developed and used in several studies by staff of Blue Cross/Blue Shield of Massachusetts, this instrument has demonstrated very good reliability as a functional measure in mental health outcome studies.

Consumer satisfaction was assessed using a modification of the form frequently used internally for quality assurance studies within in the FCHC system. The modifications included the addition of some questions focused specifically on the MCC program.

Each assessment instrument was administered twice, once at entry into the study, prior to any MCC intervention sessions, and again 6 months later. Cost data were retrieved for intervals covering the 6 months prior to entering the study and for the 6 months following enrollment. A 90-day delay in requesting fiscal data and careful scrutiny of service dates were used to insure against loss of accuracy of the cost data related to late posting of expenses.

Procedure

Once eligibility for the study was confirmed and prerandomization was complete, patients were contacted by telephone and letter to invite their participation. A research assistant met with patients at their homes, provided detailed informed consent, and conducted initial assessments. The average time elapsed from the date of diagnosis to date of study entry was 92 days. MCC intervention for the treatment group began shortly after the initial assessment. Follow-up assessments were conducted 6 months later. Patients in the MCC group were charged the customary FCHC $2 per visit copayment fee for each MCC session, so that the program would closely resemble HMO operations in all respects. Participants in the SCC group were given information on how to access FCHC's usual mental health services, should they desire to do so. All participants were eligible for full mental health benefits that are normally a part of the FCHC plan to which they subscribed.

The MCC intervention was conducted by an experienced licensed independent clinical social worker on the FCHC staff who was especially trained for this project; a treatment manual was developed and used to ensure the consistency of the intervention.[1] The manual followed the model and procedures outlined by Pollin (1994, 1995). Fidelity of the intervention was monitored regularly by reviewing case notes collected on specially designed forms and by face-to-face case discussions between the social worker and the investigators (Gerald P. Koocher and Erin Kenny Curtiss).

Results

The cancer patients in the MCC group used between 1 and 12 counseling sessions ($M = 4.04$ visits). Complete data were obtained on 20 patients receiving MCC and 18 in the SCC group. There were no significant differences between the MCC and SCC groups on mean age ($p = .30$), years of education ($p = .53$), or number of days elapsed between diagnosis and enrollment ($p = .34$). The data are summarized in Table 19.1.

Social Support

When seen at 6-month follow-up, cancer patients who received MCC reported shifts in the direction of feeling higher levels of support from their family and friends in comparison to the SCC group as measured on the CROSS ($p = .04$). They also shifted in the direction of endorsing a consumer satisfaction item (i.e., "FCHC cares about my well-being") more often than those in the control group at the time of follow-up, although this tendency did not reach statistically significant levels ($p = .06$).

Cost Data

The average cost of providing MCC services to patients in the treatment group was $398.55, but the total costs of all medical care attributed to the two groups did not

---

[1]Copies of all non-copyright protected assessment forms used in the study and the treatment manual are available from Dr. Koocher at Harvard Medical School, 300 Longwood Avenue, Boston, MA 02115.

differ significantly at follow-up, despite the average additional $398.55 cost for those in the MCC group. The average cost of mental health services (in addition to MCC) used by patients in the treatment group was $9.75. In contrast, the average cost of such services to the SCC group was $979.69.

Discussion

In view of the sample size, the data described here must be considered only a preliminary test of the efficacy of MCC. Nonetheless, several positive effectiveness outcomes are clear.

The CROSS showed some favorable shifts in perceived social support that may be related to the improved psychological status of patients who received MCC. Key elements of the MCC protocol (Pollin, 1995) include attention to enhancing personal control and mobilizing one's social support system; hence these shifts are fully consistent with hoped for outcomes.

The patients' satisfaction ratings of their HMO were particularly interesting. The cancer patients who received MCC seemed more inclined to believe that "Fallon cares about my well being" than did those in the SCC group. There is no basis to conclude that Fallon physicians spent more time or showed more attention to the MCC compared with the SCC patients. In fact, individual FCHC physicians were unlikely to know which patients had actually agreed to enroll in the study or in which group. Rather, it is highly likely that the MCC services had the effect of enhancing the favorable view of the HMO that was indirectly expressed in this way. This finding is especially noteworthy because both MCC and SCC groups had already given FCHC high satisfaction ratings from the outset.

Cost savings can be seen in the SCC group's use of more than $960 in incremental mental health costs alone. It is important to note that the data we report are only short-term (i.e., 6-month) cost data. If we consider that the MCC group may have a more enduring coping benefit or may be more compliant with their prescribed medical regimen than the SCC group, the longer term cost offset could be even better. Similarly, better social support might lead to reduced mental health service utilization or eliminate primary care physician visits driven by loneliness or other psychological factors rather than medical necessity.

The implications of these findings are highly instructive. We can conclude that MCC did indeed have beneficial effects among newly diagnosed cancer patients. We can also feel confident that MCC services do not significantly increase overall medical expenses and may actually lower other mental health service costs for some groups.

The increase in favorable perceptions of patients toward their HMO physicians is also an important finding from both clinical and business perspectives. We know that patients who feel that they have more time and concern from their physicians are also better motivated to follow medical advice. This may have significant implications for maintaining good patient health and long-range cost savings as well.

It is important to note that the 96.7-day average lag between onset of the medical crisis (i.e., cancer diagnosis) and the initiation of counseling was far less than ideal. When MCC is well-integrated in a primary care system and can be initiated swiftly, such as at the time of or shortly after initial diagnosis, the anticipated beneficial effect is far greater. In our research paradigm, with a complex recruitment and informed consent sequence, speed at initiating service was not ideal. With a more rapid initiation of intervention, the outcome would most likely be better because symptoms of emotional distress would be addressed quickly, and active coping strategies could be introduced before maladaptive behavior patterns have a chance to become entrenched.

References

Adamson, T. E., Teschann, J. M., Gullion, D. S., & Oppenberg, A. A. (1989). Physician communication skills and malpractice claims: A complex relationship. *The Western Journal of Medicine, 150,* 356–360.

Andreasen, N. J., Noyes, R., Hartford, C. E., Brodland, G. A., & Proctor, S. (1972). Management of emotional problems in seriously burned adults. *New England Journal of Medicine, 286,* 65–69.

Baron, R. A., & Bryne, D. (1981). *Social psychology: Understanding human interaction.* Boston: Allyn & Bacon.

Bersheid, E., & Walster, E. H. (1978). *Interpersonal attraction.* Reading, MA: Addison-Wesley.

Caplan, G. (1960). Patterns of parental response to the crisis of premature birth: A preliminary approach to modifying the mental health outcome. *Psychiatry, 23,* 365–374.

Carter, R. E., Carter, C. A., & Prosen, H. A. (1992). Emotional and personality types of breast cancer patients and spouses. *American Journal of Family Therapy, 20,* 300–309.

Cassilith, B. R., & Hamiliton, J. N. (1979). The family with cancer. In B. R. Cassilith (Ed.), *The cancer patient: Social and medical aspects of care.* Philadelphia: Lea & Febiger.

Derogatis, L. R. (1992). *Brief Symptom Inventory: Administration, scoring, and procedures manual–II.* Baltimore: Clinical Psychometric Research.

Derogatis, L. R., & Melisaratos, N. (1983). The Brief Symptom Inventory: An introductory report. *Psychological Medicine, 13,* 595–605.

Dunkel-Schetter, C., Folkman, S., & Lazarus, R. S. (1987). Correlates of social support receipt. *Journal of Personality and Social Psychology, 53,* 71–80.

Ell, K. O., Nishimoto, R. H., Mantell, J. M., & Hamovitch, M. H. (1988). Psychological adaptation to cancer: A comparison among patients, spouses, and nonspouses. *Family Systems Medicine, 6,* 335–348.

Faden, R. R., Becker, C., Lewis, C., Freeman, J., & Faden, A. I. (1981). Disclosure of information to patients in medical care. *Medical Care, 19,* 718–733.

Ganz, P. A., Schag, C. C., Polinsky, M. L., Heinrich, R. L., & Flack, V. F. (1987). Rehabilitation needs and breast cancer: The first month after primary therapy. *Breast Cancer Research & Treatment, 10*(3), 243–253.

Gotay, C. C. (1984). The experience of cancer during early and advanced stages: The views of patients and their mates. *Social Science and Medicine, 18,* 605–613.

Koocher, G. P., Curtiss, E. K., Pollin, I. S., & Patton, K. (in press). Medical crisis counseling in a health maintenance organization. *Professional Psychology: Research and Practice.*

Koocher, G. P., & O'Malley, J. E. (1981). *The Damocles syndrome: Psychosocial consequences of surviving childhood cancer.* New York: McGraw-Hill.

Lichtman, R. R., Taylor, S. E., & Wood, J. V. (1987). Social support and marital adjustment after breast cancer. *Journal of Psychosocial Oncology, 5,* 47–74.

Liss-Levinson, W. S. (1982). Clinical observations on the emotional responses of males to cancer. *Psychotherapy: Theory, Research and Practice, 19,* 325–330.

Mason, J. H. (1995). *CROSS users guide.* Boston: Blue Cross and Blue Shield of Massachusetts.

McDaniel, S. H., Hepworth, J., & Doherty, W. J. (1992). *Medical family therapy: A biopsychosocial approach to families with health problems.* New York: Basic Books.

McDaniel, S. H., Hepworth, J., & Doherty, W. J. (Eds.). (1997). *The shared experience of illness: Stories of patients, families, and their therapists.* New York: Basic Books.

Minuchin, S., & Fishman, H. C. (1981). *Family therapy techniques.* Cambridge, MA: Harvard University Press.

Neale, A. V., Tilley, B. C., & Vernon, S. W. (1986). Marital status, delay in seeking treatment and survival from breast cancer. *Social Science and Medicine, 23,* 305–312.

Pollin, I. (1994). *Taking charge: Overcoming the challenges of long-term illness.* New York: Times Books.

Pollin, I. (1995). *Medical crisis counseling: Short-term therapy for long-term illness.* New York: Norton.

Sarason, I. G., Levine, H. M., Basham, R. B., & Sarason, B. R. (1983). Assessing social support: The Social Support Questionnaire. *Journal of Personality & Social Psychology, 44,* 127–139.

Seligman, M. E. P. (1975). *Helplessness: On depression, development, and death.* San Francisco: W. H. Freeman.

Shapiro, D. E., & Koocher, G. P. (1996). Goals and time considerations in outpatient medical crises intervention. *Professional Psychology: Research and Practice, 27,* 109–120.

Shapiro, T. E., Boggs, S. R., Melamed, B., & Rodriguez, J. M. (1992). The effect of varied physician affect on patient recall, anxiety, and perceptions in women at risk for breast cancer: An analogue study. *Health Psychology, 11,* 61–66.

Spiegel, D. (1990). A psychosocial intervention and survival time of patients with metastatic breast cancer. *Advances, 7,* 10–19.

Spiegel, D. (1992). Effects of psychosocial support on patients with metastatic breast cancer. *Journal of Psychosocial Oncology, 10,* 113–120.

Suls, J., & Fletcher, B. (1985). The relative efficacy of avoidant and nonavoidant coping strategies: A meta-analysis. *Health Psychology, 4,* 249–288.

Waitzkin, H. (1985). Information giving in medical care. *Journal of Health & Social Behavior, 26,* 81–101.

Wrightsman, L. S., & Deaux, K. L. (1981). *Social psychology in the 80's.* Monterey, CA: Brooks & Cole.

CHAPTER 20

Speculations on the Relationship of Behavioral Theory to Psychosocial Research on Cancer

Howard Leventhal

Sasha Carr

O ur overall objective is to persuade the reader that social psychological theory can play a critical role in improving the understanding of the behavioral issues surrounding detection, control, treatment, and recovery from cancers. In addition, we hope to make the following, more specific points. First, we believe that the relationship between behavioral research on cancer and "basic" psychological theory is a two-way street, in which each side informs and influences the other. Thus, we do not believe that behavioral research on cancer is merely an applied endeavor in which investigators use "basic" psychological theory to understand behaviors related to cancer. Rather, we believe that behavioral research in the cancer domain makes important contributions to basic, psychological theory.

Second, we argue that a multilevel self-regulation model is needed for the science of modeling and the practice of influencing behaviors in the cancer domain. A fully specified, self-regulation model of this type will capture people's perceptions of cancer (e.g., its perceived symptoms, causes, consequences, time frames, control) and their perceptions of the procedures for controlling the threat of cancer, and it will conceptualize the relationships of these perceptions to the individual's personal and sociocultural context. We propose further that sociocultural variables and personal characteristics are contextual factors or moderators whose primary effects on behavior are through their influence on the perception of disease threats and the procedures used for threat management (Leventhal, Diefenbach, & Leventhal, 1992; Leventhal, Leventhal, & Cameron, in press), although we do not rule out the

We thank Andrew Baum for his encouragement and helpful comments. The work was supported by Grants AG12072 and AG03501 from the National Institute on Aging.

possibility of direct effects on behavior from these factors. For example, Hispanic cultures may encourage their members to adopt a fatalistic view of disease, leading them to see cancer as an uncontrollable entity (i.e., nontreatable) that causes pain and death, and these beliefs may reduce willingness to detect or treat cancer (Meyerowitz, Richardson, Hudson, & Leedham, 1998; Meyerowitz, Williams, & Gessner, 1987). On the other hand, other cultural factors such as respect for authority may lead the very same individuals to accept a physician's recommendation for mammography and treatment of a detected breast cancer, thereby canceling out the effects of cancer-specific beliefs conditioned by cultural fatalism.

Our third specific task is to persuade the reader that good science is compatible with clinical practice. Indeed, we take this position a step further and suggest that a powerful conceptual model both captures and deepens the understanding of the human side of suffering, hope, personal realization, and growth that is so often identified in the clinical literature.

The basic assumption underlying the self-regulation approach is that people coping with cancers are commonsense medical scientists whose formulation or representation of this disease guides their coping procedures, that is, their efforts at cancer control (Leventhal, Meyer, & Nerenz, 1980). This assumption holds whether we examine an individual's consideration of the detection of genetic risk, the detection of early stages of disease, treatment of the disease, or posttreatment rehabilitation. Exposing the mechanisms underlying this phenomenology and the overt actions associated with it is the primary goal of psychological science. The practical outcome of achieving this goal is to provide the tools needed to encourage adoption of behaviors for cancer prevention screening and early detection, acceptance of the need for treatment, a rational approach to choice of treatment, and the reduction of distress and improvements in quality of life during treatment, posttreatment rehabilitation, and terminal care. Sound theory can improve the effectiveness in achieving health-promotive values in each of these stages, and it can do so in an effective and humane way.

The Need for an Integrative Framework

Our brief survey of recent publications of behavioral research in cancer and the progress reports given by investigators at the 1997 meeting at the University of Pittsburgh Cancer Center provide a picture of a growing number of exceptionally active and sophisticated investigators working on varied projects of great interest. Diverse psychological models have been used to generate research in these areas. For example, interventions designed to reduce cancer risk by preventing the development of cigarette smoking in school children have used social skills training to resist peer pressure (Flay, 1985; Leventhal, Baker, Brandon, & Fleming, 1989) and anticipatory regret as a potential deterrent to smoking (Leventhal, Fleming, &

Wagstaff, 1989). Measures of peer group identification (Mosbach & Leventhal, 1988; Sussman et al., 1990) and measures assessing the perception of the personal characteristics of smokers have been used to identify youngsters at risk for smoking (Chassin, Presson, Sherman, Corty, & Olshavsky, 1984; Dinh, Sarason, Peterson, & Onstad, 1995), and studies of smoking cessation have used classical conditioning to develop aversion to cigarettes, along with self-regulation through self-monitoring to develop relapse prevention skills (Baker et al., 1988; Condiotte & Lichtenstein, 1981; Marlatt & Gordon, 1980). Studies of cancer screening have used risk perception models to understand willingness to take genetic tests for breast cancer (Lerman & Croyle, 1994); studies of fear in response to occurrence and recurrence of cancer have used the illness representation models (Easterling & Leventhal, 1989) and have examined the effects of temporal models of cancer on worry (Silverman, 1999). In addition, classical conditioning models have proven useful in studies of the development of symptoms during cancer chemotherapy treatments (Andrykowsky, Redd, & Hatfield, 1985; Bovbjerg et al., 1992; Burish & Redd, 1994; Nerenz, Leventhal, Easterling, & Love, 1986; Redd, 1995).

Studies of adaptation to cancer have been conducted in the framework of personality and social psychological theories; examples include studies of the moderating role of personality factors such as monitoring and blunting (S. M. Miller, 1987) and the role of social comparison to bolster self-esteem and a sense of well-being (Taylor, Lichtman & Wood, 1984; Wood & VanderZee, 1997). Important contributions have been made in understanding the role of level of functioning in specific life domains and the importance of these domains as determinants of quality of life both during cancer treatments and recovery (Cella et al., 1993; see Cella, this volume, chapter 4). There is intense interest in the role of social psychological factors, such as group support, in strengthening physiological responses that may increase survival (see Andersen, this volume, chapter 7; Fawzy et al., 1990; Speigel, Bloom, Kraemer, & Gottheil, 1989). Moreover, one should not ignore advances in the seemingly mundane techniques such as regular patient telephone contacts that can be used by health care systems to improve treatment adherence (Rimer, 1994).

This cursory scan of behavioral research provides an awareness of the variety of models at work in cancer control. Such a variety in the absence of an overall framework within which we can nest specific constructs and methods does, however, create a sense of fragmentation. Fragmentation often seems to be endemic to productive work; competitive pressures and the enormous amount of complex material that must be digested to conduct quality research creates barriers to communication among laboratories actively pursuing specific projects within different areas. There are, however, at least three other reasons for fragmentation that require attention. First, as our cursory review suggests, the arena for behavioral research is vast, ranging from studies of behavioral factors in cancer prevention (epidemiological studies of cancer causation, studies of intervention to change risky behaviors, and studies of interventions to encourage early detection), to studies of response to cancer treatment

(treatment and disease-related pain, emotional status, and quality of life; interventions to reduce pain and stress and extend longevity), to studies focused on adaptation to or "living" with cancer and cancer treatment.

Second, the research in each of these areas is often nested in separate divisions within comprehensive, clinical cancer centers, some falling under outreach, others under cancer control, and still others under clinical trials. They are divided yet again as to whether they are focused on one or another specific cancer (e.g., breast, prostate, lung). We have seen these divisions in the research carried out in the comprehensive cancer centers with which we are familiar, even though the directors of these centers have made substantial efforts to encourage interdisciplinary involvement in both science and practice so as to insure the rapid translation of basic research findings into effective practice systems.

Finally, we believe that fragmentation has been generated by the promotional efforts and profit orientation of managed care. Managed care organizations assign specific working groups to generate solutions to particular behavioral problems such as cancer prevention, quality of life, and treatment adherence and are often unaware of or unconcerned with the interconnectedness of these problems.

Variation Within a Common Paradigm

The different insights emerging from behavioral research across different types of cancer and from prevention to posttreatment recovery can encourage new insights and speed the solution of practical problems if there is cross-fertilization. Cross-fertilization is frequent in cellular biology because investigators usually share a common, underlying paradigm. For example, they all share the following basic paradigm: Cancer cells survive the normal process of apoptosis, and their unregulated multiplication causes the eventual death of their host. The genetic paradigm underlying this breakaway process is common to all cancers. It provides, therefore, a framework for all investigators whether they are interested in breast, colon, or lung cancer and whether they are focused on environmental pathogens such as cigarette smoke, viruses, or diet as the initiators of the carcinogenic process. The commonality is based in the molecular biology of the communications conducted by RNA between nucleic acids of the underlying DNA code and the proteins necessary for life. This framework allows investigators to share hypotheses respecting the mechanisms involved in the generation of cancer and provides a common set of research tools that allows for fairly rapid adoption and testing of ideas from one area of research to another. It has also provided a framework for communicating to practitioners and the public. Genes are everyday topics in the media and public conversation, where they are attributed awesome, sometimes absolute, power in determining physical appearance, susceptibility to illness, and complex behaviors. This often grossly oversimplified model has a major impact on public opinion, policy, and funding.

Unfortunately, no such framework has come into play on the behavioral side of the table. Its absence reflects, in part, the relative newness of the behavioral sciences. Lest we forget, it took 50–100 years (i.e., from the late 1800s to the mid-to-late 1900s) for the molecular paradigm to develop and displace other viewpoints, such as the protein paradigm (Kaye, 1993). The problem-focused approach of the comprehensive cancer centers offers an opportunity for the development of a common framework. Whereas the divisions within the cancer centers can often create barriers to communication, it is also true that, as we have already mentioned, their goal of integrating laboratory research with clinical and behavioral research to better serve their communities provides an institutionally grounded, problem-centered framework that can encourage integration. Although important, this institutional grounding is not sufficient: What is also needed to insure cross-fertilization is an overarching theoretical vision. Self-regulation theories can provide this vision, because they are susceptible to the conceptual differentiation needed to integrate efforts across both research and practice domains (Carver & Scheier, 1981, 1982; Leventhal, Leventhal, & Contrada, 1998; Leventhal et al., 1980; Nerenz & Leventhal, 1983; Petrie & Weinman, 1997; Skelton & Croyle, 1991).

Why Is a Framework Important?

There are many reasons for recommending self-regulation theory as a framework within which to pursue behavioral research in cancer control. First among these is the already-stated need for a framework to facilitate cross-fertilization among behavioral investigations in the various domains of cancer control. A second, equally important although less clearly recognized role is that an understandable and valid behavioral model can serve in the public domain as an alternative and barrier to the many false behavioral nostrums offered by charlatans seeking their fortune at the expense of cancer patients. Finally, we believe that the self-regulation framework provides the details needed to link behavioral factors to feedback and feedforward mechanisms involved in the biology of cancer. Drawing such links can be a step toward eliminating the opposition to preventive interventions that results from a reductionistic, purely biomedical perspective.

The Public View of Cancer

The overview of cultural conceptions of cancer in Patterson's (1987) exceptional historical review of *The Dread Disease* provides important insights into how the public's commonsense perspectives and emotional needs have affected behavior in every domain of cancer control. The absence of a theoretically sound, empirically based competitor to shape public perception of cancer allows many irrational commonsense views and fears to dominate the behavioral landscape. These views have shaped the public's image of the nature of cancer and the availability and efficacy of methods for prevention, detection, and treatment. Patterson introduces us to our cultural view of cancer as a uniquely evil and powerful disease by describing the press and public response to the illness and death of General Ulysses S. Grant, on July 23, 1885, from cancer of the mouth. Because of the terror and mystique surrounding cancer, Grant's doctors and the press avoided any mention of the dread disease during the months leading up to his death. Speculation at that time as to cancer's cause ranged from emotional distress; injuries from sharp objects and blows to the body; and in Grant's case, smoking, because he was an inveterate cigar smoker. Frightful images and metaphors abounded of this disease, which doctors and laymen alike saw as "an alien and living invader that gave little or no warning before 'eating' into people" (Patterson, 1987, p. 30) that could not be prevented or cured; "when it came, it stayed, 'lurking' as an evil and surreptitious monster on the prowl [and] carried off its victims with . . . unerring certainty" (p. 31).

This two-millennia-plus representation of cancer as a multiply caused (stress, diet, blows, smoking, etc.) painful path to a certain death, a disease that cannot be controlled by medical practitioners, is a view that creates a profound sense of dread and a desire to avoid direct contact with this disease. It is a perspective that has helped to open the door to a host of medical charlatans. For example, Norman Baker advertised that cancer is curable and opened hospitals in Laredo, Texas, and Muscatine, Iowa (Patterson, 1987, p. 106). Harry Hoxsey "touted his Hoxide Treatment as a cure for malignant tumors," and his Dallas clinic took in $1.5 million in a single year. Neither Baker nor Hoxsey are figures from a remote past: Baker's advertising campaign occurred between 1929 and 1932, and Hoxsey earned his $1.5 million in 1956; the Food and Drug Administration shut him down 4 years later (p. 106). The alternative treatments recommended by these and other charlatans have included vinegar injections, chlorophyll shots, radioactive sperm cells, salt, seaweed and nitrates, hourly drinks of vegetable and calf's liver juice, coffee enemas six times a day, and Krebiozen, a combination of mineral oil and horsemeat (pp. 162–165). The existence of this panoply of absurdities is intelligible given the popular belief that existent medical treatments (surgery, chemotherapy, and radiation) are possibly worse than the disease. It is also intelligible given the public representation of the causes of cancer. If cancer can be caused by carcinogens in food, is it not reasonable that it can be cured by ingesting substances that cleanse the body of these dangerous agents? A mysterious, magical disease can only be cured by a similarly mysterious treatment. The presence of a clear and valid biomedical view of cancer, linked to a clear and valid view of the way in which behavior is related to cancer's cause, progression, treatment, and control, is a needed alternative.

Reductionism as a Barrier to Prevention

Barriers to the development of this alternative conceptual framework exist, however, in biomedicine. The reductionistic perspective of experts who resist acknowledging the value of behavioral interventions and believe that prevention and treatment can only succeed if we have "magic bullets" facilitates the growth of the desperation that allows charlatans to prey on those seeking help. Lewis Thomas (1977), the former president of Sloan-Kettering Cancer Center, illustrated this viewpoint. With regard to the prevention of cardiovascular disease and cancer, he wrote

> Cardiovascular disease: . . . lacks any decisive, conclusive technology with the power to turn off, reverse or prevent disease. . . . It is believed in some quarters that dietary lipids are an etiological factor . . . that lack of exercise, excessive emotional stress, and various usually un-stipulated environmental influences are somewhat implicated in pathogenesis. The evidence for these beliefs is still inconclusive. In any event, intervention to correct them would involve grand-scale, societal reforms of living habits.

He concluded that until "the actual pathological events which cause the coronary lesions . . . are elucidated in some detail, a direct approach to coronary disease must await the future" (pp. 38–39). Although he believed that prevention of cancer is possible for a few types, given exposure to "known environmental carcinogens, e.g., cigarettes, asbestos and certain industrial chemicals," for the majority of cancers he concluded that "prevention in the sense of eliminating the biological steps involved in the transformation of cells is not yet feasible" (p. 39).

The contrast between the oversimplification and false hope espoused by Baker and Hoxsey on the one hand and the pessimistic reductionism of Thomas on the other points to the need for a framework or model that can represent the behavioral factors involved in various aspects of cancer control and connect these factors to the biological processes involved in cancer prevention, treatment, and recovery. In short, the framework must resolve the mind–body problem by respecting the science at both the psychological and biological levels and by suggesting ways of linking the two descriptions. Without such a resolution, that is, without a rational view as to how the mind and the body are connected, we lack an accepted, culturewide model to serve as a barrier to false nostrums such as those offered to patients and families that cancer can simply be cured by strategies such as hypnosis, visualization, and "positive thinking." In summary, we need to provide both experts and laypersons with an understandable model for thinking about the relationship between the mind (i.e., behavior) and the body in prevention and treatment. It is the basic conceptual structure that counts, not the details. In the absence of such an understanding, we are left with a division among both experts and nonexperts, some of whom believe anything about the effects of the mind and behavior on health and disease and others of whom believe nothing.

Self-Regulation Models: An Integrative Paradigm for Response to Cancer

We have stated that self-regulation models can serve as a framework for the integration of findings across multiple levels of analysis and provide a language for effective communication among scientists, practitioners, cancer patients, and the public. Self-regulation models examine the processes that mediate between the possible or the actual impact of disease and behavior: They describe the perceptions of cancer (i.e., its representations and the goals for action established by these representations), the procedures selected for reaching goals (e.g., mammography for breast cancer detection), the appraisal of behavioral outcomes, and the emotional reactions that interact with these processes. Thus, the representations of cancer, including perceptions and beliefs about its cause, time for onset, and diagnostic cues, establish goals for acting to prevent, detect, and treat the disease and affect outcomes ranging from quality of life and depression to physiological parameters that may affect disease progression and survival.

Self-regulation models are central to studies of quality of life during and after cancer treatment (see Scheier & Carver, this volume, chapter 2), investigation of changes in risk perception following counseling for genetic risk for breast cancer (see Schwartz, Lerman, & Rimer, this volume, chapter 15), analysis of the effects of social support on the processing of information that is consistent or inconsistent with existent schemata of the self and the world (see Lepore, this volume, chapter 6), and studies of monitoring styles on the processing of information about disease progression (see Miller, Fang, Diefenbach, & Bales, this volume, chapter 18). Self-regulation concepts are also at work—sometimes explicitly, sometimes implicitly—in the studies of the impact of supportive groups upon sense of belonging, self-esteem, and self-efficacy, because these factors affect both adjustment and potential longevity in patients with cancer (Fawzy, 1994; Helgeson & Cohen, 1996; Spiegel et al., 1989).

Special Properties

Three properties of self-regulation models justify our optimism regarding their utility in providing a framework for behavioral research in the cancer domain: (a) their representation of the patient–actor, (b) their representation of the disease, and (c) their treatment of the context within which the interaction of person and disease unfolds. Although self-regulation models borrow from and are similar to utility, stage, and social learning models, they differ from them in significant ways. We point to such differences where relevant.

Representation of the Actor

At the heart of all self-regulation models is the premise that the individual is an active problem solver (Kelly, 1955). Thus, people are seen as being actively involved in constructing representations in order to understand their worlds and themselves. This includes constructing commonsense models of disease threats and strategies for avoiding such threats, such as through prevention and treatment for cure or control of the disease (Lacroix, 1991; Leventhal et al., 1980; Petrie & Weinman,

1997; Skelton & Croyle, 1991). It also includes the experience of emotional reactions elicited by these changing pictures of self and world and efforts to avoid or modulate their impact (Carver, Scheier, & Weintraub, 1989; Lazarus, 1966; Lazarus & Launier, 1978; Leventhal, 1970).

The feedback mechanism, the test–operate–test–exit (TOTE) that is at the core of self-regulation models, is highly abstract; for example, it specifies a criterion (test), a response to close the gap between the current situation and the criterion (operate), and a decision as to whether the response has closed the gap (test); if the gap is closed, regulative behavior stops (exit), and if not, it repeats (Figure 20.1). The mechanism is nested within a hierarchy of similar TOTE units, with those above setting the criteria or set point for regulation for those below (Austin & Vancouver, 1996). These higher level TOTEs can reflect characteristics of the person, such as trait optimism (Scheier & Carver, 1985, 1992) or features of the social context. In

FIGURE 20.1

The test–operate–test–exit (TOTE) is a control system in which a disturbance (e.g., a somatic sensation) is converted into a symptom (input function) and compared with a reference value (e.g., throat is more or less sore than before), and then it generates an output function or plan leading to behavior (take an aspirin and get rest) to reduce the discrepancy between the input signal and the reference value (in simpler terms, to remove the symptom). The TOTE is content free and can describe the thermostat controlling the temperature of one's house as well as one's response to a sore throat.

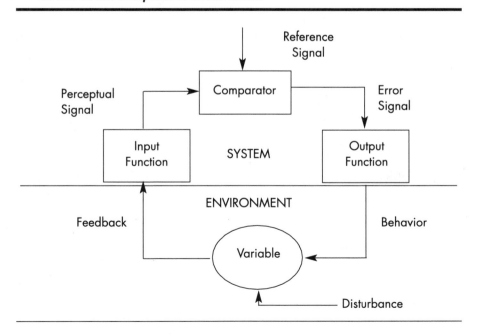

summary, the self-regulative TOTE units provide a dynamic representation of the context for action, the characteristics of the actor, the specifics of the situation within which action takes place, and the temporal unfolding of behavioral episodes. Attributes of the self can be represented as higher order TOTE units that set criteria for evaluating response outcomes and for evaluating the consequences of specific coping procedures. By stressing the ongoing nature of the self-regulation process, these models differ from the static, cross-sectional view of decision making presented by utility models and their variants, such as the theory of planned behavior (Ajzen, 1988; Ajzen & Fishbein, 1980). Distinctions from social learning models (Bandura, 1977) primarily center around the greater attention given to goal setting and higher order factors affecting goal setting.

Perception and Cognition in Representations of Illness Threats

The feedback loops pictured in the majority of self-regulation models lack specific content: They do not define specific sets of variables involved in the representation of disease threats, specific procedures for threat management, and rules for the appraisal of outcomes. Thus, they do not define the variables composing representation of cancer; the cues as to its presence (symptom identity); its causes, time line for development, and time to death; specific consequences (e.g., pain and disfigurement); the perception of it as a controllable or uncontrollable disease; and the procedures that seem effective for prevention, detection, and treatment (Leventhal et al., 1992; Leventhal et al., 1980). Content is also missing from the depiction of higher order loops; for example, there are no higher order loops to represent beliefs about vulnerabilities within the self such as perceiving oneself at high risk for heart disease and low risk for cancer or believing that one is sensitive to and risks harm from use of medication. Perceived vulnerabilities and beliefs about tolerance for treatment will condition readiness to engage in preventive and treatment actions. These are specific, higher order TOTE units that can be expected to moderate lower level control systems.

Just as advances in the science of chemistry built on the substance of the periodic table, content must be added to self-regulation theory if it is to model the mechanisms underlying behaviors relevant to health risks and the control of ongoing illness threats. Self-regulation theory cannot satisfy its scientific or practical objectives in the absence of substantive constructs that capture the phenomenal experience of cancer patients and people coping with the threat of cancer. Nearly three decades ago, when we proposed that the processing of cognition and the processing of affect were parallel and largely independent processes (Leventhal, 1970), it was clear that research was needed to identify the cognitive factors that motivated self-protective behavior. Existent models such as the theory of reasoned action (Fishbein & Azjen, 1975), which later evolved into the theory of planned behavior (Ajzen, 1988), lacked substantive constructs. Utility models such as the health belief model (Becker &

Maiman, 1975; Rosenstock, 1974) and protective motivation theory (Rogers, 1983), which included substantive constructs such as perceived vulnerability to disease, treated these variables as abstract factors that were assessed in individuals by having people rate their vulnerability on 10-point or percentile scales. As it became clear that self-reported ratings of vulnerability captured only a small portion of feelings of vulnerability (Hochbaum, 1958; Leventhal, Rosenstock, Hochbaum, & Carriger, 1960), another approach was needed.

The commonsense model of illness was proposed as a possible solution to the content problem (Leventhal et al., 1997). It spoke to the need to identify specific, substantive domains to understand how people view cancer, how they come to see themselves as being at risk, and the resources they bring to bear for risk reduction. It assumed that these substantive factors determined how people process information about health threats, cancer, and cancer treatments, including how such information is shared and elaborated upon in social discourse and whether information from health authorities would motivate behaviors to prevent, detect, and treat cancer. Failure to identify the commonsense beliefs underlying the processing of information about the threat of cancer separates public health practitioners and cancer specialists from those who are at greatest risk.

Research based on the commonsense version of self-regulation theory identified five domains or attributes of illness representations: identity (disease label and symptoms), time line (time to onset, to cure, to death), cause, controllability (Lau & Hartman, 1983), and consequences (Leventhal et al., 1980). Studies also showed that the specific attributes within each of the five domains were bi-level, that is, illness attributes were represented both as abstract cognition and as concrete percep- tions (Meyer, Leventhal, & Gutmann, 1985). This was true of every attribute (Figure 20.2). We believe that it is important to understand the implications of this bi-level representation of attributes. Specifically, if an illness is represented by its name (abstract cognition) and by its symptoms (concrete perception), either one of these features can set the goals or criteria for self-regulation. Hypertensive individuals, for example, could consistently use their prescribed medication in keeping with their abstract knowledge that high blood pressure is a chronic condition, or they could use medication sporadically to treat their symptoms, or concrete experience (Meyer et al., 1985).

Additionally, the bi-level nature of illness attributes can be represented by Scheier and Carver's (1985, 1992) model of the TOTE. A pair of TOTEs would suffice, with one representing the name, or abstract, conceptual level, and another symptoms, at the concrete-perceptual level (as in Figure 20.3), with separate action systems and criteria for evaluating response efficacy. This dual representation raises a problem, however, because a decision must be made respecting the relationship between the two TOTEs. The hierarchical structure in Figure 20.3, which is one way in which chronic illnesses such as cancer or arthritis are represented, depicts a system in which the ability to modulate symptoms implies that one is modulating

FIGURE 20.2

The parallel response model adds content to the test–operate–test–exit (TOTE). The cognitive, input function (the upper arm of the model), or the representation of the somatic sensation, has multiple attributes; that is, it is given a complete identity (symptom and label); an expectation regarding its outcome, time frame, and susceptibility to control; and a perceived cause. The representation generates a plan for action (coping procedure or output function), and its effects are evaluated and feedback is generated to alter the input stimulus or its representation. The upper right box of the model indicates that the representation may be differentiated (e.g., a person with arthritis can learn to control the symptoms of the condition although the underlying disease itself is unalterable). Emotional states, the input function for the lower arm, can be brought into play by the somatic sensation, by feedback from failed coping procedures (e.g., one may fear a more serious, underlying cause if aspirin and rest do not reduce a sore throat), and by external, non-health-related stimuli. It is important to note that the emotion and cognitive inputs can be more or less simultaneous and interact with one another, including competing for response outputs. The model defines specific content domains but does not fully represent all features of the TOTE; for example, it does not represent the comparator.

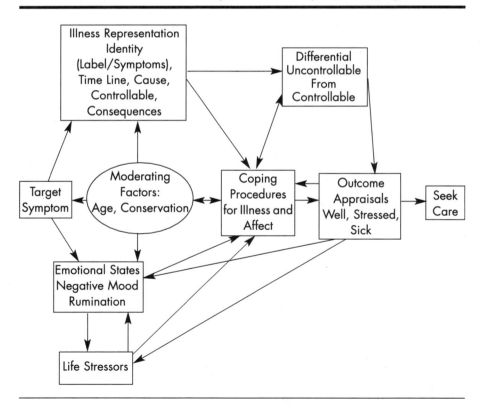

FIGURE 20.3

Hierarchical arrangement of test–operate–test–exit (TOTE) units. The hierarchical system is designed to control the somatic disturbance creating the input, success implying control of the disease. Failure to control the symptom (i.e., the lower level comparator detecting a discrepancy) activates the upper level system, which senses a continued discrepancy and continues to provoke symptom directed behavior from the lower system.

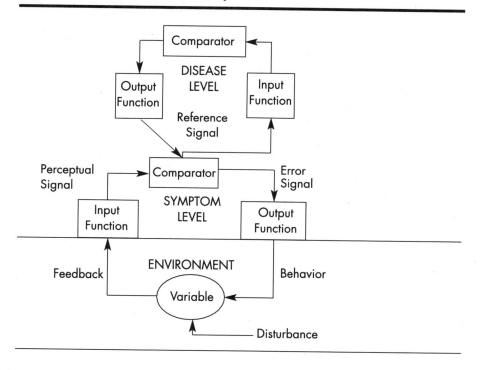

the underlying disease. Thus, if a treatment eliminates the symptom, it is assumed to have cured the disease. Figure 20.4, on the other hand, pictures separate TOTE units for the disease and its symptoms. From this perspective, a treatment that modulates symptoms may have no effect on the underlying disease.

The difference between a hierarchical and a parallel arrangement of the abstract and perceptual TOTE units is not trivial, because the different relationships that they depict between these levels predict sharply different outcomes in behavior and adjustment. For example, Affleck, Tennen, Pfeiffer, and Fifield (1987) found that people with rheumatoid arthritis reported higher levels of emotional upset the more they saw their coping efforts as being directed at controlling the disease itself. The first, hierarchical arrangement of the TOTE units, with the disease unit setting the criterion for the symptom level unit, would represent those patients who see their efforts to control symptoms as a direct indicator of their ability to control the disease.

FIGURE 20.4

A parallel arrangement of test–operate–test units allows separate regulative functions by the conceptual (disease label) and symptom-based systems. The symptom-based system can function and achieve goals, that is, symptom reduction, independent of success for the output function for the disease system (biological cure or control). The parallel system provides the better representation of "learning to live with a chronic illness," that is, managing symptoms and going about daily life in the absence of cure. Vancouver (1996) provides detailed diagrams and discussions of the interrelationship of TOTE units.

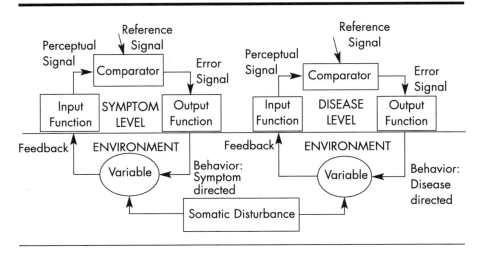

It is no surprise that they are distressed; their symptoms never disappear because arthritis is incurable. By contrast, high levels of positive affect ware reported by patients whose coping efforts were directed at symptom control. Thus, treating symptoms and disease as separate targets, as depicted in the parallel arrangement of the TOTE units, allowed for positive feedback as patients could establish a certain degree of control in the perceptual (i.e., symptom) domain. The TOTE unit is the dynamic component in the self-regulatory system; the attributes identified in the commonsense representation of illness are the content, or criteria, selected as targets for regulation.

The commonsense model points, however, to yet another complexity in the TOTE system. Specifically, the control response also has its own representation. That is, the goal or target of a procedure does not fully specify its attributes (e.g., aspirin is used to reduce pain and is defined as a pain killer, but it may have additional attributes such as a medication that can upset the stomach, as working only for mild and not severe headaches, and as removing pain quickly but only for short periods of time). Specific cancer treatments also have complex attributes above and beyond the set defined by their treatment objectives. Thus, radiation to treat a lymphoma is not simply defined by its ability to destroy tumors; it is also defined by concerns about its mode of operation (burning), its side effects (symptoms and consequences), its time line (time to eliminate the cancer, duration of effectiveness, etc.), and ideas respecting whether it removes the cancer from the body. Thus, control procedures have identities, that is, labels and experienced symptoms, time lines, consequences, perceived routes of action, and expectations respecting disease control or efficacy. Comparisons among the attributes of a disease representation and the representations of available treatment procedures, and the emotional reactions associated with these alternatives, are critical factors in treatment decisions. For example, choosing between chemotherapy and radiation to treat lymphoma, or surgery versus radiation to treat breast cancer, involves comparisons of the expected symptomatic impact, treatment time lines, relative strength of fears of being cut versus burned, and considerations of the long-term consequences of each of the treatment alternatives relative to their perceived efficacy in controlling a similar array of attributes of the disease. We can better understand prevention and treatment decisions by representing both disease threats and procedures within their respective, representational frameworks.

Representing the Context

Culture, community, family, and practitioner contacts shape the individual's representation of illness threats and the procedures used to control them. Self-regulation models' representation of the impact of these contextual factors differs from the way in which they are represented in other models. For example, the theory of planned behavior posits that the final, psychological endpoint prior to taking action, that is, intention to engage in a protective or treatment action, is affected by the actor's beliefs about other people's favorableness toward the action and the importance of these other people to the actor. Self-regulation models posit a far wider range of contextual effects. The cultural and social context are a source of fundamental beliefs or schemata respecting the nature of disease, such as whether diseases, or a particular disease, are believed to be caused by heredity, infection, or lifestyle behaviors, and the appropriate source for treatment, such as whether traditional or Western medical authorities are selected for care. For example, the commonsense representation of high blood pressure demonstrates how the language of a culture can shape expectations regarding the symptoms (and perhaps the causes) of this disease, in that the term *hypertension* suggests that one experiences hyperactivity and emotional tension. Dread of cancer is enhanced by the image of cancer as a crab: an ugly, disfiguring, painful, and life-denying disease, incurable once one is in its claws. This culturally embodied visual image combined with the label, cancer, shapes the individual's representation of cancer and gives this disease the affective qualities that define it as the "dread disease" (Patterson, 1987). Contact with individuals dying of cancer at their homes and at hospitals when in treatment provide an additional, interpersonal source of imagery to define the representation of this disease.

Patients' representations of their illnesses may differ from those held by family members, a disparity that can negatively affect quality of life (Heijmans, deRidder, & Bensing, 1999). Patient representations of an illness can also differ from those held by their doctors. When doctor and patient disagree about the concrete referent for an illness—that is, when a doctor tells a hypertensive patient that his illness is asymptomatic, and the patient disagrees, believing that his hypertension is symptomatic and that effective treatment should remove his symptoms—the disagreement can result in the patient dropping out of treatment (Meyer et al., 1985). Doubts about the efficacy of a treatment can also generate uncertainty, disagreement, and doctor shopping. For example, a patient may be dismayed by reports that treatment has shrunk his tumor by 60% when he expected complete remission, whereas his physician is pleased and attributes much of the remaining mass to scar tissue. Because the patient had no prior knowledge that treatment would create scar tissue, he has more difficulty accepting this explanation for an outcome that is less than the expected 100% remission. In summary, the physician can believe a prescribed treatment has been effective, the patient not. Differences in public and practitioner representations of the treatments for major depression provide perhaps the most vivid examples of the adverse consequences of patient–practitioner discrepancies. Psychiatrists and internists believe medications are effective treatments for depression, but nonadherence to medication is extremely common. Noncompliance is less surprising when we consider the public view of antidepressants: More than 90% of survey respondents in the United Kingdom expressed reservations about the use of antidepressants because they believed them to be addictive (Priest, Vize, Roberts, & Tylee, 1996). Beliefs about cancer treatment also may deter detection and treatment. For example, slightly more than half of the elderly, White retirement community residents (53%) we interviewed and somewhat less than half of the elderly African American women (40%) living in the greater New Brunswick area whom we questioned, believed the treatment for breast cancer was either worse than or no different from the disease itself (H. Leventhal & Crouch, 1997).

Unlike many attitude models (e.g., the theory of planned behavior; Ajzen & Fishbein, 1980), which emphasizes the valence of people's beliefs respecting specific treatment procedures, the commonsense view of the self-regulation process makes clear that the substantive details of patients' views of treatment procedures are more important than whether these views are positive or negative. Knowing that a severely depressed woman holds negative opinions of antidepressants or that a patient has negative attitudes toward radiation treatment for cancer provides few if any suggestions as to how to encourage adherence to treatment regimens. Knowing that the patient believes that antidepressants are addictive or that radiation can cause sterility does. Representing this knowledge is good science and good practice.

How people represent the self affects the procedures they gravitate toward at every step of cancer control, from prevention through posttreatment rehabilitation. The need to assess the physical self (i.e., how well one is managing disease and treatment) can motivate social comparisons. Comparisons with women with breast cancer who are doing less well than oneself can bolster self-esteem and enhance well-being (Taylor et al., 1984; Wood & VanderZee, 1997). Other types of social comparisons provide opportunities for acquiring skills for disease management (Tennen & Affleck, 1997) and hope respecting treatment outcomes (Kulik & Mahler, 1997).

The self-appraisal process takes on a different character when placed within a self-regulation framework. Behavioral output, that is, one's physical, emotional, and psychological functioning, become indicators or targets for self-appraisal and possible corrective action. The type of action taken varies depending on the perceived source of the behavioral output and higher order strategies for self-management. For example, chest pain, vigor, and energy level are monitored by many cardiac patients in their efforts to evaluate their physical status. The experience of pain or the absence of vigor is a signal of disease threat for these patients. Conservation, that is, limiting activity, reducing uncertainty, and lowering emotional distress, are strategies for moderating these signals and protecting one's physical well-being (E. A. Leventhal & Crouch, 1997). In this framework, therefore, both symptoms and emotions are unimportant as antecedent, determinants or causes of illness, or as direct consequences of illness; their significance is that of an indicator of risk. Individuals monitor and use these indicators as signals for adaptive action, such as specific tactics that would fall under the general heading or strategy of resource conservation. Belief in the need for conservation is but one way of looking at resource management. Thinking of the body as a machine that needs to kept in "fine tune," an outlook that might be termed *use it or lose it*, is another.

Conservation and fine-tuning are but two of an undoubtedly wider range of representations of the physical self that affect preventive and treatment decisions. Many older people believe that their bodies are particularly sensitive to medication (Horne, 1997; Horne & Weinman, 1999), that they have "sensitive somas"; others believe that they are resistant to illness and do not need preventive inoculations, that they have "powerful somas." These self-construals tune the individual to particular somatic events and give these events meaning, that is, they convert somatic symptoms, affective reactions, and functional changes into signals or indicators of vulnerabilities and availability of resources. As such, they are critical goals or targets for behavior, and changes in these targets are interpreted as signs of increased or decreased risk of physical harm. We suspect that the role played by emotions and physical and psychological function as indicators of well-being, resource availability, and success in resource management is a far more significant aspect of their function in behavior and the control of cancer than their function as a direct source of physiological, disease-inducing change.

Self-Regulation and Communication

We believe that the self-regulation model can provide a powerful tool for communicating with the public, patients, practitioners, and biomedical scientists. It should help us to speak with clarity to laypersons and facilitate communicating with physicians and biomedical scientists. To be effective, however, the connections must go beyond the superficial level of "conceptual similarity," that is, of using terms that sound alike.

Communicating to Laypersons

Successful communication with laypersons depends on the ability both to connect our ideas to people's preexistent belief systems and to reshape their beliefs to conform more closely with valid, biomedical knowledge. A primary reason for believing that the commonsense version of self-regulation theories will achieve this goal is that its constructs are based upon people's commonsense thinking. The model focuses on the individual's ways of representing cancer and cancer treatment at both the abstract conceptual and the concrete perceptual levels. When health professionals recognize and attend to patients' concrete experience as well as to their words, it should help to convince them that they are understood and that their concerns are being addressed. Trust emerges from such understanding. Unfortunately, information is not always available regarding how specific behaviors affect experience. For example, whereas data are available on the substantive experiences that discourage adherence to exercise among older adults (e.g., joint pain and feelings of breathlessness), much less is known about the experiences that encourage adherence. Similarly, we know that worry about breast cancer is promoted by experiencing an array of vague, somatic symptoms in combinations with feeling vulnerable to this disease (Easterling & Leventhal, 1989), but we do not know which combination of factors encourage regular use of mammography or the adoption of low-fat diets.

Second, the notion of self-regulation intrinsic to these models can appeal to people's beliefs and hopes that they can exert control over their lives. Yet this does not free the professional from responsibility for those diagnostic and treatment procedures that only she or he can perform: Patients are not abandoned; they are respected as individuals. Third, by defining a specific set of cognitive domains and their associated affective experiences, the commonsense model provides for discussion of that which is noxious (symptoms of treatment) and feared (ability to tolerate treatment; treatment induced disease) and the time and effort needed to manage both disease and treatment as well as hoped-for outcomes. Setting up a comprehensive framework for evaluating action provides ways of thinking and acting to allow prevention and treatment to go forward in the presence of momentary setbacks.

Communicating With Practitioners and Scientists

The self-regulation framework and its constructs offer a potentially powerful framework for communicating with medical practitioners. The reasons for this are twofold. First, the distinction between representation and procedure; the domains of identity, time line, consequences, control, and causal route within each; and the concrete, perceptual complements to the abstract, verbal structures used in communication are what they hear from patients. The model provides, therefore, a framework for capturing and organizing conversation and planning preventive, diagnostic, and treatment procedures. Second, the bi-level nature of these substantive domains directs practitioners to explore facets of patient experience that might otherwise be unmentioned. Symptom attribution and time line provide ready examples. Which symptoms do patients attribute to their conditions and which to their treatments? What expected time frames do they have for changes in the underlying disease, in symptoms, and for the impact of medication? The anticipated time lines for symptomatic relief prove critical for adherence (Meyer et al., 1985) and emotional distress (Heijmans et al., 1999; Silverman, 1999), as do beliefs regarding the relationship between alleviation of symptoms and cure of the underlying condition (Affleck et al., 1987). It is necessary to train people to think and use the model to explore patients' beliefs about their illnesses, their prescribed treatments, and the various alternatives they adopt as part of their self-care routines. How they appraise the efficacy of these procedures is an important step in improving adherence to prescribed treatments and avoidance of risky alternatives when engaging in the daily chores of managing chronic conditions. Clarification of time frames and criteria for evaluating efficacy are important for insuring effective treatment and increasing trust.

Communication with biomedical investigators is challenged by their investment in the magic-bullet approach to prevention and treatment so well illustrated in the 1977 quotation from Lewis Thomas. That there has been little change in this reductionistic outlook in the subsequent 20 years is illustrated by Ostrow's reply to Ferrando's (1998) request for information about the plans for the next International Conference on Biopsychosocial Aspects of HIV Infections: "There are no plans to add behavioral or Psycho-social tracks to this conference" (Ostrow, March 1998, cited in Ferrando, 1998, p. 308). Comments of this nature are made in the face of data showing that nonadherence to medication (a behavior) is a serious problem in treating HIV infection, as it is in virtually all areas of medicine (Ferrando, 1998), and that behavioral interventions have the potential of reducing HIV infection at the population level, an impact than can save hundreds of lives and millions of health care dollars (National Institute of Mental Health Multisite HIV Prevention Trial Group, 1998). Thus, whereas the effect of behavioral interventions may be modest in terms of percentage influenced by an intervention program in comparison with unexposed control patients, the effects for a population may be enormous. Effective or not, behavioral approaches do not appeal to the reductionistic mindset of the typical bioscientist: These approaches seem too simplistic and dissociated from the biological mechanisms of their interest.

Although it is unclear that self-regulation models could help us to overcome the propensity of biomedical investigators to ignore behavioral factors, there are reasons to hope that they could help. First, the appeal of self-regulation models may be enhanced by their focus on the feedback and feedforward units, because these representations are similar at a formal level to the mechanisms identified in biological systems. Second, the differentiation between labels and words (a deliberative reasoning system) and perceptual experience (an automatic, or implicit, level of function) may add to the appeal of these models as physiological systems operate automatically and intrude into awareness, permitting a degree of direct, behavioral control. Third, the self-regulative mechanisms can be seen as another level of defense; they can be included as a higher order feature in the hierarchy of the body's defense systems. Behaviors can avoid or bring one into contact with disease-inducing agents, skin and peripheral mechanisms can prevent entry into the body, and a variety of biological mechanisms exist for attacking a pathogen once it penetrates these outer defenses. Behaviors can also facilitate or disrupt these other, lower level defenses by maintaining access with pathogens, introducing manufactured agents to destroy pathogens, or facilitating the attacker by recruiting powerful adreno-cortocotropic reactions that down-regulate immune defenses when they are most needed.

The final, and we hope the most persuasive, avenue for recognizing the importance of self-regulation models is the basic premise that people practice a common-sense form of biomedicine when they self-regulate (Kaptchuk & Eisenberg, 1998). Quite simply, this signifies not only that individuals make up their own minds, but that biomedicine had best recognize that the degrees and claims of science do not hold sufficient power. Authority and scientific magic are insufficient to persuade a skeptical public whose everyday experience with health and illness, life and death, includes very little if any direct experience with molecular or cellular events and only slightly more encounters with cellular-level constructs.

Conclusion

The behavioral and biological sciences are approaching the threshold of a new and important chapter in the advance of science: a time for synthesis (Wilson, 1998). The synthesis we are urging needs to satisfy a set of extremely complex scientific and cultural demands. At the scientific side the objective is the integration of biological and behavioral theories. The nature of this integration should not be misunderstood; it does not call for one level of science to explain another (i.e., for biological constructs to explain psychological and sociological constructs). Simplistic reductionism is not the goal. What is hoped for is that differentiated models of behavior can be linked to differentiated models of organismic biology. We believe this linkage can be more easily achieved in selected domains, such as the world of cancer research. The advantages of working within a domain are multiple. First, the various cancers generate specific anatomic, physiological, and functional change, and these changes are experienced in a various ways by the behaving organism. These experiences generate more complex representations and action plans at the behavioral level, providing a vivid picture of the biobehavioral processes affected by the disease and a contrast of these processes with "normal" or predisease processes. Thus, the many relationships between biological (disease) and behavioral (prevention, detection, treatment, living with disease) processes are made salient by the impact of cancer.

Successful synthesis, however, requires conceptual detail backed by empirical data. Specific findings are needed respecting how the perception and representation of cancer affects procedures for cancer control and how these procedures affect, directly and indirectly, the disease process. Behavioral constructs backed by data can then be connected to data-linked constructs at the biological level. True synthesis, that is, cross-disciplinary consilience, requires the linkage of empirically based, conceptual structures (Wilson, 1998).

Synthesis of science and culture is our other major theme. Scientists often despair at the poverty of scientific training and knowledge among the general public. These deficits are real: Large segments of the population have no or limited understanding of the complexities of scientific theory and empirical data. More important yet is the lack of understanding that science is a quest involving the framing of answerable questions, hypotheses respecting possible answers, and the creation of methods for generating empirical evaluations of these hypotheses. Despite these deficits, there is at least one important reason for believing that the communication problem is not insurmountable. Natural selection has gifted humans with a complex brain that seeks explanations and generates models of the world in which we live. These culturewide models are typically biological, psychological, and social. They connect lifestyles with psychological states and psychological states with disease; the "stress–illness" model is but one example: It suggests particular behaviors for health promotion and the avoidance and treatment of disease. Although many (although not all) of these culturewide commonsense models are biologically wrong, they are evidence of the need—and the desire—for fuller understanding of the links between what humans are biologically, our vulnerabilities to pathogens, and how we live as individuals and members of institutional and social communities.

In summary, we are left with the following, important questions. Can we integrate psychological and biological models? Can a simply stated self-regulation model that has biological and behavioral integrity displace fraudulent visions of the relationship of disease and behavior? Can we further reduce the impact of those who build personal fortunes on the fear and despair of those who are ill? Can we enhance communication between practitioners and patients, between the public and practitioners, and between biomedical investigators and practitioners and the public? The many excellent chapters in this volume provide encouragement that integration and enhanced communication are possible and that a model connecting cancer and behavior can help to construct a valid cultural model of biology and behavior that will encourage and justify appropriate behaviors to prevent, treat, and recover from cancer. Researchers at the various comprehensive cancer centers and affiliated faculty are in the forefront of this development.

References

Affleck, G., Tennen, H., Pfeiffer, C., & Fifield, J. (1987). Appraisals of control and predictability in adapting to a chronic disease. *Journal of Personality and Social Psychology*, *53*, 273–279.

Ajzen, I. (1988). *Attitudes, personality, and behavior*. Homewood, IL: Dorsey Press.

Ajzen, I., & Fishbein, M. (1980). *Understanding attitudes and predicting social behavior*. Englewood Cliffs, NJ: Prentice Hall.

Andrykowski, M. A., Redd, W. H., & Hatfield, A. K. (1985). Development of anticipatory nausea: A prospective analysis. *Journal of Consulting and Clinical Psychology*, *53*, 447–454.

Austin, J., & Vancouver, J. (1996). Goal constructs in psychology: Structure, process, and content. *Psychological Bulletin*, *120*, 338–375.

Baker, T. B., Zelman, D., Brandon, T., Zinser, M., Baker, L. J., & Leventhal, H. (1988). Smoking cessation: Effective cognitive–behavioral interventions. In N. B. Oldbridge & D. H. Schmidt (Eds.), *Cardiac rehabilitation and clinical exercise programs: Theory and practice* (pp. 239–244). Ithaca, NY: Mouvement Publications.

Bandura, A. (1977). Self-efficacy: Toward a unifying theory of behavioral change. *Psychological Review*, *84*, 191–215.

Becker, M. H., & Maiman, L. A. (1975). Sociobehavioral determinants of compliance with health and medical care recommendations. *Medical Care*, *13*, 10–24.

Bovbjerg, D. H., Redd, W. H., Jacobsen, P. B., Manne, S. L., Taylor, K. L., Surbone, A., Crown, J. P., Norton, L., Gilewski, T. A., Hudis, C. A., Reichman, B. S., Kaufman, R. J., Currie, V. E., & Hakes, T. B. (1992). An experimental analysis of classically conditioned nausea during cancer chemotherapy. *Psychosomatic Medicine*, *54*(6), 623–637.

Burish, T. G., & Redd, W. H. (1994). Symptom control in psychosocial oncology [Review]. *Cancer*, *74*(Suppl. 4), 1438–1444.

Carver, C. S., & Scheier, M. F. (1981). *Attention and self-regulation: A control-theory approach to human behavior*. New York: Springer-Verlag.

Carver, C. S., & Scheier, M. F. (1982). Control theory: A useful conceptual framework for personality-social, clinical, and health psychology. *Psychological Bulletin*, *92*, 111–135.

Carver, C. S., Scheier, M. F., & Weintraub, J. K. (1989). Assessing coping strategies: A theoretically based approach. *Journal of Personality and Social Psychology*, *56*, 267–283.

Cella, D. F., Tulsky, D. S., Gray, G., Sarafian, B., Linn, E., Bonomi, A., Silberman, M., Yellen, S. B., Winicour, P., Brannon, J., Eckberg, K., Lloyd, S., Purl, S., Blendowski, C., Goodman, M., Barnicle, M., Stewart, I., McHale, M., Bonomi, P., Kaplan, E., Taylor, S., IV, Thomas, C. R., Jr., & Harris, J. (1993). The Functional Assessment of Cancer Therapy scale (FACT): Development and validation of the general measure. *Journal of Clinical Oncology*, *11*(3), 570–579.

Chassin, L., Presson, C., Sherman, S. J., Corty, E., & Olshavsky, R. W. (1984). Predicting the onset of cigarette smoking in adolescents: A longitudinal study. *Journal of Applied Social Psychology, 14,* 224–243.

Condiotte, M. M., & Lichtenstein, E. (1981). Self-efficacy and relapse in smoking cessation programs. *Journal of Consulting and Clinical Psychology, 49,* 648–658.

Dinh, K. T., Sarason, I. G., Peterson, A. V., & Onstad, L. E. (1995). Children's perceptions of smokers and nonsmokers: A longitudinal study. *Health Psychology, 14,* 32–40.

Easterling, D. V., & Leventhal, H. (1989). The contribution of concrete cognition to emotion: Neutral symptoms as elicitors of worry about cancer. *Journal of Applied Psychology, 74,* 787–796.

Fawzy, F. I. (1994). Immune effects of a short-term intervention for cancer patients. *Advances, 11*(3), 32–33.

Fawzy, F. I., Kemeny, M. E., Fawzy, N. W., Elashoff, R., et al. (1990). A structured psychiatric intervention for cancer patients: II. Changes over time in immunological measures. *Archives of General Psychiatry, 47,* 729–735.

Ferrando, S. I. (1998). Behavioral research on AIDS-protease inhibitors and the new millennium: Comment on Kelly, Otto-Salaj, Sikkema, Pinkerton, and Bloom. *Health Psychology, 17*(4), 307–309.

Fishbein, M., & Azjen, I. (1975). *Belief, attitude, intention, and behavior.* New York: Wiley.

Flay, B. R. (1985). Psychosocial approaches to smoking prevention: A review of findings. *Health Psychology, 4,* 449–488.

Heijmans, M., deRidder, D., & Bensing, J. (1999). Dissimilarity in patients' and spouses' representations of chronic disease: Explorations of relations to patient adaptation. *Psychology and Health, 14,* 451–466.

Helgeson, V. S., & Cohen, S. (1996). Social support and adjustment to cancer: Reconciling descriptive, correlational, and intervention research. *Health Psychology, 15,* 135–148.

Hochbaum, G. M. (1958). *Public participation in medical screening programs: A sociopsychological study.* Washington, DC: U.S. Government Printing Office.

Horne, R. (1997). Representations of medication and treatment: Advances in theory and measurement. In K. J. Petrie & J. A. Weinman (Eds.), *Perceptions of health and illness: Current research and applications* (pp. 155–188). Amsterdam: Harwood Academic Publishers.

Horne, R., & Weinman, J. (1999). Patients' beliefs about prescribed medicines and their role in adherence to treatment in chronic physical illness. *Journal of Psychosomatic Research, 47*(6), 555–567.

Kaptchuk, T. J., & Eisenberg, D. M. (1998). The persuasive appeal of alternative medicine. *Annals of Internal Medicine, 129,* 1061–1070.

Kaye, L. E. (1993). *The molecular vision of life: Caltech, the Rockefeller Foundation and the rise of the new biology.* New York: Oxford University Press.

Kelly, G. A. (1955). *The psychology of personal constructs.* New York: Norton.

Kulik, J. A., & Mahler, H. I. (1997). Social comparison, affiliation, and coping with acute medical threats. In B. P. Buunk & F. X. Gibbons (Eds.), *Health, coping, and well-being: Perspectives from social comparison theory* (pp. 227–261). Mahwah, NJ: Erlbaum.

Lacroix, J. M. (1991). Assessing illness schemata in patient populations. In J. A. Skelton & R. T. Croyle (Eds.), *Mental representation in health and illness* (pp. 193–219). New York: Springer-Verlag.

Lau, R. R., & Hartman, K. A. (1983). Common sense representations of common illnesses. *Health Psychology, 2*, 167–185.

Lazarus, R. S. (1966). *Psychological stress and the coping process.* New York: McGraw-Hill.

Lazarus, R. S., & Launier, R. (1978). Stress related transactions between person and environment. In L. A. Pervin & M. Lewis (Eds.), *Perspectives in interactional psychology* (pp. 287–327). New York: Plenum Press.

Lerman, C., & Croyle, R. T. (1994). Psychological issues in genetic testing for breast cancer susceptibility. *Archives of Internal Medicine, 154*, 609–616.

Leventhal, E. A., & Crouch, M. (1997). Are there differences in perception of illness across the lifespan? In K. J. Petrie & J. A. Weinman (Eds.), *Perceptions of health and illness: Current research and applications* (pp. 77–102). Amsterdam: Harwood Academic Publishers.

Leventhal, H. (1970). Findings and theory in the study of fear communications. *Advances in Experimental Social Psychology, 5*, 119–186.

Leventhal, H., Baker, T. B., Brandon, T., & Fleming, R. (1989). Intervening and preventing cigarette smoking. In T. Ney & A. Gale (Eds.), *Smoking and human behavior* (pp. 313–336). Oxford, England: John Wiley & Sons.

Leventhal, H., Benyamini, Y., Brownlee, S., Diefenbach, M., Leventhal, E. A., Patrick-Miller, L., & Robitaille, C. (1997). Illness representations: Theoretical foundations. In K. J. Petrie & J. A. Weinman (Eds.), *Perceptions of health and illness: Current research and applications* (pp. 19–45). Singapore: Harwood Academic.

Leventhal, H., & Crouch, M. (1997). [Beliefs about cancer among elderly white and African-American women]. Unpublished raw data.

Leventhal, H., Diefenbach, M., & Leventhal, E. A. (1992). Illness cognition: Using common sense to understand treatment adherence and affect-cognition interactions. *Cognitive Therapy and Research, 16*, 143–163.

Leventhal, H., Fleming, R., & Wagstaff, D. (1989). Prevention of smoking in children. In P. F. Lovibond & P. Wilson (Eds.), *Clinical and abnormal psychology* (pp. 167–176). North Holland, The Netherlands: Elsevier Science.

Leventhal, H., Leventhal, E. A., & Cameron, L. (in press). Representations, procedures and affect in illness self regulation: A perceptual–cognitive model. In A. Baum, T. Revenson, & J. Weinman (Eds.), *Handbook of health psychology.* Hillsdale, NJ: Erlbaum.

Leventhal, H., Leventhal, E. A., & Contrada, R. (1998). Self regulation, health, and behavior: A perceptual–cognitive approach. *Psychology and Health, 13,* 717–733.

Leventhal, H., Meyer, D., & Nerenz, D. (1980). The common sense representation of illness danger. In S. Rachman (Ed.), *Medical psychology* (Vol. 2, pp. 7–30). New York: Permagon Press.

Leventhal, H., Rosenstock, I. M., Hochbaum, G. M., & Carriger, B. K. (1960). Epidemic impact on the general population in two cities. In I. M. Rosenstock, G. M. Hochbaum, & H. Leventhal (Eds.), *The impact of Asian influenza on community life* (pp. 53–77). Washington, DC: U.S. Government Printing Office.

Marlatt, G. A., & Gordon, J. R. (1980). Determinants of relapse: Implications for the maintenance of behavior change. In P. O. Davison & S. M. Davidson (Eds.), *Behavioral medicine: Changing health lifestyles* (pp. 410–452). New York: Brunner/Mazel.

Meyer, D., Leventhal, H., & Gutmann, M. (1985). Common-sense models of illness: The example of hypertension. *Health Psychology, 4,* 115–135.

Meyerowitz, B. E., Richardson, J., Hudson, S., & Leedham, B. (1998). Ethnicity and cancer outcomes: Behavioral and psychosocial considerations. *Psychological Bulletin, 123,* 47–70.

Meyerowitz, B. E., Williams, J. G., & Gessner, J. (1987). Perceptions of controllability and attitudes toward cancer and cancer patients. *Journal of Applied Social Psychology, 17,* 471–492.

Miller, S. M. (1987). Monitoring and blunting: Validation of a questionnaire to assess styles of information-seeking under threat. *Journal of Personality and Social Psychology, 52,* 345–353.

Mosbach, P., & Leventhal, H. (1988). Peer group identification and smoking: Implications for intervention. *Journal of Abnormal Psychology, 97,* 238–245.

National Institute of Mental Health Multisite HIV Prevention Trial Group. (1998). The NIMH Multisite HIV Prevention Trial: Reducing HIV sexual risk behavior. *Science, 280*(5371), 1889–1894.

Nerenz, D. R., & Leventhal, H. (1983). Self-regulation theory in chronic illness. In T. G. Burish & L. A. Bradley (Eds.), *Coping with chronic disease: Research & applications* (pp. 13–37). New York: Academic Press.

Nerenz, D. R., Leventhal, H., Easterling, D. V., & Love, R. R. (1986). Anxiety and drug taste as predictors of anticipatory nausea in cancer and chemotherapy. *Journal of Clinical Oncology, 4,* 224–233.

Patterson, J. T. (1987). *The dread disease: Cancer and modern American culture.* Cambridge, MA: Harvard University Press.

Petrie, K. J., & Weinman, J. A. (1997). *Perceptions of health and illness: Current research and applications.* Amsterdam: Harwood Academic.

Priest, R., Vize, C., Roberts, A., & Tylee, A. (1996). Lay people's attitudes to treatment of depression: Results of opinion poll for Defeat Depression Campaign just before its launch. *British Medical Journal, 313,* 858–859.

Redd, W. H. (1995). Behavioral research in cancer as a model for health psychology. *Health Psychology, 14,* 99–100.

Rimer, B. K. (1994). Interventions to increase breast screening. Lifespan and ethnicity issues. *Cancer, 74*(Suppl. 1), 323–328.

Rogers, R. W. (1983). Cognitive and physiological processes in fear appeals and attitude change: A revised theory of protection motivation. In J. T. Cacioppo & R. E. Petty (Eds.), *Social psychophysiology* (pp. 153–176). New York: Guilford Press.

Rosenstock, I. M. (1974). Historical origins of the health belief model. *Health Education Monographs, 2,* 1–8.

Scheier, M. F., & Carver, C. S. (1985). Optimism, coping, and health: Assessment and implications of generalized outcome expectancies. *Health Psychology, 4,* 219–247.

Scheier, M. F., & Carver, C. S. (1992). Effects of optimism on psychological and physical well-being: Theoretical overview and empirical update. *Cognitive Therapy and Research, 16,* 201–228.

Silverman, C. (1999). *The effects of temporal models of cancer on worry.* Unpublished dissertation, University of Illinois, Champaign-Urbana.

Skelton, J. A., & Croyle, R. T. (1991). *Mental representation in health and illness.* New York: Springer-Verlag.

Spiegel, D., Bloom, J. R., Kraemer, H. C., & Gottheil, E. (1989). Effect of psychosocial treatment on survival of patients with metastatic breast cancer. *Lancet, 2,* 888–891.

Sussman, S., Dent, C. W., Stacy, A. W., Burciaga, C., Raynor, A., Turner, G. E., Charlin, V., Craig, S., Hansen, W. B., Burton, D., & Flay, B. R. (1990). Peer-group association and adolescent tobacco use. *Journal of Abnormal Psychology, 99,* 349–352.

Taylor, S. E., Lichtman, R. R., & Wood, J. V. (1984). Attributions, beliefs about control, and adjustment to breast cancer. *Journal of Personality and Social Psychology, 46,* 489–502.

Tennen, H., & Affleck, G. (1997). Social comparison as a coping process: A critical review and application to chronic pain disorders. In B. P. Buunk & F. X. Gibbons (Eds.), *Health, coping, and well-being: Perspectives from social comparison theory* (pp. 263–298). Mahwah, NJ: Erlbaum.

Thomas, L. (1977). On the science and technology of medicine. In J. H. Knowles (Ed.), *Doing better and feeling worse: Health in the United States* (pp. 35–46). New York: Norton.

Vancouver, J. (1996). Living systems as a paradigm for organizational behavior: Understanding humans, organizations, and social processes. *Behavioral Sciences, 41*(1), 165–204.

Wilson, E. O. (1998). *Consilience: The unity of knowledge.* New York: Knopf.

Wood, J. V., & VanderZee, K. (1997). Social comparisons among cancer patients: Under what conditions are comparisons upward and downward? In B. P. Buunk & F. X. Gibbons (Eds.), *Health, coping, and well-being: Perspectives from social comparison theory* (pp. 299–328). Mahwah, NJ: Erlbaum.

Author Index

A

Aaronson, N. K., 38, 41, 51, *53, 54,* 57, 59, 61, 63, *70,* 72, 330, *333*
Abbey, A., 86, *91*
Abbott, R. A., *35*
Abeloff, M. D., 221, 224, 228, *233*
Adams, M., 158, *172*
Adamson, T. E., 367, *373*
Adelman, M. B., 101–102, *113*
Adler, A., 331, *333*
Adler, N. E., 21, *34*
Aebersold, P., *211*
Affleck, G., 21, *32, 33,* 387, 391, 393, *396, 400*
Afifi, R., 347, *357*
Agran, L., 322, *334*
Ahmedzai, S., *70*
Aickin, M., *333*
Aiken, L., 347, *357*
Ajzen, I., 384, 390, *396, 397*
Albano, A. M., 84, *93*
Albeck, M., *320*
Alberola-Ila, J., 187, *189*
Alberts, D., *333, 338*
Albrecht, T. L., 101, 101–102, *113*
Ali, E., *210*
Ali, N., 238, *262*
Allain, A. N., 85, *96*
Allegrante, J. P., *338*
Allen, B., 350, *361*
Allen, S., *33*
Alter, C. L., 81, 82, *90,* 100, *113,* 148, 156, 158, 163, *167*
Altman, D., 348, *361*
Alumbaugh, M. J., 241, *265*
Alvarez, E., *264*
Alvarez, W., 126, *129,* 238, 293, *302*
Alvord, W. G., *191*
Amar-Costesec, A., *209*
American Cancer Society, 262, 269, 284, 287, *301*
American Psychiatric Association, 81, 82, *90,* 99, *113,* 149, 156, *167*
Amerman, R. T., *93*

Amkrant, A., 258, *266*
Anderman, C., 290, *302*
Andersen, B., 163, 166, *167*
Andersen, B. L., 22, *30,* 38, *53,* 78, 83, *90, 94, 96,* 99, 108, *113,* 120, 121, 122, 123, 126, *127, 128, 129,* 161, 223, 227, 283, 284, 310, 312, *316,* 330, 331, *333*
Anderson, A. B., *71*
Anderson, B., 106, *115,* 163, *167*
Anderson, D. E., 307, *316*
Anderson, D. M., 287, *301*
Anderson, I., 79, *93*
Anderson, J., *171*
Anderson, N. R., 133, *141*
Anderson, S., 227
Andreason, N. J., 366, *373*
Andrews, M., *316*
Andrykowski, M. A., 15, *32,* 59, *70,* 78, 81, *90, 91, 96, 113,* 122, 123, *128,* 156, 159, 163, *167, 168, 170,* 377, *396*
Angell, K., 217, *228, 230*
Angelopoulou, K., 195, *208*
Angoff, W. H., *70*
Anisman, H., 258, *266*
Antoni, M., *170,* 311, *317, 317, 336*
Antoni, M. H., *231, 339, 340*
Antonovsky, A., 19, *30*
Apostolopoulos, V., *190*
Appels, A., *360*
Arathuzik, D., 239, *262*
Arendt-Nielsen, L., 311, *320*
Armstrong, W. T., *265*
Arndt, L. A., 22, *32,* 144, *169,* 223, 228, 235, *263,* 331, *335*
Arnetz, B. B., 310, *316*
Arnold, C. B., 326, *340*
Arpin, K., 217, *228*
Arthey, S., 327, *333*
Ashley, J. D., *336*
Askelof, P., 207, *209*
Aspinwall, L. G., 20, 25, *30, 35*
Atkinson, J. W., 16, *30*
Atwood, J. R., 326, *333*
Audrain, J., 288, 289, 297, 298, *301, 302, 304, 317*

Austin, J., 383, *396*
Axelrod, A., *90, 113, 167*
Azavedo, E., 325, *338*

B

Bachen, E. A., 331, *337*
Baden, H., 350, *358*
Bahr, G. R., *230*
Baider, L., 79, *90,* 148, *172,* 238, *262*
Baile, W. F., 326, *339*
Bailey, D. E., 131, 135, *138*
Bailey, W. C., *335*
Baker, F., 21, *31*
Baker, L. J., *396*
Baker, S. M., *304*
Baker, T. B., 376, 377, *396, 398*
Bal, D. G., 321, 329, *333*
Bales, B. F, 135, *138*
Bales, C., *360*
Ballard-Barbash, R., 123, *128*
Balshem, A., 301, *303,* 329, *336, 337,* 348, 350, *359*
Balshem, A. M., 88, *94, 171, 318*
Balthrusch, H. J. F., 331, *335*
Bandura, A., 20, *30,* 344, 347, *357, 396*
Banks, P. J., 37, 43, *54*
Barakat, L. P., *93*
Baranowski, J., *334*
Baranowski, T., *334*
Barber, T., *304*
Bard, M., *333*
Bargh, J. A., 97, *116*
Barillari, G., 204, *209*
Barlow, C. E., 324, *336*
Barlow, D., 84, *90*
Barlow, D. H., 101, *114,* 153, *170*
Barlow, W. E., 290, *302*
Barnicle, M., 72, *396*
Barofsky, I., 41, *53, 56*
Baron, R. A., 366, *373*
Barraclough, J., *317, 319*
Barratt-Boyes, S. M., *128, 190*
Barre, P. E., *54*
Barry, B., 132, *138*
Barsevick, A., *359*
Bartal, D., *91*
Baruch, J. D. R., *264, 265*
Basham, R. B., 365, *374*
Basoglu, M., *93*
Bastianutti, L. M., 137, *139*
Bateman, A., 313, *316*
Baum, A., 5, 6, *11, 12,* 73, 83, 86, *90, 91,* 101, *113,* 144, 147, 149, 150, 154, 155, 163, *167, 168, 169, 170,* 310, *317, 319,* 323,

328, 330, 331, *333, 334, 335, 336, 338, 359*
Baum, M., 78, *92,* 222, 228
Baxter, J. S., *338*
Bayliss, M. S., 75
Bazin, J. C., 331, *339*
Bazzini, V. R., 331
Bean, K., 72
Beck, A. T., 242, *262*
Beck, N. C., 225, 227
Becker, C., 367, *373*
Becker, M. H., 384–385, *396*
Becker, Y., 198, *208*
Beckmann, J., 54, 72
Bell, D., 242, *263*
Bell, M., 333
Bell, M. C., *190*
Benedict, J., 333
Ben-Efraim, S., 331, 333
Ben-Eliyahu, S., 259, *262,* 331, 333
Benight, C., *170, 317, 336*
Benike, C., *210*
Benkendorf, J. L., *303*
Bennett, J. M., 224, *230*
Benotsch, E. G., *316*
Benschop, R. J., 312, *316*
Bensing, J., 390, *397*
Benson, H., 220, *229*
Benson, P., 239, *263*
Benyamini, Y., *398*
Berek, J. S., *230*
Bergenmar, M., *263*
Berglund, G., 242, *262*
Bergman, B., 59, *70, 71*
Bergner, M., 61, *70, 75*
Berkman, L. F., 227
Berkowitz, L., *95, 115, 359*
Berlin, M., *304*
Berman, S., 143, 156, *168*
Bernard, T. M., 347, *358*
Bernhard, J., 68, *71*
Bernstein, G., *230*
Bernstein, L., 287, *303,* 324, *334*
Berntson, G. G., *316*
Berrenberg, J., 346, *357*
Berry, D. R., *128*
Berry, H., *334*
Bersheid, E., 366, *373*
Besedovsky, H. O., 193, *209*
Besselman, L., *266*
Bevington, D. J., *94, 171, 265*
Bhartiya, V. R., 159, *173*
Bianchi, R., *334*
Biassoni, R., *210*

Bice, T. W., 66, *71*
Biddison, W. E., *210*
Biesecker, B., 299, *302, 303*
Bijlsma, W. J., *316*
Billings, J. H., *265*
Binik, Y. M., *54*
Birbaumer, N., *318*
Birenbaum, L., *359*
Birsell, J. M., 327, *334*
Biswas, A., 181, *190*, 225, *230*
Bizzini, V. R., *339*
Bjerring, P., 311, *320*
Bjordal, K., *71*
Bjork, S., *71*
Black, W. C., 6, *11*
Blackwood, M. A., *316*
Blair, S. N., 324, *336*
Blair, V., 291, *302*
Blake, D. D., 84, *93*
Blake, S., 26, *36*, 78, *97*
Blalock, S., 347, *357*
Blanchard, C., 240, *262*
Blanchard, E., 85, *90*, 155, 165, *168*
Bleiker, E., *320*
Blendowski, C., *72, 396*
Bliss, J. M., *264, 265*
Blomke, M., 323, *339*
Bloom, E. T., 310, *318*
Bloom, H., 144, *172*
Bloom, J., 272, 273, *285, 286*
Bloom, J. R., 24, *35*, 37, 38, 40, 41, 43, 52,
    53, 54, 55, 129, 181, *191*, 217, 222, 223,
    224, 228, 232, 235, 237, 241, *262, 266*,
    270, *286*, 323, *333, 339*, 377, *400*
Blumberg, B., *359*
Blumberg, H. H., 131, *139*
Bluming, A. Z., *97, 173*
Bobbitt, R. A., *70*
Boca, S., 86, *96*
Bodmer, W. F., 307, *316*
Bogaards, M., 311, *320*
Boggs, S. R., 367, *374*
Bohrnstedt, G. W., 57, *71*
Boi, S., *333*
Bolden, S., 119, *128*, 321, *338*
Bole, G. G., 225, *229*
Bolund, C., 242, *262, 263*
Bondy, M. L., 290, *302*
Bonica, J. J., *96*
Bonita, J. A., 135
Bonito, J. A., *138*
Bonne, O., 83, *96*, 154
Bonneau, R. H., *317*
Bonnell, G., *265, 318*

Bonney, G., *318*
Bonomi, A., *396*
Bonomi, A. E., 57, 59, 60, 61, 63, *71, 72*
Bonomi, P., *72, 396*
Bookwala, J., 22, *35*
Boon, C., 19n, *35, 101, 116*
Boon, T., 196, 200, 201, *209*
Bootzin, R. R., 102, *113*
Borgen, P., *316, 320*
Borkovec, T. D., 88, *90*, 349, *357*
Borland, R., 328, *334, 336*
Bornand, T., *209*
Borysenko, J., 220, *229*
Bos-Branolte, G., 243, *262*
Bossio, L. M., 21, *34*
Bostrom, A., 295, *302*
Bottazzi, B., 195, *210*
Bottino, C., *210*
Bottomley, A., 241, *263*
Bouchard, T. J., 132, *138*
Boucher, Y., 203, *209*
Bourassa, M. G., *285*
Bourne, T. H., 349, *362*
Bovbjerg, D., *97*, 156, *170, 173*, 310, *316*
Bovbjerg, D. H., 78, 79, *91, 96*, 304, 309, 311,
    314, 315, *316, 317, 320*, 377, *396*
Bowcock, A. M., *128*
Bowden, C. J., *210*
Bower, J. E., 124, *128*
Bowles, C. A., 310, *319*
Boyce, A., *359*
Boyd, N. F., 69, *71*
Boyd, S., *266*
Boyle, P., *319*
Bradley, C., 241, *263*
Bradley, E. L., *210*
Bradley, L. A., *399*
Brady, M. J., 59, 60, 63, *70, 71*
Braitman, L., 63, *71*
Branch, L. G., 39, *55*
Brand, A., *210*
Brand, R. J., *265*
Brandberg, Y., 237, *263*
Brandon, T., 376, *396, 398*
Brandstadter, J., 20, *30*
Brandstatter, H., *140*
Brannon, J., *72, 396*
Branstetter, A. D., 309, *319*
Brantley, B., 158, 161, *171*
Brasure, J., 324, *340*
Breast Cancer Linkage Consortium, 302
Breitbart, P. K., *35*
Brenn, T., 324, *340*
Brenner, S. O., *316*

Breslow, D. M., 322, *334*
Breslow, L., 322, *334*
Brewin, C., 101, *113*
Brewin, C. R., 86, *90*
Bridge, L. R., 239, *263*
Bridges, M. W., 21, 22, 25, *31, 34, 35*
Briner, W., *265, 318*
Brinton, L. A., *302*
Brisson, J., 38, *55,* 224, *231*
Brittenden, J., 194, *209*
Britton, K., 259, *264*
Broadbent, R., *190*
Brodland, G. A., 366, *373*
Brodsky, I., 314, *320*
Brody, D. S., 348, 350, 351, *360*
Brody, L. C., *304*
Bromet, E., 83, *93*
Bronstein, B. R., *340*
Brook, R. H., 57–58, *75*
Brooks, R., 61, *71*
Broste, S. K., *75*
Brown, B., 216, *230*
Brown, G., 242, *262*
Brown, J. D., 272, *286*
Brown, K., 287–288, *304, 320*
Brown, L. L., *91*
Brown, M., *264*
Brown, S. A., *336*
Brown, S. E., *265*
Brown, V., 131, 137, *139, 140*
Browne, G., 216, *230*
Browne, G. B., 217, *228*
Brownlee, S., *398*
Brownson, R. C., 321, *333*
Bryant, B. K., *167*
Bryant, R., 155, *168*
Bryne, D., 366, *373*
Buchanan, W. W., *72*
Buchannan, R., 78, *93*
Budd, M., 220, *229*
Budman, D. R., 123, *128*
Bukowski, R. M., *190*
Buller, D., B., 328, *334*
Buller, M. K., 328, *334*
Buller, R. E., 106, *115*
Bullinger, M., *70*
Bulman, R. J., 19n, *31*
Bunney, W., *266*
Bunston, T., 20, *31*
Bunting, P. S., 195, *208*
Burciaga, C., *400*
Burgess, C., 163, *172, 266*
Burgess, P., 83, *91,* 102, *113,* 155, *168*
Burish, T. G., 223, *228, 263,* 377, *396, 399*

Burke, M. A., 323, *334*
Burleson, B. R., 101, *113, 138*
Burleson, M. H., *316*
Burnell, G. M., 52, *54,* 237, *262*
Burnell, L. D., 288, *302*
Burnish, T. G., 239
Burton, D., *400*
Burton, R., *232*
Bush, J. W., 68, *71, 74*
Buunk, B. P., 25, *31, 35,* 273, 284, *398, 400*
Buzaglo, J. S., *360*
Byar, D. P., *302*
Byrd, G., *266*

C

Cabrera, T., *211*
Cacioppo, J. T., 312, *316, 318, 319,* 399
Caddell, J. M., 83, *93,* 102, *114,* 149, *170*
Cain, E. N., 223, *228*
Caldwell, C., *336*
Calenoff, E., *209*
Calhoun, L. G., 27, *36*
Callahan, R., 204, *209*
Callmer, E., *336*
Calman, K. C., 40, *54*
Calnan, M., 347, *357*
Calzone, K., *316*
Calzone, K. A., *302*
Camacho, L. M., 131, 134, 135, *138, 140, 141*
Cameron, L., 375, *398*
Campbell, A., 40, *54*
Campbell, D. T., 57, *71*
Campbell, H. S., 327, *334*
Campbell, J. P., *139*
Campbell, R. J., *139*
Campbell, S., *362*
Campeau, L., *316*
Campion, M. A., 135, *141*
Canadian Erythropoietin Study Group, 69, *71*
Cancer and Leukemia Group, The, *93*
Canellos, G. P., 79, *93, 171*
Canfield, D., 328, *337*
Cantor, N., 20, *32*
Caplan, G., 364, *373*
Caplan, R., *209*
Caplan, R. D., 216, *233*
Caputo, C., *303, 337*
Carbone, D. P., *209*
Carey, T. E., *211*
Carkhuff, R. R., 282, *284*
Carlson, K., *12*
Carlson, R. W., 181, *190,* 225, *230*
Carnike, C. L., Jr., 224, *228, 230*
Carpenter, J. K., *264*

Carpenter, J. S., 123, *128*
Carrigan, L., 156, *172*
Carriger, B. K., 385, *399*
Carroll, E. M., 84, *92*
Carroll, J. S., *91*
Carter, C. A., 366, *373*
Carter, L., 177, *189*
Carter, R. E., 366, *373*
Carter, W. A., 314, *320*
Carter, W. B., *70*
Carver, C. S., 16, 17, 18, 19, 20, 21, 22, 25, 26, 27, *31, 34, 35,* 84, 88, *90,* 164, *168,* 344, 347, 351, *357, 361,* 379, 383, 385, *396, 400*
Cascione, R., *33*
Casey, J. T., 136, *139*
Casey, R., *93*
Cassileth, B. R., 78, *91,* 323, *334,* 350, *357,* 366, *373*
Catane, R., *320*
Cavalli, F., 68, 69, *73*
Cella, D., 60, 62, 64, 65, 66, 72, *74, 76,* 100, *113,* 159, 160, 163, *168,* 297, 298, *301, 304*
Cella, D. F., 40, 41, 51, *54, 56,* 57, 58, 59, 60, 61, 62, 63, 64, 71, 72, 73, 79, *91, 93,* 163, 164, 165, *168, 171,* 242, *263,* 377, *396*
Centers for Disease Control and Prevention, 324, *334*
Cerottini, J. C., *209*
Chaiken, S., 329, 332, *337*
Chaliki, H., 299, *302*
Chambers, H., *169*
Chambers, L. W., 61, *72*
Champion, V., 344, *357*
Chang, A. E., *211*
Chang, C. H., 62, 64, *72*
Chang, E. C., *35*
Chang, L. J. C., *336*
Chany, C., 331, *339*
Chapin, C. C., *75*
Chapko, M. K., 80, *91, 97*
Charles, K., 323, *339*
Charlin, V., *400*
Chassin, L., 377, *397*
Cheang, M., 226, *230*
Cheever, M. A., 196, *209*
Chen, A. E., *208*
Chen, C. C., 322, *334*
Chen, H. L., *209*
Chen, M., 68, *71*
Chen, W., 196, *209*
Cherin, E., 79, *171*

Cherin, E. A., 57, 58, 72, *93*
Chetty, U., *336*
Chi, F. S., *12*
Chochinov, H. M., 216, *228*
Choppin, B., 66, *72*
Christ, G., 223, *233*
Christ, M., 204, *209*
Christakis, D. A., 82, *93, 96*
Christensen, A. J., 311, *316,* 350, 352, *358*
Christianson, S., *170*
Christman, N. J., 21, *31,* 156, *168*
Chwalow, A. J., 61, *72*
Ciborowski, P., *128*
Cinciripini, P. M., *339*
Cirrincione, C. T., *128*
Clark, K. C., *31, 90, 168,* 357
Clark, L. A., 103, *116,* 275, *286*
Clark, L. F., 18, *31,* 87, *91,* 101, 102, *113*
Clarke, V. A., 327, *333*
Classen, C., 83, *93,* 148, *171,* 217, 221, *228*
Claus, E. R., 290, 291, *302*
Clinch, J., 61, 72, *75*
Clinch, J. J., *228*
Cline-Elsen, J., 239, *263*
Coates, D., 86, *91,* 102, *113,* 273, *284*
Cobleigh, M., *71*
Cocker, K., 242, *263*
Cohen, J., 235, 262, *263*
Cohen, L., 86, *90,* 101, *113,* 150, 155, *167,* 328, 330, 331, *333, 334, 338*
Cohen, R. D., *32*
Cohen, S., 26, *32,* 41, *53,* 58, 73, 79, *96, 99,* 108, 112, *114,* 124, *129,* 144, *169,* 269, 271, 278, 279, 280, 281, *284, 285,* 310, *317,* 331, 337, 382, *397*
Cohen, S. G., 131, 135, *138*
Cohen, S. J., *335*
Cohn, L., *338*
Colditz, G. A., *340*
Coligan, J. E., 180, *189*
Collette, L., 19, *33*
Collins, R. L., 15, 25, *31,* 273, *284*
Collins, W., 349, *362*
Colotta, F., 195, *210*
Combs, C., 353, *360*
Comegno, A., *12*
Commings, B. J., *71*
Compas, B., 100, *114*
Comstock, G. W., 78, *91*
Conaway, M., *304*
Concha, A., *211*
Condiotte, M. M., 377, *397*
Connolly, T., 135–136, 137, *139*
Connors, K. F., *75*

Conran, P., 311, *319*
Consensus Development Panel, 327, *334*
Conti, E., *338*
Contrada, R., 379, *398*
Conway, T., *318*
Cook, E. F., 69, *75*
Cook, M., *54, 55*
Coombes, C., 350, *361*
Coons, H. L., 79, *94*
Cooper, A. F., 39, *54*
Cooper, C., *93*
Cooper, E. J., *336*
Cooper, M. L., *115*
Cooper, M. R., *93*, 102, *115*
Cooper, R., *171*
Cooper, W. H., 137, *139*
Coopersmith, S., 242, *263*
Copeland, L. J., 122, *127*
Cordova, M. J., 81, 84, *90, 91*, 100, *113*, 122,
    128, 156, 158, 159, 163, *167, 168*
Corey, P., 217, *228*
Corle, D. K., *302*
Cornell, C. E., *94, 171, 265*
Corty, E., 377, *397*
Coscarelli, A., *54, 59*, 60, 61, *73*
Coscarelli Schag, C. A., *73*
Coskun, H., 137, *139*
Costanza, M., 346, *361*
Cotton, J. L., 135, *139*
Couch, F. J., 307, *316*
Counte, M. A., 40, *56*
Courtney, M., *127*
Cousins, N., *32,* 123–124, *128*, 223, 226, *228,*
    229, 241, 244, 246, 259, *263, 264, 284*
Cox, D. R., 68, *72*
Cox, R., 272, *285*
Coyne, J., 87, *91*
Coyne, J. C., 283, *284*
Cozzarelli, C., 21, *31*, 102, *115*
Crabtree, R. J., *94, 171, 265*
Craig, K. J., 155, *168, 169*, 310, *317*
Craig, S., *400*
Craig, T. J., 78, *91*
Craig, T. K., *231*
Craig, T. K. J., *338*
Crane, L. A., *230*
Creamer, M., 83, 85, 86, *91*, 102, *113*, 155,
    168
Creekmore, S. P., *191*
Cristiano, R. J., 206, *211*
Cristinzio, S., *359*
Cristofolini, M., 330, 331, *334*
Crockett, S., *338*
Croft, M., 177, *189*

Crooks, D., 216, *230*
Cross, D., 326, *338*
Cross, P. A., *91*
Crouch, M., 390, 391, *398*
Crowley-Nowick, P. A., *190*
Crown, J. P., *396*
Crowther, D., 158, 161, *168, 169*
Croyle, R., 350, *358*
Croyle, R. T., *359*, 377, 379, 383, *398, 400*
Csikszentmihalyi, M., 136, *139*
Cueller, D., *266*
Cuerdon, T., 220, *231*
Cull, A., 38, *53, 70*
Cullen, J., 235, 262, *263*
Cummings, C., 80, *91, 97*
Cummings, N., *339*
Cummings, N. A., 220, *228*
Cundick, K. E., 352, *358*
Cunningham, A. J., 241, 242, *263*
Cunningham, H. T., *209*
Cunningham, L., *128*
Curbow, B., 21, *31*
Curran, S. L., 123, *128*
Currie, V., *97*
Currie, V. E., *396*
Curry, S. J., 290, *302*, 323, 330, *334*
Curti, B. D., *191*
Curtiss, E. K., 368, *374*
Cutrona, C. E., 281, *284*
Cyranowski, J. C., 122, *127*
Czerwinski, D., *210*

D

Dadds, M. R., 79, *96*
Dakof, G., 219, *232*
Dakof, G. A., 25, *31, 273, 284*
Dalgleish, R., 101, *113*
Dalgleish, T., 86, *90*
Daly, M., 84, 88, *94, 96, 171*, 289, 293, 294,
    299, *303, 304, 318*, 337, 347, 348, 349,
    350, 351, *359, 361*
Daly, M. B., 288, *302, 361*
d'Angelo, T., 331, *337*
Daniels, M., 310, *318*
Danks, J. H., *73*
D'Avanzo, B., *338*
David, A. S., *334*
Davidson, J. R. T., 84, 85, *91*
Davidson, J. E., *139, 172*
Davidson, L. M., 83, *91*, 145, 147, 150, 155,
    168, 169
Davidson, S. M., *399*
Davies, A. R., 41, *54*
Davies, M. F., 131, *139*

Davis, D. M., *190*
Davis, H., *334*
Davis, J. D., 137, *139*
Davis, J. H., *140*
Davis, T., 349, 350, *358*
Davison, P. O., *399*
Dawson, J. L., *334*
Dawson, N. V., *75*
Dean, C., 160, 161, 162, 166, *168*
Deasy, S., *71*
Deaux, K. L., 366, *374*
Debatin, K. M., *211*
DeBruin, A. F., 61, *72*
Decarli, A., *319, 334, 338*
Decker, T., 239, *263*
DeCosimo, D., 156, *169*
Degner, L. F., 350, *358*
de Graeff, A., *340*
de Haes, C. J. M., 61, *72, 73*, 99, *113*
de Haes, J. C., *70*
de Jongh, A., 349, 352, 353, *361*
de Keijser, J., 283, *285*
Delahanty, D., 330, *334*
Delahanty, D. L., 147, 155, 165, *168*, 310, *317*
Delaney, R., *33*
Delmoor, E., *303, 337*
DeLongis, A., 283, *284*
DeMuth, J., 162, *173*
Dennis, A. R., 137, *139*
De-Nour, A., 148, 166, *169, 172*
De-Nour, A. K., 238, *262*
Dent, C. W., *400*
De Plaen, E., *209*
deProsse, C., 163, *167*
deRidder, D., 390, *397*
de Rijk, R., 189, *191*
Derlega, V. J., *116*
Derogatis, L., 160, *168*
Derogatis, L. R., 216, 221, *228*, 238, *263*, 288, *302, 308, 317, 370, 373*
de Ruiter, J., 99, *113*
Deschenes, L., 38, *55,* 224, *231*
Deshano, M. L., *316*
De Urics, M. J., *340*
Devadas, R., 135, *139*
DeVellis, R., 238, *266*, 347, *357*
Devine, E. C., 220, *228*
Devins, G. M., 40, 45, *54*
Devlen, J., 158, 161, *168, 169*
de Vries, H., 326, *340*
de Vries, M. J., *231*
de Vries, S., 88, *95*
De Witte, L. P., 61, *72*
Dhabhar, F. S., *128*

Diamandis, E. P., 195, *208*
Diamond, S., 217, *230*
Dickey, D., 311, *319*
Diederiks, J. P., 61, *72*
Diefenbach, M., *359, 360, 375, 398*
Diefenbach, M. A., 346, 347, 348, 351, *360, 361*
Diehl, M., 135, 136, *139*
Difede, J., 156, *172*
Diggle, P. J., 68, *73*
Diller, L., *264*
Dillman, R. O., 207, *209*
Dimsdale, J. E., *73*
Dinh, K. T., 377, *397*
Disis, M. L., 195, *209*
Ditto, P. H., 58, *73*
Dobbs, J., *334*
Docherty, J., *266*
Dodd, G. D., 322, *334*
Doerfler, L., 156, 157, *169*
Doherty, W. J., 364, *374*
Dolan, N. C., 6, *12,* 347, *358*
Doll, R., 321, *334*
Domel, S. B., 326, *334*
Domenech, N., *190*
Donegan, W. L., *233*
Donnerberg, R., *265, 318*
D'Onofrio, C., 38, *55*
Donovan, M. I., 164, *168*
Dopp, J. M., *316*
Dorfman, S. F., *335*
Dorvitch, A., 330, *339*
Dosik, G. M., *97, 173*
Dougall, A. L., 155, *168, 169*, 310, *317*
Dougherty, J., 87, 8f8, *94*, 99, *115*
Dow, K. H., 15, *32*
Drake, D. A., *266*
Drijfhout, J. W., *210*
Droppleman, L., 38, *55,* 59, *74,* 239, 265, 293, *303*
Druley, J. A., *72*
Dubinett, S. N., *210*
Dubois, P., 260, *264*
Ducey, C., 152, *173*
Dudovitz, B., *334*
Duez, N. J., *70*
Duffy, K., 287, *301*
DuHamel, K., 83, *91, 94, 97*
DuHamel, K. N., 82, 83, 84, *91, 92, 96, 97*
Duivenvoorden, H., 243, *262*
Duivenvoorden, H. J., 119, *129*
Dunkel-Schetter, C., *31,* 87, *92,* 153, *173,* 236, *263,* 330, *335,* 365, *373*
Dunn, D., 19n, *32*

Dunn, S. M., 236, *265*
Duout, Y., *72*
Dura, J. R., 310, *318*
Dusser, D., *72*
Dutton, R. W., 177, *189*
Dwyer, J., *337*
Dyer, C. S., *336*
Dzindolet, M. T., 131, 134, 135, 136, *140*
D'Zurilla, T. J., 296, *302*

E

Eads, N., *303*
Eakes, G., 161, 166, *169*
Earnest, D., *338*
Earp, J. A., 224, *233*
Earp, J. L., 79, *97*
Easterling, D., 161, *171*
Easterling, D. V., 377, *397, 399*
Easterling, F., 79, *94*
Easton, D. F., 307, *317*
Easton, D. T., *302*
Ebbeson, E. B., *267*
Eckberg, K., *72, 396*
Edgar, L., 243, *263*
Edmonds, C. V. I., 242, *263*
Edwards, A., 314, *317*
Edwards, D. L., *316*
Edwards, P. W., 350, *358*
Eika, S., *76*
Eisenberg, D. M., 394, *397*
Eisenthal, S., 225, *228*
Elashoff, R., *32, 128, 228, 229, 263, 264, 284, 335, 397*
Elashoff, R. M., *336*
Elder, E., 180, *190*
Elder, G., 152, *171*
Ell, K., 224, *228, 373*
Ell, K. O., 365, *366*
Ellard, I. H., 87, *94*
Elliott, R. L., 331, *336*
Ellwin, L., 322, *334*
Elmer, P. J., *338*
Emery, G., 242, *262*
Emery, R., 225, *228*
Emmelkamp, P. M., *231*
Emmons, K. M., 323, 330, *334*
Emmons, R. A., 20, *32*
Eneroth, P., *316*
Engleman, E. G., *210*
Engstrom, P., *303, 318, 337*
Engstrom, P. F., 301, *303, 329, 336, 337, 339, 359, 361*
Enns, M., *228*
Ensoli, B., 204, *209*

Epping-Jordan, J. E., 100, *114*
Epstein, D., *74*
Epstein, N., 242, *262*
Epstein, S., 100, *114*
Epstein, S. A., *169, 309, 317*
Erblich, J., 309, *317*
Eremin, O., 194, *209*
Eriksen, E., *326*
Eriksen, M., *340*
Ersek, M., 19n, *32*
Espindle, D., 122, *127*
Essex, M. J., 20, *34*
Eth, S., 83, *96, 154, 172*
EuroQOL, 61, *74*
EuroQol Group, the, 61, *73*
Evans, D. G. R., 288, 291, 295, 300, *302*
Ever-Hadani, P., 148, *172*
Everson, S. A., 22, *32*
Eyfjord, J. E., *320*
Ezrachi, O., *264*

F

Faden, A. I., 367, *373*
Faden, R. R., 367, *373*
Fagerberg, J., 207, *209*
Fagnoni, F., *210*
Fahey, J., 310, *319*
Fahey, J. L., *32, 124, 128, 229, 284, 335*
Fahs, M., *232*
Fahy, T., *334*
Fairbank, J., 85, *94*
Fairbank, J. A., 84, 91, 152, *169*
Falcini, F., *338*
Falk, A., 313, *319*
Falk, W., *211*
Falke, R. L., 236, *263, 277, 286, 330, 335*
Fallowfield, L. I., 78, *92, 222, 228*
Fan, D., *210*
Farber, J., 226, *230*
Farrar, W., 122, *129*
Farrar, W. B., *127*
Fawzy, F., *228*
Fawzy, F. I., 22, 23, *32, 80, 97, 123, 123–124, 124, 128, 144, 169, 223, 225, 226, 229, 235, 241, 244, 246, 259, 263, 264, 265, 270, 271, 284, 311, 317, 323, 331, 333, 335, 377, 382, 397*
Fawzy, N. W., 22, *32, 128, 144, 169, 223, 228, 229, 235, 240, 263, 264, 284, 311, 317, 331, 335, 397*
Fearon, D. T., 176, *190*
Feather, N. T., 16, *32*
Feeny, D., 63, *75*
Feinstein, L., 330, *335*

Feinstein, L. G., 236, *263*
Feldstein, M., *333*
Felten, D. L., 313, *319*
Felton, B. J., 224, *229*
Fentiman, I. S., *231, 338*
Ferguson, K., 225, *229*
Ferlic, M., 223, *229*
Ferrando, S. I., 393, *397*
Ferree, C. R., *128*
Ferrell, B. R., 15, 19n, *32*
Festinger, L., 101, *114*, 132, *139*
Fetting, J., *168, 228*
Fetting, J. H., 224, *233*
Fiedman, A., *316*
Fields, K. K., *170*
Fifield, J., 387, *396*
Filiberti, A., *70, 338*
Filipp, S. H., *92*
Fink, A., 41, *55*
Fink, D., *333*
Finke, J. H., 187, *190*
Finn, O. J., *128, 129*, 179, 180, 181, *190*
Finnegan, J. R., *338*
Fiore, M. C., 324, *335*
Fischoff, B., 295, *302*
Fishbein, M., 384, 390, *396, 397*
Fisher, B., *209, 229*
Fisher, E. R., 200, *209*
Fisher, J. D., 322, *335*
Fisher, L., 310, *318*
Fisher, L. M., 83, *93*
Fisher, S. P., *211*
Fisher, W. A., 322, *335*
Fishkin, S. A., 329, *339*
Fishman, H. C., 364, *374*
Fisk, B., *210*
Fiske, D. W., *71*
Fisler, R., 152, *173*
Fitch, M., 217, *228*
Fitzgerald, T. E., 21, *32,* 348, *358*
Fitzpatrick, R., *72*
Flack, V. F., 366, *373*
Flamer, D. P., *54, 55*
Flay, B. R., 376, *397, 400*
Flechtner, H., *70*
Fleischman, S. B., *70*
Fleiss, J., 78, *92*
Fleiss, J. L., *229*
Fleming, I., 147, 150, *167, 169*
Fleming, R., 376–377, *398*
Fletcher, A. I., *72*
Fletcher, B., 26, *35,* 365, *374*
Fletcher, M., *170, 336*
Fletcher, M. A., *317*

Flum, H., 89, *96*
Foa, E. B., 83, 84, 85, 86, *91, 92,* 150, 151, 155, 159, *169, 172,* 354, 356, *358*
Fobair, P., 38 , *55,* 272, *285*
Foerster, S. B., 321, *333*
Foley, K. M., *96*
Folkman, S., 19, *33,* 149, *171,* 245, 247, 258, *265,* 281, *285, 337,* 344, *359,* 365, 373
Folsom, A. R., 324, *338*
Fontana, A., *33,* 83, *92,* 209
Ford, D., 287, *302,* 307, *317*
Ford, R. E., 80, *92*
Forester, B., 78, *92,* 223, 225, *229*
Forlenza, M. J., 5, *12*
Forman, M. R., 123, *128*
Forneris, C., *168*
Fosle, D. W., 57
Foster, D., 229
Foster, R., 346, *361*
Fotopolis, S., *54, 55*
Fox, B., 254, 258, *264, 266*
Foy, D. W., 84, 89, *92,* 148, *170, 172*
Frances, A. J., 83, *95,* 156, *172*
Franceschi, S., *319, 338*
Francis, K., 324, *335*
Frank, R. G., *227*
Franks, C. M., 120, *129*
Frasure-Smith, N., 282, *285*
Fred, C., *54, 55*
Freedman, L. S., 307, *319*
Freeman, J., 367, *373*
Frei, E. III, *128, 264*
Freidenbergs, I., *264*
French, L. E., *209*
Freud, S., 87, *92,* 152, *169*
Friedenreich, C. M., 324, *335*
Friedman, H., *316*
Friedman, H. S., *34,* 327, *336*
Friedman, K., *339*
Friedman, L. L., 15, *36*
Friedman, L. N., 330, *335*
Friedman, M., 153, *169*
Friend, S. H., 307, *317*
Frieze, I. H., *91,* 150, 153, *170*
Frist, W. H., 22, *33*
Fritz, H. L., 58, *73*
Fromm, K., 15, *32*
Frueh, B. C., 83, *92*
Fullerton, C. S., 155, 159, *168, 173*
Fulmore, C., *318*
Funch, D. P., 322, 323, *335*
Futterman, A. D., 79, *96*
Futterman, R., *338*

G

Gaard, M., 324, *340*
Gabrilovich, D. I., 203, *209*
Gadd, M. A., *12*
Gafni, A., 217, 228
Gail, M. H., 287, 290, *302*
Gaines, J. G., 21, *31*
Gaiser, J., 161, *169*
Gale, R., 259, *262*
Gale, R. P., 331, *333*
Gale, Z., *398*
Gallagher, M., 239, *263*
Galleli, K., 83, *94*
Gallo, R. C., 204, *208*
Gallupe, R. B., 137, *139*
Gamace, M., 227
Ganer, W., *336*
Gangeri, L., *71*
Ganguly, A., *316*
Ganz, P., 60, 61, *73*
Ganz, P. A., 38, 39, 40, 41, 50, *54, 55,* 59, 61,
    75, 223, *229,* 366, 373
Garber, J., *116,* 297, 298, *301, 304*
Garber, J. E., *302*
Garber, R. A., *285*
Gard, D., 350, *358*
Gardiner, J., 327, *339*
Garfinkel, L., 3, 4, *12,* 321, 322, *335*
Garrido, F., *211*
Garssen, B., *340*
Gates, C., *54, 55*
Gattuso, S. M., 348, 353, *358*
Gautaum, S., 350, *358*
Geden, E. A., 227
Geenen, R., *316*
Gehde, E., 331, *335*
Geiser, P. B., 78, *91*
Gelber, R. D., 68, 69, 71, *73*
Geller, A. C., 329, *337*
Gellert, G. A., 225, 226, *229, 231*
Genest, M., 8, *12*
Gerardi, R. J., 85, *90*
Gerin, W., *320*
Germain, R. N., 195, *209*
Germino, B. B., 20, *34,* 158, *172*
Gerrard, M., 273, *285*
Gessner, J., 376, *399*
Gettys, C. F., 136, *139*
Gianola, F. J., 41, *56*
Gibbons, F. X., 273, *285, 398, 400*
Gigone, D., 136, *139*
Gilbar, O., 166, *169*
Gilewski, T. A., *396*
Gill, R. F., 204, *211*

Giller, E. L., 97, 146, *171, 173,* 330, *340*
Gillin, J. C., 330, *336*
Gilmore, S. L., *316*
Gilson, B. S., *70*
Girgis, A., 328, *335*
Girgis, K. R., *209*
Girodano, L., *333*
Given, B. A., 15, *32, 36,* 224, *229*
Given, C. W., 15, 20, 22, *32, 36,* 224, *229*
Glanz, K., 99, *114*
Glaser, R., 5, *12,* 120, 123, *127,* 265, 310,
    311, 312, *316, 317, 318,* 330, *333, 336*
Glasgow, R. E., 309, *319,* 322, 324, *337*
Glass, A., 224, *229*
Glass, D. C., 330, *335*
Glass, G. V., 220, *231*
Glassman, B., 301, *304*
Glassman, M., 99, *115*
Gleser, G. C., 84, *92*
Gloeb, B. D., *338*
Godaert, G. L. R., *316*
Godenberg, B., *113*
Gold, K., *318*
Goldberg, D. E., *32*
Goldbert, H., *93*
Goldenberg, B., *90, 95, 167*
Golden-Kreutz, D., *127*
Goldgar, D. E. *302*
Goldhirsch, A., 68, 69, *73*
Goldin, B., *337*
Golding, T., 328, *335*
Goldman, A., 223, *229*
Goldman, L., *75*
Goldman, S., *340*
Goldsmith, D., 101, *113*
Goldstein, A., 307, *319*
Goldstein, L., *303, 318, 337, 359*
Goldstein, M. G., *335*
Gollock, J., *336*
Gollwitzer, P. M., 18, *36*
Gomez, O., *211*
Gomez-Caminero, A., *301, 303, 318*
Gonin, R., 62, 64, 72, *73*
Goodkin, K., 323, *334, 340*
Goodman, M., *72, 396*
Goodman, P. S., 135, *139*
Goodwin, J. S., 219, *229*
Gorbach, S., *337*
Gordon, J. R., 377, *399*
Gordon, W. A., 236, 238, 241, *264*
Gore, S. M., *72*
Gorman, A., 236, *265*
Gotay, C. C., 119, *128,* 366, *374*
Gottheil, E., *35, 129,* 144, *172,* 181, *191,* 222,
    223, *232,* 235, *266,* 270, *286,* 323, *339,*
    377, *400*

Gottlieb, B., *114*
Gottlieg, A., *171*
Gould, K. L., *265*
Goulmy, E., 311, *320*
Goydos, J. S., 180, *190*
Grace, M. C., 84, *92*
Gradman, A., *33*
Grady, M. J., 81, *90*
Graham, S., 324, *340*
Gramzow, R. H., 107, *115*
Grant, I., *264, 336*
Graves, K., *338*
Gray, G., *72, 396*
Grayson, H., 205, *211*
Greaves, C., 218, 219, *233*
Green, B., 153, 154, 156, 159, 160, *169*
Green, B. L., 84, 85, *92*
Green, M. R., *128*
Green, S. B., *302*
Green, V., *360*
Greenberg, J., 29, *34*
Greenberg, M., 101, *114*
Greenberg, M. A., 86, *92*, 102, *114*
Greenhalgh, R., 291, *302*
Greenlee, R. T., 119, *128*
Greenwald, P., 322, 323, 325, *335*
Greenwood, D., *170*, 317, *336*
Greer, H. S., *55, 78, 95*, 224, 231, 236, *265*
Greer, S., 26, 27, *32, 34, 36*, 38, 78, *97*, 163,
    172, 217, 221, 223, 229, 233, 235, 242,
    264, 265, 266, 331, *335, 338*
Gress, R. E., *209*
Grillo-Lopez, A., *210*
Gritz, E. R., 324, *335, 339*
Grobois, B., *90, 113, 167*
Grohr, P., 310, *319*
Groner, B., *209*
Grossbart, T. A, 329, *337*
Gruber, B., 260, *264*
Gruber, B. L., 238, *264*
Grudberg, S. C., *12*
Grunberg, N. E., 323, 330, *335*
Gulasekaram, P., 15, *32*
Gullion, D. S., 367, *373*
Gump, B., 147, 148, 164, *169*
Gunning, J., *230*
Gustafson, J., 223, *229*
Gustafsson, U., 242, *262*
Gutherie, D., *128*
Guthrie, D., *32, 229*, 264, 284, *335*
Gutmann, M., 385, *399*
Guttman, R. D., *54*
Guyatt, G., 63, *73*
Guyatt, G. H., 63, *73*

H

Haas, G. P., *210*
Hadicke, A., *319*
Hadley, D., *303*
Hahne, M., 203, *209*
Hailey, B. J., *74*, 309, *319*
Hakes, T., *171*
Hakes, T. B., *396*
Halabi, S., 290, *302*
Hall, A., 222, *228*
Hall, L., 6, *12*
Hall, M., 86, *90*, 101, *113*, 150, 155, *167*
Hall, M. H., 330, *333, 338*
Hall, N., 260, *264*
Hall, N. J., *338*
Hall, N. R. S., *264*
Hall, W. J., *302*
Hallett, C. D., 287, *301*
Halper, M., 343, *358*
Halper, M. S., 6, *12, 143, 170*, 303, 308, *318*
Hamersma, E., *72*
Hamilton, J. N., 366, *373*
Hammer, A. L., 20, *36*
Hammer, J. S., *232*
Hamovitch, M., 224, *228*
Hamovitch, M. H., 365, *373*
Hanau, C., *334*
Hanisch, R., 324, *334*
Hanjani, P., 303, *337, 359*
Hanna, D. M., *170*
Hanquet, P., *71*
Hansen, W. B., *400*
Haraphongse, M., *358*
Harber, K., 101, *116*
Hare, A. P., 131, *139*
Harkness, L., 146, *171*
Harlow, R. E., 20, *32*
Harrell, F. E., *75*
Harris, H., *90, 113, 167*
Harris, J., *72*, 350, *358, 396*
Harris, J. R., 306, 307, *317*
Harris, R., 226, 230, 240, *265*
Harris, S. D., *31, 90*, 168, *357*
Harris, W. J., 41, *54*
Hartford, C. E., 366, *373*
Hartge, P., *304*
Hartman, K. A., 344, 347, *358*, 385, *398*
Harvey, A., 155, *168*
Harwood, A., 61, *73*
Hastie, R., 136, *139*
Hatfield, A. K., 377, *396*
Hauger, R., 259, *264*
Hawken, L., *168*
Haynes, K. N., 20, *35*

Haynes, L. T., *230*
Hays, R. D., 41, *55,* 58, *73,* 109, *116*
Hayward, M., *168*
Head, J. F., 331, *336*
Healy, J. N., *114*
Heasman, K. Z., *71*
Heber, D., 326, *336*
Heggan, T., *303, 318, 337, 359*
Heijmans, M., 390, 393, *397*
Heijnen, C. J., *316, 340*
Heinrich, 366
Heinrich, R., 38, *55*
Heinrich, R. L., 61, *75,* 366, 374
Heinrichs, M., *168*
Heitjan, D. F., 290, *302*
Helgeson, V. S., 26, 28, 29, *32,* 58, *73,* 99,
        100, 102, 104, 108, 109, 110, 111, 112,
        114, 115, 144, *169,* 269, 271, 275, 278,
        279, 280, 283, *285,* 382, *397*
Hellman, C. J., 220, *229*
Helm, C. W., *303*
Helm, W., 348, *361*
Helzlsouer, K., *301*
Hendersen, E., *171*
Henderson, B. E., 324, *334*
Henderson, I. C., *128,* 325, *336*
Henderson, M. M., *340*
Henderson, R., 205, *211*
Henderson, R. A., *128,* 179, 181, *190*
Hendrick, C., *140*
Henrichs, M., *228*
Henriques, B., 350, *358*
Henry, J. P., 313, *317*
Henry, S. M., 18, *31*
Hepworth, J., 364, *374*
Herberman, H., *168,* 193, *209,* 331, *333*
Herberman, R., 331, *336, 337*
Herberman, R. B., *230*
Herbert, M., *35*
Herbert, T. B., 87, 92, 124, *129,* 310, *316, 317*
Herd, R. M., 329, 330, *336*
Hermanson, K., 217, *230*
Hernandez, E., *303*
Hersen, M., *93*
Hersey, P., 314, *317*
Hersh, S., 260, *264*
Hertog, J., *338*
Hewstone, M., *140*
Heyman, R. B., *335*
Heys, S. D., 194, *209*
Hibbard, M., *264*
Hickey, S. S., 20, *33*
Hickling, E., *168*
Higgins, E. T., 16, *35,* 132, *140*

Hilgard, E. R., 223, *230*
Hilgard, J. R., 223, *230*
Hill, D., 327, 328, 330, *334, 336, 338, 339*
Hillman, G. G., 200, *210*
Hiltbold, E. M., *128*
Hines, K. L., *209*
Hinrichsen, G. A., 224, *229*
Hippe, E., *76*
Hirji, K., *54, 55, 73*
Hjalmar, M. L., *336*
Hjorth, M., *76*
Ho, E., *333*
Hoagland, A. C., 224, *230*
Hochbaum, G. M., 385, *397, 399*
Holahan, C. K., 20, *33*
Holbrook, J., *335*
Holland, J., *35, 55,* 217, *230, 316, 343, 358*
Holland, J. C., 6, *12, 54,* 57, 58, *73,* 74, 78,
        79, 80, *91, 92, 94, 116,* 143, 156, 162,
        166, *170, 171, 173,* 237, *264, 285,* 288,
        295, *303, 304,* 308, *316, 318, 320, 333*
Holland, J. F., *264*
Holland, P. W., *70*
Holliday, J., *265, 336*
Hollingdale, R. J., *34*
Hollingshead, A. B., 135, 137, *138, 140*
Hollingsworth, C. E., *264*
Holm, L. E., 325, *336, 338*
Holman, E. A., 107, *116*
Holman, H. R., 220, *230*
Holmberg, E., *76*
Holmberg, L., 216, *231*
Holomby, D. J., *54*
Honeyman, M., 314, *317*
Hooker, K., 21, *33, 35*
Hoppe, R. T., 272, *285*
Hopwood, P., 288, 291, *302*
Horne, R., 391, *397*
Horowitz, M., 100, *114,* 126, *129,* 150, 151,
        152, 153, 154, 158, 163, *170, 171, 173,*
        238, *264,* 293, *302,* 344, 348, *358*
Horowitz, M. J., 85, 87, *93,* 100, 101, *114*
Hosaka, T., 241, *264*
Hoskins, K. F., 287, 290, *302*
Hoskins, W., *171*
Hospers, H., 301, *304*
Houbiers, J. G., 196, *210*
Houghson, A. V., 39, *54*
Houghton, A. N., 195, *211*
House, J. S., 219, *230*
Houskamp, B., 82, *96*
Houts, P. S., 290, 301, *302*
Howell, A., 288, 291, *302*
Howell, D. C., 100, *114*

Howells, J. G., *265*
Hoyert, D. L., 4, *12*
Hsu, F. J., 206, *210*
Huang, H., *170, 317, 336*
Huang, M., 200, *210*
Hudis, C. A., *396*
Hudson, S., 122, *129*, 376, *399*
Hughes, C., *302, 303, 318*
Hughes, J., *317*
Hughes, J. E., 78, *93*, 162, 166, *170*
Hughes, M., 83, *93*
Hughson, T. L. G., 135, *139*
Hunt, J., 15, *32*
Hunt, J. W., 59, *70*, 81, *90*
Hunt, S., 61, *73*
Hunt, W. C., 219, *229*
Hunter, J. A., *336*
Hunton, S., 241, *263*
Hurley, K., 88, *95*, 343, 344, 345, 346, 351, *361*
Hursting, S., *338*
Hutchinson, C., 21, *33*
Hutchinson, T. A., *54*
Hwang, L., *190*
Hyde, R. T., 324, *338*
Hyer, L., 151, *170*
Hyun, C. S., *32, 128, 229, 264, 284, 311, 317, 335*

I

Ilnyckyj, A., 226, *230*
Inayat, Q., *266*
Institute for the Future, 11, *12*
Insull, W., Jr., *340*
Ioannides, C. G., 196, *210*
Ironson, G., 155, 163, *170*, 310, 311, *317, 330, 336, 339*
Irvine, D., 216, 224, *230*
Irwin, M., 259, *264, 265*, 310, *318*, 330, *336*
Itano, J., 224, *230*
Ituarte, P. H. G., 99, *115*

J

Jaccard, J., *168*
Jacob, T. C., 353, *358*
Jacobs, R., 312, *319*
Jacobsberg, L., 83, *95*, 156, *172*
Jacobsen, M., *35*
Jacobsen, P., *320*
Jacobsen, P. B., 78, *93*, 156, 163, *170, 396*
Jacobson, N. S., 63, *73*
Jaén, C. R., *335*
Jaeschke, R., 63, *73*

Jain, R. K., *209*
James, J., *303, 318, 337, 359*
Jamieson, G., *190*
Jamison, K. R., 78, *93*, 224, *230*, 283, *285*
Janigian, A. S., 19n, *36*
Janis, I. L., 8, *12*, 133, 136, *139*
Janoff-Bulman, R., 100, 102, *114*, 149, 150, 151, 152, 153, 158, *170*, 224, *233*
Jarrett, S. R., 221, *230*
Jendteg, S., *71*
Jenkins, F. J., *168*, 310, *317*, 330, *334*
Jenkins, G., 242, *263*
Jenkins, P. L., 79, 80, *93*
Jenkins, R. A., 239, *263*
Jepson, C., *337, 359*
Jerome, K. R., *129, 190*
Jeschke, M., *209*
Jochimsen, P. R., 38, *53*
Johnson, J. E., 8, *12, 333*
Johnson, P. D., 102, *114*
Johnston, M., 37, 43, *54, 359*
Jonasson, J. G., *320*
Jones, D., *31*
Jones, D. R., *72*
Jones, J., *209*
Jones, J. C., 101, *114*, 153, *170*
Jones, J. S., 350, *358*
Jones, L., 241, 259, *263, 264*
Jones, S., 102, *115*
Jones-Webb, R. J., 39, 52, *54*
Joseph, S., 86, *90*, 101, *113*
Juhlin, C., *190*
Juliano, M. A., 78, *96*
Juneau, M., *285*
Jung, S., 196, *210*

K

Kaasa, S., 38, *53, 76*
Kahana, B., 97, 146, 330, *340*
Kahn, B., *54, 73*
Kahn, D., 15, *33*
Kaizer, L., *74*
Kakar, F., *338*
Kalechman, Y., *320*
Kalichman, S. C., *230*
Kampert, J. B., 324, *336*
Kantz, M. E., 41, *54*
Kao, T. C., 155, 159, *173*
Kaplan, C. P., *230*
Kaplan, E., 71, 72, *396*
Kaplan, G. A., *32*, 224, *231*
Kaplan, H. I., *285*
Kaplan, R. M., 68, *74*
Kaplan, S., *90, 95, 113, 167*

Kaptchuk, T. J., 394, *397*
Karanikas, V., 180, *190*
Karau, S. J., 137, *139*
Karlsson, S., *209*
Kash, K., 143, *171, 173,* 308, *316, 318,* 329,
    337, 343, 347, 348, 349, 350, *358, 359*
Kash, K. M., 6, *12,* 143, *170,* 288, 289, 295,
    298, 300, *303, 304,* 308, *318, 320*
Kasprisin, C. A., *92*
Kast, W. M., *210*
Katon, W., 217, 233
Kaufman, B., *320*
Kaufman, R. J., *396*
Kavanaugh, D., *209*
Kay, D. R., *227*
Kaye, L. E., 379, *397*
Kazak, A. E., 82, *93, 96*
Keane, T., 85, *94*
Keane, T. M., 83, 84, 85, *93,* 102, *114,* 149,
    151, 165, *170*
Keefe, F., 158, 161, *171*
Keel, E., 161, *169*
Keesling, B., 327, *336*
Keintz, M. K., 329, *339*
Kellen, J. A., 195, *208*
Kelly, G. A., 382, *397*
Kelly, G. M., *266*
Kelly, J. A., 223, *230*
Kelly, J. R., 137, *139*
Kelsey, J. L., 287, *303*
Kemeny, M., 78, 310, *319*
Kemeny, M. E., 27, *32, 34, 35, 93,* 99, 124,
    128, 223, 226, 228, 229, 244, 263, 264,
    284, 397
Kemeny, N., 87, *94, 115*
Kenady, D. E., 81, *90, 91, 113,* 122, *128,* 168
Kenemans, P., *210*
Kennedy, B. J., 223, *229*
Kennedy, S., 310, *317, 318*
Kent, M. V., 131, *139*
Kerber, R. A., 287, *304*
Kerner, J., *303*
Kerner, J. D., 187, *189*
Kerns, R., *33*
Kessler, H. B., 329, *339*
Kessler, L., 37, 38, *54*
Kessler, R. C., 83, *93*
Ketcham, A. S., *31, 90, 168, 357*
Key, C. R., 219, *229*
Keyes, C. L. M., 20, *34*
Khalil, H., 238, *262*
Kidman, A., 242, *263*
Kiecolt-Glaser, J. K., 5, *12,* 120, 123, *127,* 260,
    265, 310, 311, 312, *316, 317, 318, 319,*
    330, 330–331, 331, 333, *336*

Kiessling, R., *190*
Kindt, M., 348, *361*
King, D. W., 148, *170*
King, E., 301, *303*
King, E. S., 329, *336*
King, L. A., 20, *32,* 148, *170*
Kipnis, V., 123, *128*
Kirkeeide, R. L., *265*
Kirkwood, J., *230*
Kirscher, E., *338*
Klas, C., *211*
Klein, E., *190*
Klein, M., 329, *340*
Klein, R., *338*
Klein, T., *316*
Kleinmann, A., *73*
Kliewer, W. L., 102, 107, *114*
Klimas, N., *170, 317, 336*
Klock, S., 21, *33*
Knapp, J. E., 22, *35*
Knapp, M. L., *113*
Knowles, J. H., *400*
Kobasa, S. C., 19, *33*
Kochanek, K. D., 4, *12*
Kogon, M. M., 181, *190,* 225, *230*
Koh, H. K., 329, 330, *337*
Kohl, H. W. III, 324, *336*
Kohorn, E. I., 223, *228*
Kok, G., 326, *340*
Kolb, L., 85, *90,* 153, *171*
Koob, J. J., *230*
Koocher, G. P., 363, 368, *374*
Koopman, C., 83, 89, *93,* 148, *171,* 217, 228,
    230
Korn, E. L., 68, *74*
Kornblith, A. B., 57, 58, *74,* 79, *93,* 163, 166,
    171
Kornfeld, D., 78, *92*
Kornfeld, D. S., 223, *229*
Kosinski, M. A., *75*
Kosten, T., 146, *171*
Kosty, M. P., *93*
Kottke, T., *335*
Kowalski, R., 132, *139*
Kozak, M. J., 83, 84, 85, 86, *92,* 354, 356,
    358
Kraag, G., *72*
Kraemer, H., 63, *74*
Kraemer, H. C., *35, 129,* 181, *191,* 223, 232,
    235, *266,* 270, 278, *285, 286,* 323, *339,*
    377, *400*
Kraemer, J., 144, *172*
Krailo, M., 225, 232, 237, *266*
Kraines, R. G., 220, *230*

Kral, T., 313, *316*
Kramer, M. M., 324, *337*
Kramer, T. J., 136, *140*
Krammer, P. H., *211*
Krantz, D., *359*
Kreitler, J., 85, *94*
Kreitler, S., 85, *94*
Krinsley, K. E., 83, *93*
Kriss, R. T., 278, *285*
Kristal, A. R., *340*
Krohne, H. W., *90*
Kronish, L. E., *170*
Kruglanski, A. W., *140*
Krupnick, J., 153
Krupnick, J. L., *169, 171*
Kuchemann, C. S., *94, 171, 265*
Kudoh, S., *190*
Kulik, J. A., 283, *285, 353, 358,* 391, *398*
Kulkarni, A. B., *209*
Kuller, L. H., 6, *12,* 322, *338*
Kumar, N. B., 326, *339*
Kunkel, A. W., *138*
Kunz, J. F., *264*
Kurtz, J. C., 15, *32, 33*
Kurtz, M. E., 15, *32, 33, 36*
Kushi, L. H., 324, *338*
Kutz, L. A., *127*
Kuyken, W., *74*
Kverno, K. S., *264*
Kyle, M. J., 323, *339*

L

Lacroix, J. M., 382, *398*
Lai, P., 187, *190*
Lam, J. S., *210*
Lamas, G. A., *75*
Lamdan, R., *304*
Lamkin, L., *230*
Lander, S., *228*
Landis, K. R., 219, *230*
Landmann, R., 313, *318*
Lando, H. A., *335*
Lang, P., 151, *171*
Lang, P. J., 84, *94,* 309, *318*
LaPerriere, A., *170, 317, 336*
Larcombe, I., 328, *338*
Larey, T. S., 131, *140, 141*
Larsen, K., 106, *115*
Larson, L., *339*
Laszlo, J., 224, *230*
Latimer, J. J., 5, *12*
Latimer, K., 223, *228*
Latreille, J., *74*
Lau, R., 344

Lau, R. R., 347, *358,* 385, *398*
Lauder, S., 302
Launier, R., 383, *398*
LaVecchia, C., *319, 338*
Law, M., *75, 265*
Law, M. G., *264*
Lawler, C., *12*
Lawless, J., 250, *265*
Lawrence, J. W., *12,* 335, *340*
Lawton, W., 349, *358*
Lazare, A., 225, *228*
Lazarus, R., 245, 247, 258, *265,* 344, *359*
Lazarus, R. S., 20, *35,* 149, *171,* 330, *337,*
    365, *373,* 383, *398*
Leaf, D. A., *336*
Leandri, S., *339*
Leary, M. R., 132, *139*
LeBaron, S., 223, *233*
Lebovitz, A., 78, *92,* 156, *170,* 232
Lederberg, M., *35*
Ledford, G. E., 138, *138*
Lee, A. M., 6, *12,* 347, *358*
Lee, E. G., *94, 171, 265*
Lee, J., 230, 250, *265*
Lee, K., 152, *171*
Lee, T. H., *75*
Lee, Y. H., 20, *34*
Lee, Y. T., 224, *230*
Leedham, B., 22, *33,* 122, *129,* 376, *399*
Lefebvre, R. C., *35*
Legro, M. W., 21, *31*
Lehman, D. R., 87, *94,* 101, *114*
Lehrer, P. H., *95*
Leibowitz, R. L., *97, 173*
Leigh, S., 15, *32*
Leinbach, A., 348, *360*
Leitman, S., *211*
Lemon, S. J., *318*
Lenhard, R. E., *12,* 335, *340*
Lenihan, W. M., *211*
Lenoir, G., *318*
Leonard, A., *92*
Leonard, S. B., *334*
Leone, L., *171*
Lepore, J., *171*
Lepore, S. J., 86, 87, 88, *94,* 99, 100, 101,
    102, 103, 104, 105, 106, 107, 108, 110,
    111, *114, 115,* 136, *139,* 283, *285,* 315,
    318
Lerman, C., 84, 88, *94, 96,* 99, *114,* 143, 158,
    171, 288, 289, 292, 293, 294, 295, 297,
    298, 299, 300, 301, *302, 303, 304,* 308,
    308–309, 309, *317, 318, 319,* 323, 329,
    330, *337,* 343, 347, 348, 349, 350, 351,
    352, *358, 359, 361,* 377, *398*

Lerman, C. L., 291, 292, *303*, 309
Lerner, H., *229*
Lerner, M. J., *92*
Lesko, L., *95*, 216, *231*
Lesko, L. M., 79, 80, *94, 96*, 272, *285*
Lesperance, F., *285*
Lessan, G., 346, *361*
Levenkron, J., *302*
Leventhal, E., 347, *360*
Leventhal, E. A., 375, 379, 391, *398*
Leventhal, H., 8, *12,* 79, *94*, 161, *171*, *337*,
    344, 347, 348, *359, 360*, 375, 376, 377,
    379, 382, 383, 384, 385, 390, *396, 397,
    398, 399*
Levi, L., *316*
Levine, A. M., 225, 232, 237, *266*
Levine, H. M., 365, *374*
Levine, J., 26, *33*
Levine, J. M., 131, 132, 133, 134, *139, 140*
Levine, L., *264*
Levine, S., 40, *54*
Levitsky, K., 41, *54*
Levitt, M., *75*, 228
Levy, J. S., 315, *318*
Levy, R., *210*
Levy, S., 331, *337, 339*
Levy, S. M., 222, *230*
Lew, R. A., 329, *337*
Lewis, C., 367, *373*
Lewis, C. E., *317, 319*
Lewis, F. M., 20, *33,* 38, 44, *55*
Lewis, M., *398*
Liang, K. Y., 68, *73*
Liang, L. P., 236, *265*
Libet, J. M., 83, *92*
Lichmann, R. R., 366
Lichtenstein, E., 322, 324, *337*, 377, *397*
Lichtman, R. R., *97, 173*, 273, 277, *286, 374,
    400*
Lidbrick, E., *336*
Lieberman, M. A., 273, *285*
Liebeskind, J., 259, 262, 331, *333*
Lienard, D., 209
Liff, D., 223, *233*
Lightner, R., 123, *128*
Liles, T. M., *210*
Lin, E. H., 217, *233*
Lin, T. H., 297, 298, *301, 304, 317*
Lindgren, B., *71*
Lindy, J. D., 84, *92*
Linn, B. S., 226, *230*, 240, *265*
Linn, E., *72, 396*
Linn, M. W., 226, *230*, 240, *265*
Linville, P., 18, *33*

Lipetz, P. D., 5, *12*
Lipkins, R., *264*
Lipkus, I., *304*
Lippman, M., 331, *337*
Lippman, M. E., 306, *317*
Liss-Levinson, W. S., 367, *374*
Litt, M., 353, *360*
Litt, M. D., 21, *33, 348, 358*
Little, B. R., 20, *34*
Litwin, M. S., 41, 51, *55*
Litz, B. T., *115*
Livingston, A., 79, *93*
Livingston, R. B., *209*
Llewellyn-Thomas, H. A., 350, *361*
Lloyd, S., 62, 64, *71, 72, 73, 396*
Lloyd, S. R., 62, *71, 72*
Locksley, R. M., 176, *190*
Lockwood, G. A., 242, *263*, 350, *361*
Loescher, L. J., 328, *334*
Logan-Young, W., *302*
Lombard, D., 328, *337*
Lomenech, N., *129*
Long, B. C., 20, *33*
Longcope, C., 325, *337*
Longo, D. L., *190, 191*
Loos, W., *168*
Lorig, K., 220, *230*
Lorr, M., 38, *55, 59, 74,* 239, *265,* 293, *303*
Loscalzo, M. J., *35*
Loseth, D., *171*
Lotze, M. T., 180, *190, 211*
Love, R. R., 79, *94,* 161, 166, *171,* 377, *399*
Lowman, J. T., *333*
Lu, J. F. R., 61, *74*
Lubaroff, D. M., *316*
Lubeck, D., 220, *230*
Lubin, M. B., *316*
Lucas, V., Jr., 224, *230*
Luchterhand, C. M., 79, *94*
Lucido, D., *264*
Ludwick-Rosenfeld, R., 353, 354, *360*
Lum, J. L., *230*
Lund, E., 324, 325, *340*
Lurie, A., *72*
Lurquin, C., *209*
Lusk, E. J., *91*
Lustbader, E., *171, 303, 318, 337, 359*
Lustbader, E. D., 290, *302*
Lutgendorf, S., 106, *115*, 311, *317*
Ly, J., 15, *32*
Lydon, N., *209*
Lyles, J. N., 223, *228,* 239, *263*
Lyman, G. H., 326, *339*
Lyna, P., *304*

Lynch, H., *318*
Lynch, H. T., 309, *319*
Lynch, J., *303, 318*
Lynn, J., *75*
Lyonfields, J. D., 88, *90,* 349, *357*
Lyons, J. S., *232*

M

MacCallum, R., *127*
MacDonald, D. J., *12*
Macdonald, L. A., *72*
MacElwee, N., *359*
MacGillis, D. R., 194, *210*
Mackall, C. L., *209*
Mackie, A., 20, *31*
MacLennan, I. C. M., 176, *190*
MacLeod, C., 151, *173*
Madden, K. S., 313, *319*
Maddi, S. R., 19, *33*
Maddox, W. A., 327, *340*
Magarian-Blander, J., *190*
Magnusson, I., *190*
Magovern, G. J., *35*
Maguire, G. P., *75,* 78, *92, 94,* 158, 161, *171,* 222, 228
Maguire, P., 38, *55,* 158, 161, *168, 169,* 236, 265
Maguire, T., *358*
Mahler, H. I., 391, *398*
Mahler, H. I. M., 283, *285*
Mahon, S. M., 164, *168*
Maiman, L. A., 384–385, *396*
Main, D., *318*
Major, B., 102, 107, *115*
Malarkey, W., *317, 319*
Malarkey, W. B., 312, *316, 318*
Malec, I. F., 78, *97*
Malkoff, S., 310, *318*
Malloy, P., 85, *94*
Maloney, D. G., 207, *210*
Malt, U. F., 159, *173*
Maluish, A., 331, *337*
Mamakos, J., *320*
Mandel, F., *90, 95, 113, 167*
Mandelboim, O., *190*
Mangan, C. E., 86, 88, *95,* 349, 350, *360, 361*
Manis, M., 281, *286*
Manne, S., 83, 86, 87, 88, *91, 94,* 105, 106
Manne, S. L., 99, *115, 396*
Manning, C., 136, *139*
Manson, L. A., 204, *210*
Mansson-Brahme, E., *263*
Mantell, J., 224, *228*
Mantell, J. M., 365, *373*

Mantovani, A., 195, 204, *210*
Mantovani, G., *190*
Manuck, S. B., 331, *337*
Manuel, G., 158, 161, *171*
Mao, J. T., *210*
March, J. S., 85, *94*
March, V., 350, *357*
Marcus, A. C., 224, *230,* 287, *301*
Margolese, R., *229*
Mark, M. M., 121, *129,* 144, *172,* 271, *285*
Marks, R., 330, *336, 339*
Marlatt, G. A., 377, *399*
Marlenga, B., 327, *337*
Marshall, J. R., 322, 323, *335*
Martin, G., *359*
Martin, L., 235, *263*
Martin, R. L., *262*
Mascovic, A. *264*
Maser, J., *171*
Mashberg, D., 80
Mashberg, D. E., 80, *94, 95*
Masny, A., 84, 88, *94, 96,* 289, *303, 304,* 347, 348, 350, *359, 361*
Masny, M., *303*
Mason, A., *264, 265*
Mason, J., 146, 147, 153, *171*
Mason, J. H., 370, *374*
Massie, M. H., *285*
Matchar, D. B., *75*
Mathews, A., 151, *173*
Matsuda, M., *190*
Matthews, K. A., *35,* 147, 148, 164, *169,* 316
Matzinger, P., 202, *210*
Matzky, S., *211*
Maunsell, E., 38, *55,* 224, *231*
Maxwell, R. M., 226, *229*
Mayberry, S. D., 314, *320*
Mayman, M., 281, *286*
McAdams, M., *304*
McArdle, C. S., 39, *54*
McArdle, S., 147, *169*
McBride, C., 290, *302*
McCabe, M., *74*
McCallion, P., 240, *262*
McCann, I. L., 100, *115*
McCarthy, W. H., 314, *317*
McCarthy, W. J., *336*
McCartney-Francis, N. L., *209*
McCaul, K. D., 309, *319*
McClelland, D. C., 220, 220
McClure, J. B., *339*
McCorkle, R., *35,* 164, *171*
McCormack, G., 350, *358*
McCoy, J. L., 331, *336*

McDaniel, S. H., 364, *374*
McDermott, M. M., 6, *12,* 347, *358*
McEwen, B. S., *128*
McEwen, J., *73*
McFarlane, A. C., 80–81, 83, 89, *95,* 97, 148, 155, 159, *171, 172, 173*
McFeeley, S., 6, *12, 230*
McGinnis, M. C., 200
McGlynn, E., *209*
McGrady, A., 311, *319*
McGrath, J. E., 137, *140*
McGrath, P., *128, 168*
McGrath, P. C., 81, *90, 91, 113*
McHale, M., *72, 396*
McHorney, C. A., 59, 60, 61, 65, 66, *74, 75*
McIntosh, D. N., 19n, *33,* 86, *95*
McIntosh, J., 350, *360*
McKelvey, L., *316*
McKenna, S. P., *73*
McKenzie, I. F. C., *190*
McKinnon, W., 310, *319*
McLanahan, S. M., *265*
McLaren, A., *336*
McLaughlin, G., *209*
McMahon, T., *266*
McMurray, A., *75*
M .ʌair, D., 239, *265,* 293, *303*
McNair, D. M., *74*
McNair, P. M., 38, *55,* 59
Meadows, A. T., *93*
Mechanic, D., *359*
Mecklenberg, R., *335*
Meeske, K., *93*
Meichenbaum, D., 8, *12,* 88, *95,* 349, 354, 356, *360*
Meissner, H., *210*
Melamed, B., 367, 368, *374*
Melief, C. J., *210*
Melisartos, N., 221, *228,* 370, *373*
Mellstedt, H., *190,* 207, *209*
Meny, G. M., *209*
Merajver, S. D., *302*
Mermelstein, H. T., 216, *231*
Mermelstein, R. J., 327, *337*
Mesquita, B., 86, *96*
Messick, G., *265, 318*
Meyer, D., 376, 385, 390, 393, *398, 399*
Meyer, T. J., 121, *129,* 144, *172,* 271, *285*
Meyerowitz, B. E., 22, 26, *33,* 39, *55,* 122, *129,* 156, 161, 166, *172,* 236, *265,* 329, 332, *333, 337,* 376, *399*
Meyers, B., *90, 95, 113, 167*
Meyskens, E., *333*
Meyskens, F. L., 326, *338*

Mezzetti, M., 308, *319*
Micciolio, R., *334*
Michell, M., *334*
Michelson, H. *263*
Mihm, M. C., Jr., *340*
Miles, H. J., 315, *318*
Millar, K., 309, *319*
Millar, M. G., 309, *319*
Miller, A. H., *128*
Miller, D., *316, 320,* 343, *358*
Miller, D. G., 6, *12,* 143, *170, 173,* 288, 295, *303,* 304, 308, *318, 320*
Miller, D. M., 327, *340*
Miller, D. R., 329, *337*
Miller, D. S., *91*
Miller, G. E., *316*
Miller, G. R., *113*
Miller, L. Y., 309, *319*
Miller, S., 289, 293, *303,* 304, 337, *359*
Miller, S. M., 26, *33,* 84, 86, 88, *95, 96, 171,* 301, *303,* 343, 344, 345, 346, 347, 348, 349, 350, 351, 352, 353, *359, 360, 361,* 377, *399*
Miller, T., 156, *167*
Milligan, M., 223, *233*
Millner, L., *337*
Mills, M., 343, *361*
Mills, P. J., *316*
Mingari, M. C., *210*
Mings, D., 20, *31*
Mink, P. J., 324, *338*
Minuchin, S., 364, *374*
Mischel, W., 343, 345, 351, 352, *360, 361*
Mita, S., 200, *210*
Mizel, D. E., *209*
Mizoguchi, H., *190, 191*
Mo, F., *71*
Modan, B., 322, *338*
Modlin, R., *210*
Moe, R., *209*
Moffat, F. L. Jr., *31, 90, 168,* 357
Moinpour, C. M., 61, *74*
Moller, P., *211*
Momberg, F., *210*
Monahan, D., 21, *33*
Montada, L., *92*
Montecillo, E., *210*
Montella, M., *338*
Moore, K. A., *73*
Moore, P. J., 21, *34*
Moorey, S., *264, 265*
Moos, R. H., 221, *231*
Moran, P. J., 349, *358*
Morasco, B. J., *91*

Moreland, R. L., 131, 133, *139, 140*
Moretta, A., 194, *210*
Moretta, L., *210*
Morgan, M. G., *230*
Morganstern, M., 322, *334*
Morgenstern, H., 225, *231*
Morrell, C., 223, *231*
Morrill, A., *337*
Morris, T., 27, *32, 34,* 38, *55,* 78, *95,* 221, 224, *229, 231,* 236, *265,* 331, *335, 338*
Morrow, G., *168*
Morrow, G. R., 223, 224, 228, *230, 231*
Morton, D., *32, 128,* 228, *229, 263, 264, 284*
Morton, D. L., *32, 229, 264, 284, 335*
Morvay, T., 224, *228*
Mosbach, P., 377, *399*
Moskowitz, J. T., 19, 27, *33*
Moskowitz, M., *340*
Mowchun, N., *228*
Moyer, A, 39, 53, *55*
Mueller, P. M., *115*
Muenz, L., *54*
Muirhead, J., 22, *33*
Mulder, C. L., 223, *231, 340*
Muldoon, M. F., 331, *337*
Mullan, P., 327, *339*
Mullen, B., 26, *34*
Mullen, P. D., *335*
Mullis, R. M., *338*
Mulvihill, J. J., *302*
Mumford, E., 220, *231*
Mumma, G. H., 80, *94*
Munster, A., 156, *172*
Muraoka, M. Y., 119, *128*
Murdoch, P., 133, *140*
Muris, P., 88, *95,* 348, 349, 352, 353, *361*
Murowski, B., *54, 55*
Murphy, A. E., *209*
Murphy, D. A., *230*
Murphy, G. P., *12,* 335, *336, 340*
Murphy, S. L., 4, *12*
Murray, T., 119, *128*
Musngi, G., 83, *95,* 156, *172*
Muss, H. B., *128*
Mussen, R., *128*
Myers, D. G., 133, *140*
Myers, R. E., 329, *338*

N

Nadaf, S., *209*
Nader, K., 79, *96*
Nagacomi, H., 187, *190*
Nagar, D., 131, *140, 141*
Nakashima, Y., 200, *210*

Naliboff, B. D., *316*
Namir, S., 241, 244, 247, *264, 265*
Narod, S., 309, *318, 319*
Narod, S. A., *302*
National Institute of Mental Health Multisite HIV Prevention Trial Group, 393, *399*
Nayfield, S. G., *74*
Neale, A. V., 365, *374*
Nease, R. F., Jr., 6, *11*
Negri, E., 325, *338*
Neijt, J. P., 61, *73*
Nelson, C. B., 83, *93*
Nemeth, C., *12*
Nemeth, C. J., 134, *140*
Nerenz, D., 161, *170,* 376, *398*
Nerenz, D. R., 377, 379, *399*
Nett, L. M., *335*
Nettesheim, K. M., 224, *233*
Neubauer, T. E., 328, *337*
Neufeld, R. W., 353, 354, *360*
Neuhausen, S., *320*
Newberry, B., *266*
Newcomb, P. A., 323, *339*
Ney, T., *398*
Nicholson, R. A., 152, *169*
Nietzsche, F., 15, *34*
Nijhawan, M., 350, *358*
Nijman, H. W., *210*
Niles, B. L., 83, *93*
Nilsson, B., 325, *336, 338*
Nishimoto, R., 224, *228*
Nishimoto, R. H., 365, *373*
Nixon, D. W., 321, *333*
Nolte, S., *303,* 337, *359*
Nord, E., 61, *74*
Nordevang, E., 325, *336, 338*
Nordic Myeloma Study Group, *75*
Noriega, V., *31, 90, 168, 357*
Norman, G., 63, *73*
North, W. R., *231*
North, W. R. S., *338*
Northouse, L. L., 79, *95,* 224, *231*
Norton, L., *128, 396*
Novaco, R. W., 242, *265*
Nowlis, D., 243, *263*
Noy, S., 328, *334*
Noyes, R., 366, *373*
Nuber, G., *232*
Nunnerly, H., *334*
Nye, C., 353, *360*

O

O'Brian, C. A., *210*
Ochoa, A. C., *190, 191*

O'Connor, A. P., 20, *34, 158*, 164, *172*
Odegaard, V., 350, *362*
O'Fallon, J., 68, *74*
Offit, K., 287–288, *304*, *320*
Offner, A. K., 136, *140*
Ogawa, M., 200, *210*
Ogmundsdottir, H. M., *320*
Ogrocki, P., *336*
Ohman, A., *318*
Ohuchi, N., 204, *209*
O'Keefe, M., 150, *168*
Olafsdottir, G., *320*
Old, L. J., 195, 200, *210*
Oldbridge, N. B., *396*
O'Leary, A., *361*
O'Leary, S., 343
Olshavsky, R. W., 377, *397*
O'Malley, J. E., 363, *374*
Omne-Ponten, M., 216, *231*
Ong, C. S., *190*
Onstad, L. E., 377, *397*
Opetz, G., 205, *211*
Oppenberg, A. A., 367, *373*
Orley, J., *74*
Ormel, J., 217, *233*
Ornish, D., 235, *265*
Ortaldo, J., 331, *336*
Ortega, A. H., 131, *140*
Ortega, S., *339*
Ortiz-Reyes, R., *210*
Osborn, A. F., 133, 135, *140*
Osborne, M., *173, 316, 320*
Osborne, M. P., 288, 295, *303, 304, 320*
O'Shea, J. J., *190*
Oskin, D., 102, *114*
Osoba, D., 59, 61, *74*
Ostfeld, A. M., 225, *231*
Ostroff, J., 80, 272, *285*
Ostroff, J. S., 80, 82, 84, *91, 94, 95*
Ostroff, R., 146, *171*
Ostrow, D., 393
Osuch, J., *32*
O'Sullivan, C., *317, 319*
O'Sullivan, J., 350, 351, 352, *361*
Owens, J. F., *35*
Oxley, N. L., 136, *140*
Oye, R. K., *75*
Ozer, D., *114*

P

Paddison, P. L., *232*
Paffenbarger, R. S., 324, *338*
Paik, S. M., *209*
Palmer, A. G., 158, 163, *172*

Palva, I., *76*
Palys, T. S., 20, *34*
Panerai, A. E., 189, *190*
Papadopoulos, E., 82, 83, *91, 92, 97*
Pape, S., 88, *94*
Papp, E., *73*
Parent du Chatelet, I., *72*
Park, C. L., 21, *34*
Parker, J. C., *227*
Parker, S. L., 321, 323, 324, 328, *338*
Parkes, C. M., 100, *115*
Parpinel, M., *338*
Pasnau, R. O., 22, *32, 78, 93*, 144, *169*, 223, 224, *228, 230*, 235, *263, 264*, 283, 285, 331, *335*
Patenaude, A. F., 79, *95*
Pater, J., *74*
Patrick, C., 220, *231*
Patrick, D. L., 68, *71*
Patrick-Miller, L., *398*
Patterson, D. R., 156, *172*
Patterson, J. T., 379, 380, 389, *399*
Patterson, S. M., 330, *338*
Patterson, T., *264, 336*
Pattison, P., 83, *91*, 102, *113*, 155, *168*
Patton, K., 368, *374*
Paul, G. L., 120, *129*
Paul, W. E., 176, 177, *190*
Paulen, A., 162, *173*
Paulus, P. B., 131, 133, 134, 136, 137, *138, 139, 140, 141*
Pazmany, L., *190*
Pbert, L., 156, *169*
Peace, D. J., 196, *209*
Peacock, E. J., 20, *34*
Pearl, D., 181, *190*, 225, *230, 319*
Pearlman, L. A., 100, *115*
Pearson, J., *190*
Pecher, G., *190*
Pee, D., 38, *54*
Pelcovitz, D., 79, 81, 84, *90, 95, 113, 167*
Penati, B., *93*
Pende, D., *210*
Penman, D., 38, 52, *54, 55*, 228
Penn, G., *336*
Penn, N. E., 353, *358*
Pennanen, M., *301*
Pennebaker, J. W., 61, *74*, 87, *95*, 101, 102, *115, 116*, 136, *141*
Pequignot, E., 314, *320*
Peretz, T., 148, 164, *172*
Perez-Ayala, M., *211*
Perlmutter, R., 187, *189*
Pernet, A., 349, *362*

Pernet, A. L., *362*
Perrson, U., *71*
Perry, S. P., 83, *95*, 156, 157, *172*
Pervin, L. A., *398*
Peshkin, B. N., *302*
Peters, A. M. G., *211*
Petersen, L., *54, 55, 73*
Peters-Golden, H., 273, *285*
Peterson, A. V., *397*
Peterson, C., 20, 21, *34*
Petersson, M., *190*
Peto, J., 307, *317*
Petrie, K. J., 379, 382, 397, 398, 399
Petrini, B., *316*
Pettingale, K. W., 27, *32, 34*, 163, 166, *172*, 221, *229, 231*, 331, 335, *338*
Petty, R. E., *399*
Pfeffer, M., *91*
Pfeiffer, C., 387, *396*
Philipport, T., 86, *96*
Phillips, P., 158, 161, *168, 169*
Phillips, R. S., *75*
Piasetsky, S., *168, 228*
Pickering, T. G., *320*
Pietersz, G. A., *190*
Pietroni, P. C., 239, *263*
Pillemer, D., 151, *172*
Pirie, P., *338*
Pitman, R., 148, *172*
Pitts, J., 19n, *36*
Pliske, R. M., 136, *139*
Plotkin, D., *229*
Poggi, A., *210*
Poletes, G., 134, *140*
Polinsky, M. L., *54, 55*, 366, *373*
Pollin, I., 364, 365, 367, 371, 372, *374*
Pollin, I. S., *374*
Pontes, J. E., *210*
Pope, L. K., 20, *35*
Portenoy, R., *171*
Ports, T. A., *265*
Posluszny, D. M., 6, *12*
Pot-Mees, C., 79, *95*
Potter, J. D., 326, *338*
Powers, G. C., *191*
Pozo, C., *31, 90, 168, 357*
Pransky, G. S., 21, *32*
Pratt, A., 79, *91*
Prentice, R. L., 326, *338, 340*
Presson, C., 377, *397*
Pretlow, T. P., *210*
Preto, R., 321, *334*
Price, A. A., 22, *35*
Priest, R., 390, *399*

Priest, R. G., 239, *263*
Primomo, J., 224, *231*
Prince, R. H., *285*
Proctor, S., 366, *373*
Prosen, H. A., 366, *373*
Pross, H. F., 194, *210*
Provencio, M., 259, *264*
Pruitt, B. T., 237, *266*
Pruyn, J., 223, *233*
Pukkala, E., *32*
Puri, R. K., *210*
Purl, S., 72, *396*
Pynoos, R. S., 79, *96*
Pyszczynski, T., 29, *34*

Q

Quadrel, M. J., 295, *302*
Questad, K. A., 156, *172*
Quinlan, D. M., 223, *228*
Quint-Benoliel, J., 164, *171*

R

Raatgever, J. W., *72*
Rabin, B. S., 331, *337*
Rabinowich, H., *190*
Rabkin, J., 258, *266*
Rachman, S., 87, *95*, 100, *116*
Raczek, A., *75*
Raczek, A. E., 59, *74*
Ragan, J. D., 102, *115*
Rageb, N. E., 39, *55*
Rakfal, S., 161, *169*
Ramirez, A. J., 219, 221, *230, 231*, 322–323, 323, 331, *338*
Ramsay, J. O., 65, *74*
Ramsey, J. O., *74*
Raphael, B., 225, *231*
Rassaby, J., 328, *338*
Raynor, A., *400*
Reading, A. E., *230*
Rebbeck, T., *316*
Rebbeck, T. R., *302*
Rectanus, E., 147, *169*
Redd, W. H., 78, 79, 82, 83, 84, *91, 94, 96*, 97, 112, *113, 116*, 156, *168, 170*, 377, *396, 399*
Redmond, C., *229*
Redondo, M., *211*
Reed, G. M., 27, *34*
Reed, M. R., *303*
Rees-McGee, S., *333*
Reichman, B. S., *396*
Reidbord, S., 154, *170*

Reinhardt, J., *338*
Reis, T. J., 273, *285*
Reizenstein, P., 322, *338*
Reker, G. T., 20, *34*
Renner, G., 20, *30*
Reno, R., 347, *357*
Repetti, R. L., 26, *34, 308, 320*
Resch, N., *359*
Resnick, H., 146, 148, *172, 173*, 330, *340*
Resnick, H. S., 84, *92*
Resnick, L. B., 132, *140*
Resnicow, K., 326, *338*
Retsky, M. W., 205, *211*
Revenson, T. A., 224, *229*
Revicki, D. A., 65, 66, *74*
Reyburn, H., 176, *190*
Reynier, J., 331, *339*
Reynolds, C. P., 310, *319*
Reynolds, P., 224, *231*
Rhone, A., *319*
Richards, C., 102, *115*
Richards, M. A., 221, *230*
Richardson, J., 122, *129*, 376, *399*
Richardson, J. L., 225, 226, 232, 237, 254, *266*
Richardson, S. L., *338*
Richter, S., *319*
Ricker, D., *265, 318*
Ricketts, P., 82, *96, 97*
Riecken, H. W., 101, *114*
Riesenberg, L. A., 327, *337*
Riessman, F., 219, *232*
Rijpma, S. E., 23, *36*
Rijshouwer, Y., 243, *262*
Riley, P., *334*
Rimer, B., 86, 88, *96*, 101, *116, 171*, 301, *303,*
    304, 359
Rimer, B. K., 291, 292, 293, 294, 297, 298,
    299, *301, 302, 303, 304, 317, 329, 336,*
    337, 339, 377, 399
Rimoldi, D., *209*
Ringborg, U., *263*
Risch, N., 290, *302*
Ritenbaugh, C., *333*
Rivier, W., 259, *265*
Rizzo, E., *230*
Roberts, A., 390, *399*
Roberts, F. D., 323, *339*
Roberts, G., 241, *263*
Roberts, J., 216, *230*
Robertson, B., *75, 266*
Robertson, B. M., *264, 265*
Robinson, D. S., *31, 90, 168, 357*
Robinson, J. K., 329, *339*
Robinson, L., *335*

Robinson, R., 156, *172*
Robitaille, C., *398*
Roca, R., 156, 157, *172*
Rockette, H., *209*
Rodin, J., 225, 232, *339*
Rodoletz, M., 86, 88, *95*, 349, 352, *361*
Rodriguez, J. M., 367
Rodriguez, M., *170, 317, 336*
Rodriguez, R., *35*
Rogentine, G., 258, *266*
Rogers, R. W., 385, *399*
Rogers, W. H., *75*
Rohan, T. E., 324, *335*
Romero, P., *209*
Romisher, S., *265, 318*
Romsaas, E. P., 78, *97*
Rooney, B., *338*
Rosan, J. R., 329, *339*
Rosberger, Z., 243, *263*
Rosen, L., *91, 97*
Rosenberg, J., *210*
Rosenberg, M., 44, 48, *55*
Rosenberg, P. P., 273, *285*
Rosenberg, S. A., 41, *56, 206, 211*
Rosenblatt, J., *266*
Rosenheck, R., 83, *92*
Rosenman, K. D., 327, *339*
Rosenstock, I. M., 385, *399, 400*
Ross, E., 290, *302, 337*
Ross, J., 194, *209*
Ross, R., *55*
Ross, R. D., 52, *54*, 237, *262*
Ross, R. K., 324, *334*
Rosser, R. M., *72*
Rossi, P. H., *71*
Roth, J. A., 206, *211*
Roth, S., 158, 161, *171*
Rothbaum, B. O., 83, *92*, 150, 155, 159, *169,*
    172
Rothman, A. J., 329, 332, *339*
Roussi, P., 348, 349, *361*
Routhieaux, R. L., 135–136, *139*
Rovira, D. K., 196, *209*
Rowden, L., *264, 265*
Rowland, J., 78, *92*, 217, *230*
Rowland, J. H., *94, 99, 116*, 156, *169, 170*
Rowley, P. T., *302*
Roy, C., *336*
Royle, G. T., 78, *93*
Rubens, R. D., *231, 338*
Rubin, S., *75*
Ruco, L., 195, *210*
Ruehlman, L. S., 20, *34*
Ruiz-Cabello, F., 202, *210*

Rusalem, R., 78, *92*, 156, *170*
Rush, A. J., 242, *262*
Rutter, D., 347, *357*
Ryan, J. C., 194, *211*
Ryff, C. D., 18, 20, *34, 35*

S

Sacerdote, P., 189, *190*
Sadock, B. J., *285*
Salonen, J. T., *32*
Salovey, P., 329, *339*
Samet, J. M., 219, *229*
Sandfort, T. G., *231*
Sandler, R., 347, *357*
Sands, C., *171*, 293, 294, *302, 303, 304, 318, 337, 347, 349, 350, 359*
Sands, S., *359*
Sanson-Fisher, R. W., 328, *335*
Sanson-Fisher, S., 328, *335*
Santor, D. A., 65, *74*
Sarafian, B., *72*, 242, *263, 396*
Sarason, B. R., 365, *374, 397*
Sarason, I. G., 365, *374*, 377
Sarell, M., 79, *90*
Sarna, L., 40, *55*
Sartorius, N., 61, *75*
SAS Institute Inc., 250, *266*
Sata, P., *230*
Satariano, W. A., 39, 53, *55,* 79, *97*
Savage, E., *230*
Savage, H. E., *211*
Sawyer, K., 136, *139*
Scarborough, R., *359*
Schachter, S., 101, *114*
Schaefer, J. A., 221, *231*
Schag, C., 366, *373*
Schag, C. A. C., 38, 39, *54, 55,* 61, *73, 75*
Schain, W., 45, *55*
Schain, W. S., 78, *93*
Schairer, C., *302*
Schantz, S. P., *211*
Schapira, D. V., 326, *339*
Schatzkin, A., 307, *319*
Schaumberger, M., *358*
Schedlowski, M., 312, 313, *319*
Scheier, M. F., 16, 17, 18, 19, 20, 21, 22, 25, 27, *31, 34, 35,* 88, *90, 96, 168,* 344, 347, *357, 361,* 377, *383, 385, 396, 400*
Scherg, H., 323, *339*
Scherwitz, L. W., *265*
Schilter, L., 80, *91*
Schipper, H., 57–58, 61, *75*
Schlesinger, H. J., 220, *231*
Schlien, B., 331, *337*

Schlom, J., 204, *209*
Schluchter, M. D., 68, *75*
Schluesener, H. J., 196, *210*
Schmale, A., *168*
Schmale, A. M., *228*
Schmidt, D. H., *396*
Schmidt, R. E., *319*
Schmitz, J. B., *168,* 330, *334*
Schmoll, H. J., 312, *319*
Schmutte, P. S., 20, *34*
Schneider, P., 209
Schneider, S. G., *35*
Schneider, S. K., 135–136, *139*
Schneiderman, N., 8, *12, 170,* 317, 322, *336, 339*
Schneidler, J., *97*
Schreiber, H., *190*
Schreier, M., *209*
Schrimshaw, E. W., *97*
Schroeder, C. M., 86, 88, *95, 303,* 349, *361*
Schroeder, D. M., 309, *319*
Schroter, M., *209*
Schulman, K., *318*
Schulz, R., 22, 26, *32, 35,* 112, *114,* 269, 278, *285*
Schut, H. A. W., 283, *285*
Schwartz, G., *33*
Schwartz, J. L., 322, 324, *339*
Schwartz, L. S., 83, *92*
Schwartz, M., 288, 293, *303,* 309, *318,* 347, 352, *361*
Schwartz, M. D., 84, 86, *96,* 289, 294, 295, 296, 297, 298, *302, 304,* 309, *319, 320, 359*
Schwartz, P. E., 223, *228*
Schwartzentruber, D. J., *211*
Sciacchitano, A. M., *115*
Seaman, W. E., 194, *211*
Seay, J., 301, *303,* 329, *336, 359*
Seder, R. A., 176, 177, *190*
Sedlacek, T. V., 86, 88, *95,* 349, *360, 361*
Seeman, T., 308, *320*
Segerstrom, S. C., 310, *319*
Seigal, J., *304*
Seipp, C. A., *211*
Selesznick, M., 220, *230*
Seligman, M. E. P., 20, 21, *34, 35, 116,* 367, *374*
Sellers, T. A., 324, *338*
Sellick, S. M., 323, 329, 330, *339*
Sendo, F., 193, *209*
Septimus, A., *90, 113*
Sgoutas-Emch, S. A., 313, *319*
Shafer, D., 353, *360*

Shah, J., 16, *35*
Shalev, A. Y., 83, *96,* 148, 154, 155, *172, 173*
Shani, A., *320*
Shapiro, D. E., 363, *374*
Shapiro, T. E., 367, *374*
Sharma, S., *210*
Shattuck, A. L., *340*
Shaw, B. F., 242, *262*
Shedler, J., 281, *286*
Sheehan, E., *333*
Sheley, J., 346, *361*
Shelton, D. R., 225, 232, 237, *266*
Shephard, R. J., 324, *339*
Sheppard, L., *338*
Sheppard, S., *265, 318*
Shepperd, J. A., 135, *141*
Sherbourne, C. D., *74,* 275, *286*
Sherman, S. J., 377, *397*
Sherwood, J. J., 137, *139*
Sheu, E. G., *190*
Shibata, H., *229*
Shiffman, S., *335*
Shifren, K., 21, *33, 35*
Shiomoto, G., *71*
Shivers, N., *227*
Shoda, Y., 88, *95,* 343, 344, 345, 346, 351, 354, *361*
Shoptaw, S. J., 277, *286*
Shover, L. R., 38, *55*
Showers, C. J., 18, *35*
Shrapnell, K., 26, *36, 78, 97*
Shuttleworth, E. C., *336*
Sieber, W. J., 331, *339*
Siegel, B. S., 225–226, 226, *229, 231*
Siegel, J., 148, *173*
Siegler, M., *75*
Siejak, K. K., *303*
Silberman, M., *72, 396*
Silver, R. C., 19n, *33, 35,* 86, *94, 95, 97,* 101, 102, 107, *115, 116*
Silver, R. L., 101, 102
Silver, R. T., *93, 171*
Silverfarb, P. M., 78, *96*
Silverman, C., 377, 393, *400*
Sim, M. S., *54*
Simmonds, M. A., 290, *302*
Simms, S. L., *360*
Singer, J., 63, *73*
Singer, J. E., 323, 330, 333, *335*
Singer, P., 63, *75*
Singh, A., 313, *316*
Sipprelle, R. C., 84, *92*
Sjoden, P. O., 216, *231,* 242, *262, 263*
Skaar, K. L., 324, *339*

Skelton, J. A., *359, 379, 383, 398, 400*
Skinner, C. S., 301, *304*
Sklar, L., 258, *266*
Skokan, L. A., 15, *31*
Slattery, M. L., 287, *304*
Slavin, J., *338*
Sloan, D., *128, 168*
Sloan, D. A., 81, *90, 91, 113*
Sloan, J. A., 350, *358*
Smedley, B. D., *11*
Smith, B. L., 6, *12*
Smith, C. A., 20, *35*
Smith, D., *359*
Smith, D. C., 39, *54*
Smith, D. W., 83, *92*
Smith, E., *227*
Smith, K., 79, *96,* 272, *285*
Smith, M., *91, 92*
Smith, M. Y., 82, 83, 84, *91, 96*
Smith, R. D., 85, *91*
Smith, S., *33*
Smith, T. L., 310, *318,* 330, *336*
Smith, T. W., 352, *358*
Smucker, W. D., *73*
Smyth, M., *334*
Snaith, R. P., 241, *267*
Snider, P. R., 21, *35,* 78, *96,* 158, 161, 166, *172,* 242, *263*
Snowden, L. R., 39, 52, *54*
Snyder, C., *318*
Snyder, C. R., 20, *31, 35*
Snyder, E. L., *92*
Snyder, M. P., *338*
Snyder, S., *232*
Snyder, S. L., 239, *263*
Sobel, H. J., 246, *266*
Solares, M. E., *336*
Soloman, G., 258, *266*
Solomon, G. F., 310, *316, 319*
Solomon, L., 346, *361*
Solomon, S., 313, *316*
Solomon, Z., 89, *96*
Somerfield, M. R., 21, *31*
Sondik, E. J., 322, 323, 325, *335*
Sonnega, A., 83, *93*
Soreide, J. A., 159, *173*
Sorenson, S., 59, *70*
Sorosky, J. I., 106, *115*
Souba, W. W., *12*
Soukup, J. R., 69, *75*
Southwick, S. M., *97*
Sozzani, S., 195, *210*
Spangers, M. A. G., 38, *53*
Sparks, F. C., 39, *55*

Speicher, C. E., 5, *12*, 265, 310, *318, 336*
Speith, L. E., *358*
Speizer, F. E., *340*
Spence, R., *172*
Spencer, P., 308, *317*
Spencer, R. L., *128*, 156
Spencer, S. M., 22, 26, 30, *35*
Sperner-Unterweger, B., *71*
Spertus, I. L., *169*
Spiegel, D., 24, 25, 28, *35, 83, 93*, 119, 121, 123, *129*, 144, 148, *170, 172, 181, 190, 191*, 217, 219, 220, 221, 222, 223, 225, 228, *230, 232*, 235, 241, 243, *262, 266*, 270, 271, 273, 278, 281, 282, 286, 323, 331, *339, 365, 374, 377, 382, 400*
Spiegelhaler, D. J., *72*
Spielberger, C. D., 242, *266*
Spieth, L. E., 353
Spiker, A. V., 119, *129*
Spilker, B., 61, *72, 75*
Splett, P., *338*
Spratt, J. S., *233*
Sprent, J., 176, *191*
Springer, T. A., 176, *191*
Sredni, B., 313, 314, *320*
Srivastava, P. K., 198, *211*
Stacy, A. W., *400*
Stadil, F. 350, *358*
Stallman, D., 350, *358*
Stampfer, M. J., *340*
Stanley, J., *190*
Stanton, A. L., 21, *31, 35*, 78, *96*, 158, 161, 166, *172*
Stasser, G., 136, *141*
Steakley, C., *169*
Steenbakkers, M., 326, *340*
Steer, R. A., 242, *262*
Steeves, R., 15, *33*
Stefanek, M., 143, *171*, 297, 298, *301, 304*, 308, *317, 318*, 329, 337, 348, 349, *359*
Stefanek, M. E., 309, *320*, 343, 347, *361*
Steffens, R., *301*
Stein, J. A., 331, *333*
Steinberg, A., 348, *361*
Steinberg, M. D., 78, *96*
Steinberg, S. M., *211*
Steinitz, M., 207, *209*
Steinmayer, K., *97*
Steketee, G., 83, *92, 169*
Stellato, T., *210*
Stephens, R. E., 5, *12*
Steptoe, A., 350, 351, 352, *360, 361*
Stern, N. M., *169*
Sternberg, R. J., *139*

Sterns, E., 194, *210*
Stevens, M. J., 135, *141*
Stevenson, L. Y., *230*
Stewart, A. J., *114*
Stewart, A. L., 40, *55*, 57–58, 58, *73, 75*, 109, 116
Stewart, D. D., 136, *141*
Stewart, G. L., 132, *138*
Stewart, I., *72, 396*
Stewart, S. L., 37, 38, 43, *54, 55*
Stewart, T., 205, *211*
Stewart, T. H., 205, *211*
Stiles, W. B., 102, *116*
Stitzer, M. L., *335*
Stocker-Kreichgauer, G., *140*
Stocking, C., *75*
Stockton, P., *169*
Stoddard, E., 353, *360*
Stommel, M., *32*
Stone, A., 310, *316*
Stones, M. H., 19n, *35*, 101, *116*
Stopfer, J., *316*
Stopfer, J. E., *302*
Storer, B. E., 323, *339*
Stout, J., 265, *318*
Strachey, J., *92, 169*
Strain, E., *265*
Strain, J. J., 220, *232*
Strassmann, G., *320*
Stratmann, G., *319*
Strauch, G., *72*
Strauss, E., *232*
Strauss, L., 346, *361*
Strayer, D. R., 314, *320*
Strecher, V. J., *301, 304*
Streuning, E., 258, *266*
Strigo, T. S., 299, *304*
Strobl, S. L., *191*
Stroebe, M. S., 283, *285*
Stroebe, W., 135, 136, *139, 140*
Strominger, J. L., *190*
Strouse, T. B., *91*
Strudler-Wallston, B., 238, *266*
Struewing, J. P., 287, *304*
Stuart-Harris, R., 236, *265*
Stuber, M. L., 79, 81, 82, *93, 96*
Studts, J., *128*, 156, *167*
Sugarbaker, P. H., *56*
Sullivan, K. M., 80, *91, 97*
Sullivan, M., 59, *70*
Sullivan-Halley, J., 324, *334*
Suls, J., 26, *34, 35*, 365, *374*
Suls, J. M., 132, *141*
Summerton, J., 350, 351, *360*

Surbone, A., *396*
Sussman, S., 377, *400*
Sutcliffe, I., 350, *361*
Sutherland, D. J., 195, *208*
Sutherland, H. J., *71*, 350, *361*
Sutker, P. B., 85, *96*
Sutton-Smith, K., 350, *357*
Svane, G., 325, *338*
Swain, M. A., 224, *231*
Swain, S. L., 177, *189*
Swanson, G. M., 39, *55,* 327, *339*
Swanson, M., 324, *340*
Syme, S. L., *11,* 227
Syrjala, K. L., 80, *91, 97*

T

Taidi, B., *210*
Tait, B., *190*
Tait, R., 86, *97,* 101, 102, *116*
Takaki, S., *189*
Takatsu, K., 200, *210*
Talamini, R., *319, 338*
Tambor, E. S., 299, *304*
Tanabe, P., *230*
Tanjasiri, S. P., 329, *340*
Tanner, M. A., 78, *97*
Taplin, S. H., 290, *302*
Tarr, K., *265*
Tasch, E., *75*
Taupin, J.-L., *190*
Taylor, A., *168,* 259, *262*
Taylor, A. N., 331, *333*
Taylor, D. M., 18, *31*
Taylor, I., 78, *93*
Taylor, K., 87, 88, *94*
Taylor, K. L., 79, *96,* 99, *115,* 289, *304, 396*
Taylor, S., 219, 330, *335*
Taylor, S. E., 15, 20, 21, 25, 27, *30, 31, 34, 35,* 78, *97, 124, 128,* 134, *141,* 152, 153, 161, 164, *173,* 232, 236, *263,* 272, 273, 277, *284, 286,* 308, *320,* 366, *374,* 377, 391, *400*
Taylor, S., IV, *72, 396*
Tedeschi, R. G., 27, *36*
Telch, C. F., 121, *129,* 223, 232
Telch, M. J., 121, *129,* 223, 232
Tellegen, A., 103, *116,* 275, *286*
Temoshok, L., *266*
Temoshok, L. R., 193, *209,* 221, 232, 258
Tempelaar, R., 99, *113*
Tenaglia, A. N., *91*
Tennen, H., 21, *32, 33,* 387, 391, *396, 400*
ter Horst, G., 349, *361*
Teschann, J. M., 367, *373*

Testa, M., *115*
Tewes, U., 312, *319*
Thaler, H., *171*
Theobald, T., 330, 331, *336, 339*
Thoits, P., 87, *97*
Thomas, C. R., Jr., *72, 396*
Thomas, L., 381, *400*
Thompson, L., 133, *140,* 381, 393
Thompson, S. C., 19n, *36*
Thompson, W. D., 290, *302*
Thompson, W. O., *334*
Thorlacius, S., 307, *320*
Threatt, B. A., 79, *97,* 216, 233
Thune, I., 324, 325, *340*
Thynne, G., *190*
Tian, H., *209*
Tichler, T., *320*
Till, J. E., 350, *361*
Tilley, B. C., 365, *374*
Timko, C., 224, 233
Timmerman, M. M., *304*
Tjemsland, L., 159, *173*
Tjosvold, D., 134, *141*
Tocco, E. K., 241, *263*
Tommasello, A. L., *335*
Tong, T., 321, *338*
Tonin, P., *318*
Topalian, S. L., *211*
Tormey, D., 162, *173*
Torrance, G., 63, 69, *75*
Torrance, G. W., 69, *75*
Torrey, W., 152, *171*
Toseland, R., 240, *262*
Tosteson, A. N., 6, *11*
Trakowski, J. H., *168*
Trask, O. J., 310, *318*
Trauth, B. C., 197, *211*
Traversari, C., *209*
Trentham-Dietz, A., 323, *339*
Trijsburg, R. S., 22–23, *36,* 119, *129*
Trinchieri, G., 314, *319*
Triozzi, P. L., 206, *211*
Tripodi, D. A, 328, *335*
Tritchler, D. L., *71,* 350, 361
Trock, B., *318,* 329, 337, 349, *359*
Tross, S., 59, *72,* 79, *91, 93,* 100, *113,* 159, 160, 163, *168, 170*
Truax, P., 63, *73*
Tryggvadottir, L., *320*
Tsai, S. C., 205, *211*
Tschopp, J., 209
Tsevat, J., 69, *75*
Tsoh, J. Y., *339*
Tubbs, R. R., *190*

Tucker, M. A., *304*
Tucker, S., 158, *171*
Tugwell, P., 72
Tulsky, D. S., 41, 51, *54, 71*, 72, *396*
Tuma, A., *171*
Tunder, J., 329, *340*
Tunmore, R., *265*
Tuomilehto, J., *32*
Turk, D. C., 8, *12*
Turner, C. W., 352, *358*
Turner, G. E., *400*
Turner, M., *140*
Turner, R. A., 21, *34*
Turner, R. J., 225, *233*
Turns, D. M., 223, *233*
Turvey, C., 329, *339*
Tylee, A., 390, *399*

U

Uchino, B. N., *319*
Uddo-Crane, M., 85, *96*
Udin, H., 225, *228*
Udono, H., 198, *211*
Uleman, J. S., *97, 116*
Ullman, S., 148, *173*
Umberson, D., 219, *230*
Urba, W. J., *191*
Urban, N., *340*
Urist, M. M., 327, *340*
Ursano, R. J., 155, 159, *168, 173*
Uyemura, K., *210*
Uziely, B., 238, *262*

V

Vaillant, G., 152, *171*
Valacich, J. S., 137, *139*
Valdimarsdottir, H. B., 143, *173*, 288–289,
      289, *304*, 308, 309, 311, 314, 315, *316*,
      317, 320
Vale, W., 259, *265*
Vales-Gomez, M., *190*
van Assema, P., 326, *340*
Vance, K., 155, *173*
Vancouver, J., 383, 388, *396, 400*
van den Borne, B., 223, *233*
VandenBos, G. R., 167, 220, *228*
van den Bout, J., 283, *285*
Van Den Eynde, B., *209*
van der Berg, S. H., *210*
Van Der Bruggen, P., *209*
van der Burg, M. E. L., 72
van der Hart, O., 100, *116*
van der Kolk, B. A., 100, *116*, 151, 152, 153,
      173

van der Pompe, G., *316*, 323, *340*
VanderZee, K., 377, 391, *400*
van de Velde, C. J., *210*
van de Vijver, F. A., *231*
van Houwelingen, H. C., 311, *320*
Van Kammen, D., *266*
van Knippenberg, F. C. E., 22–23, *36*, 61, *73*
Van Pel, A., *209*
Van Rood, V. R., 311, *320*
Van Yperen, N. W., 25, *31*, 273, *284*
Van Zee, K., *320*
van Zuuren, F., *95*, 348, 349, *361*
van Zuuren, F. J., 88, *95*
Varghese, A., 272, *285*
Vaughan, H., *190*
Vena, J. E., 324, *340*
Venot, A., 72
Ventafridda, V., *96*
Verma, S., 205, *211*
Vernon, S. W., 365, *374*
Veronesi, U., 306, *317*
Verrier, P., *285*
Veugeiers, P. J., *231*
Vickburg, S., 80, 89, *91, 96*
Vickburg, S. M. J., 82, 83, 84, *91, 92, 96, 97*
Viergutz, G., 162, *173*
Vijayasaradhi, S., 195, *211*
Villego, L., *335*
Vinciguerra, V., *95*
Vinokur, A. D, 79, *97*, 216, *233*
Vinokur-Kaplan, D., 79, *97*
Visscher, B. R., 27, *34, 210*
Viswanath, K., *338*
Vitale, M., *210*
Vitaliano, P. P., 80, *97*
Vittinghoff, E., 19, *33*
Vize, C., 390, *399*
Vlamis, V., *171*
Vlock, D. R., 195, 204, *211*
Vogel, V. G., 290, 297, 298, *301, 302, 304*
Voigts, A., 350, *358*
Von Korff, M., 217, *233*
Vroom, V. H., 16, *36*

W

Wacholder, S., *304*
Wagner, T. O. F., *319*
Wagstaff, D., 376–377, *398*
Wahl, S. M., *209*
Wainer, H., *70*
Waitzkin, H., 367, *374*
Wake, F. R., 328, *338*
Waldichuk, C., *210*
Waletzky, L. R., *264*

Waligora-Serafin, B., *266*
Walker, S. R., *72*
Wallace, L., *359*
Wallston, K. A., 238, *266*
Walsh, W. P., 350, 351, *359*
Walster, E. H., 366, *373*
Walter, S., 63, *73*
Walter, S. D., 225, *230, 231*
Wan, G. J., 40, *56*
Wandersman, A., 143, 156, *168*
Wang, H., 204, *211*
Wang, H. J., 27, *34*
Wang, J., *210*
Ward, J. M., *209*
Ward, S., 162, *173*
Wardle, F. J., 349, *362*
Ware, J., 344, *358*
Ware, J. E., 40, 41, 44, 47, 48, 49, 50, *54, 55, 56, 57–58, 59*, 60, 61, 74, 75, 109, *116*, 275, *286*
Warr, D., *74*
Warram, J., *337*
Warren, R., 158, *172*
Warrenburg, S., *33*
Wasserman, J., *316*
Watkins, I. K., 39, *55*
Watkins, L. O., 350, 353, *362*
Watson, A., 328, *335*
Watson, A. C. H., *336*
Watson, D., 103, *116*, 275, *286*
Watson, J. P., *231, 338*
Watson, M., 26, *36, 61*, 75, 78, *93, 97*, 223, *233*, 241, *264, 265, 266*, 331, *338*
Watts, F. N., 151, *173*
Wayment, H. A., 86, *94*, 101, *115*
Weaver, L., 350, *362*
Weber, B. L., *302, 316*
Weeks, M. O., 204, *209*
Wegner, D. M., 102, *116*
Wei, W. Z., 204, *211*
Weichselbaum, R., *75*
Weiland, M., *230*
Weinberg, G. B., 6, 12, 290, *302*
Weinblatt, M., *95*
Weiner, H., 310, *318*
Weinerman, B., 226, *230*
Weinman, J., 221, *230*, 397
Weinman, J. A., 379, 382–383, *397, 398, 399*
Weinstein, M. C., 68, *75*
Weinstein, N. D., 153, *173*
Weinstock, M. A., 327, *340*
Weintraub, J. K., 344, *357*, 383, *396*
Weir, D., 180, *191*
Weisberg, J. H., 325, *340*

Weisman, A., 78, *97*
Weisman, A. D., 20, *36, 235*, 236, 245, 246, *266, 267*
Weiss, D., 163, *173*
Weiss, R. B., *93, 128, 171*
Weiss, S. M., *264*
Weisse, C. S., 310, *319*
Weissfeld, J. L., 6, *12*
Wellisch, D. K., 78, 80, *93, 97*, 224, *230*, 241, *264, 283, 285*
Wells, C. L., 324, *337*
West, M. A., 133, *141*
West, S., 347, *357*
Westin, J., *76*
Wetter, D. W., *339*
Wewers, M. E., *335*
Wharton, J. T., *210*
White, D. E., *211*
White, E., 326, *340*
White, P., 38, *55*, 78, *95*, 224, *231, 236, 265*
White, V., *336*
Whitehead, M. I., *362*
Whiteside, T., *339*
Whiteside, T. L., 180, *190*
Whitman, H., 223, *229*
Whittaker, I. A., 79, *93*
WHOQOL (World Health Organization QOL) Group, 61, *76*
Wicker, C. A., 20, *34, 158, 172*
Wicklund, R. A., 18, *36*
Widows, M. R., *170*
Wieand, H. S., *229*
Wiebe, J. S., *316*
Wigzell, H., 207, *209*
Wiklund, I., 61, *75*
Wilckens, T., 189, *191*
Wilcox, P., 309, *320, 343*, 347, *361*
Wilcox, P. M., 224, *233*
Willard, K., *304*
Willems-Groot, J., *71*
Willett, W., 306, *317*
Willett, W. C., *340*
Williams, A. F., 101, *114*
Williams, C. L., 326, *340*
Williams, G. M., 325, *340*
Williams, J., *73*
Williams, J. G., 376, *399*
Williams, J. M. G., 151, *173*
Williamson, G. M., 22, *35*
Williger, D., *265*, 318
Willison, J., *303*
Wills, T., *335*
Wills, T. A., 132, *141*, 273, 281, *284, 286*
Wilner, N., 126, *129, 238, 264*, 293, *302*

Wilson, E. O., 394, 395, *400*
Wilson, J., *303*
Wilson, K. G., *228*
Wilson, S., *97*
Wiltrout, R. H., *190*
Winett, R. A., 328, *337*
Wing, A. L., 324, *338*
Wingard, J. R., 21, *31*
Wingo, P. A., 119, *128*, 321, *338*
Winicour, P., 72, 242, *263*, *396*
Winkel, G., *91*
Winston, T., 102, *113*, 273, *284*
Winter, J. P., 136, *140*
Wise, L., 78, *96*
Wisloff, F., 59, *76*
Wojtkowiak, S. L., 290, *302*
Wolberg, W. H., 78, *97*
Wolchik, S. A., 20, *34*
Wolcott, D. L., 80, *97*, 241, 244, *264*, *265*
Woler, J., *229*
Wolf, C., *264*
Wolf, G. T., *211*
Wolf, T., *337*
Wolfson, C., *285*
Wollman, J., *210*
Wollman, K., *338*
Wolmark, N., *229*
Wolter, J., *229*
Wong, G., *171*
Wong, P. T. P., 20, *34*
Wood, J. V., *97*, *173*, 273, *286*, 366, *374*, 377, 391, *400*
Wood, P. E., 223, *233*
Wood, W. C., *128*
Woodbeck, H., 323, *339*
Woods, M., *337*
Woods, M. N., *340*
Woods, N. F., 79, *97*, 224, *231*, *233*
Woods, X. A., 122, *128*
Woodward, C., 347, *357*
Woolfolk, R. L., *95*, *360*
Worden, J., 78, *97*, 346, *361*
Worden, J. W., 20, *36*, 236, 246, *266*, *267*
World Health Organization, 61, *76*
Worth, R., 20, *36*
Wortman, C. B., 19n, *31*, *33*, 86, 87, *91*, *94*, *95*, 101, *114*, *115*, *116*, 153, *170*, *173*
Wright, B. D., 62, *72*
Wright, J. D., *71*
Wrightsman, L. S., 366, *374*
Wu, Y., 6, *12*
Wyatt, G., 15, *33*, *36*
Wyllie, A. H., *129*
Wynder, E. L., 326, *338*, *340*
Wynings, C., *170*, 317, *336*

Wynne, B. E., 137, *139*
Wyszynski, A. A., 225, *233*

X

Xing, P. X., *190*

Y

Yager, J., 241, *264*
Yalom, I., 24, *35*, 217, 220, 223, *232*, *233*, 273, *286*
Yalom, I. D., 121, *129*, 218, 219, 221, *233*, 241, *266*
Yalom, V., 220, *233*
Yancey, A. K., 329, *340*
Yang, J. C., *211*
Yarnall, K., *304*
Yasko, J., 26, *32*, 112, *114*, 269, 278, *285*
Yasuda, P., 79, *96*
Yates, B. C., 224, *231*
Yehuda, R., 80–81, 82, 83, 84, 89, *97*, 146, 147, 153, *172*, *173*, 330, *340*
Yellen, S. B., 58, 60, 72, *76*, 242, *263*, *396*
Yin, R. K., *203*
Yirmiya, R., 259, 262, 331, *333*
You, S. G., *209*
Younes, E., *210*
Young, J., *266*
Yurek, D., 122, *129*

Z

Zachariae, R., 311, *320*
Zakowski, S. G., 308, *320*, *338*
Zea, A. H., 187, *190*, *191*
Zee, B., *74*
Zeger, S. L., 68, *73*
Zeidner, M., 20, *36*
Zelman, D., *396*
Zeltzer, L., 223, *233*
Zhu, Z., 327, *339*
Zielezny, M., 324, *340*
Zielstra, E. M., 243, *262*
Zigmond, A., 241, *267*
Zilberg, N., 163, *173*
Zimbardo, P., *267*
Zimmering, R. T., 83, *93*, 102, *114*, 149, *170*
Zimmerman, B. L., 216, *233*
Zinbarg, R., 155, *169*
Zinser, M., *396*
Zittoun, R., *71*
Zubeck, J. M., 102, *115*
Zuckerman, E., 79, *93*, *171*
Zumiani, G., *334*
Zupkis, R. V., 350, *357*
Zuroff, D. C., 65, *74*

Subject Index

A

Acceptance, in coping process, 26–27
Accommodation, 100
Adaptive immunity, 176, 177, 195–196
Adherence
  to breast cancer screening guidelines, 289
  to exercise, 392
  to medical treatment, 224–225
  See also Compliance problems
Adverse responses, from interventions, 25–26
Affect
  cancer-relevant, 345, 348–350
  exploration of, 218
Affective state, 247
Affector mechanisms, 193, 197–199
African American women
  and distress from breast cancer, 39
  and genetic counseling intervention, 300, 301
  and intrusiveness of cancer experience, 52
  and mammography adherence, 309
Age
  and cancer risk, 3, 322
  and quality of life, 40
  and sun exposure, 327, 328
Antigen-presenting cells. See APC
Antigens, tumor, 177, 178–179, 181, 185, 206–207
  and B cells, 198
  heterogeneity of expression of, 202
  identification of, 200
  targeting of, 201
  and T-cell responses, 197
  and vaccines, 178
  See also MUC1 protein
Anxiety
  in cancer patients, 216, 349
  about death, 221
  in psychoeducational intervention, 247, 248, 249
Anxiety disorder
  fear networks in, 151
  among women with breast cancer, 217
APC (antigen-presenting cells), 176, 178–179, 197

deficiencies in, 187
"professional," 197, 202
Assessment
  computerized and practical, 64–65
  disease-specific vs. generic, 40, 60
  in MCC (medical crisis counseling), 367–368
  See also Measurement
Assimilation, 100
Assumptive world model, 151, 152–153
Attentional style. See Blunting; Monitoring
Autonomy, for support groups, 135
Avoidance, 86, 87–88, 151–152
  in cognitive processing of traumatic events, 100–101
  as method of coping, 245–246
  status quo maintained by, 365

B

BCRC (breast cancer risk counseling), 289–295, 300
Beck Depression Inventory, IRT approach to, 65
BE (β-endorphin) effect, 189
Behavioral factors, cancer affected by, 10
Behavioral interventions, 331–332
  and diet, 325–326
  and exercise, 324–325
  vs. reductionistic perspective, 380–381, 393
  and screening or surveillance, 328–330
  self-regulation model of, 375, 376 (see also Self-regulation model)
  stress management, 330–331
  and sun exposure, 326–328
  and tobacco use, 324
Behavioral research in cancer, 376–378
  fragmentation of, 377–378
  and psychological theory, 375
  self-regulation model for, 379
Behavioral sciences, synthesis of, 394–395
Behavioral self-regulation
  goal-striving model of, 16–19
  See also Self-regulation model
Behavioral training, 238–240

Behavior change
  as prevention, 322
  as public health development, 11
Behavior Therapy: Appraisal and Status
    (Franks), 120
Beliefs, cancer-relevant, 345, 347–348
Bereavement issues
  and women with cancer in family history,
    308
  See also Grieving
Biobehavioral model for psychological
    interventions, 119–120
  and change mechanisms, 123–124
  and effectiveness of interventions, 120–121,
    124–125
  experiment on (Stress and Immunity Breast
    Cancer Project), 125–127
  and individuals receiving treatment,
    121–122
  and problems to be treated, 122–123
Biological models of trauma, 153
Biological sciences, synthesis of, 394–395
Blunting, 345–346, 377
  and C-SHIP model, 347–352
  and tailoring of psychosocial interventions to
    attentional style, 353–354
BMT (bone marrow transplantation)
  mothers of children undergoing, 89
  and psychosocial problems, 79–81
  PTSD or PTSD symptoms, 80, 82, 84
Breast cancer, 287
  antigen for (MUC1), 180–185
  and exercise, 324
  and health behaviors, 308
  and immunosuppression, 204–205
  and mammography, 6 (see also
      Mammography adherence or utilization)
  psychological impact of, 272–273
  in quantity-of-life studies, 225–226
  risk factors for, 287
  and estrogen, 325
  family history, 287, 305, 306, 306–307
    (see also Risk for cancer)
  and schematic vs. conceptual memories, 346
  Stress and Immunity Breast Cancer Project,
    125–127
  threat appraisal in adjustment to, 216
  in women under age 50, 37
  women at increased risk for
  breast cancer risk counseling (BCRC) for,
    289–295, 300
  distress among, 288–289, 305, 307–308
  and family history, 287, 314
  future directions for interventions with,
    300–301

  genetic counseling interventions for,
    298–300
  perceived risk and adherence among, 288,
    289
  psychoeducational interventions, 295–298
  worry and distress over risk of, 158
  See also Cancer
Breast cancer patients
  anxiety disorders among, 217
  in cognitive-behavioral therapy, 241, 242
  coping strategies of, 217
  depression in, 216
  group-intervention study on, 272–282
  optimism and distress in, 21, 88
  physical difficulties of, 39
  psychosocial issues for, 235–236
  quality of life of
  and distress, 38–39, 216, 349
  study on, 42–53
  Spiegel study on psychotherapeutic group
    for, 270, 282
  traumatic stress reactions among, 158–159,
    162
Breast cancer risk counseling (BCRC),
    289–295, 300
Breast cancer survivors, 37
  aversive side effects for, 78–79
Breast Cancer in Young Women: A Population-
    Based Approach (project), 42

C

Cancer, 4
  behavioral or psychosocial factors in, 10
  contextual aspects of, 124
  early detection of, 322 (see also Screening
    activities)
  as health problem, 3–5, 321
  individuals with family histories of, 314–315
  individual's representation of, 389
  public view of, 379–380
  risk factors for, 322, 323 (see also Risk for
    cancer)
  as stressful, 143–145, 146–149, 156
  and traumatic stress, 145, 155–156, 157
  and disease severity, 162–163
  and end of treatment, 161–162
  and immediate stressors, 160–161
  and PTSD, 156–160, 162, 163–164,
    165–166, 166
  research needed on, 166–167
  and stressors associated with cancer,
    146–149
  and subsequent stressors, 164–165

and traumatic vs. nontraumatic stress,
145–146
See also Breast cancer
Cancer diagnosis
coping with, 217
as disruption of hope, 18
and immunosuppressive environment, 178
as loss of control, 272
and normalcy, 363
psychosocial consequences of, 215–217
as stressful, 144, 147, 216
vs. more immediate stressors, 160
as traumatic stressor, 148, 155, 163–164
sudden vs. gradual, 146
varying reactions to, 15
Cancer patients
adjustment problems of, 99, 146, 166
numbers of, 119
psychosocial problems among, 215–217
and PTSD, 148, 157–160, 162, 163–164,
165–166, 166
See also Breast cancer patients
Cancer prevention, 321–322
difficulty of, 323
evaluation of intervention for, 323
modification of behavioral sources of risk
and diet, 325–326
and exercise, 324–325
and screening or surveillance, 328–330
stress management, 330–331
sun exposure, 326–328
tobacco use, 324
reductionism as barrier to, 380–381
scope of, 322–323
CAncer Rehabilitation Evaluation System
(CARES), 38, 59
Cancer-relevant affects and emotions, 345,
348–350
Cancer-relevant encodings and self-construals,
345, 346–347
Cancer-relevant expectancies and beliefs, 345,
347–348
Cancer-relevant self-regulatory and coping
strategies, 345, 351–352
Cancer-relevant values and goals, 345,
350–351
Cancer survivors
adjustment problems of, 77
and PTSD symptoms, 79, 80–83, 89 (see
also PTSD)
stress and trauma history, 164
number of, 235
and pessimism, 22
types of, 119–120

Cancer treatment
concerns arising from, 7
defining attributes of, 388–389
distress or stress associated with, 78–80,
155, 160–161
and immune system, 175 (see also Immune
system)
patients' adherence to, 224–225 (see also
Adherence)
CAP (cognitive-affective preparation)
procedure, 354–356
Caregivers, optimism of, 22
CARES (CAncer Rehabilitation Evaluation
System), 38, 59
Cellular biology, cross-fertilization in, 378
Cellular response, 200, 201
Clinical practice, and science, 376
Clinical significance, and QOL measurement,
63
Cognitive-affective preparation (CAP)
procedure, 354–356
Cognitive-behavioral interventions, 305,
315–316
and immune system, 311
Cognitive-behavioral therapy, group, 241–242
Cognitive coping methods, active, 245
Cognitive-processing model, 99–101
and predispositional factors, 88–89
social modulation in, 101–102
of trauma reactions, 85–88, 89
Cognitive-social health information-processing
(C-SHIP) model, 344–346
cancer-relevant affects and emotions, 345,
348–350
cancer-relevant encodings and self-
construals, 345, 346–347
cancer-relevant expectancies and beliefs,
345, 347–348
cancer-relevant self-regulatory and coping
strategies, 345, 351–352
cancer-relevant values and goals, 345,
350–351
Commonsense model of illness, 385
Commonsense view of self-regulation process,
390, 392
Communication
framing of, 329, 332, 353–354
and MCC (medical crisis counseling), 365
with physicians, 222
and self-regulation model, 391–394
tailored print messages, 300–301
Communications theory, fear arousing, 309
Community implementation, as research issue,
284

Community intervention trials, for diet change, 326
Comparisons, social. See Social comparison
Completion hypothesis, 112
Completion tendency, 100
Compliance problems, 123
  and stress, 330
  See also Adherence
Computer based interaction, 137
Computerized adaptive testing (CAT), 65
Conceptual memories, 346
Conditioned responses, in Hodgkin's disease survivors, 79
Conditioning model, for PTSD, 83–85, 151
Control by patient
  and group-intervention study, 275, 276, 279
  loss of, 272
  and medical system, 367
  and promising psychotherapies, 223
  and therapy group participation, 225
Coping
  and acceptance, 26–27
  and group sharing, 258
  in intervention with women at high risk for breast cancer, 295
  problem-focused vs. emotion-focused, 281
Coping assistance, 87
Coping patterns or styles, 236
  differences in within relationships, 366
Coping skills
  as intervention component, 23, 245–247
  in psychotherapy programs, 218
  and support groups, 282
Coping skills intervention, single-session, 297–298
Coping strategies, 88, 221
  in C-SHIP model, 345, 351–352
  and psychosocial support, 217
Corticosteroids, 189
Cost-effectiveness
  of group therapy, 220
  as research issue, 284
Cost-utility approach, in health status measurement, 69
Counseling approach, to genetic counseling, 299
Cross-cultural validity, in QOL measurement, 61–63
CROSS (Customer Reported Outcomes and Satisfaction Scales), 370
C-SHIP. See Cognitive-social health information-processing model
CTL (cytolytic T lymphocytes), 177–178, 180, 193, 197

MUC1-specific, 180, 183–184
Culture
  and distress from breast cancer, 38–39
  and intrusiveness of cancer exprience, 52
  and QOL measurement, 61–63
  synthesis of with science, 395
Customer Reported Outcomes and Satisfaction Scales (CROSS), 370
Cytokines, 176, 177, 189, 193, 199, 204, 205–206
  measuring production of, 184–186
Cytolytic T lymphocytes (CTL), 177–178

D

Damocles syndrome, 363
"Danger" model of the immune system, 202–203
Death anxiety, 221
Decentering, 61
Denial, 26–27, 152
Dependency, as impediment to optimal functioning, 366
Depression
  and breast cancer study, 47, 50
  in cancer patients, 216
  and distress of breast cancer patients, 38, 78
  and optimism, 22
  in psychoeducational intervention, 247, 248, 249
  and purpose in life, 20
Desensitization, 86, 90
Desensitization hypothesis, 112
Detoxifying dying, 221
Diagnostic and Statistical Manual of Mental Disorders. See at DSM
Diet, and cancer risk, 325–326
Differential item functioning, 67
Disease, "shifting burden of," 11
Disease outcomes, 179, 180
  vs. immunological outcomes (MUC1 antigen), 180–181
Disease-specific assessment, vs. generic assessment, 40, 60
Dispositional factors, in cognitive processing, 88–89
Distress
  and BCRC (breast cancer risk counseling) intervention, 293
  of breast cancer patients, 38, 78
  and optimism, 21, 88
  and breast cancer screening, 308–309
  and cancer treatment, 78–80
  and immune system, 305, 312–313
  and outcomes, 4

in PTSD, 163
    among relatives of cancer patients, 288–289
    in women with family histories of breast
        cancer, 307–308
    See also Stress; Traumatic stress
DSM-III, 149
DSM-III-R, 149
DSM-IV
    and cancer as PTSD stressor, 81
    and PTSD, 156

E

Education, hope or optimism from, 23
Educational approach, to genetic counseling,
    299
Educational group, vs. support group, 26
Educational interventions, 23, 218, 237–238
    and cost-effectiveness, 284
    effectiveness of, 271
    in group-intervention study, 273, 275, 276,
        278, 279
    and hope, 29
    and problem-focused coping, 281
    See also at Psychoeducational
Effector mechanisms, 178–180, 193, 196–197,
    199
Electronic support groups, 137–138
Emotional expression, 220–221
    and peer-discussion group, 278
Emotional isolation, 365–366
Emotional support, 23
    desirability of, 280
    in group sessions, 258
    and stage of treatment, 281
Emotional suppression, 217–218
Emotions, cancer-relevant, 345, 348–350
Encodings and self-construals, cancer-relevant,
    345, 346–347
EORTC Quality of Life Questionnaire,
    emotional functioning scale of, 59
Ethnicity
    and distress from breast cancer, 38–39
    and intrusiveness of cancer experience, 49,
        52
Exercise, and cancer risk, 324–325
Expectancies, cancer-relevant, 345, 347–348
Expectancy-value models of motivation, 16, 18

F

Facilitation, immune, 203–205
FACT–B (Functional Assessment of Cancer
    Therapy–Breast) Measurement
    System, 59, 60

Fallon Community Health Care (FCHC)
    system, MCC (medical crisis counseling)
    study at, 368–373
Family support, 222
    emotional support in, 280
    and search for meaning, 87
    and support group attendance, 277–278
Fear arousing communications theory, 309
Fear of death, 221
Fear networks, 85, 151
Feedback, response to. See Cognitive-social
    health information-processing model
Feedback, and self-regulation framework, 379
Flexible assessment length, 66
Framing of information, 353–354. See also
    Message framing
Freedom of movement, loss of, 366
Freud, Sigmund, on traumatic neurosis, 152
Friends
    emotional support from, 280
    and search for meaning, 87
    and support group attendance, 277–278
Functional Assessment of Cancer
    Therapy–Breast (FACT–B) Measurement
    System, 59, 60

G

Generic measures of quality of life (QOL),
    40–41, 44, 60
Genetic counseling, divergent responses to,
    343
Genetic counseling interventions, 298–300
Genetic testing, 289
Gimme 5 program, 326
Goal engagement, 16
    benefits of, 22
    and interventions, 24
    and optimism, 19
Goals
    abandonment of, 366
    in behavioral self-regulation, 16–19
    cancer-relevant, 345, 350–351
    letting go of, 29
    See also Purpose
Granzymes, 197
Grieving, among group members, 221
Group cognitive-behavioral therapy, 241–242
Group interventions for cancer patients, 23,
    269–270
    group therapy, 218–220
    outcomes of, 223
    research on, 270–272
    research issues on, 279–280, 282–284
    study on, 272–282

See also Support groups
Group processes
    and coping, 258
    in health and well-being, 131
    in support groups, 132–136
    improvement of, 136–138
Group psychotherapy, supportive, 247, 258
Groups
    and communication with physicians, 222
    research on, 131
Group therapy, 218–220. See also Group
        interventions for cancer patients;
        Support groups
Groupthink, 136

H

Health
    group factors in, 131
    and purpose or hope, 19–22
Health behaviors, and breast cancer, 308
Health care, changes in, 11
Health education, as intervention component,
        244
Health habits, and psychoeducational
        intervention, 254
Helper T cells, MUC1-specific, 184, 185
Helper-therapy principle, 219, 273
HIV
    behavioral interventions toward, 393
    and cancer patient interventions, 8
    and preventive behavior modification, 322
HMOs
    and changes in health care, 11
    medical crisis counseling in (Fallon
        Community Health Care system),
        368–373
Holocaust
    and distress from cancer diagnosis, 164
    and distress from current stressors, 148
Hope or hopefulness
    and goal striving, 16
    and health or well-being, 19, 20–22
    holding on to, 29
    from interventions, 23–24, 30
    and purpose, 27–29
    in response to cancer, 15–16
    See also Optimism
Humoral response, 200, 201

I

I Can Cope program, 270
Illness
    as obstacle to goal attainment, 18

patient representations of, 390
Illness threats, representations of, 384–389
Immune surveillance vs. immune facilitation,
        203–205
Immune system, 175, 193
    and cognitive-behavioral interventions, 311
    factors in enhancement of, 259–260
    and fear or distress, 305, 312–313
    and psychoeducational intervention model,
        250, 252, 253
    and psychosocial interventions, 181, 193
    and NK activity, 196
    and stress, 178, 181, 187, 189, 310–313,
        331
    and family history of cancer, 314–315
    mediators of change in, 313
    and tumor-specific immunity, 175–178
    effector mechanisms in responses, 178–180
        (see also Effector mechanisms)
    measurement of responses in patients
        undergoing intervention, 181–186,
        187,
        188
    and MUC1 breast cancer antigen, 180–185
    and stress or stress reduction, 187, 189
    See also Tumor immunology
Immunity
    innate vs. adaptive, 176, 177, 194–196
    Stress and Immunity Breast Cancer Project,
        125–127
Immunological outcome, 179
    vs. disease outcome (MUC1 antigen),
        180–181
Immunology, 124
Immunotherapy, nonspecific vs. specific,
        205–207
Information, hope or optimism from, 23
Information-processing model, for PTSD, 83,
        85, 150–151, 152
Innate immunity, 176, 177, 194–195, 196
International Conference on Biopsychosocial
        Aspects of HIV Infections, 393
Interpersonal relationships
    and cognitive-emotional processes of
        adaptation to cancer, 107–108
    differences in coping styles within, 366
    in emotional adjustment to cancer, 99
    See also Family support; Friends; Social-
        cognitive processing model of
        emotional adjustment to cancer; Spouse
Interpretability, and QOL (quality of life)
        measurement, 63
Intracellular cytokine staining, 184
Intrusive thoughts

and adherence to mammography regimes, 349
in cognitive processing of traumatic events, 100
and group-intervention study, 275, 278
from intervening stressors, 165
and social processing in adjustment, 103–107
from traumatic event, 150, 155, 165
in traumatic neurosis, 152
among women with family history of breast cancer, 308
Isolation, as impediment to optimal functioning, 365–366
Item bank(ing), 66
advantages and disadvantages of, 66–67
Item characteristic curve, 65
Item response theory (IRT) measurement model, 65

K

Know Your Body program, 326

L

Learning theory, and PTSD-like syndromes, 151
Life priorities, reordering of, 221–222
Literacy, and QOL assessment, 62
Longitudinal data, quality and quantity in analysis of, 67–70
Loss of control, in medical system, 367
Losses, as impediment to optimal functioning, 366

M

Macrophages, 175–176, 176–177, 184, 193, 194–195, 197, 198, 199, 204
Mammography adherence or utilization
BCRC (Breast cancer risk counseling) impact on, 294
and distress, 289, 309
and individualized breast cancer risk information, 291
and intrusive thoughts, 349
and psychoeducational intervention, 296
and women at high risk levels, 6
Managed care
and fragmentation of research, 378
See also HMOs
Mastectomy, 39, 42, 43, 78
MCC. See Medical crisis counseling
Meaning

in negative event, 19n
and traumatic experience, 102
Meaningfulness, and sense of coherence, 19
Measurement
of cytokine production, 184–186
of immune responses
nonspecific, 187, 188
tumor-specific, 181–186
of quality of life (QOL), 40–42
aggregated vs. disaggregated scores in, 58–60
in breast cancer study, 43–47, 47–51
disease-specific vs. generic assessment in, 40, 60
emerging research issues in, 60–70
See also Assessment
Medical crises, intervention during, 363
Medical crisis counseling (MCC), 363
assessment in, 367–368
basic assumptions of, 364–365, 367
and impediments to optimal functioning, 365–367
study on, 368–373
Medical system, loss of control in, 367
Medical treatment adherence, 224–225
Memories
conceptual, 346
schematic, 346
traumatic, 152
Mental health
and breast cancer study, 44, 46, 48, 49, 50
among cancer patients, 160, 162
and physical health, 59
Message framing, 332
for screening, 329
See also Framing of information
Mind-body problem, 381
Missing data, in QOL (quality of life)/data analysis, 67–68
Monitoring, 88–89, 345–346, 377
and C-SHIP model, 347–352
and tailoring of psychosocial interventions to attentional style, 353–354
MOS SF-36 (MOS Short Form-36) Scale, 41, 45, 48, 50, 51
MUC1 protein, 180–181
MUC1-specific antibodies, 182
MUC1-specific CTL (cytolytic T lymphocytes), 180, 183–184
MUC1-specific helper T cells, 184, 185
Multicomponent interventions, 121
Multilingual QOL (quality of life) instruments, 61

N

Natural killer cells. See NK cells
Negative downward comparisons, in group-intervention study, 276–277
Neurosis, traumatic, 152
NK (natural killer) cells, 175–176, 179–180, 193, 194, 196, 197
  and breast cancer project, 126
  deficiencies in, 187
  and family history of cancer, 314
  and innate vs. adaptive debate, 196, 199
  interferon produced by, 184
  and prior activation, 176
  and relaxation training, 311
  and stress, 6, 312–313, 331
Noncompliance with treatment, 123. See also Adherence
Nonspecific immunotherapy, 205–207

O

Observational studies, 30
Oncology, psychosocial and behavioral, 3
Optimal functioning, impediments to, 365–367
Optimism
  as coping ingredient, 245
  and distress over breast cancer, 21, 88
  and expectancies, 347
  and goal engagement, 19
  and health or well-being, 20
  from interventions, 23–24
  of patient caregivers, 22
  and reactions to negative events, 88
  and upward/downward social comparisons, 25
  See also Hope or hopefulness
Outcome measures, in MCC (medical crisis counseling) study, 369–370
Outcomes
  immunological vs. disease, 179, 180–181
  of psychosocial interventions, 235
  of psychotherapeutic intervention, 223–226

P

Patient, skills demanded of, 367
Patient-actor, 382–384
Patient-physician relationship, 226
Patient-spouse relationship, 283
Peer discussion intervention, in group-intervention study, 273–275, 276–278, 279, 280, 284
Peer dyad intervention, 283
Perforin, 197

Personal characteristics, and behavior, 375–376
Personal relationships. See Interpersonal relationships
Personal resources, and group-intervention study, 279
Pessimism
  and cancer survival, 22
  and reactions to negative events, 88
  and upward/downward social comparisons, 25
Physical appearance, adverse changes in, 366
Physical functioning, and breast cancer, 39
Physical health, and mental health, 59
Physical self, representations of, 390–391
Physicians
  communication with, 222
  patients' relationship with, 226
POMS (Profile of Mood States), 59, 239
Post-diagnosis interventions, 7
Post-diagnosis phase of cancer, 6
Post-traumatic stress disorder. See PTSD
Predictors, of response to treatment, 223–224
Print communications, tailored, 300–301
Prior life history, in cognitive processing, 88–89
Prior trauma, and distress from current stressors, 148
Problem-solving and supportive therapy, 240–244
Problem-solving techniques
  as intervention component, 245–247
  in interventions, 23
Problem-solving training (PST), 296–297, 298
Processing style. See Blunting; Monitoring
Profile of Mood States (POMS), 59, 239
Project Omega, 246
Psychiatric history, and cognitive processing of negative life events, 89
Psychoeducational intervention(s), 121, 238
  for women at high risk for breast cancer, 295–298
  See also Educational interventions
Psychoeducational intervention model, structured, 244
  conceptual model for, 260, 261
  experimental design and model components of, 244
  coping skills (problem-solving techniques), 245–247
  health education, 244
  stress management, 244–245
  supportive group psychotherapy, 247, 258
  presumed mechanisms in, 254, 258–260

results in, 247–254, 255–257
Psychological interventions, biobehavioral
    model for, 119–120
and change mechanisms, 123–124
and effectiveness of interventions, 120–121,
    124–125
experiment on (Stress and Immunity Breast
    Cancer Project), 125–127
and individuals receiving treatment,
    121–122
and problems to be treated, 122–123
Psychological theory, and behavioral research
    in cancer, 375
Psychological trauma, 149–150
adjustment to, 154–155
and PTSD, 150–154 (see also PTSD)
See also at Trauma
Psychoneuroimmunology (PNI), 124
Psychosocial and behavioral oncology, 3
Psychosocial factors, cancer affected by, 10
Psychosocial interventions for cancer, 3
adverse effects from, 25–26
and biomedical intervention, 215
considerations in, 29–30
face-to-face contact in, 137
as fostering hope and purpose, 16
hope and optimism augmented in, 23–24,
    30
and immune system, 181, 193
measurement of responses, 181–186, 187,
    188
and NK activity, 196
and individual's response, 344
medical crisis counseling (MCC), 363–373
as multifaceted, 22–23
need for, 215–217
as nonspecific immunotherapeutics, 205,
    207
observational studies for, 30
outcomes of, 235
overlapping areas of, 10–11
and patient's attentional style, 352–356
and previous mental health research, 7–9
psychotherapeutic methods, 217–218
group therapy, 218–220
themes in, 220–223
psychotherapeutic outcomes, 223–226
purpose augmented in, 24–25, 30
question of relative effectiveness of
    components in, 271
and relative importance of purpose and
    hope, 27–29
and social-cognitive processing theory,
    108–110, 111

as spanning several stages, 6–7
stressors addressed in, 144
structured psychoeducational model,
    244–260
coping skills (problem-solving techniques),
    245–247
health education, 244
stress management, 244–245
supportive group psychotherapy, 247, 258
types of
behavioral training, 238–240
educational, 237–238 (see also Educational
    interventions)
problem-solving and supportive therapy,
    240–244
variables in design and implementation of,
    7, 8
Psychosocial interventions for women with
    increased breast cancer risk
breast cancer risk counseling (BCRC),
    289–295, 300
future directions in, 300–301
genetic counseling interventions, 298–300
psychoeducational interventions, 295–298
and risk comprehension, 289
Psychosocial issues on cancer and cancer
    treatment, 235–237
research on, 5–9
Psychosocial problems
among BMT (bone marrow transplantation)
    recipients, 79–81, 82, 84
among cancer patients, 215–217
Psychotherapeutic interventions
methods of, 217–223
outcomes of, 223–226
as public health development, 11
PTSD (posttraumatic stress disorder)
from cancer diagnosis, 156
and cancer patients, 148, 157–160, 162,
    163–164, 165–166, 166
in cancer survivors, 79, 80–83, 89
decline in symptoms of over time, 155
etiology of
conditioning model of, 83–85, 151
information-processing model of, 83, 85,
    150–151, 152
factors in explanation of, 83
and intrusive thoughts about breast cancer,
    308
in medical patients, 156–157
and prior psychopathology, 89
and psychological trauma, 150–154
Public view of cancer, 379–380
Purpose

and health or well-being, 19–20
from interventions, 24–25, 30
and hope, 27–29
in response to cancer, 15–16
See also Goals

Q

Quality-adjusted life-years (QALYs), 68
Quality-adjusted time without symptoms or
    toxicity (Q-TWiST), 68, 69
Quality of life (QOL), 39–40, 119
  of breast cancer patients
  and distress, 38–39, 216, 349
  study on, 42–53
  definition of, 40, 52, 58
  dimensions of, 58
  and emotional support, 280
  important issues on, 120
  measurement of, 40–42
  aggregated vs. disaggregated scores in,
    58–60
  in breast cancer study, 43–47, 47–51
  clinical significance, 63
  disease-specific vs. generic assessment in,
    40, 60
  emerging research issues in, 60–70
  and passage of time, 270
  and post-diagnosis interventions, 6
  and terminal patients, 240
  and value of intervention, 57
Quantity of life
  and group psychotherapy, 225–226
  as measure, 57
Quantity of life data analyses, in combination
  with quality of life, 67–70

R

Reach to Recovery program, 270
Reality, shared, 132, 134
Reductionism
  as barrier to prevention, 380–381
  vs. behavioral approaches, 393
Relationships. See Interpersonal relationships
Research
  behavioral, 375–379
  conceptual model for, 260, 261
  on groups and group interventions, 131,
    270–272
  importance of, 5
  obstacles to, 4
Research issues
  on group interventions, 279–280, 282–284
  individual differences in treatment response,
    122

in QOL (quality of life) assessment, 60–61
  combining quality with quantity in
    longitudinal data, 67–70
  computerizing practical assessment, 64–65
  cross-cultural validity, 61–63
  interpretability and clinical significance, 63
  item banking, 66–67
  standardizing scores across common
    instruments, 64
  test brevity risks, 65–66
  on traumatic stress from cancer, 166–167
Response to treatment, predictors of, 223–224
Risk for cancer, 322
  behavioral sources of, 323
  diet, 325–326
  and exercise, 324–325
  and screening or surveillance, 328–330
  stress, 330–331 (see also Stress)
  sun exposure, 326–328
  tobacco use, 324
  for breast cancer
  and breast cancer risk counseling (BCRC),
    289–295, 300
  factors in, 287, 305, 306, 306–307, 325
  over- and under-estimation of, by high-risk
    women, 288
  and heredity, 305
  perceived and objective, 346–347
  psychological aspects of, 6
Role flexibility, 222

S

Schemas, 151
Schematic memories, 346
Science
  and clinical practice, 376
  synthesis of with culture, 395
Screening activities
  for breast cancer, 308–310
  and cancer risk, 328–330
  and risk perception or distress, 289
  stress as interfering with, 6, 7, 308–310
Secondary stressors, 150
Self, patient's representation of, 390–391
Self-appraisal process, 391
Self-construals, cancer-relevant, 345, 346–347
Self-efficacy expectations, of monitors vs.
  blunters, 348
Self-esteem, and group-intervention study,
  273, 274, 276, 279
Self-image
  in breast cancer patients, 49, 53, 272–273
  and education intervention, 276
Self-managing teams, 135

"Self-nonself" model, 202, 203
Self-regulation
  goal-engagement and acceptance in, 29
  goal-striving model of, 16–19
  and hope, 20
Self-regulation model, 375, 376, 379, 381–382
  appeal of, 393–394
  and communication, 391–394
  contextual factors in, 389–391
  questions on accomplishments of, 395
  representation of illness threats in, 384–389
  representation of patient-actor in, 382–384
  theoretical vision from, 379
Self-regulation techniques or skills, 218, 223
Self-regulatory strategies, cancer-relevant, 345,
    351–352
Self-selection, into intervention group,
    270–271
Sexual functioning
  and breast cancer patients, 38, 216
  mastectomy patients, 236
  and individual differences in treatment
    response, 122
Sharing process, in therapeutic support groups,
    131–138
"Shifting burden of disease," 11
Significance, clinical, and QOL (quality of life)
    measurement, 63
Smoking
  interventions against, 376–377
  as risk factor, 324
Social-cognitive processing model of emotional
    adjustment to cancer, 99
  and cognitive processing, 99–101
  empirical studies on, 102–108
  mechanisms involved in, 111–113
  and psychosocial interventions, 108–110,
    111
  and social environment, 101–102
Social comparison
  and assessment of physical self, 390–391
  and group intervention study, 273
  and peer discussion, 276–277
  upward/downward, 25
Social modulation of cognitive processing,
    101–102
Social network, and support group attendance,
    277–278
Social processing, 87, 89
Social psychological factors, 377
Social psychological theory, and behavioral
    research in cancer, 375
Social reality, 132
Social stigma, attached to cancer, 4

Social support, 23
  in group therapy, 219
  hope or optimism from, 23
  and hope or purpose, 28–29
  and MCC (medical crisis counseling), 365,
    371
  and need for intervention, 224
  in psychoeducational intervention, 258
  and PTSD, 83
  as therapeutic theme, 220
  See also Support groups
Sociocultural variables, and behavior, 375–376
Sociodemographic factors, in women's
    response to cancer diagnosis, 38
Socioeconomic status, and cancer, 3
Specific immunotherapy, 205–207
Spouse, as source of support, 283
"Standard gamble" approach, 69
Standardizing, of QOL (quality of life) scores,
    64
Stress, 330
  as barrier to breast cancer screening,
    308–310
  cancer development and progression from,
    4–5, 322–323
  from cancer diagnosis, 144, 147, 160, 216
  in cancer patients, 143–145, 146–149, 156
  cancer recurrence from, 219
  and cancer risk, 330–331
  from viewing oneself as cancer risk, 6, 7
  and compliance, 330
  and "danger" model, 202
  and disease, 143
  and immune system, 178, 181, 187, 189,
    310–313, 331
  and family history of cancer, 314–315
  mediators of change in, 313
  and medical outcome, 227
  physiological systems in, 123
  and psychoeducational intervention, 254,
    258
  and social support, 225
  traumatic vs. nontraumatic, 145–146
  See also Distress; Traumatic stress
Stress and Immunity Breast Cancer Project,
    125–127
Stress management, as intervention
    component, 244–245, 330–331
Structured psychoeducational intervention
    model. See Psychoeducational
  intervention model, structured
Sun exposure, and cancer risk, 326–328
Support groups, 270
  distinguishing between effects of, 112–113

vs. educational group, 26
group processes in, 132–136
improvement of, 136–138
individual variation in benefit from, 132, 278–279
patients reluctant to join, 277
question of advisability of, 282
as reason for living, 24–25
and social-cognitive processing model, 108–110, 111
and treatment adherence, 224–225
of women with support deficits, 281
See also Group interventions for cancer patients; Social support
Support intervention, research issues on, 283
Supportive-expressive group therapy, 121, 223, 282
Supportive group psychotherapy, 247, 258
Supportive therapy, 240–244
Surveillance, and cancer risk, 328–330
Surveillance, immune, 203–205
Survival analyses, 67
Survival time, as measure, 57. See also Quantity of life
Symptom control, 222–223
Synthesis
in behavioral and biological sciences, 394–395
of science and culture, 395

T

Tailored print communications, 300–301
Talking, and emotional adjustment, 101
T-cell receptors (TCRs), 195
Teamwork, as organizational strategy, 134–135
Telephone contacts, 377
Telephone counseling, 290, 300, 301
Test brevity, risks of, 65–66
Test-operate-test-exit (TOTE) mechanism, 383–384, 385, 386, 387–388
T_H (T helper lymphocyte) activity, 199–201
Therapeutic support groups. See Support groups
Time management, for medical crisis clinicians, 368
Time tradeoff approach, 69
Tobacco use. See Smoking
TOTE (test-operate-test-exit) mechanism, 383–384, 385, 386, 387–388
Trauma
and cognitive-processing model, 85–88
predispositional factors in, 88–89
and conditioning model, 83–85
and information-processing model, 83, 85

Traumatic events, 149
Traumatic neurosis, 152
Traumatic stress, 149–150
adjustment to, 154–155
and cancer, 145, 155–156, 157–160
and disease severity, 162–163
and end of treatment, 161–162
and immediate stressors, 160–161
vs. nontraumatic stress, 145–146
and PTSD, 156–160, 162, 163–164, 165–166, 166
research needed on, 166–167
and stressors associated with cancer, 146–149
and subsequent stressors, 164–165
and secondary stressors, 150
See also Stress
Treatment phase, concerns arising in, 7. See also Cancer treatment
Trial Outcome Index (TOI), 60
Tumor antigens. See Antigens, tumor
Tumor immunology, 193–194, 208
and "effector" vs. "affector" mechanisms, 196–199 (see also Affector mechanisms; Effector mechanisms)
and immune surveillance vs. immune facilitation, 203–205
and innate vs. adaptive immunity, 194–196
and nonspecific vs. specific immunotherapy, 205–207
"self-nonself" vs. "danger" model in, 201–203
and T_H (T helper lymphocyte) activity, 199–201
Tumor-specific immunity, 175–178
effector mechanisms in responses, 178–180 (see also Effector mechanisms)
and MUC1 breast cancer antigen, 180–181
and psychosocial intervention, 181
and cytokine production, 184–186
and MUC1-specific antibodies, 182
and MUC1-specific CTL (cytolytic T lymphocytes), 183–184
and MUC1-specific helper T cells, 184, 185
and other tumor antigens, 185
and stress or stress reduction, 187, 189

U

Us Too, 270
Utility approach, to health status measurement, 68–70

V

Vaccines, 178, 179, 180, 206
Values, cancer-relevant, 345, 350–351

W

Well-being
   group factors in, 131
   and purpose or hope, 19–22
Well-years, 68
"Work of worrying," 8
Worry
   cancer patients' areas of, 236
   from viewing oneself as cancer risk, 6, 7

About the Editors

Andrew Baum received his BS in psychology from the University of Pittsburgh in 1970 and his PhD from the State University of New York at Stony Brook in 1974. He is currently deputy director for Cancer Control and Population Sciences of the University of Pittsburgh Cancer Institute (UPCI). He is also the director of Behavioral Medicine and Oncology, interim director of the African American Cancer Program at the UPCI, and professor of psychiatry and psychology at the University of Pittsburgh. Since 1972 he has studied chronic stress and long-term consequences of traumatic or persistent stressors such as cancer and has focused more specifically on mental health and psychological and physical symptoms of victims of disasters, motor vehicle accidents, and chronic illnesses. Dr. Baum also studies the effects of stress on immune system activity and psychosocial and biobehavioral aspects of cancer. He has edited, coedited, or coauthored more than 30 books and authored or coauthored more than 125 scientific and professional publications.

In 1992, Dr. Baum received a Centennial Award from the American Psychological Association (APA) for activities on behalf of the Science Directorate, and in 1985 and 1997 he received awards for outstanding contributions to health psychology from the APA Division of Health Psychology (Division 38). He was also recognized for outstanding service to the division in 2000. Dr. Baum was president of the Division of Health Psychology in 1989 and is currently treasurer of the Academy of Behavioral Medicine Research and secretary–treasurer of the Council of Directors of Health Psychology Training. He is a Fellow of several professional societies including the Academy of Behavioral Medicine Research, the Society of Behavioral Medicine, the APA, and the American Psychological Society. He is editor of the *Journal of Applied Social Psychology* and coeditor of the APA book series *Application and Practice in Health Psychology*. He also serves on several editorial boards, including *Health Psychology*. Dr. Baum lives in Fox Chapel, Pennsylvania, with his wife Carlene and two children, Jesse, age 10, and Callie, age 7.

Barbara L. Andersen is a professor in the Department of Psychology at the Ohio State University. She is a Fellow of Divisions 12 and 38 (Health Psychology). She received her PhD in clinical psychology from the University of Illinois in 1980 and completed her postdoctoral studies at the Neuropsychiatric Institute at UCLA. She has published two books and over 120 papers on behavioral medicine. She has chaired the American Cancer Society's (ACS) Grant Panel for Psychosocial Research, as well as similar panels for the National Institutes of Health and the Department of Defense Army Breast Cancer Research Program. Dr. Andersen has served on several editorial boards and was associate editor for the *Journal of Consulting and Clinical Psychology*, *Health Psychology*, and the *Annals of Behavioral Medicine*. In 1995, she was one of 50 women scientists invited to the White House for a briefing on the Clinton administration initiatives in science and technology.

Dr. Andersen conducts research in two areas: biobehavioral responses to cancer and sexual self-concept (schema) and sexual dysfunction. One of her current projects is a clinical intervention trial for women with breast cancer, funded by the ACS, the National Institute of Mental Health, and the Army. Dr. Andersen resides in Upper Arlington, Ohio, with her two children, Christina, age 11, and Anthony, age 7.